Manual of
Emergency Care

Manual of Emergency Care

Fifth Edition

Susan Budassi Sheehy, RN, MSN, MS, CEN, FAAN

Director of Nursing
Emergency Services
Brigham & Women's Hospital
Boston, Massachusetts

Gail Pisarcik Lenehan, EdD, RN, CS

Editor
Journal of Emergency Nursing
Hingham, Massachusetts

with 361 illustrations

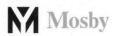 Mosby

St. Louis Baltimore Boston Carlsbad Chicago Minneapolis New York Philadelphia Portland
London Milan Sydney Tokyo Toronto

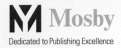
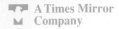

Dedicated to Publishing Excellence

A Times Mirror
Company

Publisher: Nancy L. Coon
Managing Editor: Lisa Potts
Developmental Editor: Aimee E. Loewe
Project Manager: John Rogers
Associate Production Editor: Mary Turner
Manufacturing Supervisor: Karen Boehme
Book and Cover Design: Yael Kats

FIFTH EDITION

Copyright © 1999 Mosby, Inc.

Previous editions copyrighted 1979, 1984, 1990, 1995

Composition by the Clarinda Company
Printing/binding by R.R. Donnelley & Sons Company

Mosby, Inc.
11830 Westline Industrial Drive
St. Louis, Missouri 63146

Library of Congress Cataloging in Publication Data

Sheehy, Susan Budassi, 1948-
    Manual of emergency care / Susan Budassi Sheehy, Gail Pisarcik
Lenehan. — 5th ed.
      p.   cm.
    Includes bibliographical references and index.
    ISBN 0-323-00304-4
    1. Medical emergencies—Handbooks, manuals, etc.   2. Emergency
nursing—Handbooks, manuals, etc.   I. Lenehan, Gail Pisarcik.
II. Title.
    [DNLM: 1. Emergency Medical Services handbooks. 2. Emergency
Nursing handbooks. 3. Emergency Medicine.   WX 39S541m 1998]
RC86.8.S54   1998
616.02′5—dc21
DNLM/DLC
for Library of Congress   98-8531
                                        CIP

98 99 00 01 02 / 9 8 7 6 5 4 3 2 1

Contributors

Joan Elaine Begg-Whitman, RN, CEN

Staff Nurse
Emergency Center
Cape Cod Hospital
Hyannis, Massachusetts

Nancy M. Bonalumi, RN, MS, CEN

Nurse Manager
Emergency Department
Pinnacle Health Hospitals
Harrisburg, Pennsylvania

Anne Phelan Bowen, MS, RN

Trauma Outreach Nurse
Children's Hospital
Boston, Massachusetts

Suzanne L. Brown, RN, BSN, CEN, SANE

Coordinator
Sexual Assault Nurse Examiner Program
Inova Fairfax Hospital
Falls Church, Virginia

Peggy Cass, EMT-Paramedic, MEd

Former Paramedic Services Coordinator
South Shore Hospital
South Weymouth, Massachusetts

Donna E. Chase, RN, BS

Director of Education
South Shore Hospital
South Weymouth, Massachusetts

Debra DeLorenzo, RN, BS

Nurse Manager, Oncology
Education and Training
South Shore Hospital
South Weymouth, Massachusetts

Kathy M. Dolan, RN, BS, CEN

Staff Nurse
Mercy Trauma Center
Cedar Rapids, Iowa

Faye P. Everson, RN, CEN, EMT-M

Staff Nurse
Emergency Center
Cape Cod Hospital;
Clinical Coordinator for Paramedic Training
Emergency Medical Teaching Services, Inc.
Hyannis, Massachusetts

Mary Dahlgren Gunnels, RN, MS, CHES, CEN

Trauma Coordinator
Oregon Health Sciences University
Portland, Oregon

Deborah Parkman Henderson, PhD, RN

Assistant Professor
UCLA School of Medicine
Harbor-UCLA Medical Center
Torrance, California

Robert D. Herr, MD, MBA, FACEP

Clinical Associate Professor of Surgery
Division of Emergency Medicine
University of Utah Medical School
Salt Lake City, Utah

Stephen H. Johnson, MD

Attending Neurosurgeon
South Shore Hospital
South Weymouth, Massachusetts

Diane Panton Lapsley, RN, MS, CS

Cardiovascular Research Nurse
Department of Veterans Affairs
Brockton/West Roxbury VAMC
West Roxbury, Massachusetts

Louise LeBlanc, RN, BScN, ENC(c)

Manager of Nursing Practice—Emergency
Emergency Department
Scarborough General Hospital
Scarborough, Ontario
Canada

Genell Lee, RN, MSN, JD

Nurse Attorney
Hauth & Lee, L.L.C.
Birmingham, Alabama

Anne Marie E. Lewis, RN, BSN, BA, MA, CEN

Resource Specialist/Educator
Department of Emergency & Ambulatory
  Services
Sturdy Memorial Hospital
Attleboro, Massachusetts

Anne P. Manton, RN, PhD, CEN

Assistant Professor
Fairfield University
School of Nursing
Fairfield, Connecticut;
Staff Nurse
Emergency Department
Hospital of St. Raphael
New Haven, Connecticut

Benjamin E. Marett, RN, MSN, CEN, COHN-S

Clinical Nurse Specialist
US Healthworks NC-SC
Rock Hill, South Carolina

Susan Mathias, RN, BSN, CEN

Clinical Research Coordinator
Emergency Medicine Association of Pittsburgh
Pittsburgh, Pennsylvania

Lisa B. McCabe, MS, CCRN, ARNP

Nurse Practitioner
Department of Surgery
Dartmouth-Hitchcock Medical Center
Lebanon, New Hampshire

Margaret McCarthy-Mogan, MS, RN, CEN

Nursing Education Department
Brigham & Women's Hospital
Boston, Massachusetts

Jessie M. Moore, RN, MSN, CEN

Clinical Nurse Specialist
Emergency Department
Midstate Medical Center
Meriden, Connecticut

Ingrid B. Mroz, MS, CCRN, ARNP

Nurse Practitioner
Dartmouth-Hitchcock Medical Center
Lebanon, New Hampshire

Marybeth Murphy, MS, RN

Instructor, Maternal Child Nursing
Education and Training
South Shore Hospital
South Weymouth, Massachusetts

Andrea Novak, RN, MS, CEN

Director
Interdisciplinary Education
Southern Regional Area Health Education Center
Fayetteville, North Carolina

Suzanne O'Connor, MSN, CS

Psychiatric Clinical Nurse Specialist
Emergency Department
Massachusetts General Hospital;
President
Healthcare Satisfaction
Boston, Massachusetts

Gail E. Polli, RN, MS, CS

Psychiatric Clinical Nurse Specialist and
  Manager
Emergency Department Psychiatric Service
South Shore Hospital
South Weymouth, Massachusetts

Kathy Sciabica Robinson, RN, CEN, EMT-P

Staff Nurse
Emergency Department
Penn State Geisinger Health System
Geisinger Medical Center
Danville, Pennsylvania

Jaye M. Sengewald, RN, MSN, CDE

Director of Diabetes Care and Education
Health-Mor Personal Care Corporation
Bradley, Illinois

Patricia M. Speck, MSN, RN, CS, FNP

Coordinator of Nursing Services
City of Memphis Sexual Assault Resource
  Center;
Adjunct Faculty
University of Tennessee—Memphis
College of Nursing
Memphis, Tennessee

Susan F. Strauss, RN, CEN, CCRN

Executive Vice President
The Consultants Gateway
Poughkeepsie, New York

Barbara A. Tilden, RNC, BSN

Instructor
Education and Training
South Shore Hospital
South Weymouth, Massachusetts

Anne Cassels Turner, RN, BA

Staff Nurse
Emergency Department
Massachusetts General Hospital
Boston, Massachusetts

Polly Gerber Zimmerman, RN, MS, MBA, CEN

Staff Nurse
Emergency Department
Swedish Covenant Hospital
Chicago, Illinois

Acknowledgments for Previous Contributions

Judith Boehm, RN, MSN

Jorda Chapin, RN, CEN

Jane deMoll, RN, CEN

Christine DiGeronimo, RN, BSN, CURN

Deborah C. Harcke, RN, BSN, CEN

Lisa Schneck Hegel, RN, BS, CEN

Linda J. Kobokovich, RNC, MSCN

Judith E. Lombardi, RN, MSN, ENP, CEN

Kelly F. Malmquist, RN, BSN

Brenda M. Moore, RN, CEN

Delberta Murphy, RN, BS, CEN

Carla Obar, RN, CSPI

Sandra Thomas Ouellette, RN, CPTC

Tracy Pike-Amato, RN, BSN, CEN

Maureen Quigley, RN, BSN, CEN

Carol Rittenhouse, RN, CCRN

Peggy Shedd, MSN, RN, CS

Daun Smith, RN, MS

Janet L. Sudekum, RN, BSN, CCRN

Geoffrey Tarbox, RN, MS

Lori Tucker, RN, CEN

Deborah Upton, RN, BSN, CEN

Kathleen Waine, RN, CEN

Mary E. Wood, RN, MS, CDE

Andrea B. Wyle, RN, ONC

Mary Young, RN, MSN

To John,
who always "makes things happen."
With much love from Goaliesma.

SBS

To Marcella and John,
whose unconditional love
was so naturally given to three
children who were their whole world. I wish they
could be here to share, and thank once again . . . and
to Joe and our three children, Patrick,
Kate, and John, who are our whole world.

GPL

Foreword

In my travels as President of the Emergency Nurses Association, I have seen this manual, now in its twentieth year, dog-eared and worn in many emergency departments across the country—the best proof of its usefulness and popularity. For almost 20 years it has provided practical information that has been used, not only in clinical settings, but also for review and study for the national CEN exam.

This fifth edition has brought together two familiar and respected names in emergency nursing, who are both personal friends and colleagues, Susan Budassi Sheehy and Gail Pisarcik Lenehan. They have obviously drawn on their extensive network to gather an impressive list of contributors with impressive expertise in the field.

The current explosion of information in nursing is even more daunting for those in a specialty that by definition is based on information from virtually every other specialty from pediatrics to geriatrics, neurology to urology, and medicine to trauma. This book, with its tightly written overview and "pearls of wisdom" from those who truly know emergency nursing, will be welcomed by both veteran and fledgling emergency nurses. It will help to remind as well as teach, and it will make a valuable addition to any emergency department library and any emergency nurse's personal library.

Mosby publishers is to be congratulated on yet another addition to its extensive offerings in emergency care.

Anne Manton, RN, PhD, CEN

Assistant Professor
Fairfield University School of Nursing;
President, Emergency Nurses Association
Fairfield, Connecticut

Preface

1999 marks the twentieth anniversary of the original publication of *Manual of Emergency Care*. The first edition was written and published to meet a need—"a basic text and technical reference for individuals engaged in the advanced skills of life support." It was written to be a resource book for emergency nurses and others who were attempting to define the specialty. We knew that we were on the brink of the birth of a new and exciting specialty, Emergency Nursing, along with Emergency Medicine and Pre-Hospital Care.

Now, two decades later, we can look back in amazement at the remarkable strides we have made. The specialty of Emergency Nursing and the certification of Emergency Nurses is recognized and respected internationally. Emergency Medicine is a recognized board certified medical specialty, and Intermediate to Advanced Level Pre-Hospital Care is the expected norm in most communities. It was not so long ago that it wasn't that way. Out of these Emergency Care specialties have grown numerous subspecialists—Flight Nurses and Flight Paramedics, Emergency Nurse Practitioners, Poison Information and Emergency Toxicology experts, Pediatric Emergency Nursing and Pediatric Emergency Medicine experts, Forensic Nurses, Sexual Assault Nurse Examiners, and many, many more. With all these subspecialties came emerging bodies of new and exciting knowledge.

Technology has expanded beyond all of our wildest imaginations. We've seen many "sacred cows" of our practice go by the wayside to make room for new and innovative technologies and techniques. Our knowledge base continues to grow and provides the foundation on which we nurture all aspects of Emergency Care.

So, here we are, 20 years later. Yet another edition of *Manual of Emergency Care* has been published for a more sophisticated Emergency Care provider. Over time and several editions we have added much information and asked many experts to teach us this new information. It is our hope that this edition will be as useful to you as the first one was.

Acknowledgments

Any monumental project, such as this, is a team effort. We are most grateful to Karen Halm, our project manager, who kept everything organized; she could probably run a Fortune-500 company. Her commitment to this project and unfailing sense of humor were invaluable. Characteristically, she made everything look easy and made this edition come to fruition.

Many new authors joined us for this fifth edition. We thank them and all of our authors and revisors, both old and new, for their efforts to make this edition outstanding. Special thanks go to Emelie Goudey for her help with photographs. The deadlines were short and our phone calls, e-mails, and faxes were plentiful. *Everyone* was a star.

We would like to thank our editorial and production crews at Mosby for working under incredible deadlines. Most notably, to Lisa Potts and Aimee Loewe for their patience, hard work, and help in meeting those short deadlines.

Most importantly, we would like to acknowledge our families, who have understood the commitment it takes to edit such a project. Our children have grown up with the understanding that "Mom has to write, so we have to be quiet now—or at least be noisy somewhere else in the house." It is truly amazing how much writing and editing can be accomplished at the ice hockey rink before a game or in the parking lot before a football game, a wrestling match, or an Irish step-dance competition.

Contents

PART THREE
Trauma Emergencies

PART FOUR
Special Populations

Basic Principles of Emergency Care

CHAPTER 1

Communicating in Crisis

Suzanne O'Connor

Imagine having a normal day suddenly interrupted by a sudden illness, accident, or social crisis and being brought to the emergency department (ED) with a condition that might change your life. Your behavior, communication, and inability to make decisions would reflect your anxiety.

Most patients enter the emergency department afraid and uncertain about their injury or illness. Surrounded by unfamiliar faces and a noisy, congested, unpredictable foreign environment, patients experience symptoms, pain, and procedures they are unfamiliar with. Further adding to patients' tension is the stress of:

- waiting for permission from their primary care provider to be seen in the emergency department
- waiting to be assessed, treated, and informed about their condition
- waiting to be sent home, or to the operating room, or up to a hospital bed

They may not understand what they are being told or may have misconceptions about that information. They may worry about the condition of other victims in the accident or family members who need to be notified. The patient sees other ill or injured patients and anxious families, and usually experiences an invasion of privacy, having to undress and being asked personal questions by unfamiliar staff. The patient's family and friends may not know the patient is there, or may be restricted to the waiting area, which adds to the patient's sense of helplessness and isolation.[1] Some emergency department patients have expressed the feeling of being a foreigner in the strange world of emergency care. As if in a foreign country, they overhear jargon and words that are difficult to comprehend, and feel isolated from the familiar sounds and people that could calm their anxiety.

A crisis occurs when an imbalance exists between the magnitude of the problem and the immediate resources available to deal with it. The goal of those who work with people in crisis is to restore them to their precrisis level of functioning.[2]

In the Press-Ganey Patient Satisfaction Survey (Table 1-1) in 1994, the top patient "satisfiers" were related to communication and caring. To establish an environment for crisis intervention, patients must be familiarized with caregivers and with their surroundings, and a rapport or connection must be established.

RECOGNIZING FEELINGS

It is helpful to validate the patient's feelings. Patients need to know that their feelings are accepted and acknowledged by emergency care personnel. Caregivers should never belittle or criticize feelings expressed by others because this would diminish effective therapeutic communication and trust. Caregivers can give verbal and nonverbal messages to communicate that they are willing to help patients understand their own feelings. Recognizing emotions can sometimes diminish the intensity of those feelings and the need to act them out. A statement may be as simple as: "I *feel* for what you are going through now. I have *felt* nervous too in similar situations." This *feel/felt* statement of staff acceptance can enhance problem-solving in the relationship between staff and patient.

It is important not to *assume* what patients are feeling, but to *ask* if what they are saying through their words, body language, and silence means that they are angry, sad, frightened, and so forth. It is important for those who work in emergency care to be aware of their own feelings and biases and how those feelings can

TABLE 1-1   Emergency Department Patients Value Most

ITEM	CORRELATION*
Staff cared about you as a person	.97
Nurses informative re treatments	.95
Nurses took problems seriously	.94
Nurses' attention to you	.94
Nurses' concern for privacy	.93
Technical skill of nurses	.93
Adequacy of info to family/friends	.92
Courtesy shown family/friends	.92
Informed about delays	.92
Likelihood of recommending	.91
Dr's informative: Rx & home care	.86
Waiting time to see doctor	.86
Doctors' concern for comfort	.85

Press-Ganey Associates: *Patient satisfaction survey of the emergency department,* Weston, Mass, August to November, 1994, unpublished data.
*n = 194

interfere with therapeutic communication. It is imperative for staff to maintain self-control and not be overwhelmed by feelings of anxiety and urgency. Self-control helps staff remain strong for those in crisis. Striving toward a climate of mutual trust and respect requires patience, knowledge, skill, and genuine caring. Acceptance of a patient is recognition without value judgment; it is the commitment to treat the person as a unique human being with specific individual needs and expectations.

THE NEED FOR THERAPEUTIC COMMUNICATION

The first encounter a person has with emergency personnel, whether on the phone or face to face, will set the tone for the entire emergency care experience. If invasive procedures must be performed immediately because of the patient's condition, verbal communication should be used briefly to explain the procedures and to gain the patient's confidence and understanding. This does not eliminate the crisis, but does make it possible for others to feel more confident in utilizing their own strengths. No therapeutic intervention should be performed without at least a brief explanation to the patient, who should know the reason for the intervention and the risks, pain, and side effects that it may cause. Even if the patient is unresponsive, attempts to state what is being done and why are important because the unconscious patient may still be able to hear.

COMMUNICATION TECHNIQUES

Support

Support is essential in helping patients maintain self-control in the presence of high anxiety. Some ways of being supportive include:
- Recognizing that the person is unique and has individual and cultural needs
- Verbalizing support
- Being available to listen when the patient appears isolated
- Listening for content and feelings
- Accepting the patient's feelings as legitimate
- "Seeking to *understand* before being understood"
- Observing and sensitively commenting on behavioral clues to the patient's feelings

- Touching the patient—hand, arm, shoulder, if it is comfortable for both the patient and caregiver.
- Initiating actions that visibly reflect a warm attitude of concern and respect

Silence

Silence may be used constructively to help conversations, allowing participants to pause to reflect and to think about what is being asked or said.
- Active listening involves being silent and aware of the speaker's need for silence.
- It can help find solutions to problems and answers to questions.
- It is a way of conveying feelings and acceptance.
- It may also indicate anxiety in both the speaker and the listener.
- It can be used for pacing, timing, resistance, or relaxation.

Listening

The ability to listen is more important than the ability to speak. "The real question is not 'What do you tell the patient?' but rather 'What does the patient tell you?' "[3]
- Encourage the patient to verbalize thoughts and feelings by such statements as: "Go on . . . I see . . . Tell me more about . . . I'm confused, and want to understand. Could you explain that again? . . . I understand how important this is."

Questions

One of the ways in which caregivers can stabilize a crisis, be helpful, and decrease patients' feelings of power-lessness is by collecting information through questions. Types of questions vary in usefulness.

Nonhelpful questions

■ **LEADING QUESTION**
"Why would you ever skip your medications?"
- This type of question contains a suggested answer.
- It restricts the respondent.
- It implies the asker's judgment.

■ **NO-CHOICE QUESTION**
"You're ready for your x-ray, aren't you?"
- This implies a command. It shows authority and may be interpreted as one-upmanship.

■ **DOUBLE QUESTION**
"Do you want something for pain? Are you allergic to morphine?"
- This type of question actually consists of two questions asked in sequence, without pausing.
- It is confusing and forces the patient to choose which question to answer.
- It allows the patient to avoid the subject.

Helpful questions

■ **LIMITED CHOICE AND HELPFUL QUESTION**
"Do you want this injection in your hip or in your arm?"
- This type of question gives the responder some control. It implies the patient's compliance in the situation.

■ **OPEN-ENDED QUESTION**
"What made you come to the hospital today?"
- These questions usually begin with "what," "where," "when," "how," or "tell me more."
- The answer to this type of question often reveals feelings and content as well as thoughts.
- It encourages the patient to elaborate, describe, and compare.
- It allows freedom of response and may need to be focused on current needs and symptoms.

■ **CLOSED QUESTION**
"Do you have headache, nausea, . . .?"
• This type of question elicits a yes/no response.
• It can narrow the focus and is best used after open-ended questions.

■ **SENSITIVE QUESTION**
"Is there any more information that may have been left out, that I need to know, to best help your loved one?"
• It provides impetus for the person to reflect on information and add missing data.
• When asked with a tone of empathy the person may be able to reveal important information or secrets that improve treatment.

Don'ts in questioning

• Don't ask too many questions. Let the patient speak as much as possible.
• Don't ask "why" questions—they cast feelings of blame (instead, say, "Tell me more about . . .").
• Don't ask double questions.
• Don't ask long, elaborate questions.

Special Communication Situations

Communicating with children

When communicating with a child, especially one who is suddenly ill or injured, a consistent, calm approach is best. Children react to illness or injury with anxiety, fear of separation, aversion to pain and needles, and fear of the unknown. Be familiar with growth and development patterns, and utilize age-appropriate language and a familiar medium for communication. Children communicate through play, so offering a child a stuffed animal or having a toy available in your pocket may be the catalyst in creating trust.

Demonstrating your physical exam or applying oxygen to a doll or teddy bear may ease the child's fears and improve his or her knowledge and cooperation with the treatment. Encourage the child perhaps by using a stuffed animal or a doll to speak openly and express feelings through the persona of the stuffed animal. When talking with the child, speak in open, direct language and use the child's familiar name. For example, when asking a seven-year-old to move her limbs, you might say, "Liz, pretend you are riding a bike." When the child asks questions, answer honestly. Speak directly and give simple instructions and acceptable choices. Use touch to aid in communication and convey warmth, friendliness, and caring.

Whenever possible encourage at least one of the parents to stay with the child. Remember that a child's way of coping with illness may be to cry, withdraw, or scream. Always remain calm, confident, and express your concern for getting the child better.

Communicating with victims of trauma

When an unexpected trauma occurs, whether minor or major, the patient often appears to be in a state of crisis (Table 1-2). Trauma patients are often in pain and terrified of death, disfigurement, and changes in their body image. They may become angry and blame themselves or someone else for the accident. They often worry about friends and family involved in the accident, worry about their condition, and fear they may be dead.

People are affected in different ways by the anxiety related to the trauma. Some people may narrow their focus to such a limited area that they are unaware of the serious nature of their problems. These people will require gentle, calm repetition and explanation to organize their perceptions of what is happening. Other people may have widened their focus of attention so much that they are overwhelmed and unable to focus on what you are saying.

Communicating with very anxious patients

• Communicate in short, simple, direct, and repetitive phrases.
• Limit extra stimulation by speaking to them quietly in a private place without distractions.

- Keep your facial expression confident and your voice tone calm, firm, and empathic. Give meaningful, important information.

Communicating with all patients

- Inform patients about what is being done and why.[4]
- Talk with patients frequently and let them know how the health care provider can be reached.
- Encourage patients to discuss their opinions and make choices even as to which arm they would like an IV started in.
- Help patients feel involved and in control.
- Help patients to verbalize frustrations, fears, and guilt.
- Although families should never be given false hope, offer any realistic hope.
- Deliver bad news in small, incremental segments. (This allows time for defense mechanisms to be employed.)

Patients may experience post-traumatic stress response following a major traumatic event. It is helpful to prepare the patient by informing him/her that it is not unusual to have flashbacks or nightmares about the event and to be obsessed with retelling the story or their survival guilt.[5] These re-experiencings of the event may be a way for the person to work through its significance. Other more serious reactions may be emotional withdrawal and numbness, followed by self-destructive thoughts and actions (substance abuse, suicide attempts, interpersonal difficulties, avoidance of the trauma location, and poor control of impulsive behavior). Patients experiencing these more serious reactions should be encouraged to seek counseling. Some responses are self-limiting, but reactions that last longer than a month and persist in severity may develop into a psychiatric condition, post-traumatic disorder.[6] This is why it is important to ensure that both patient and family receive follow-up care after their time in the emergency department and the hospital stay.

Communicating with hearing-impaired patients

To communicate with hearing-impaired patients you may have to speak in a lower tone, and speak face to face to allow them to read your lips. Finding a quiet room may allow a partially deaf person to hear you more clearly. You may need to write your questions. If sign language is most appropriate, the Americans with Disabilities Act states that an interpreter must be provided for patients upon their request.

Communicating with non-English–speaking patients

Medicaid requires that hospitals provide a trained language interpreter for those in need. Although family members can be included in helping with translation, it may not be appropriate. They may be too protective, deferential, embarrassed, or biased to translate accurately. A person's cultural background will help predict his or her responses to trauma and suggest interventions.

Communicating with survivors when a sudden death occurs

When a patient dies in the emergency care setting, staff involvement should go beyond the patient and reach out to the patient's family and friends. Staff personnel, as resource persons for the survivors, will need to provide empathic listening, support, information, and direction. Families experience a wide range of reactions, including shock, disbelief, sadness, anger, loneliness, and guilt as the realization of death sets in. Sudden death leaves families with a sense of unreality about the loss. Griefstricken and shocked by death, families may not be able to ask for help. Staff needs to anticipate their needs and guide them. An inhibition of the grief process in the emergency department can lead to survivors' difficulty in mourning their loss later on.[7]

Helpful interventions have been suggested for the onset of sudden loss. According to Fanslow, grieving spouses reported that being with the patient and able to verbalize their own anxiety, plus knowing their spouses were given all the available emergency treatment, were essential needs that facilitated their adjustment.[8] It is important to offer additional emotional supports to grieving families, for example, chaplain, psychiatric clinical nurse specialist, or social worker, and provide a quiet room with a telephone whenever possible. Survivors of patients who die suddenly should be given every opportunity to see the deceased for as long as they desire. This helps to make the death real, and begins the healing process.

TABLE 1-2 Guidelines for Assessing Patients in Crisis*

IMPACT	BEHAVIORS	EMOTIONS	COGNITION	EXAMPLES
No emotional impact				
No observable effect of the situation on the person's behavior	Questions, responses, activities are appropriate for the situation May ask questions, request information, obtain knowledge correctly Not withdrawn or anxious	Expresses that he is "all right" Feels in control of emotions Expresses concerns and reactions clearly	Evidences clear thinking Able to make decisions Plans well Is reality-oriented	Reports that "I will be OK" Reports that he can "handle it"
Mild impact				
Behavior, emotions, and cognition are only slightly affected by the situation	Questions, responses, and activities are mostly appropriate May evidence some anxiety, fear, stress May be cooperative and responsive, displays few visible signs of upset	Seems in control of emotions and is basically calm May report a little embarrassment Is able to talk about the situation	Clear, good to very good future plans	Reports some confidence that he "will be OK" Feels sure that with help "I'll handle it"
Moderate impact				
Is noticeably affected by the situation but response is not continuous or highly intense Responds to help and reassurance Can conceptualize strategies for dealing	May tear or cry a little during the examination, but visible affect or distress is minimal May display some silly or inappropriate behavior May be anxious, unable to absorb information easily, somewhat confused	May seem somewhat affected by the situation but responds to reassurance from others Expresses worry, fear, some inability to concentrate Somewhat dependent	Asks for help and has good plans and strategies for coping with the problem.	Asks for help and support Reports concern about the future impact: "Will I be OK?"

Severe impact

Is clearly affected by the situation in one or more life areas Behavioral response occurs more than once and is somewhat intense Needs reassurance, and experiences difficulty conceptualizing strategies for future planning	Is visibly upset during part of the evaluation, yet responds to reassurance; the signs of distress can be pinpointed to certain factors (the questions about incident, the examination, the outcome and future problems)	Expresses feelings of guilt, self-blame, helplessness, either by demonstrating strong emotion or verbally expressing guilt, self-blame, or helplessness	Appears confused or disoriented Is visibly upset, yet has some plans for handling problems arising from the situation	Says he is very frightened, "doesn't want to go out anymore," or states other unrealistic plans

Very severe impact

Has a strong reaction in one or more areas Is not incapacitated but highly affected by the situation Behaviors are continuous and intense Seems only somewhat responsive to reassurance and is only somewhat able to conceptualize strategies for dealing with the future	Is visibly upset during most of the examination Crying, trembling, withdrawal evident throughout the examination Responses occurring almost continuously—not focused only on the situation—generalized distress	Verbalizes strong reactions; may repeat responses with intensity Generalized fear and/or anger	Very confused, disoriented, unable to comprehend situation May deny responses No plans for the future; evidences little ability to consider alternatives or develop strategies for the future	Reports that he will "never drive again," "never look the same," or "can't go home"

Extremely severe impact

Is incapacitated by the situation; may be hospitalized for psychiatric observation or treatment Behaviors are multiple, continuous, and extremely intense Unaware of efforts to reassure	May be suicidal, catatonic, hysterical, or crying May have phobias or other psychological symptoms that indicate he is incapacitated in some way	Shows extreme nervous disorders, psychotic reactions	Is unable to deal with the situation or the future Is unable to make decisions for self	Has no awareness of what happened or where he is; out of touch with reality

*Developed by Dr. Susan Meyers Chandler, School of Social Work and Dr. Libby O. Ruch, Sociology Department and Women's Studies Program, University of Hawaii, Honolulu, Hawaii. (From Newbury L, Emergency Nurses Association: Sheehy's *Emergency nursing: principles and practice*, ed 3, St Louis, 1992, Mosby.)

Bereavement assessment and intervention

As soon as it becomes evident that a patient's death is imminent or that his or her condition is deteriorating, a member of the emergency care team should make contact with the family and remain or make periodic contact throughout the resuscitation. If the patient is not doing well, be honest and inform them specifically. Listen to what the family is saying and be aware of their body language and nonverbal communication to fully assess their needs. It may be necessary to ask open-ended questions so that the family can begin to express their fears. Gently assess family members about religious beliefs; this may be important and something that doesn't occur to them. Ask the family about the events leading to the traumatic event if they choose to discuss this. You may be the person who will ask the family about organ donation (see Chapter 39).

After the death, you may offer them the opportunity to see their loved one after they have had time to react to the news. Encourage the family to talk and support one another. Assist a family member who is alone to call someone for themselves.

Reactions to the death of a loved one may vary from crying or screaming to being quiet or talking incessantly. Encourage family members to release their emotions. Avoid giving medication unless a person's history indicates that a specific medication has been helpful. Medications can make the time surrounding the crisis cloudy, and possibly interfere with resolution. Rather than medicating for anxiety, staff may want to give sleeping pills to afford some rest. The number should be small, given the potential for suicide during crisis.

If the medical examiner deems that an autopsy is necessary, help the family to understand the legal role of the medical examiner and why the autopsy is conducted. Tell them what they need to do next in terms of contacting their funeral home and that the details will be taken care of when they have been contacted.

At one urban teaching hospital, the psychiatric clinical nurse specialist calls all bereaved families 4 to 6 weeks after a death. Most families are moved by the concern expressed on behalf of the hospital—*for them*— and they are given the opportunity to ask unanswered questions about the prehospital and emergency department experience. This phone call provides a forum to anticipate any further counseling referrals.

In summary, the value of therapeutic communication is the foundation of understanding, trust, assessment, and cooperation among colleagues, patients, and families in crisis. These communication techniques will aid in inspiring trust and fortify relationships to help others cope better. To meet this challenge, emergency care providers need to value themselves. Authentic communication will flow from staff who preserve their ability to give of themselves to satisfy those who are in crisis. The quality of that *caring relationship* is immeasurable and more essential now than ever before in health care.

REFERENCES

1. Lenehan G: Emotional impact of trauma, *Nurs Clin North Am* 21(4): 729-740, 1986.
2. Johnson B: *Psychiatric mental health nursing: adaption and growth,* ed 2, Philadelphia, 1989, Lippincott.
3. Saunders C: The moment of truth: care of the dying person. In Pearson L, editor: *Death and dying,* Cleveland, 1969, University Press.
4. Press-Ganey Associates: *Patient satisfaction survey of the emergency department,* Weston, Mass, August to November, 1994, unpublished data.
5. North American Nursing Diagnosis Association: *Classification of nursing diagnosis,* Proceedings of the Ninth Conference, Caroll-Johnson RN, editor, Philadelphia, 1991, Lippincott.
6. American Psychiatric Association: *Diagnostic and statistical manual of psychiatric disorders,* ed 3, Washington, D.C., 1987, American Psychiatric Association.
7. Mian P: Sudden bereavement: nursing intervention in the ED, *Crit Care Nurs* 10(1): 30-41, 1990.
8. Fanslow J: Needs of grieving spouses in sudden death situations, *J Emerg Nurs* 9(4): 213-216, 1983.

CHAPTER 2

Patient Assessment, Reporting, and Documentation

Peggy Cass

Rapid, accurate initial patient assessment and precise reporting and documentation, whether in the prehospital or hospital setting, are keys to effective patient care. Situations that could make assessment and/or reporting difficult are: an unconscious patient with an unknown history, poor weather or terrain conditions, loud street sounds in the prehospital setting, many patients, or an understaffed emergency department on a very busy shift.

Following patient assessment, it is crucial that the information gathered is communicated to others on the care team to ensure that care is consistent. Both the prehospital provider and hospital personnel should use common terminology. In the prehospital setting, patient information obtained will differ depending on the skill level of the prehospital provider (for example, basic emergency medical technician vs. paramedic). The information is usually reported verbally and recorded by prehospital personnel and verified by hospital personnel. In many situations, prehospital personnel function under preapproved protocols or standing orders. When the information gathered is interpreted, therapeutic intervention should be instituted. This may be necessary even when information is incomplete, to correct or prevent life-threatening events.

To assess a patient accurately, one must be an astute observer and know what to look for, using eyes, ears, nose, fingers, and hands to gather data. Before assessing the patient, the caregiver must verify that the scene is secure for caregivers and safe for the patient. Occasionally it is necessary to delay patient assessment; for example, in an unsecure shooting scene, or when a patient must be removed from a burning building or other hazardous environment. After securing rescuer and patient safety, begin the initial assessment.

STEPS IN ASSESSMENT

1. The Primary Survey (*Always* begin with the primary survey)

(All multiple trauma patients are considered to have C-spine injury until proven otherwise.) *PROTECT THE C-SPINE!*

A = Airway

Is the airway open?
  If not, open it and clear it.
  Consider OPA or NPA.

B = Breathing

Is the patient breathing? Adequately?
  Consider supplemental oxygen.
  Consider intubation.
  Consider ventilatory assistance.

What is the respiratory rate, rhythm, and depth?

Does the patient have breath sounds? If not immediately inspect the chest wall for obvious injuries, for example, flail or sucking chest wound.

C^1 = Circulation

Does the patient have a pulse? Where?

Initiate chest compressions if pulses are absent.

Consider placing the patient on a cardiac monitor.

What is the quality, rate, and rhythm of the pulse?

What can you note regarding skin color, temperature, moisture?

Is there any obvious bleeding?

Control bleeding by direct pressure, pressure points, or tourniquet *(last resort)*.

Consider using the pneumatic antishock garment (PASG) to temporarily control intraabdominal or pelvic hemorrhage.

What is the patient's blood pressure?

C^2 = C-spine

Does the patient have any C-spine tenderness?

2. The Secondary Survey (*Always* inspect visually before palpation or auscultation)
General observations

What is the patient's general appearance? Note body positioning, posture, guarding or self-protection activity.

Are there any obvious problems? Any odors?

What is the patient's level of consciousness?

How is the patient's behavior?

Can the patient walk?

Can the patient speak? Clearly?

What is the patient's temperature?

Examine the patient from head to toe.

Check for obvious injuries.

Head and face

Inspect for gross deformity, depressions, and bleeding.

Check pupils for size and reactivity to light.

Consider assessing gross visual acuity.

Palpate for scalp wounds, tenderness, deformity.

Palpate facial bones for deformity, tenderness.

Check nose for bleeding or clear discharge.

Check ears for bleeding or clear discharge.

Check mouth for bleeding, obstruction, color, hydration, absent or fractured teeth, injured or swollen tongue.

Check for asymmetrical facial expression.

Neck

Inspect the neck:

For wounds

For midline trachea and presence of subcutaneous emphysema

For jugular vein size

Auscultate carotid arteries for bruits.

Palpate C-spine for tenderness.

Chest

Inspect for deformities, flailing, and obvious injuries.
Note rate, depth, and ease of respiratory effort.
Palpate bony areas for pain, deformities, crepitus.
Auscultate for breath sounds.
Auscultate for heart sounds.

Abdomen

Inspect for obvious injuries, discoloration, distension, masses, scars, impaled objects, exposed internal organs.
Auscultate for bowel sounds.
   (One minute in each quadrant)
Auscultate for abdominal aorta bruit.
Palpate for tenderness, pain, guarding, rebound, masses.
Palpate femoral pulses and aorta.
Palpate the liver.
Compress symphysis pubis and ischial wings to check for presence of pain and instability.

Limbs

Inspect extremities for wounds, deformities, edema or ecchymosis, and for needle "track" marks.
Note distal extremity color, temperature, capillary refill, sensation.
Palpate for pain and crepitus.

Back (Log roll patient while protecting C-spine)

Check for wounds and deformities.
NOTE: Repeat vital signs after completing secondary survey.
Palpate for tenderness or pain.
Occasionally, in the prehospital setting, it may be necessary to perform therapeutic interventions en route to the hospital because of the patient's critical condition and the need to get to the hospital as quickly as possible. In field terminology, this type of situation is usually known as a "scoop and run" or a "load and go." Patients who fall into this category are those who are rapidly losing consciousness and are in severe respiratory failure or shock from trauma. In all such cases, the patient should be transported to the hospital immediately after the primary survey and initial stabilization on a long backboard. The secondary survey and additional treatment including intravenous therapy, splinting, and so on should occur en route to the hospital.

Pain assessment

If immediate transport is not necessary, perform a secondary survey at the scene. The secondary survey might include a more in-depth assessment of pain. A preferred mnemonic when assessing a patient whose chief complaint is pain is "PQRST."

P = Provokes

What provokes the pain? What makes it feel worse? Better?
What was the patient doing when the pain began?

Q = Quality

What does the pain feel like? Have the patient describe it. Words commonly used are *dull, sharp, pressure, tearing.*

R = Radiates

In what direction does the pain radiate? Is it located in one area? Does it move? Is it located in any other area?

S = Severity

How severe is the pain? On a scale of 1 to 10, with 1 being the least and 10 being the worst, ask the patient to give the pain a number.

T = Time

When did it start? How long did it last? Has the patient ever had it before? When? How long did it last? Does the pain remain constant, or does it come and go?

If the patient is a trauma patient, a head-to-toe secondary survey (see Chapter 29) is appropriate. If the patient has other chief complaints, perform assessments specific to that chief complaint (see specific topic chapters for further information).

DOCUMENTATION

Be sure to obtain and record other information about the patient, such as name, age, sex, address and phone number, any medical history or allergies, the patient's approximate build and weight, and any pertinent signs (what can be observed) or symptoms (what the patient tells you he or she feels). Remember to document positive findings as well as pertinent negatives. If you are unable to assess a certain parameter (such as blood pressure), be sure to state the reason why (such as, "both arms pinned under car"). This ensures that there is an explanation for omissions. Remember that if something is not documented, it will be assumed that it did not occur.

For prehospital personnel, an organized method of presentation for your radio report is important. One example of a report format follows:

Prehospital Unit Name
Receiving or Base Hospital Name
Request Physician/Nurse
Type of Patient (urgent, critical, nonurgent)
Location (home, doctor's office, supermarket, street)
Age (approximate)
Weight (approximate)
Sex
Problem/Chief Complaint/Injury
    Mechanism of injury/Loss of consciousness
History of present illness using findings obtained in your PQRST history and patient exam.
Pertinent History/Medications
Primary Survey Results/Secondary Survey findings, including current vital signs

In the event of a multiple patient call, tell the receiver you have X number of patients. Then proceed by giving the first report on the most seriously ill or injured patient, referring to "patient number one."

In the emergency department, be sure to record detailed nurse's notes. Include a triage note that contains the time of the patient's arrival, mode of transportation (for example, ambulance, private car), condition on arrival, initial vital signs, and the patient's statement about the chief complaint. Also include information offered by prehospital caregivers and all treatment done in the field (that is, patient arrives on long backboard, cervical collar in place, with one IV run at KVO, 18 gauge in left hand).

Record findings of the emergency department primary and secondary survey. Include descriptions of any therapeutic interventions that were performed and any response from these interventions. Accuracy is crucial when recording the time each event occurred. Save cardiac rhythm strips (labeled with patient's name, date, and time) to include in the patient's record. Record any lab values or x-ray results that are reported before written reports are available. Use standard abbreviations (Box 2-1). Also record times phone calls/pages were made to consultants and the time consultants actually arrived in the emergency department.

Flow charts are often useful, especially if the patient being treated is in critical condition and has had multiple therapeutic interventions with documentable data points.

BOX 2-1   Common Abbreviations for Radio Reports and Documentation

ALS	Advanced life support
A + O × 3	Alert and oriented to person, place, and time
ASA	Aspirin
Bicarb	Sodium bicarbonate
BLS	Basic life support
BP	Blood pressure
BSA	Body surface area
BVM	Bag-valve mask
CHF	Congestive heart failure
CNS	Central nervous system
COPD	Chronic obstructive pulmonary disease
CPR	Cardiopulmonary resuscitation
CSF	Cerebrospinal fluid
CVA	Cerebrovascular accident
D/C	Discontinue
DTs	Delirium tremens
EOA	Esophageal obturator airway
EPI	Epinephrine
ETA	Estimated time of arrival
ETOH	Ethyl alcohol
ETT	Endotracheal tube
GCS	Glasgow coma score
GI	Gastrointestinal tract
GSW	Gunshot wound
Hx	History
IM	Intramuscular
IV	Intravenous
IVP	Intravenous push
JVD	Jugular vein distended
KVO	Keep vein open
LBB	Long back board
LOC	Level of consciousness
MAE	Moves all extremities
MCI	Mass casualty incident
NKA	No known allergies
NPO	Nothing by mouth
N/V	Nausea and vomiting
NS	Normal saline
Nitro	Nitroglycerine
OD	Overdose
OPA	Oropharyngeal airway
PRN	As needed
PVC	Premature ventricular contraction
SQ	Subcutaneous
STAT	Immediately
SVT	Supraventricular tachycardia
TIA	Transient ischemic attack
TKO	To keep open
VF	Ventricular fibrillation
VT	Ventricular tachycardia

BIOMEDICAL COMMUNICATIONS

Biomedical communications is the term used to send medical information about a patient from one point (usually the location of the patient) to another (usually the base or receiving hospital) by radio, telephone, or television. All personnel involved in the process of biomedical communications must thoroughly understand the local EMS system policies, procedures, and protocols/patient care guidelines. There should be knowledge of the limits and liabilities of all caregivers. In addition, hospital personnel should have an understanding of and appreciation for the unique circumstances found in the prehospital care setting.

Be sure to keep accurate records on all communications, including any communication problems, mechanical or otherwise; have an alternative plan for communication should difficulties arise. When talking on the radio or telephone from field to hospital, speak clearly and use simple terms. Refer to Boxes 2-2, 2-3, and 2-4

BOX 2-2 Federal Communications Commission Aural Brevity Code (the "10" codes)

10-1	Signal weak		**10-21**	Call _____ by phone
10-2	Signal good		**10-22**	Disregard
10-3	Stop transmitting		**10-23**	Arrived at scene
10-4	Affirmative (OK)		**10-24**	Assignment completed
10-5	Relay to		**10-25**	Report to _____
10-6	Busy		**10-26**	Estimated time of arrival
10-7	Out of service		**10-27**	License/permit information
10-8	In service		**10-28**	Ownership information
10-9	Repeat		**10-29**	Records check
10-10	Negative		**10-30**	Danger/caution
10-11	_____ on duty		**10-31**	Pick up _____
10-12	Stand by (stop)		**10-32**	_____ units of blood needed (specify type)
10-13	Existing conditions		**10-33**	Need help quick
10-14	Message/information		**10-34**	Time
10-15	Message delivered		**10-35**	Reserved
10-16	Reply to message		**10-36**	Reserved
10-17	En route		**10-37**	Reserved
10-18	Urgent		**10-38**	Reserved
10-19	In contact		**10-39**	Reserved
10-20	Location			

BOX 2-3 Frequently Used Radio Terms

come in	Used in asking for acknowledgment of transmission.
go ahead	Proceed with your message.
repeat/say again	The message was not understood.
received	Used in acknowledging that the message is received and understood.
ETA	Estimated time of arrival.
spell out	Used in asking sender to spell out phonetically words that are unclear.
stand by	Please wait.
landline	Telephone communication.
over	End of message.
clear	End of transmission.

BOX 2-4   The International Phonetic Alphabet

A	Alpha	**J**	Juliet	**S**	Sierra
B	Bravo	**K**	Kilo	**T**	Tango
C	Charley	**L**	Lima	**U**	Uniform
D	Delta	**M**	Mike	**V**	Victor
E	Echo	**N**	November	**W**	Whiskey
F	Foxtrot	**O**	Oscar	**X**	X-ray
G	Golf	**P**	Papa	**Y**	Yankee
H	Hotel	**Q**	Quebec	**Z**	Zebra
I	India	**R**	Romeo		

---

for information to aid you in radio transmissions (Aural Brevity Code, Frequently Used Radio Terms, and The International Phonetic Alphabet). If the Aural Brevity Code is used in your system, be familiar with it. Be as brief as possible without sacrificing information about the patient. Make sure that the message is received, and use the phonetic alphabet if it is necessary to spell a word. If using a radio, always identify yourself and the unit you are addressing with each transmission in the event that multiple runs are ongoing or multiple agencies are sending and/or receiving messages. Also, be sure to sign off at the end of the complete transmission.

If cardiac rhythm strips or 12-lead ECGs are sent via telemetry or fax transmissions should be short and intermittent. On receipt, each ECG transmission should be interpreted by concurrence by both the sender and the receiver. The diagnosis of myocardial infarction cannot be made on the basis of a single lead rhythm strip in the field.

In multiple-call situations in which more than one ambulance is making contact with the hospital at the same time, it is imperative to use proper radio communication techniques. The hospital will usually control the situation. The ambulance units may not be able to hear each other. If a phone line is available, the hospital may request that one of the squads use the "landline," after first ensuring that the patient's condition is not critical and there is time to do so. In such a situation, it is essential that strict attention be paid to detail by hospital personnel on the radio. In many systems, radio traffic will be organized by a central medical emergency dispatch (CMED) dispatcher to avoid multiple ambulances on the same radio frequency at the same time. Hospital and ambulance personnel should be familiar with common terminology and abbreviations. Remaining calm and organized should result in the optimal handling of this potentially difficult situation.

SUGGESTED READINGS

Brown SK, Preston P, Smith RN: Getting a better read on thermometry, *RN* 61(3): 57-60, 1998.

Davis M et al: Designing and implementing a significant findings charting system in the pediatric emergency department, *J Emerg Nurs* 23(5): 481-486, 1997.

Harahill M: Strategies for improving trauma documentation, *J Emerg Nurs* 23(2): 187-188, 1997.

Keddington RK: A triage vital sign policy for a children's hospital emergency department, *J Emerg Nurs* 24(2): 189-192, 1998.

Mattera CJ: Principles of EMS documentation for mobile intensive care nurses, *J Emerg Nurs* 21(3): 231-237, 1995.

Merkley K, Nelson NC: Computerized charting by exception at triage, *J Emerg Nurs* 21(6): 571-573, 1995.

CHAPTER 3

Patient and Family Education*

Donna E. Chase

RATIONALE FOR PATIENT TEACHING

Patient and family education is the responsibility of every emergency nurse. The provision of information to patients and their families not only reduces anxiety, but it also leads to a greater understanding of what is happening to them and around them. Documentation of patient and family education is mandated by both quality assurance and accreditation criteria. The goal of patient and family education, as stated by the Joint Commission on Accreditation of Healthcare Organizations (JCAHO) in its 1997 standards, is to improve patient health outcomes by promoting healthy behavior and involving the patient and the family in care and care decisions. Documentation of patient teaching must include the following: date and time; who the learner is; whether he/she is a patient or family member; content and teaching method used; supplemental learning aids provided; the learner's response; and referrals and signature of nurse and patient. If the patient is unable to sign then the signature of a family member should be obtained.

Patient education materials have become more sophisticated. Gone are the days of homemade mimeographed copies of information (Figure 3-1). Today we have colorful, humorous, informative booklets and pamphlets as well as videotapes and computer assisted programs. Many hospitals use advanced technology, with their own web sites where patients and their families can obtain valuable information. Learning materials are published in languages other than English and in picture and audio format for patients with limited reading ability.

In today's health care environment the need for patient and family education has increased dramatically. The emergency department now sends the majority of patients home. Fear of litigation, cost containment, and restriction of admissions by HMOs and insurance companies account for the decline in admissions to the emergency department. The Patient Bill of Rights, first introduced in 1972 by the American Hospital Association, dramatically increased public awareness of key issues regarding patient and family education. Health care consumers are not only more informed today; they are better educated. The media has also provided enough derogatory publicity regarding errors of omission and commission of health care providers to significantly increase the number of malpractice suits. Managed care, in an effort to further reduce rising health care costs, restricts patient admissions to those persons with illnesses or injuries clearly defined in specific diagnostic related groups. The emphasis is on "wellness and prevention." We now treat episodes of illness.

The drive to reduce the use of hospital emergency rooms as a way to reduce escalating health care costs would seem to point to a decline in emergency department patients. However, the patients who do come to the emergency department have a higher acuity than those seen over the past decade. Transportation problems, financial reasons, and limited physician hours for nonemergent office visits still make the emergency department the primary access to care for some patients. Despite all of the above factors, patient and family education remains a top priority of local, state, and federal government. It is not only perceived as a patient right but also

*Portions of this chapter are from Miller MM: Patient teaching. In Sheehy SB: *Emergency nursing principles and practice,* ed 3, St Louis, 1992, Mosby.

HOW TO TAKE A CHILD'S TEMPERATURE

1. Shake the thermometer down.
2. **Oral Thermometer**
   a) Place the long, silver tip of thermometer under child's tongue.
   b) Have child close lips gently, being careful not to bite the thermometer.

Rectal Thermometer

   a) Lubricate silver end of the thermometer.
   b) Spread the buttocks so that rectum can be seen easily.
   c) Insert thermometer gently into the rectum until silver tip can no longer be seen.

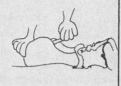

3. Hold thermometer in place for 3-5 minutes.
4. Remove the thermometer.
5. Rotate the thermometer until the wide silver line can be seen.
6. Read degree of temperature (exactly where the mercury stops). Read the temperature at the end of the silver line and write down the number.

CU/BMC 6-75

YOUR CHILD IS VOMITING

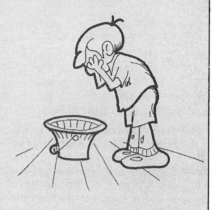

Saint Joseph Hospital
Emergency Service

YOUR CHILD IS VOMITING

Persistent vomiting — If your child cannot keep down even plain water for more than half a day, contact your physician. Vomiting causes loss of body water resulting in dehydration.

Stop: All feedings
Rest the stomach
No milk
No solid foods
Nothing by mouth for at least an hour

Infants: Start feeding sugar water* or 7-Up in a bottle or with a spoon.

*Sugar water — Add 1 teaspoon of sugar to 4 ounces (½ cup) of boiled cool water.

Older Children: Feed small quantities of cold water or ice chips.

When: The child can keep water or ice chips down, then you may give several sips OR swallows every 15 minutes of:

a. Weak tea, kool aid, sweetened
b. 7-Up
c. Gingerale

When: The child can keep down gingerale, 7-Up, or tea, you can further add other liquids such as:

a. Clear broth
b. Fruit juices — apple, pineapple, or orange
c. Jello — liquid or solid form

Medication: Do not give any medications to stop vomiting, unless ordered by your doctor.

Do Not Give Aspirin: It may increase your child's vomiting.

If your child needs medicine for fever, you may use Tylenol or Tempra in liquid form

If: your child has not vomited for 8-12 hours and feels hungry, you may give the following foods:

First Day
1. Cereal — Rice, oatmeal, cooked cream of wheat
2. Mashed potato, soft cooked rice with butter
3. Dry toast, Soda crackers
4. Apple sauce, Jello
5. Mashed ripe bananas

Second Day
1. May start 2+ or skim milk
2. Lean meat suitable for age: Chicken or Beef
3. Vegetables — Green beans, peas, carrots, spinach cooked tender
4. Vanilla ice cream or puddings, or fruit — jello

FIGURE 3-1. "Your Child is Vomiting."
(From St. Joseph Hospital Emergency Services, Omaha, NE.)

as a means to contain health care costs and prevent frivolous law suits. When we take into account these professional, governmental, and economic factors, the need for effective patient teaching by the professional emergency nurse is evident.

Providing patient and family education in the emergency department is a special challenge. There are many barriers to learning in the emergency department that are not as evident in other health care settings. The varied patient population, multiplicity of illnesses and accidents, the physician, the psychoemotionally compromised condition of patients, the various age groups, the emergency department environment, and the increased level of anxiety of emergency department patients in general make teaching patients and their families very difficult.

To minimize the constraints and to teach effectively, the emergency nurse must be familiar with the teaching and learning process. Higher knowledge must be current and he or she must be skilled in a large variety of interventions. The ability to decrease the patient and their family's anxiety level is also essential. As with the use of any process involving knowledge and skill, familiarity with the sequential steps increases ease and effectiveness. Each time the nurse does patient teaching he or she becomes more familiar with the process and confidence as well as skills improve.

The wide variety of health problems and the varied age groups of patients presenting to the emergency department means that the emergency nurse is faced with the unique problem of developing and maintaining the current knowledge and skills necessary to teach patients with multiple needs. Skills and knowledge can be updated through attendance at professional continuing education or through inservice education. The nurse can also participate in local, regional, or national professional meetings and symposiums, or through independent study courses available through nursing journals or through computer-assisted learning programs. Another excellent source of knowledge that nurses sometimes forget to take advantage of is their peers. Often these people have expertise in specific areas and can be called upon to present educational offerings, act as a reference, or serve as a preceptor or mentor for new staff or staff with less experience.

Although moderate anxiety enhances learning, high anxiety may act as a deterrent. Emergency nurses must be able to effectively reduce patients' anxiety by the use of verbal and nonverbal methods. The emergency department itself lends to increased anxiety in some patients. The bright lights, unfamiliar equipment, strange sounds, unusual sights, and bustling personnel speaking in medical jargon can add to the stress that the patient is already experiencing just from being ill. The environment itself cannot be changed. However, when the nurse is explaining procedures to the patient, the use of nonmedical terms can relieve some anxiety. Nonverbal communication, including touch, facial expressions, and body language, can be used effectively to reduce anxiety as well. Other approaches to reducing anxiety are actively listening to what the patient is saying and staying with, or allowing a relative to stay with, frightened patients. Privacy screening or simply dimming the lights can also reduce the patient's anxiety.

Patient teaching in the emergency department is an integral component of professional nursing care. Although the focus of patient teaching in the emergency department is on the immediate needs of the patient, referrals for long-term or home care must also be taken into account.

1. Identify the implied and expressed learning needs of the patient or learner.
2. Assess the learner's readiness, capabilities, and motivation.
3. Cooperatively establish realistic learning goals.
4. Select and use an appropriate teaching method based on the identified learning needs, the content to be learned, and the individual characteristics of the learner.
5. Provide time, space, necessary equipment and supplies, and teaching tools such as visual aids, videotapes, or written instructions for home care.
6. Evaluate the effectiveness of teaching.
7. Document the content taught, the method used, the home care instruction sheets provided, the learner's response, and referrals made.

To use this process effectively, the nurse and teacher must have knowledge and skills regarding the content area, astutely assess the learner, establish realistic learning goals, and communicate effectively.

IDENTIFYING LEARNING NEEDS

The initial step in the teaching process, identification of implied and expressed learning needs, is directly related to the patient's problem. For example, if the patient has a fractured arm that must be casted, the implied learning need is for measures that promote healing and prevent complications in the care of the casted arm. However, the patient may request information regarding the advisability of taking previously prescribed medications. Specific questions asked by the patient identify expressed learning needs. If these questions are ignored, the patient's anxiety about medications may block his or her ability to learn the information about cast care that you are sharing.

Categories of home care learning needs are (1) procedures or techniques and (2) general supportive care. When procedural and technical needs have been identified, the nurse teacher includes the following content: what procedures and techniques are to be performed and why; specifics of how and when to perform them; the anticipated results; a list of necessary supplies or equipment with instructions for care of the equipment; situations in which professional help is necessary; and whom to call for help. For example, a right-handed patient has a laceration on the left thumb, which has been sutured. The physician has prescribed a procedure of twice-daily suture line cleansing, application of antibiotic ointment, and reapplication of sterile dressing. The nurse explains that this procedure is necessary to prevent infection and demonstrates the procedure. To define frequency, the nurse may suggest performing the procedure in the morning and at night or relate timing to the patient's working schedule. A picture and a verbal explanation of a noninfected sutured wound identify the anticipated results. The same method can be used to illustrate an infected suture line that indicates the need for professional help. The nurse either gives the patient a prescription or provides the prescribed ointment and dressings. The patient is also given a referral card, which provides the name and phone number of the health care professional to be contacted if problems arise.

When identifying learning needs related to general supportive care, the nurse teacher selects the appropriate content from an extensive list of potential needs. Included in this broad category are hygiene, rest and nutritional requirements, elimination needs, skin and pressure-point protection, correct body alignment and position changes, oxygenation and ventilation needs, range-of-motion and activity levels, safety factors, and the scheduling of medications and prescribed therapeutic measures. Obviously the supportive needs list can be long. In the telescoped teaching time available in the emergency department, the nurse must astutely select the most pertinent content and provide referral for less pressing needs.

Patients being transferred to another unit within the agency or to another health care facility also have urgent learning needs. Specifically, these patients need to know where they are going, how they will get there, and the reason for their transfer. Explaining the reason for the transfer and the logistics of it minimizes the patient's anxiety and reduces the potential for undesirable physiologic stress responses in the patient.

ASSESSING THE LEARNER

After identifying the probable learning needs of the patient, the nurse must assess the learner's readiness to learn, capabilities, and motivation level. Numerous factors influence the patient's readiness to learn self-care measures, including the patient's age, education, culture and primary language, present anxiety level, contact with health care professionals for concomitant or previous health problems, prior experience with self-care, and self-concept. The nurse obtains this information from various sources. The patient's record indicates age, family status, nationality, and ability to finance health care. However, much necessary information is obtained from the patient interview and pertinent observation. For example, during the admission process, patients are asked about medications taken at home and current health problems. The patient's way of speaking or answering questions may indicate his or her primary language and educational level.

The patient's record indicates anticipated or completed diagnostic and therapeutic measures. This information is extremely important because the nurse must select a time for patient teaching that does not interfere with or counteract diagnostic and therapeutic measures used in treatment. To illustrate, if a patient has received a central nervous system depressant for treatment of severe pain, the stimulus of initiating patient teaching may counteract the desired effect of the medication. Questions about previous healthcare experiences can provide a helpful point of reference for teaching. Using analogies and similes to relate new content to previous experiences increases the meaningfulness of the new content.

Pertinent observations provide additional information. If the patient's basic physiologic needs are not met, his or her readiness to learn is diminished. When a person is dehydrated or has hypoxia, a full bladder, or acute pain, initiating patient teaching is unproductive. These physiologic conditions require prompt remediation. Patient behaviors and appearances that typically indicate a poor self-concept include poor hygiene, lack of eye contact, or muffled voice quality. Generally an inadequate self-concept results in a lack of the self-confidence necessary to learn new self-care behaviors. Because these patients doubt their own capabilities to learn a new behavior, the likelihood that they will attempt to learn or will successfully learn is severely limited.[1] It is equally important to observe the patient for the presence of physical limitations that prohibit the learning of some skills. Physical wholeness and dexterity are prerequisites for learning some psychomotor skills.

In assessing motivation level, look for verbal, nonverbal, and behavioral clues. Verbal clues indicating increased motivation might be specific questions the patient asks or the patient's initiation of a discussion about home self-care measures. A less direct verbal clue is a statement such as "I'm going to have to learn to do that." Nonverbal clues include changes in facial expression that indicate interest in what the nurse is doing: watching rather than turning away can be a clue. Observations of small independent behaviors such as initiating position changes indicate the patient's desire to change from the dependent, sick role to increasing independence.

Certain physical behaviors and extensive muscle tenseness can indicate excessive anxiety, which interferes with readiness and motivation to learn. Anxious persons may exhibit either excessive or decreased activity of voluntary muscles. Although some anxious persons exhibit withdrawal behaviors, such as maintaining a fetal position, covering the face, or lowering the eyes, the majority display hyperactive behaviors. For example, these persons may tense the arm, facial, or neck muscles, fidget with bed sheets, smack or purse lips, or have tremors while attempting purposeful movements. Information regarding the patient's age helps the nurse determine the patient's ability to comprehend specific learning content and adhere to self-care measures. For example, a 2-year-old child is incapable of comprehending information about sterile dressings and lacks the physical dexterity necessary to apply a sterile dressing. Therefore the parent or guardian must be taught to complete this procedure at home. Conversely, an elderly person may be able to comprehend information about dressing changes but unable to complete the task because of impaired sight and osteoarthritic finger joints.

Because of the cultural and ethnic diversity in the United States, language can present a problem. If the emergency department staff is unable to converse in the patient's language, a resource person must be obtained. This person can help not only with translation but also with knowledge of cultural factors that may enhance or detract from the patient's adherence to the home care measures being taught. In some instances home care instruction materials and other learning aids are available in the different languages prevalent in the community.

Collecting assessment data is nonsensical unless the data are used. In the teaching and learning situation, nurse teachers must build on assessed strengths and minimize or delete factors that inhibit learning.

ESTABLISHING LEARNING GOALS

The third step in the teaching and learning process is to establish realistic, individualized learning goals. Although healthcare educators advise designing both short-term and long-term learning goals, the time constraints and the emergency patient's anxiety level preclude addressing long-term teaching needs except through referral. Goals for the emergency patient, based on the learner's assessment data and time-constraints, should be realistic. For example, if the patient has a fractured tibia, concomitant diabetes, a hangnail, and a sinus problem, the emergency nurse must determine the paramount learning needs without attempting to meet all the learning needs of this patient. Because of the diverse health problems, the patient would probably be unable to comprehend all the necessary information if the nurse tried to discuss all concerns at once. Realistically the nurse might focus on two of the patient's most pressing needs. The nurse might share the identified learning needs with the patient and ask which are most important to him or her, thereby cooperatively establishing learning goals. The patient's remaining needs can be met by referral to his or her physician, a community health agency, or local groups such as the American Diabetes Association. Local phone companies and public health agencies publish listings of resources available in various communities. These lists are handy reference resources for any emergency department.

To individualize the teaching and learning process, the nurse must interview the patient regarding his or her work and home situation to discover potential problems the patient might have in adhering to prescribed home care measures. For example, a man is admitted to the emergency department with acute back pain sustained after 2 hours of sawing, lifting, and stacking logs for his fireplace. After taking vertebral radiographs, the physician diagnoses low back muscle strain and prescribes a muscle relaxant. Proper lifting and bending methods are demonstrated, and a back care instruction sheet is given to the patient for future reference. It is also appropriate to inquire about the man's occupation. If he has a desk job, his return to work the next day would not interfere with his recuperation. However, if his job involves loading trucks, which requires a significant amount of bending and lifting, return to work must be delayed until he has recuperated. For maximum effectiveness, the patient's medication schedule should be correlated with his work schedule. Absorption of medication depends on the metabolic rate; if the patient works from 4 PM to midnight, his schedule for taking the prescribed muscle relaxant will be different from that of a person working from 9 AM to 5 PM. When medications are prescribed, administration scheduling and other pertinent information regarding food and activity restrictions that enhance the effectiveness of the medication should be discussed.

In addition to considering the patient's home and work situation, the nurse can further individualize and adapt the learning experience based on the patient's previous experiences with self-care, potential work-related problems, and family or cultural taboos or expectations. If the patient has had positive experiences with self-care, his or her attitude toward learning is more positive. It is advantageous to use teaching approaches that have been successful previously. For example, if a patient finds it easy to remember to take medications at mealtime or when a specific television program begins, that approach should be used in designing a medication schedule. For other patients, keeping a record helps to ensure that medications or treatments follow the prescribed timing. When patients admit previous noncompliance, tactfully ask them why they have not adhered to prescribed home care measures. The reason may be lack of finances or failure to comprehend all the components of a procedure. In these instances referral for financial or home health assistance may be the answer. You may also discover that the patient did not learn because of the teaching approach. For example, many young people learn best by using videotaped or computer-assisted instruction, whereas an older person may prefer demonstration and discussion. Occasionally, patients state that they did not follow through with home care measures because they did not understand what was expected of them. Possibly compliance would have been increased if their preferred learning method had been used.

Some occupations, because of either the nature of the work or unusual hours, may cause problems with follow-through in home care measures. Consider, for example, the needs of a long-haul truck driver who is treated for a bladder infection. The physician prescribes 500 mg sulfisoxazole (Gantrisin) to be taken 4 times daily. Recognizing the sulfa base of this medication, the nurse must teach the patient that increased water intake prevents the formation of sulfa salt urinary stones. Because the patient is a truck driver, carrying a thermos of water in the truck may be a logical home care measure. The nurse should also discuss with the patient a list of fluids and foods that produce the desired acid ash.

In some instances the expectations of the patient or family conflict with adherence to prescribed home measures. Consider the compulsive worker who is admitted to the hospital with recurrent angina. Because of his role as family breadwinner, he states that he has to get right back to work. Obviously the nurse cannot change the patient's culturally based life-style with a single teaching opportunity in the emergency department. However, the nurse can seize this moment to explain briefly the causes and effects of angina and the anticipated results of the prescribed medications, and the nurse can refer the patient to the support group for persons with heart diseases in the community.

The objective of this step in the teaching and learning process is to elicit data and adapt the teaching approach to realistic, individualized learning goals that will help the patient adhere to prescribed self-care and prevent potential complications.

SELECTING AND USING APPROPRIATE TEACHING METHODS

The fourth step in the teaching process is to select and use the teaching method or methods appropriate to the content to be taught and the assessed capabilities and preference of the learner. Some patients require only a quick review of previously learned information or answers to specific questions. For example, consider the parent of many children, several of whom have had fractures and casts. This parent may need only a quick review of cast care and activity restrictions. Other patients, however, require a more structured teaching approach.

Types of Learning

Three types of learning are cognitive, effective, and psychomotor. Cognitive learning involves thinking and reasoning: the focus is on comprehension of content and practical application to real-life situations. Effective learning involves a change in attitude or values. In the emergency department an effective learning goal is often achieved by referring the patient to a community health agency or a support group such as an ostomy or stroke club. Psychomotor learning requires coordination of the brain and extremities to complete a task. After skills are demonstrated, the learner needs practice time before a return demonstration is given. Typically, effective learning requires more time than cognitive or psychomotor learning.

Principles of Learning

The effectiveness of learning depends on several teaching and learning principles. A major tenet of learning is that active participation by the learner increases the meaningfulness and retention of the content. For this reason, two-way discussion and demonstration followed by practice are more effective than a lecture of dos and don'ts. Both verbal and physical incentives motivate learning. Physical incentives such as lollipops, balloons, or a coloring book are effective motivators for children. Adults typically respond positively to verbal reinforcement, especially when the reinforcement is accompanied by appropriate nonverbal behaviors. Successful efforts should be noted because this recognition increases the self-confidence of the learner.

Another principle of learning is that building on past experiences makes learning new content easier and increases retention. This type of learning is enhanced by the teacher's use of analogies and similes. Providing successful experiences by starting with the easiest content and progressing to the more difficult also motivates learners. Recall the old saying, "Nothing succeeds like success." Actually, the building-step concept is the basis for our entire educational system.

Although a comfortable atmosphere promotes learning, the mild degree of anxiety prevalent in the emergency setting is not detrimental in most instances. Another principle of learning is that repetition strengthens learning, which is particularly true of psychomotor skills.

Teaching Methods

Teaching methods commonly used include discussion, question and answer, visual aids, and the lecture. The advantage of lecturing, or telling information to the patient, is speed, but the major disadvantage outweighs the primary advantage: there is no opportunity to evaluate the patient's comprehension of the content. Lecturing violates the first principle of effective teaching: participation in the process increases retention. Teaching is not complete until the learner has learned.

The advantage of discussion is that it involves two-way responsive communication. The patient and the teacher are free to question and respond to one another. The sequence leads to discussion of "what if" situations, which increase the practicality of learning. The question and answer approach is the most direct because the nurse is responding to the patient's specific learning needs.

Using visual aids as an adjunct method increases the sensory experience of the patient and gives meaning to abstract terms or concepts. For example, showing a patient the radiograph of his or her fractured bone provides a graphic description of the problem. A chart or illustration of the location of body organs aids in describing illness, defining the anticipated effects of prescribed treatments, or explaining the extent of trauma.

Demonstration is the most effective method to teach psychomotor skills. You may spend 30 minutes explaining the technique of figure-eight bandaging, but a 5-minute demonstration is more meaningful. When demonstration is used, the patient must have an opportunity to practice the skill before dismissal. This practice prevents errors in technique and provides the opportunity for active participation and repetition. Recent research has revealed that use of videotapes for skill demonstration provides accurate and consistent information in a cost-effective manner.[2,3] In addition, the visual appeal results in increased retention of the content. Another visual participative teaching technique is computer-assisted learning, which is particularly effective for patients with reading or hearing problems and for many computer-literate patients.[4] However, the use of videotapes and computer-assisted learning programs requires an initial financial investment in hardware and the purchase or development of software and also necessitates dedication of space in or adjacent to the emergency department. An extensive amount of software is available for purchase, rental, or loan. A number of pharmaceutical and medical supply companies produce and are willing to loan patient teaching videotapes and computer software programs to emergency departments.

Generally, the content and the learning goal dictate the most appropriate teaching method. In most instances more than one method is used. For example, if the patient needs to learn the technique of sterile dressing change, demonstration is the teaching approach of choice. However, an explanation of the rationale for the procedure and a discussion regarding the list of necessary supplies is also necessary. Potential problems related to bleeding and infection should likewise be discussed. A picture of both properly healing wounds and infected wounds would be helpful. This teaching scenario illustrates that in most patient teaching situations, multiple teaching methods are used to achieve a single learning goal. Planning ahead regarding essential content, necessary equipment and supplies, and potential teaching tools decreases interruptions detrimental to the teaching and learning process.

Effective communication is the one prerequisite common to all teaching methods. Recalling that the goal of communication is mutual understanding, use common, nontechnical words rather than medical jargon. When using healthcare terms, define words the patient may not comprehend. Avoid using medical abbreviations that are not generally intelligible. To emphasize the content of your message, match your tone of voice, facial expression, and body language with what you are saying. Consistency of verbal with nonverbal communication prevents the patient from receiving conflicting messages. Because enthusiasm in the learning situation is contagious, be enthusiastic about patient teaching. When the same content is taught repeatedly, sustaining enthusiasm may be difficult. Recall, however, that although this may be your fiftieth presentation of this content, it is the first for the patient. To maintain enthusiasm for teaching specific content, be creative and vary the teaching methods you use. Having a repertoire of teaching approaches benefits the learner, particularly when you are able to adapt your approach to his or her most effective learning style.

After the appropriate teaching method is implemented, provide the time, space, and necessary supplies and learning tools to permit the patient to absorb the content and practice newly learned skills. Learning new content and skills takes time. Rushing the patient's dismissal inhibits effective learning of the content and skills required for home care. Allowing time for the patient to consider practical questions and practice skills enhances retention and compliance with prescribed home care measures.

Occasional visits to the home by the nurse teacher permit the nurse to observe the patient's skill proficiency level and noncomprehension of content or technique and shows the teacher's interest in responding to the patient's questions, concerns, or fears. Also, during these visits errors in technique can be corrected before they become habitual. Occasionally a patient may ask a question you are unable to answer. When this occurs, consult another professional; then be sure to provide the answer for the patient.

When the patient obviously does not comprehend the content, try another teaching approach. In some instances, relating your personal experience is beneficial. For example, if you use a date and time calendar to keep track of medications taken, share this approach with the patient. Lack of space in an extremely busy or small emergency department can present a problem. However, to learn and retain home care measures, the patient needs a place to practice skills and to reflect on potential problems or concerns that may affect compliance. The use of an adjacent office or conference room for this purpose frees a patient treatment room and provides proximity that allows the nurse teacher to stop by to observe skills and answer questions as they arise.

EVALUATING LEARNING EFFECTIVENESS

Evaluating the effectiveness of learning is the sixth step in the teaching and learning process. The content and teaching method dictate the appropriate evaluation method. To illustrate, discussion has been used to teach home care of a casted lower arm. An appropriate evaluative question may be "To keep the cast dry, is it better to take a shower or tub bath?" If a picture has been used to depict the outcome of figure-eight bandaging that prevents elbow extension, ask the patient to identify the areas on his or her arm that require the thickest part of the bandage. Another valuable evaluation approach is to ask "what if" questions. For example, if an anticonvulsant medication has been prescribed, ask, "What will you do if you have the flu and vomit your morning pill?" Remember that the patient's ability to rephrase and respond correctly to practical questions indicates a higher level of comprehension than his or her ability to simply restate what has been said.

The most valuable way to evaluate skill learning is the return demonstration, whether the patient was taught by personal demonstration or by videotaped instructions. Recall, however, that practice should precede evaluation of skill proficiency. Many computer-assisted learning programs provide built-in evaluation. One distinctive feature of computer-assisted learning programs is that the learner progresses only after learning the essential content. Incidental observations indicating incorporation of new learning into the patient's repertoire of behaviors is another valid evaluation method. To illustrate, after teaching active ankle range-of-motion exercises to a patient with dependent edema, you pass the door of his room and observe him doing the exercises without prompting. Likewise, when a patient asks pertinent questions related to self-care measures in his or her work situation, the patient has obviously correlated new learning with his or her real-life situation. Remember that the patient must understand the content before he or she can answer questions regarding how he or she will implement instructions for home care.

In a rushed emergency department, evaluating attitudinal changes is difficult but possible. For example, a patient with newly diagnosed diabetes says he will attend the local American Diabetes Association meetings, which indicates his interest in self-help. To validate his attendance, you may phone the patient or the association to ascertain whether the referred patient did actually attend. In some instances, when referrals are repeatedly made to a specific agency, a reporting system is designed to inform emergency departments of follow-through with referred patients.

Other evaluative approaches used by some agencies are analysis of statistical data regarding readmissions for the same problem and patient callbacks, in which patients are asked about their needs for additional information regarding home care measures.

DOCUMENTATION

The final step in the teaching process is documentation. Because of hospital policy regarding discharge instructions and accreditation criteria and to prevent litigation, accurate documentation of teaching and of the patient's response is essential. As with all other nursing procedures, if the teaching is not documented, it is assumed that the teaching was not done. Complete documentation includes the following information: content taught, method

---

BOX 3-1   *Sample Patient Teaching Documentation*

7/10/98
9:45 AM
Sterile hand bandaging technique demonstrated. Instruction sheet "Sterile Bandage Changing" given to patient's husband, Jerry Howard. Correct return demonstration of sterile bandage change completed. Appointment card for stitch removal on 8/17/98 given to patient.
M. Miller, RN

used, patient response, adjunct instructions provided, date, time, and nurse's name and status. If someone other than the patient was taught the self-care measures, his or her name and relationship to the patient should be included. Box 3-1 illustrates correct documentation. In some agencies the patient also signs the form to indicate that the information was provided. Because the patient record is a legal document, precise documentation is essential.

HOME CARE REFERENCE SHEETS OR BOOKLETS

Because high anxiety levels decrease retention of newly learned content and skills, it is advisable to provide patients with home care instructional handouts. The diversity of instructional media has increased dramatically in the past decade. Whether you intend to purchase the handouts or design and publish them in-house, statistical data regarding patient admissions should be used as a guide when priorities are set for the purchase or development of these materials.

Sources other than patient care publishing companies and the hospital publication department include many national health care associations, such as the American Lung Association or American Diabetes Association, and state health departments. In some instances these publications are free; sometimes a nominal fee is charged.

If the hospital intends to publish instruction sheets, decisions regarding design, content, and personal responsibility for the project must be made. Within the emergency department, nurses with specific areas of expertise and interest can develop home care instruction material. Using the staff's special talents such as drawing, writing, and editing can be motivating; because involvement begets commitment, opinions and ideas about the final publication should be solicited from other emergency nurses. Williams and Manske[3] have suggested that when color, humor, and pictures that move or suggest movement are incorporated in the design of instructional media, the result is a more useful product. Successful patient education publishing companies have incorporated these elements in their design of information booklets.

Home care instructions should be brief and clearly stated. They should be written in simple, nontechnical language. For example, if the patient prescription reads, "Bacitracin oint. To suture line, b.i.d.," the patient instructions should read: "After cleaning stitches with peroxide, apply antibiotic ointment to suture line in AM and PM." If dressings are to be reapplied, instruction for reapplication should be included.

As shown in Figure 3-2, pictures can provide graphic directions. These pictures are particularly beneficial for patients who do not speak English or for those with poor reading skills. A graphic or a listing of objective signs and symptoms that indicate the need to contact a physician or the emergency department should also be included in a home care instruction sheet. When a language other than English is predominant in a community, providing instruction sheets in that language is beneficial. In some areas of the country all instruction sheets are available in both Spanish and English. In addition, some pharmaceutical companies are now producing patient handouts in languages other than English.

To ensure accuracy of information, institute a trial use period before reproducing large quantities of teaching tools developed in-house. In some instances minor refinements of content placement or wording result in a more practical and accurate teaching tool. (See Box 3-2 for examples of discharge instructions.) Some agencies color-code the various patient instruction sheets to increase visibility. Store the instruction sheets in an easily accessible space.

Development of a teaching plan file benefits the teaching nurses who are newly employed or work as needed, as well as those who may be unfamiliar with the teaching needs of specific types of patients, especially those with rarely seen conditions. Typically contained in a looseleaf notebook or card file, the teaching plan outline should include the following information: patient problem and diagnosis; potential resulting problems; therapeutic, restorative, and preventive home care measures; specific content to be taught, in logical order; list of necessary equipment and supplies; and suggestions for teaching and evaluation methods.

To ensure inclusion of patient teaching as an essential component of patient care, the process of patient teaching and a review of the learning tools available should be included in the orientation of new employees and presented as an annual in-service educational program for experienced staff. In most agencies a policy and procedure for patient teaching is incorporated in the agency and department policy and procedure manuals.

COPING WITH DIGESTIVE PROBLEMS

If you are one of the millions of people who suffer from acid-related gastrointestinal discomfort, there are things you can do to improve your health and enhance the quality of your life.

1 Avoid spicy, acidic, and tomato-based foods like fruit juices and Mexican and Italian food (eg, pizza).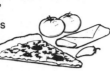

6 Don't exercise too soon after eating.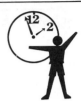

2 Avoid fast-food hamburgers and other fatty foods. Chocolate in any form should also be avoided by people with gastric reflux.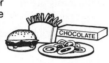

7 Avoid bedtime snacks and eat meals at least 3 to 4 hours before lying down.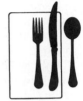

3 Limit your intake of coffee, tea, alcohol, and cola.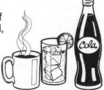

8 Stop (or at least cut down on) smoking.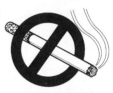

4 Watch your weight. (Being overweight increases pressure in the abdominal area, which can aggravate reflux.)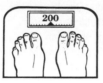

9 Elevate the head of your bed with wooden blocks. (*Don't* elevate your head by using extra pillows; this can increase abdominal pressure.)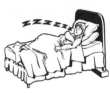

5 Don't gorge yourself at mealtime. Eat moderate amounts of food.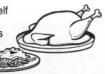

10 See your physician if you are taking antacids three or more times a week.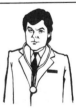

Provided in the interest of good health by: **Glaxo Pharmaceuticals**™
DIVISION OF GLAXO INC.
Research Triangle Park, NC 27709

FIGURE 3-2. "Coping with Digestive Problems."
(Reproduced with permission of Glaxo Wellcome Inc., Research Triangle Park, N.C.)

BOX 3-2   Examples of Discharge Instructions

Urinary tract infection
1. Drink plenty of fluids (at least 8 glasses a day).
2. Take antibiotic exactly as directed until you have finished the prescription.
3. See your private doctor or return to ED if you develop
    a. fever over 101.5 or shaking chills
    b. severe pain
    c. vomiting
    d. worsening symptoms or your present symptoms are not improved in 3 days
4. See your private doctor to have your urine rechecked after you finish your antibiotic.

Nosebleed
1. Do not pick your nose or insert anything in it.
2. Do not blow your nose and if you have to sneeze, expel the sneeze through your open mouth.
3. Avoid stooping or strenuous activity.
4. Do not lie flat for 2 days.
5. Do not take aspirin.
6. If bleeding starts again, sit up with your head slightly forward and squeeze the lower half of your nose firmly between your thumb and forefinger.
7. Return to ED if you feel faint or bleeding does not stop in 25 minutes.
8. If packing was placed in nose, it must be removed in 24 to 48 hours.

Sore throats/colds
Sore throats are usually caused by a virus for which antibiotics are not helpful. If a culture was taken, you will be notified in 24 to 48 hours if it is positive, so that you may begin antibiotics.
1. Drink plenty of fluids.
2. Appropriate dose of Tylenol for fever every 3 to 4 hours.
3. You may use lozenges or sprays for temporary relief.
4. Return to ED if you develop difficulty swallowing or breathing.
5. If symptoms are unimproved in 3 to 4 days, see your personal doctor.

Wound care/burn care
1. Leave dressing in place for 24 hours (unless otherwise directed). Change dressing daily or as often as is necessary to keep bandages and wound clean and dry.
2. Wash gently with warm water daily. Then, REAPPLY antibacterial ointment (neosporin or Bacitracin) and re-bandage.
3. Return to the ED if wound becomes red, swollen, shows pus or read streaks, or if you develop a fever over 100.5 F.
4. Elevate the wound and do not use the injured area. This will help reduce pain and swelling.
5. Return to the ED for suture/staple removal or wound check in _____ days.
6. Please note the date you received a tetanus booster.

Donna Chase: *Examples of Discharge Instructions,* South Weymouth, Mass, 1997, South Shore Hospital.

Documentation of patient teaching is one of the elements listed in quality assurance criteria and in some instances is included in staff performance evaluation criteria.

Even though home care instruction tools have improved significantly in the past decade, they are only an adjunct to the individualized teaching approach selected by the nurse teacher.

SUMMARY

To ensure adherence to prescribed therapeutic, restorative, and preventive measures, the emergency department nurse is responsible for providing effective, individualized instruction regarding home care measures and the process involved in emergency care. This responsibility necessitates familiarity with the sequential steps in the teaching and learning process. The process includes identifying learning needs, assessing the learner, establishing realistic goals, selecting and using appropriate teaching methods, allowing for learning time, evaluating the results, and documenting the instruction. Application of learning and communication principles are prerequisite to effective teaching. Because all emergency department nurses must be familiar with the process involved in carrying out their professional role as nurse teacher, content regarding the patient teaching process is included in orientation and in-service educational programs. In addition, patient teaching is a criterion of quality assurance and clinical ladder or performance evaluation.

Home care instruction sheets or booklets are worthwhile teaching tools. These tools can be purchased from patient education publishing companies or designed and published in-house. These tools should be selected based on the typical patients seen in the emergency department. For inexperienced personnel and for atypical patient conditions, development of a teaching plan file can provide a handy reference.

Because knowledge of home care is a patient's right and also benefits the emergency department by reducing the number of callbacks and return visits, patient teaching can be considered an integral component of emergency patient care.

REFERENCES

1. Merritt S: Patient self-efficacy: a framework for designing patient education, *Focus Crit Care* 16(1):68, 1989.
2. Taylor JE: *Recall and retention of adult patients using videotaped versus written discharge instructions in a hospital emergency department.* Presented at 1989 Emergency Nurses Association Scientific Assembly, Sept 8, 1989, Washington, D.C.
3. Williams M, Manske P: Efficacy of audiovisual tape versus verbal instructions on crutch walking: a comparison, *JEN* 13(3):156, 1987.
4. Luker K, Caress AL: Rethinking patient education, *J Adv Nurs* 14:711, 1989.

SUGGESTED READINGS

Loring, K: *Patient education: a practical approach,* St Louis, 1992, Mosby.
Nelson D, Coleman K, Walker J: Why are you waiting? formulating an information pamphlet for use in the accident and emergency department, *Accid Emerg Nurs* 5(1):39-41, 1997.
Logan PD, Schwab RA, Salomone JA 3rd et al: Patient understanding of emergency department discharge instructions, *South Med J* 89(8):770-774, 1996.
Jolly BT, Scott JL, Sanford SM: Simplification of emergency department discharge instructions improves patient comprehension, *Ann Emerg Med* 26(4):443-446, 1995.

Basic Life Support

Barbara A. Tilden

More than 650,000 people die from myocardial infarction each year in the United States. Almost half of these people die within the first 2 hours of the infarction. The national trend has been to educate the public regarding the warning signs of impending myocardial infarction, to train lay personnel in the skills and knowledge of basic life support, and to train paramedical and medical personnel in the skills of both basic and advanced life support. These training programs have improved the survival rate from out-of-hospital myocardial infarction that results in cardiopulmonary arrest.

THE COMPONENTS OF BASIC LIFE SUPPORT

Basic life support is the first component of advanced life support. It is the area that may be taught to all levels of personnel, from lay persons to highly skilled medical practitioners. It consists of recognizing unconsciousness, opening the airway, and maintaining the airway. The rescuer then checks for the presence or absence of breathing. If breathing is present, the rescuer must assist in maintaining an open airway. If breathing is not present, the rescuer must begin artificial respiration by giving two *slow* breaths. The rescuer must then check for the presence or absence of circulation by checking for the presence of a carotid pulse. If a pulse is present, the rescuer must continue to maintain an open airway and breathing. If a pulse is not present, the rescuer must also provide chest compressions.

Airway Management

The currently accepted method for early airway management in the patient *not* suspected of having concurrent cervical spine trauma is the **head tilt/chin lift** method (Figure 4-1). The head is tilted back with one hand, and the chin is lifted with the fingers of the other hand. In the case of a suspected cervical spine injury, the **jaw thrust** maneuver is applied, in which the head remains in a neutral position and the jaw is thrust forward using the fingers of both hands at the angle of the jaw (Figure 4-2).

Breathing

Once the airway is established, you must ensure that breathing is present. If the patient is not breathing spontaneously (one cannot see or feel the chest rising and cannot hear or feel air movement), you must assist the patient's breathing. The most rapid method of doing this is by **mouth-to-mouth** breathing, where you use your own mouth to deliver air to the patient's lungs. Instructions for this procedure follow. In an adult, place your mouth over the mouth of the patient, and pinch off the patient's nose. Forming a tight seal, force air into victim's mouth and lungs using two *slow* breaths initially of 1½ to 2 seconds each with a brief pause in between to allow for exhalation (Figure 4-3). This provides a volume of oxygen before proceeding to the next step of basic life support. When breathing into the victim's mouth, you should meet no resistance and should see the victim's chest rise.

 If you cannot perform mouth-to-mouth breathing, you may elect to perform mouth-to-nose breathing; hold the patient's mouth closed and breathe into the patient's nose. In either mouth-to-mouth or mouth-to-nose

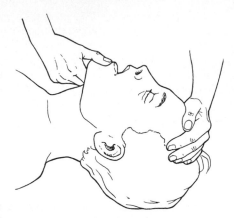

FIGURE 4-1. Head tilt/jaw thrust maneuver. Pull mandible forward using thumb and forefingers.

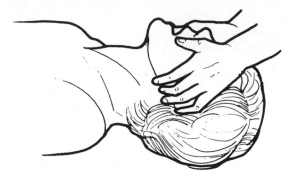

FIGURE 4-2. Jaw thrust maneuver.

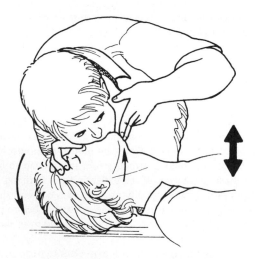

FIGURE 4-3. Mouth-to-mouth breathing. Blow into victim's mouth while observing chest rise.

breathing, you must remove your mouth from the patient's mouth or nose to allow for passive exhalation. Breathe for the patient once every 5 seconds, or in accordance with ratios determined when doing one-person or two-person CPR.

Rescuers in the field may choose or be required to use a barrier device during mouth-to-mouth ventilation. Whatever device is used, it is critical to ensure an adequate seal without air leak.

If a lone rescuer is reluctant to initiate mouth-to-mouth ventilation, for fear of the risk of disease transmission, the rescuer should activate the EMS system, open the airway, and perform chest compressions until another rescuer arrives who is willing to ventilate.

Obstructed airway

When the rescuer attempts to breathe for a patient and finds that the patient's airway is obstructed, an attempt must be made to remove the obstruction. The rescuer should first reposition the patient's head and attempt to ventilate the patient once again. If this is unsuccessful, the rescuer must perform five abdominal thrusts (also known as the subdiaphragmatic abdominal thrust maneuver). (Chest thrust is recommended for victims in advanced pregnancy or if the patient is markedly obese.) To accomplish this maneuver when the patient is prone, straddle the patient and apply the fleshy part of the palm two finger breadths below the tip of the xiphoid process, or one finger breadth above the umbilicus, at the midline. Place the other hand on top of the first, and administer a rapid inward and upward motion (Figure 4-4, *A*). Repeat 5 times. To see if the maneuver was successful, open the patient's mouth by grasping the tongue and lower jaw between the thumb and fingers and lift the mandible. Perform a finger sweep by inserting the index finger of the other hand down along the inside of the cheek, sweeping deeply into the throat. Then reposition the head and attempt to ventilate the patient once again. If unsuccessful, repeat the five abdominal thrusts and follow the sequence as many times as necessary to establish an open and unobstructed airway. The Heimlich maneuver may also be accomplished if the patient is not yet unconscious or is unconscious and slumped over in a chair. Proceed as follows: place both arms around the victim's waist, make a fist with one hand, and place the thumb side of the fist against the victim's abdomen below the xiphoid process and above the umbilicus; place the other hand on top of the fist, and administer a quick inward and upward motion (Figure 4-4, *B*). The Heimlich maneuver causes a sudden increase in intrathoracic pressure and may dislodge the foreign body if there is a total airway obstruction.

Circulation

Once airway and breathing are ensured, you must check for the presence of a pulse. Check for a pulse in the carotid area. Do *not* attempt to initiate circulation before ensuring the presence of an airway and breathing and determining the absence of a pulse. When you cannot detect a pulse, provide circulation by performing chest compressions. Ensure proper body position and hand placement before beginning chest compression. Follow this procedure: Slightly separate your knees and keep them close to the patient; keep your shoulders parallel with the axis of the patient's body. Locate the xiphoid process and place the heel of one hand two finger breadths above the xiphoid. Position the heel of the other hand on top of the first hand, locking the fingers of both hands together and ensuring that your fingers do not touch the chest. Keep your arms straight and elbows locked. Begin compressions with a smooth downward motion, compressing the sternum (Figure 4-5). The ratio of downward to upward motion should be 1:1. Avoid sharp, jabbing motions, and compress at a depth of 1½ to 2 inches or to a depth sufficient to produce a palpable carotid or femoral pulse. The ratio of compressions to breaths is 15:2 when doing one-person CPR and 5:1 when doing two-person CPR. The compression rate should be approximately 80 to 100 per minute in both one-person and two-person CPR. In two-person CPR **pause between compressions when giving the breath.** (See Tables 4-1 and 4-2.)

When initiating chest compression during cardiopulmonary resuscitation, be sure that the patient is on a firm surface. You may have to remove the victim from a bed and place him or her on the floor or another firm surface, or you may place a cardiac board under the victim in the bed. If this is not done, pressure exerted to compress the chest will be transmitted into the soft surface, and very little chest compression will occur.

Approximately 80% to 90% of adult victims of cardiac arrest are in ventricular fibrillation. Basic CPR cannot convert this rhythm. Defibrillation is the definitive treatment. The earlier in the arrest this intervention is

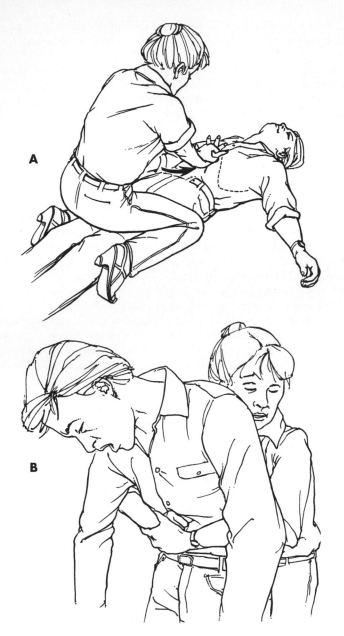

FIGURE 4-4. Heimlich maneuver.
(Reproduced with permission from American Heart Association: *Textbook of basic life support for healthcare providers,* 1997, American Heart Association.)

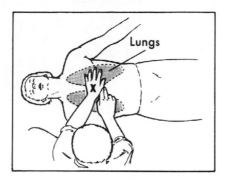

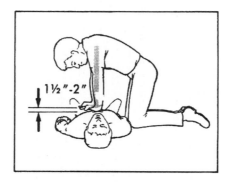

FIGURE 4-5. Body position for CPR. Rescuer should be kneeling with knees slightly separated and elbows in straight, locked position.

TABLE 4-1   Comparison of One-Person and Two-Person CPR

	ONE-PERSON CPR	TWO-PERSON CPR
Initial Breaths	2	2
Compression Rate	80 to 100/min	80 to 100/min
Compression:Breath Ratio	15:2	5:1
Other		Pause for breath

performed, the more successful the survival rate. The American Heart Association Task Force on Early Defibrillation has recommended that instruction on automatic external defibrillation be included in all levels of their classes.

■ **THERAPEUTIC INTERVENTION IN INFANT CPR**

Rescuer procedure

Establish unresponsiveness.

Position the infant on its back, supporting the head and neck (Figure 4-6).

Open the airway, using the head tilt/chin lift method.

Do not hyperextend the neck because it will cause airway obstruction posteriorly.

Check for breathing by looking for chest rise, listening for air movement, and feeling the chest rise and air movement against your face.

If breathing is absent, make a seal over the infant's nose and mouth with your mouth and give two *slow*

TABLE 4-2 Differential Diagnosis in Cardiopulmonary Arrest

There are many causes of cardiopulmonary arrest in addition to primary cardiac abnormalities. It is important for the rescuer to be familiar with these causes and to be alert to their signs and symptoms, as identification of these may modify the type of therapeutic intervention given. Listed below are some of the conditions that may lead to cardiopulmonary arrest that are not primary cardiac abnormalities. *All therapeutic interventions listed are in addition to basic and advanced cardiac life support measures.*

CAUSES	SPECIFIC	SIGNS AND SYMPTOMS	THERAPEUTIC INTERVENTION	NOTES
Metabolic	Hypoglycemia	Physical signs of insulin or oral hypoglycemic agent usage; tachydysrhythmias; seizures; aspiration	Dextrose, 50%	Consider this a strong possibility in patients who have a history of diabetes
	Hyperkalemia	ECG: prolonged Q-T interval; peaked T waves; loss of P waves; wide QRS complexes	Calcium chloride; sodium bicarbonate	Often seen in hemodialysis and renal failure patients; also seen in patients on Aldactone
Drug-induced	Tricyclic antidepressants (e.g., Elavil, Triavil, Tofranil, Etrafon, Sinequan, Vivactil)	Tachydysrhythmias	Sodium bicarbonate (to keep pH at 7.5)	Causes direct cardiac toxicity; often delayed toxicity in adults
	Narcotics	Bradydysrhythmias; heart blocks	Naloxone (Narcan)	There is a question of direct cardiac toxicity
	Propranolol	Cardiac: Heart blocks Bradydysrhythmias, PVCs	Isuprel Atropine	PVCs may be rate-related
		Respiratory: Bronchospasm	Aminophylline	
		Metabolic: Hypoglycemia	Dextrose, 50%	
Pulmonary (any disease causing severe hypoxia)	Asthma	Severe bronchospasm causing hypoxia and respiratory acidosis; ECG: tachydysrhythmias (especially ventricular fibrillation)	Endotracheal intubation and ventilatory support	Abuse of sympathomimetic inhalants

Cause/Etiology	Signs	Treatment	Pathophysiology/Comments
Pulmonary embolus	Pleuritic chest pain; shortness of breath in high-risk patients (e.g., postoperative, birth control pills); syncope (recent study shows 63% have syncope as part of initial complaint); tachydysrhythmias	Good ventilatory support	Pathophysiology: acute hypoxia and cor pulmonale leading to tachydysrhythmias
Tension pneumothorax	Distended neck veins; tracheal deviation; asymmetric chest expansion; ECG: often electrical mechanical dissociation	Needle thoracotomy; chest tube	Often seen in patients with blunt chest trauma; often occurs during CPR because of chest compressions (especially in patients with COPD)
Neurogenic — Increased intracranial pressure from any cause (e.g., subarachnoid hemorrhage; subdural hematoma)	Central neurogenic breathing; dilated pupil(s); decerebrate decorticate posturing; ECG: wide range of dysrhythmias, especially heart blocks	Central neurogenic hyperventilation (causes respiratory alkalosis, which causes cerebral vasoconstriction); steroids; diuretic agents; surgery	Pathophysiology: damage to brainstem and autonomic centers
Hypovolemic — Anything that causes volume loss such as GI bleeding, severe trauma with organ damage, ruptured ectopic pregnancy, dissecting/leaking aneurysm	Tachycardia; decreasing blood pressure; skin cool, clammy, pale; obvious signs of external blood loss	IV fluids; pneumatic antishock garment (PASG); shock position; surgery	A major cause of cardiopulmonary arrest that may be unrecognized
Other cardiac causes — Pericardial tamponade	Distended neck veins; decreasing blood pressure; distant heart sounds; ECG: electrical mechanical dissociation or bradydysrhythmias; widening pulse pressure	IV fluids; PASG; atropine; Isuprel; pericardiocentesis; thoracotomy	Look for it, especially in patients with blunt chest trauma or prolonged CPR efforts

SPECIAL NOTE FOR PREHOSPITAL CARE: Consider early transport for young patients in cardiac arrest because definitive therapeutic intervention will most likely include procedures not performed in the field situation.

Reprinted from Budassi SA: Differential diagnosis in cardiopulmonary arrest, JEN 7(2): 79, 1981, Emergency Nurses Association.

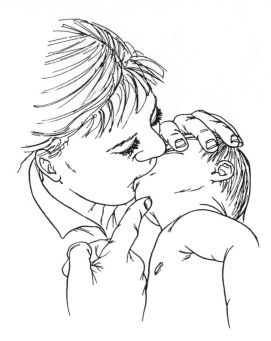

FIGURE 4-6. Infant mouth-to-mouth breathing. Place infant's head and neck in a sniffing position. Do not hyperextend infant's neck.
(Reproduced with permission from American Heart Association: *Textbook of basic life support for healthcare providers,* 1997, American Heart Association.)

breaths 1 to 1½ seconds per breath, observing for chest rise. Allow for passive exhalation between breaths.

Check for a brachial pulse.

Feel for a pulse in the upper arm (in the brachial area) for 5 to 10 seconds. If pulses are *present,* continue to maintain the airway and breathing at 20 breaths per minute. If pulses are *absent,* prepare for chest compressions. Imagine a line between the nipples, and place two fingers one finger width below this imaginary line. Compress the chest ½ to 1 inch in an equal compression:relaxation ratio at a rate of at least 100 per minute (Figure 4-7, *A, B*). Compression to ventilation ratio should be 5:1, ensuring a pause for ventilations. Check for the return of a pulse after 1 minute. If apnea and pulselessness persist, continue CPR.

If the airway is obstructed: Reposition the head and attempt to breathe once again. If unsuccessful, place the infant head dependent and face down, and administer five blows to the back. Turn the infant supine, and administer five chest thrusts in the midsternal region. Do a jaw lift, and observe for (and remove, if present) a foreign body. Reposition the head, and attempt to ventilate. Repeat the entire procedure until the airway is unobstructed.

Notes on resuscitation of newborns. Remember that newborns are obligate nose breathers.

The American Academy of Pediatrics and the American Heart Association recommend suctioning the mouth first, then the nose. This is done to prevent the infant from aspirating if the infant gasps when the nose is suctioned.

If a newborn is *not* breathing spontaneously, and the heart rate is over 110 beats per minute:

Suction the airway and stimulate the infant. Most infants will then begin to breathe spontaneously.

If there is still no breathing:

Begin ventilation by giving two *slow* breaths, pausing between each to allow for exhalation.

The newborn will probably begin to breathe.

If not, continue breathing for the child and check for a pulse.

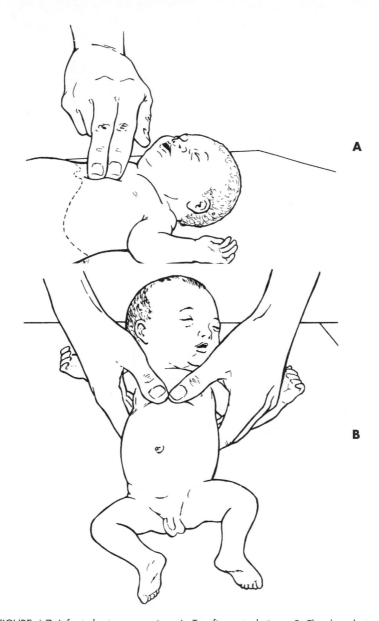

FIGURE 4-7. Infant chest compression. A, Two-finger technique. B, Thumb technique.

Use supplemental oxygen when breathing for the child, and insert an endotracheal tube when possible.
Breaths should continue to be given at a rate of 20 to 30 per minute.
If breathing is absent or labored and the pulse rate is less than 110 beats per minute:
    Open the airway.
    Suction the airway.
    Ventilate.
If respirations and heart rate continue to decrease:
    Continue to ventilate the child.

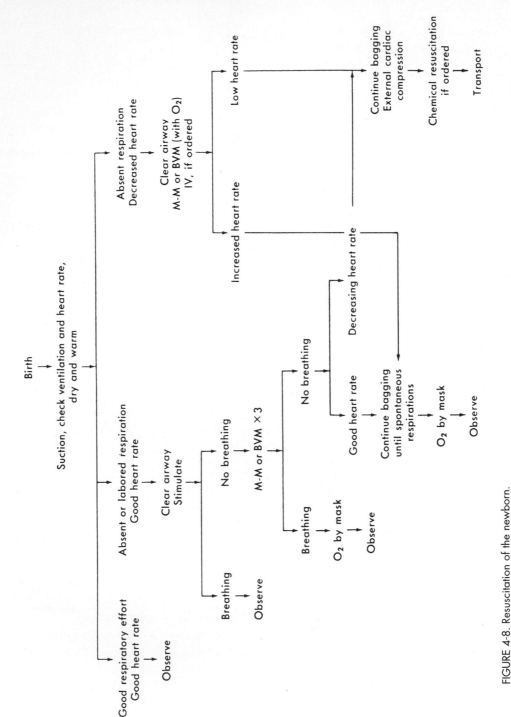

FIGURE 4-8. Resuscitation of the newborn.
(From Melker R: Resuscitation of neonates, infants and children. In Auerbach PA, Budassi SA, editors: *Cardiac arrest and CPR*, ed 2, Rockville, Md, 1983, Aspen.)

If a pulse cannot be palpated:

Begin chest compressions at a rate of at least 100 per minute.

Institute advanced life support measures.

The initial steps in the resuscitation of a newborn (Figure 4-8) are:

1. Airway management
2. Breathing with supplemental oxygen
3. Circulation
4. Establishment of an IV line (usually via the umbilical vein)
5. Administration of epinephrine (0.1-0.3 ml/kg of a 1:10,000 solution)
6. If epinephrine is not effective, a volume expander and/or sodium bicarbonate. Administration of sodium bicarbonate (2 mEq/kg diluted 1:1) by push

Remember that hypothermia can be detrimental to the resuscitation of newborns, infants, and children of all ages. *Keep the patient warm.*

■ **CHILD CPR**

Rescuer procedure. These guidelines are for children under 8 years of age. If the child is 8 years old or older, use the adult procedure for CPR.

Establish unresponsiveness.

Position the child on its back.

Open the airway using the head tilt/chin lift or jaw thrust method.

Assess for breathing by looking for chest rise, listening for air movement, and feeling for chest rise and air movement against your face. If breathing is *present,* maintain an open airway. If breathing is *absent,* make a seal over the child's mouth with your mouth and pinch off the nose. Then administer two slow breaths, 1 to 1½ seconds per breath.

Check for a pulse in the carotid area.

If a pulse is *present,* maintain an airway and breathing. If a pulse is *absent,* kneel by the child's shoulders and prepare to administer chest compressions. Place the heel of one hand two finger widths above the end of the sternum. Compress the chest at a rate of at least 100 per minute; compress 1 to 1½ inches. Ensure that the compression and relaxation phases are equal.

The compression:ventilation ratio should be 5:1 in one-person CPR, or two-person CPR. In two-person CPR, be sure to allow for a pause in chest compressions while giving the breath.

Reassess the pulse after 1 minute of compressions and ventilations.

If the airway is obstructed: Reposition the child's head and attempt to ventilate again. If unsuccessful, kneel at the child's feet and place the heel of one hand against the child's abdomen just above the umbilicus and well below the xiphoid. Place the second hand on top of the first hand. Press inward and upward quickly five times. Check for a foreign body by performing a jaw lift and attempting to visualize the foreign body. If unable to visualize, reposition the head and attempt to ventilate. Continue to repeat the procedure until the airway is unobstructed. If airway obstruction is not relieved after 1 minute, activate the EMS system.

SUGGESTED READINGS

American Heart Association: Adult basic life support, *JAMA* 268(16):2184, 1992.

American Heart Association: *Basic life support for healthcare providers,* Chicago, 1997, American Heart Association.

American Heart Association: Pediatric basic life support, *JAMA* 268(16):2251, 1992.

American Heart Association: *Textbook of neonatal resuscitation,* Chicago, 1996, American Heart Association.

Cayten CG et al: Basic life support vs. advanced life support for injured patients with an injury severity score of 10 or more, *J Trauma* S 35(3):460, 1993.

Lauder GR et al: Basic life support training, *Anesthesia* 47(11):1000, 1992.

Seidel JS et al: Education in pediatric basic and advanced life support, *Ann Emerg Med,* 22(2):489, 1993.

CHAPTER 5

Advanced Life Support

Margaret McCarthy-Mogan

Sudden cardiac death, or unexpected death that occurs within 1 hour of the onset of signs and symptoms of the event, accounts for approximately 400,000 deaths per year in the United States. Most sudden deaths reflect underlying coronary artery disease. The majority of persons who die suddenly initially experience ventricular tachycardia, which subsequently degenerates into ventricular fibrillation over a variable period of time.

The key to improving survival from sudden cardiac arrest is activation of a particular series of response events as rapidly as possible. Specialized knowledge and skills must be developed in all four links of this "chain of survival"[1] (Figure 5-1).

Weakness in any link lessens the chance of survival and condemns the efforts of emergency medical services to poor results. This chapter describes the care associated with the links of early defibrillation and early advanced care. The victim can survive neurologically intact if CPR is delivered within 4 minutes and defibrillation within 10 minutes of collapse. For every minute that passes without resuscitation, there is a 7% to 10% decrease in probability of patient survival even if defibrillation is achieved. *Time is of the essence.*

AIRWAY MANAGEMENT

Of supreme importance in an emergency situation are the ABCs—airway, breathing, and circulation. Because the basic positions of head tilt and chin lift for airway management have been discussed earlier, this section deals with adjuncts for airway management.

Usual Airway Adjuncts

Oropharyngeal airway

The oropharyngeal airway is a curved piece of equipment constructed of plastic, rubber, or metal (Figure 5-2). It is inserted over the tongue and into the posterior pharyngeal area. Its primary use is to prevent the tongue from slipping back into the posterior pharyngeal area, thereby occluding the airway. It should be positioned either by inserting it upside down with the curved portion lying on the tongue, and then rotating it 180 degrees as it is advanced into the posterior pharyngeal area, or by using a tongue blade or similar piece of equipment to depress and displace the tongue while the airway is inserted right side up.

Remember that if the oropharyngeal airway is not positioned properly, it may actually cause airway obstruction. This airway is recommended for use in the unconscious patient who has an adequate respiratory effort. It should not be used in the conscious patient with an intact gag reflex. Once the airway is in place, strict attention must be paid to maintenance of proper head tilt, chin lift, or jaw thrust maneuver.

Nasopharyngeal airway

The nasopharyngeal airway (trumpet tube) is a soft rubber tube about 6 inches long (Figure 5-3). It is inserted through a nostril, using a topical anesthetic lubricant. Then it is gently slid backward (behind the tongue) in line with the base of the ears, with the bevel against the septum, to the posterior pharyngeal area. If inserted too deep, the tip may stimulate laryngospasm or enter the esophagus. This airway is tolerated by the alert, ori-

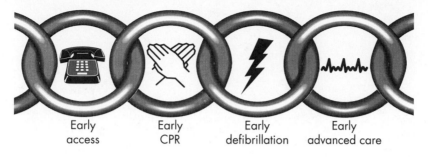

Early
access

Early
CPR

Early
defibrillation

Early
advanced care

FIGURE 5-1. Chain of survival.

(Modified from American Heart Association: *Guidelines for cardiopulmonary resuscitation and emergency cardiac care*, Dallas, 1997, American Heart Association.)

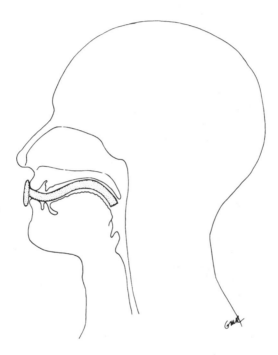

FIGURE 5-2. Oropharyngeal airway.

ented patient and is particularly useful when there has been considerable facial trauma. Potential complications include epistaxis, laryngospasm, and vomiting.

Endotracheal intubation

An endotracheal tube is passed directly into the trachea (Figure 5-4). Endotracheal intubation requires a great deal of technical skill and may be accomplished in the prehospital situation (in accordance with state laws) or in the hospital by trained, skilled individuals. The endotracheal tube is open at both ends.

■ **EQUIPMENT**

Cuffed tube with a standard 15-mm adapter for use with a bag-valve or other type of resuscitation device
Malleable stylet

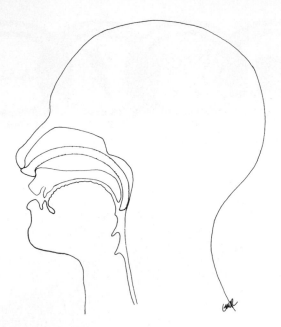

FIGURE 5-3. Nasopharyngeal airway.

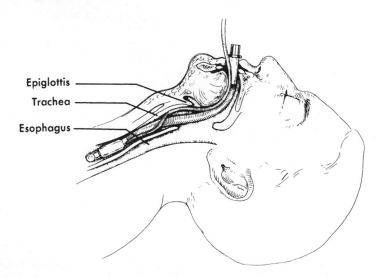

Epiglottis ————
Trachea ————
Esophagus ————

FIGURE 5-4. Endotracheal tube in place.

Laryngoscope handle with curved or straight blade
Suction equipment

■ **INSERTION**
    1. Prepare the equipment.
       a. Inflate the cuff of the tube to make sure it is intact, then deflate the cuff.
       b. Insert the malleable stylet into the tube and shape it to the configuration desired, ensuring that the stylet does not slip beyond the end of the tube.

    c. Prepare the laryngoscope by connecting the blade to the handle, ensuring that the batteries are charged and the light is working.

    d. Ready the suction equipment.

    e. Ready the bag-valve device or respirator.

2. Remove the patient's dentures.
3. Hyperventilate the patient with 100% oxygen.
4. Align the three axes of the mouth, pharynx, and trachea to allow for visualization of the vocal cords by placing the patient's head in a "sniffing position." Put a small pillow under the occiput of the patient. (Do *not* hang the head over the end of the bed or table.)
5. Using the left hand, insert the laryngoscope blade just to the right of the midline into the mouth, following the natural curves of the upper airway.
6. Lift up on the laryngoscope to elevate the tongue and shift it to the left side of the mouth. The blade should be in the midline position.
7. Advance the laryngoscope until the glottic opening can be seen by placing the curved laryngoscope blade into the space between the base of the tongue and the epiglottis (the vallecula) or by placing the straight laryngoscope blade under the epiglottis. Do *not* use the teeth as a fulcrum.
8. Advance the endotracheal tube with the right hand from the right side of the mouth into the trachea until the cuff rests just below the vocal cords.
9. Remove the laryngoscope carefully.
10. Inflate the balloon and blow into the airway to check proper positioning; observe to see that the chest rises symmetrically and auscultate the epigastrum. Auscultate right and left lung fields at the apices and anterior bases.
11. Attach an end-tidal CO_2 detector and confirm proper positioning of the tube. Confirm tube placement using a lighted stylet.
12. Attach the tube to the bag-valve device or the respirator.
13. Secure the tube to the patient's face, using adhesive tape, umbilical tape, or a device designed for this purpose.
14. Insert an oropharyngeal airway or bite block.
15. Obtain a portable anterior/posterior chest x-ray film to ensure proper positioning of the tube. If the tube is found in the right mainstem bronchus, pull back on the tube slightly.

If the patient has had spontaneous respirations for 8 hours, and the arterial blood gases are at an acceptable level, the patient may be weaned from the ventilator, and the endotracheal tube removed.

■ **REMOVAL**
1. Suction the tube and the patient's mouth and posterior pharyngeal area.
2. Deflate the cuff.
3. Withdraw the tube. (*Never* withdraw the tube without deflating the cuff.)
4. Always have a suction apparatus ready.
5. Monitor the patient for cardiac dysrhythmias.

■ **ADVANTAGES**
The tube provides control of the airway.
The patient is protected from aspiration.
Intermittent positive pressure breathing with 100% oxygen can be given.
The trachea is easy to suction.
It causes less gastric distension.
Chest compressions can be continued after insertion.
It provides access for drug administration.

■ **DISADVANTAGES**
The tube can easily pass into the esophagus.
A skilled technician is required to place it.

It may cause hypoxia during prolonged insertion. (Patient should be unventilated for no longer than 15 to 20 seconds.)

Chest compressions must be interrupted during insertion.

Tactile endotracheal intubation

Tactile or digital endotracheal intubation is an alternative method of intubation that may be used when the vocal cords are visually obstructed or there is a strict need to maintain the head and neck in alignment. Do not use this method unless the patient is deeply comatose.

1. Prepare the endotracheal tube by inserting a stylet and making an open-ended "J" at the end of the tube.
2. Face the patient. Insert the index and middle finger of the gloved, nondominant hand along the side of the patient's tongue, moving the tongue out of the way as the fingers are advanced to the anterior pharyngeal region.
3. Advance the fingers until the epiglottis or opening of the trachea can be palpated.
4. Grasp the endotracheal tube in the dominant hand and insert it into the patient's mouth.
5. Advance the tube to the posterior pharyngeal area until the tip of the tube can be felt by the fingers of the nondominant hand.
6. Slip the tube into the larynx.
7. Remove the stylet and advance the tube simultaneously.
8. Force air into the tube, observing for chest rise and listening for breath sounds bilaterally.
9. Proceed with the remaining steps to secure the tube, as in any other type of intubation procedure.

Alternate invasive airways

Endotracheal intubation is the preferred method of managing the airway invasively during cardiopulmonary arrest. But in some settings endotracheal intubation is not permitted, or practitioners have little experience with it. Alternative airways in use that involve blind passage are (1) the esophageal obturator airway (EOA), (2) the esophageal gastric tube airway (EGTA), and (3) the pharyngotracheal lumen (PTL) airway. With all of these there is increased risk of complications compared to endotracheal intubation. Problems seen with esophageal airways include:

Esophageal laceration and rupture

Inadvertent placement into the trachea

Inadequate seal at the face

If the patient arrives with one of these alternative invasive airways in place, it should be removed as soon as possible. Because emesis often occurs on removal of the alternate airway, an endotracheal tube should first be inserted.

■ **REMOVAL OF THE ESOPHAGEAL AIRWAY**

1. Have suction apparatus available and functioning.
2. If the patient is unable to maintain his or her own respirations, insert an endotracheal tube around the esophageal airway. If the patient has effective spontaneous respirations and a gag reflex, turn the patient on his or her side. (This is not necessary if an endotracheal tube is in place.)
3. Deflate the cuff.
4. Withdraw the airway. (*Never* withdraw it without first deflating the cuff.)

Techniques for Managing the Difficult Airway

Difficulty in obtaining an airway can lead to direct airway trauma and morbidity from hypoxia and hypercarbia. The American Society of Anesthesiologists recommends use of a specific algorithm for management of the difficult airway[2] (Figure 5-5). Three of these techniques are described.

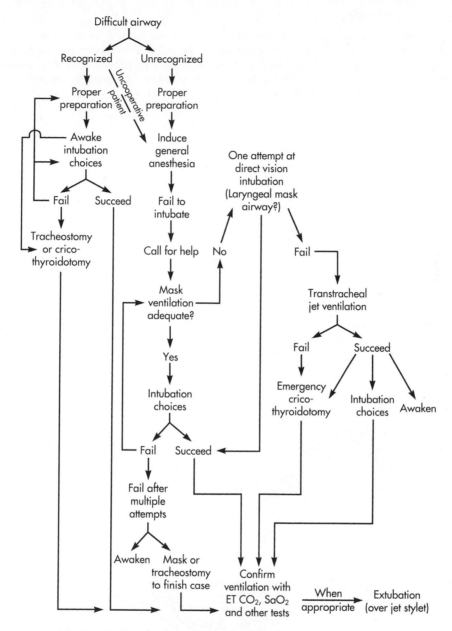

FIGURE 5-5. Algorithm for managing the difficult airway.
(From Benumof JL: Management of the difficult airway, *Anesthesiology* 75:1090, 1991.)

Laryngeal mask airway

The laryngeal mask is a new device that is intermediate in design and function between a mask/oropharyngeal airway and an endotracheal tube (Figure 5-6). It provides a safe and swift airway by sealing the outside of the laryngeal inlet with an inflatable cuff. Although the larynx does not need to be visualized for insertion, its use of the laryngeal mask requires considerable training and skill. It can only be inserted when reflexes are sufficiently depressed and stomach contents are not present.

■ **EQUIPMENT**

 Laryngeal mask
 Lubricant
 Syringe
 Gauze sponges

■ **PROCEDURE**

 1. Make sure that the mask is fully deflated.
 2. Lubricate the mask well.
 3. Place the nondominant hand underneath the patient's head; using this hand extend the head and flex the neck forward. Keep the hand in place under the head during insertion.

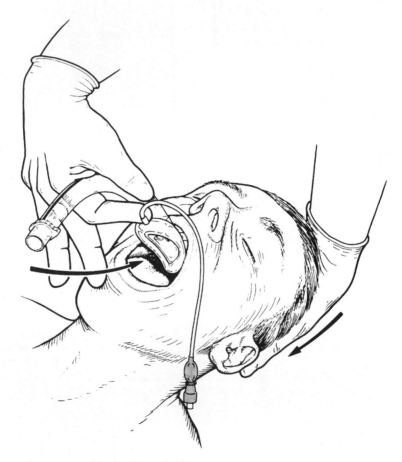

FIGURE 5-6. Technique for insertion of laryngeal mask airway.
(From Brain AJ: *The Intavent laryngeal mask instruction manual,* Berkshire, UK, 1992, Brain Medical Ltd.)

4. Have an assistant place several fingers on the patient's lower jaw to open the mouth.
5. Insert the mask tip into the patient's mouth with the dominant hand, pressing the mask against the hard palate to flatten it.
6. Advance the mask into the pharynx using the index finger while pressing upward until resistance (upper esophageal sphincter) is felt.
7. Grasp the tube with the other hand and withdraw the index finger.
8. Inflate the mask with the recommended volume of air.
9. Ventilate the patient.
10. Use rolled gauze sponges as bite blocks and place on either side of the tube in the patient's mouth.
11. Tape the tube and gauze in place.

■ **ADVANTAGES**

The laryngeal mask provides rapid access when the trachea cannot be intubated with an endotracheal tube. It is inserted blindly without direct visualization of the airway.
The patient can breathe spontaneously through the tube or be ventilated continuously.

■ **COMPLICATIONS**

Laryngeal spasm
Aspiration of stomach contents
Incorrect placement causing obstruction

Percutaneous transtracheal ventilation (needle cricothyrotomy)

If the airway is obstructed, a rapid means of access to the airway is via needle cricothyrotomy (Figure 5-7). Ventilation by this method should not continue longer than 1 to 2 hours.

■ **EQUIPMENT**

14-gauge (or larger) over-the-needle catheter
3 ml syringe
Alcohol swabs

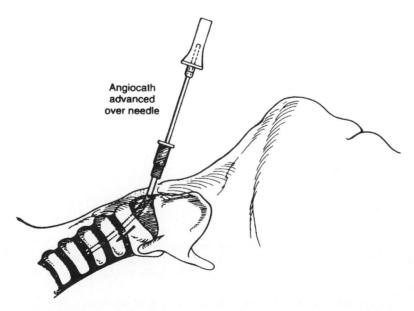

FIGURE 5-7. Technique for insertion of catheter-over-needle for percutaneous transtracheal ventilation.
(From Wilkins E: *Emergency medicine scientific foundations and current practice,* Baltimore, 1989, Williams and Wilkins.)

3.0 or 3.5 endotracheal tube tapered adapter
High pressure oxygen source

■ **PROCEDURE**

1. Locate the cricothyroid membrane.
   a. It extends from the thyroid cartilage to the cricoid cartilage.
   b. Palpate by placing a finger on the cricoid cartilage and moving the finger upward 2 cm.
2. Prepare the area with alcohol or other antiseptic solution.
3. Stabilize the larynx with the nondominant hand.
4. Perforate both skin and membrane with the over-the-needle catheter attached to the syringe, directing the catheter down and toward the feet at a 45-degree angle.
5. To verify entrance into the trachea, aspirate air with the syringe.
6. Remove the syringe and needle while manually stabilizing the catheter. Advance the catheter as needed.
7. Attach the catheter to the narrow tip of the endotracheal tube adapter.
8. Connect the wider end of the adapter to a bag-valve device or a high-pressure oxygen delivery device (preferred) and oxygenate the patient.
9. Secure the catheter in place.

NOTE: Secretions in the patient's upper airway are blown out of the mouth and nose during insufflation, so stand back and wear protective garb.

■ **ADVANTAGES**

Percutaneous transtracheal ventilation is simple and relatively safe to perform. It provides rapid access to the airway when the patient cannot be intubated or ventilated by mask.

■ **COMPLICATIONS**

Subcutaneous and/or mediastinal emphysema
Hemorrhage
Posterior tracheal wall or esophageal perforation
Kinking or blockage of catheter
Aspiration

Surgical cricothyrotomy

Surgical cricothyrotomy is an alternate method of rapid access to a blocked airway in which a scalpel or other such instrument is used to perforate the cricothyroid membrane to create an opening into the airway.

■ **EQUIPMENT**

Antiseptic solution
Scalpel and blade
Tracheal dilator or hemostat
Suction device
Small airway tube (or other such instrument)

■ **PROCEDURE**

1. Identify the cricothyroid membrane.
2. Prepare the skin with antiseptic solution.
3. Spread the overlying skin to make it taut.
4. Using the scalpel, make a small incision over the membrane through the skin.
5. Once the skin is invaded, make a horizontal puncture hole through the cricothyroid membrane into the trachea (Figure 5-8). (A little bleeding may occur, but usually it is not excessive.) Listen and feel for air flow.
6. Enlarge the space with the scalpel handle, a tracheal dilator, or hemostat.
7. Insert a small tube, such as a No. 6 tracheostomy tube, into the opening. (If a tube is not available, use whatever means are available to maintain an opening.)

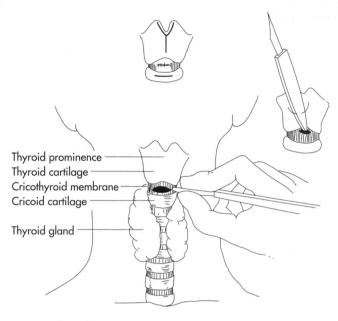

FIGURE 5-8. Cricothyrotomy incision, frontal view.
(From Miller RH, Cantrey JR: *Textbook of emergency medicine,* St Louis, 1975, Mosby.)

Thyroid prominence
Thyroid cartilage
Cricothyroid membrane
Cricoid cartilage
Thyroid gland

8. Supply oxygen via the opening. (If the patient is apneic, there is need for a cuffed tracheostomy tube and positive pressure breathing.)

■ **ADVANTAGES**

Surgical cricothyrotomy provides rapid entrance into an obstructed airway. A cuffed tracheostomy tube can be placed quickly for the apneic patient. An endotracheal tube can be placed while the patient is being ventilated continuously.

■ **COMPLICATIONS**

Hemorrhage
Laceration of the esophagus or trachea
Incorrect tube placement
Subcutaneous and/or mediastinal emphysema
Vocal cord injury
Aspiration
Infection
Tracheal stenosis (later)

Tracheostomy

Tracheostomy is performed when other attempts at ventilation have failed and when one has been unable to obtain control of the airway, usually because of laryngeal edema, foreign body, or tumors.

Tracheostomy is rarely performed in the emergency department; it is usually done in surgery, in a controlled environment.

■ **EQUIPMENT**

Tracheostomy tube of appropriate size (available in French sizes 13 to 38 and Jackson sizes 00 to 9)
Tracheostomy tape
20-ml syringe
Scalpel handle and blade

Kelly clamp with rubber-coated tips

Scissors

Hemostats

Vein retractor

Suture materials

Tissue forceps

Sterile 4 × 4-inch gauze

Sterile drapes

Suction

Gloves, mask, gown, goggles, and cap

Antiseptic solution

Crash cart (including monitor and defibrillator)

■ **PROCEDURE**

1. Position the patient with a pillow under his or her shoulders and the neck in extension.
2. Ventilate the patient via an endotracheal tube, cricothyrotomy, or other method.
3. Prepare the skin (chin to nipples).
4. Drape the patient.
5. Locate the area for the incision, usually the third or fourth tracheal ring in an adult.
6. Make an incision into the skin. It may be a flap, or a horizontal or vertical incision; usually a vertical incision is used to avoid arteries, veins, and nerves on the lateral borders of the trachea.
7. Control the bleeding.
8. Dissect down through the subcutaneous fat and platysma muscle.
9. Retract the midline muscle.
10. Expose the tracheal rings. Retract the thyroid isthmus cephalad.
11. Inject local anesthesia into the tracheal lumen to decrease the cough reflex.
12. Create a stoma by removing 1 square centimeter of cartilage.
13. Continuously suction to remove blood and secretions.
14. Insert the tracheostomy tube.
15. Ensure correct tube position by checking for air movement.
16. Attach the tube to a ventilation device.
17. Auscultate the lungs.
18. Inflate the cuff.
19. Suture the corners of the incision loosely.
20. Secure the tube with tracheostomy tape.
21. Dress the wound.
22. Obtain a follow-up chest x-ray film.

■ **ADVANTAGES**

Tracheostomy reduces physiologic dead space.

It allows for prolonged positive pressure breathing.

There is direct access to the respiratory tract for secretion removal.

■ **COMPLICATIONS**

Inaccurate tube placement

Laceration of arteries, veins, and nerves

Hemorrhage

Pressure necrosis from cuff

Perforation of the esophagus

Subcutaneous emphysema

Mediastinal emphysema

Oxygen Therapy Devices

Several different devices are available for the delivery of oxygen to a patient. One should be familiar with the various types and be able to select the proper device for an individual patient's needs (Table 5-1).

Nasal cannula

The nasal cannula is the most commonly used oxygen delivery device. It can be used on the patient who is breathing spontaneously. If the oxygen flow rate is adjusted to 2 to 6 L/min, one can achieve an oxygen concentration of 24% to 44%. Its value is reduced if the person is a mouth breather.

Face mask

Face masks are tolerated fairly well by most individuals, except those who are experiencing severe dyspnea, when the face mask may make them feel as if they are suffocating (Figure 5-9). This device must also be used on the spontaneously breathing patient. At a flow rate of 5 to 10 L/min, an oxygen concentration of 40% to 60% can be achieved.

Partial rebreather mask

The face mask is attached to a reservoir bag that allows the patient to inhale the oxygen-rich air from the bag (Figure 5-10). It can provide 50% to 80% oxygen concentration with the flow at 8 to 12 L/min to patients who have adequate spontaneous respirations.

Nonrebreather mask

The nonrebreather mask is similar to the partial rebreather mask except that (1) a one-way valve lies between the mask and reservoir bag, preventing exhaled air from entering the bag, and (2) one-way valves on the side exhalation ports allow gas to leave the mask during exhalation and prevent room air from entering during inspiration (Figure 5-11). Increase the oxygen flow rate between 12 and 15 L/min to keep the reservoir bag inflated during maximal inspiration and expiration. With this mask, it is possible to deliver a high oxygen concentration of 85% to 100%. Make sure that the reservoir bag is not pinched off or the inhalation valve obstructed, for then carbon dioxide can accumulate.

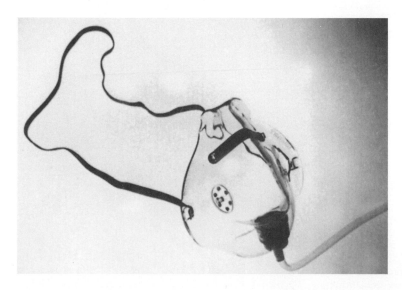

FIGURE 5-9. Oxygen face mask.

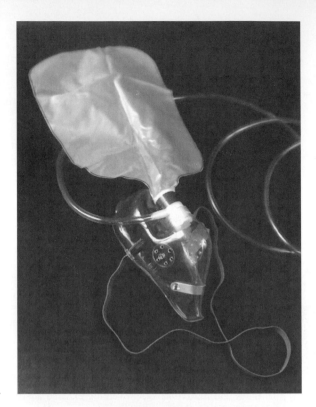

FIGURE 5-10. Partial rebreather mask.

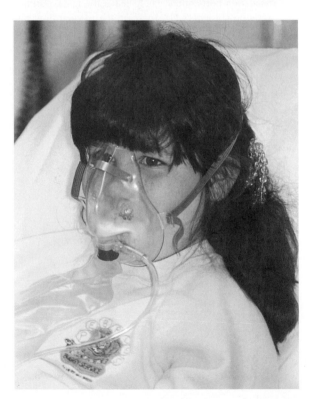

FIGURE 5-11. Nonrebreather mask.
(Courtesy Emilie Goudey, Lenox, Mass.)

TABLE 5-1   Summary of Oxygen Therapy Devices

TYPE OF BREATHING DEVICE	OXYGEN FLOW RATE	OXYGEN CONCENTRATIONS	ADVANTAGES	DISADVANTAGES
Nasal cannula	2-6 L/min	24%-44%	No rebreathing of expired air	Can only be used on patients breathing spontaneously; actual amount of inspired oxygen varies greatly.
Face mask	5-10 L/min	40%-60%	Higher oxygen concentration than nasal cannula	Not tolerated well by severely dyspneic patients; can only be used on patients who are breathing spontaneously
Partial rebreather mask	8-12 L/min	50%-80%	Higher oxygen concentration than nasal cannula or face mask	Must have tight seal on mask; can only be used on patients breathing spontaneously; actual amount of inspired oxygen varies greatly
Nonrebreather mask	12-15 L/min	85%-100%	Highest oxygen concentration available by mask	Must have tight seal on mask; do not allow bag to collapse; can only be used on patients breathing spontaneously
Venturi mask	2-12 L/min	24%-50%	Oxygen concentration can be adjusted	Can only be used on patients breathing spontaneously
Pocket mask	10 L/min	50%	Avoids direct contact with patient's mouth; may add oxygen source; may be used on apneic patient; may be used on children; can obtain excellent tidal volume	Rescuer fatigue
Bag-valve-mask	Room air 12 L/min	21% 40%-90%	Quick; oxygen concentration may be increased; rescuer can sense lung compliance; may be used on both apneic and spontaneously breathing patients	Air in stomach; low tidal volume; difficulty obtaining a leak-proof seal
Oxygen-powered breathing device	100 L/min	100%	High oxygen flow, positive pressure; improved lung inflation	Gastric distension; overinflation; standard device cannot be used in children without special adapter; requires an oxygen source

Venturi mask

If a victim has a history of chronic obstructive lung disease and is currently experiencing respiratory distress, one should consider using the Venturi mask, which allows for delivery of a fixed concentration of oxygen (Figure 5-12). For example, at 2 L/min oxygen flow rate, the oxygen concentration is 24% with a blue dilutor cap in place (Baxter Airlife Percento Mask). Using various caps and flow rates oxygen concentration can be increased stepwise by 4% to 5% increments up to an inspired oxygen concentration of 50%. The proper method for using this device is to initiate the flow at the 24% oxygen concentration setting and then to observe the patient closely. If respiratory depression is not present, one may elect to increase the oxygen concentration to 28% and repeat the observation, continuing to increase the oxygen concentration as long as the patient tolerates the previously lower concentration well.

Pocket mask

A pocket mask is used to perform mouth-to-mask artificial ventilations (Figure 5-13). In this way mouth-to-mouth contact is avoided. The mask fits snugly onto the victim's face, covering the nose and the mouth. The victim's head should be tilted back, using the chin lift or jaw thrust maneuver. The rescuer can then blow into

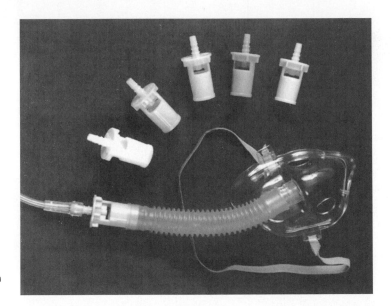

FIGURE 5-12. Venturi mask and oxygen regulator caps.

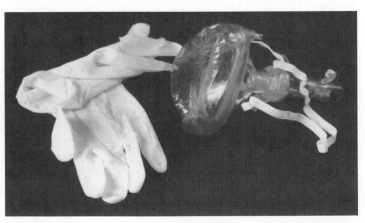

FIGURE 5-13. Pocket mask.

the tube on top of the mask. If one adds supplemental oxygen and regulates the oxygen flow at 10 L/min, a delivered oxygen concentration of about 50% is achieved. A one-way valve diverts the victim's exhaled air, protecting the rescuer from exposure to infectious diseases. Masks are available in a variety of sizes and configurations.

Bag-valve mask

The bag-valve-mask unit includes a self-inflating bag, a nonrebreathing valve, and a face mask (Figure 5-14). It can deliver 21% oxygen (room air) to a victim. By adding a supplemental oxygen source of 12 L/min, one can achieve an oxygen concentration of 40%. By adding a reservoir with an open end, one can obtain about a 90% oxygen concentration.

The mask of the bag-valve-mask unit is applied in the same way as the resuscitation mask, obtaining a tight seal around the nose and the mouth. One-person ventilations using the bag-valve-mask device are less effective than two-person techniques in which both hands are used to get a seal (Figure 5-15). It is appropriate to use an oropharyngeal or nasopharyngeal airway in conjunction with the bag-valve-mask device. Without the mask, the bag can be used to perform ventilations via an endotracheal tube. Bags are available in adult and child sizes.

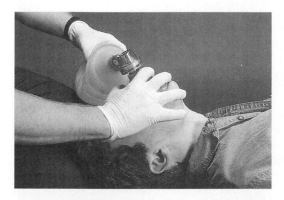

FIGURE 5-14. Bag-valve-mask device.
(From Stoy, Center for Emergency Medicine: *Mosby's EMT-basic textbook*, St Louis, 1996, Mosby.)

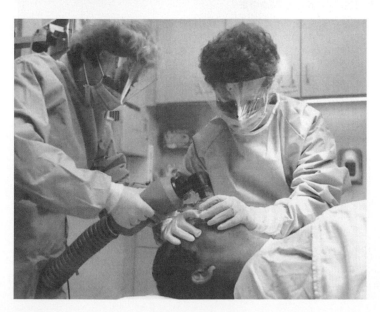

FIGURE 5-15. Use of bag-valve-mask device with oxygen reservoir.
(Courtesy Emilie Goudey, Lenox, Mass.)

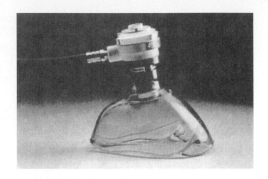

FIGURE 5-16. Oxygen-powered breathing device.

Although there are many brands of bag-valve-mask devices on the market, a transparent mask is recommended so that one may observe and intervene rapidly should emesis occur.

Oxygen-powered devices

Oxygen-powered devices can deliver 100% oxygen at a rate of 100 L/min to a resuscitation mask, an attached mask, an endotracheal tube, or a transtracheal catheter insufflation device (Figure 5-16). Timing and length of oxygen delivery are left up to the operator. This device should *not* be used in children under 12 years of age. The rescuer must be trained in its proper use.

CARDIAC DYSRHYTHMIAS

When the normal rhythm from the sinus node fails or its conduction is disturbed, a dysrhythmia occurs. On the basis of current knowledge, there are two categories of dysrhythmias:

Abnormalities of conduction caused by conduction block, reentry, or reflection.

Abnormalities of impulse initiation caused by altered automaticity or triggered activity.

The reader is referred to cardiac textbooks for explanation of these phenomena.

Dysrhythmias Originating in the Sinus Node
Normal sinus rhythm

Rate	60 to 100 beats/minute
Rhythm	Regular
P waves	Present
QRS complex	Present; normal duration
P/QRS relationship	P wave preceding each QRS complex
PR interval	Normal

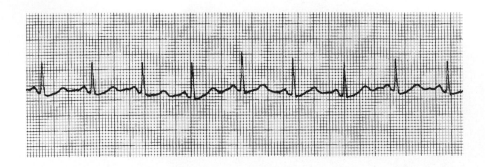

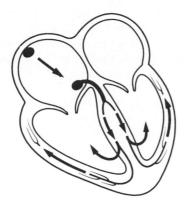

Impulse travels from
SA to AV node through
bundle of His to Purkinje
fibers

■ **SIGNIFICANCE**

The SA node is the normal pacemaker of the heart; it is influenced both by the parasympathetic and the sympathetic branches of the autonomic nervous system.

■ **THERAPEUTIC INTERVENTIONS**

None required.

Sinus tachycardia

Rate	100 to 180 beats/minute
Rhythm	Regular
P waves	Present, may merge with T wave
QRS complexes	Present, normal duration
P/QRS relationship	P wave preceding each QRS complex
PR interval	Normal

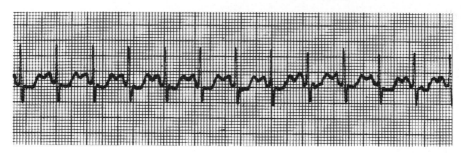

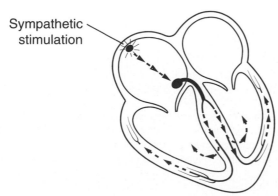

Sympathetic
stimulation

SA node originates
impulses at regular
rate of greater than
100 / minute

■ **SIGNIFICANCE**

The normal pacemaker of the heart is firing at an increased rate because of anxiety, fever, pain, exercise, nicotine, caffeine, hyperthyroidism, heart failure, volume loss, or other reasons that may cause increased tissue oxygen demands. This condition may also be caused by decreased vagal tone (parasympathetic decrease), which allows the sinus node to increase its rate.

■ **THERAPEUTIC INTERVENTIONS**

Treat the cause. There is no specific drug given for sinus tachycardia except that with increased sympathetic discharge in a myocardial infarction a beta-blocker may be used. If sinus tachycardia is the dysrhythmia seen following cardiopulmonary arrest, a Swan-Ganz catheter should be placed, and the wedge pressure should be maintained at 15 to 18 mm Hg.

Sinus bradycardia

Rate	<60 beats/minute
Rhythm	Regular
P waves	Present
QRS complexes	Present; normal duration
P/QRS relationship	P wave preceding each QRS complex
PR interval	Normal

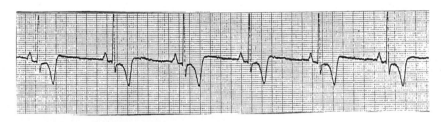

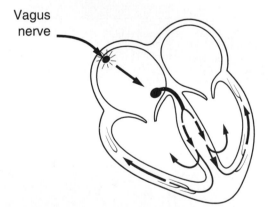

Vagus nerve

SA node originates impulses at a regular rate of less than 60 / minute

■ **SIGNIFICANCE**

The normal pacemaker, the SA node, is slowed by increased vagal tone (parasympathetic stimulation). Causes include sleep, a normal athletic heart, anoxia, hypothyroidism, increased intracranial pressure, acute myocardial infarction, and vagal stimulation (such as vomiting, straining at stool, carotid sinus massage, or ocular pressure). It may also be caused by medications, such as digitalis, verapamil, or beta blockers, or may occur after cardioversion.

■ **THERAPEUTIC INTERVENTIONS**

Observe the patient for symptoms of decreased cardiac output, such as a decrease in blood pressure, decreasing level of consciousness, syncope, shock, or acidosis.

1. Hold digitalis, beta blocker, or verapamil.
2. Administer oxygen.
3. Keep patient supine if symptomatic.
4. Treat with atropine or a transcutaneous pacemaker if the patient develops symptoms (e.g., severe hypotension, syncope).
5. Administer IV infusion of dopamine or epinephrine if severe symptoms. (See Figure 5-27 on p. 97.)

Sinus arrhythmia

Rate	60 to 100 beats usually; may increase with inspiration and decrease with expiration
Rhythm	Irregular
P waves	Present
QRS complexes	Present; normal duration
P/QRS relationship	P wave preceding each QRS complex
PR interval	Normal

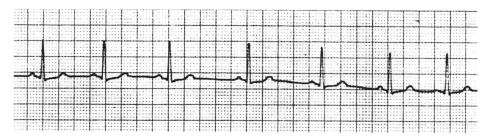

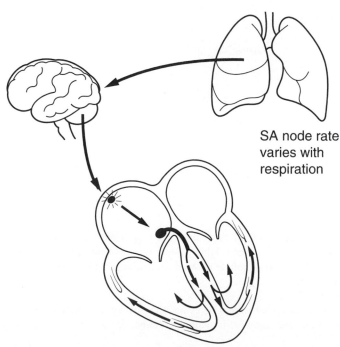

SA node rate
varies with
respiration

■ **SIGNIFICANCE**

This dysrhythmia is a normal finding in children and young adults because of parasympathetic influence. It often varies with the respiratory cycle, but this is not always true. For this variance to be considered a dysrhythmia, the variation must exceed 0.12 seconds between the longest and shortest cycles.

■ **THERAPEUTIC INTERVENTIONS**

None required.

Dysrhythmias Originating in the Atria

Premature atrial complex (PAC)

Rate	Usually 60 to 100 beats/minute
Rhythm	Irregular due to early beats
P waves	Present, but premature P wave may appear different in configuration (because it did not originate in the SA node)
QRS complexes	Present; normal duration; noncompensatory pause
P/QRS relationship	P wave preceding each QRS complex, though if it appears quite early, QRS may not follow
PR interval	Usually normal

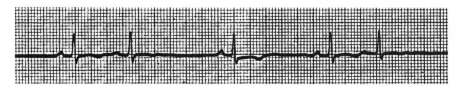

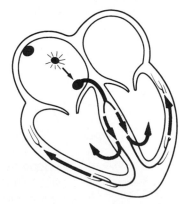

Atrial origin of abnormal impulse

■ **SIGNIFICANCE**

PACs are the result of an irritable ectopic focus that may be caused by emotions, fatigue, alcohol, caffeine, nicotine, digitalis toxicity, congestive heart failure, electrolyte imbalance, hypoxia, or ischemia; sometimes the etiology is unknown. They may be a prelude to atrial fibrillation, atrial flutter, atrial tachycardia, or paroxysmal supraventricular tachycardia (PVST).

■ **THERAPEUTIC INTERVENTIONS**

Treatment is usually unnecessary but should be given if the patient is symptomatic. Drugs that could be used are quinidine, procainamide, and digitalis. If alcohol, caffeine, or nicotine is the cause, advise the patient to eliminate it.

Atrial flutter

Rate	Atrial rate of 230 to 350 beats/minute, ventricular rate usually 150 to 170 beats/minute
Rhythm	Regular or irregular
P waves	Sawtoothed pattern of flutter waves
QRS complexes	Present; normal duration
P/QRS relationship	Because of rapid atrial rate, there may be two or more flutter waves for every QRS; it may be regular or irregular
PR interval	Flutter to R wave interval may be fixed or variable

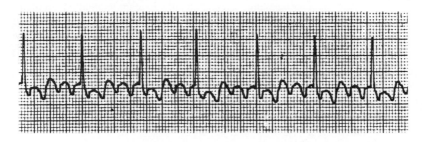

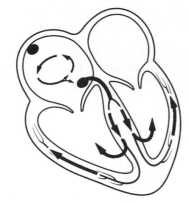

Reentry circuit in right atrium; block present in AV node

■ **SIGNIFICANCE**

A single reentry circuit within the right atrium is thought to be responsible for this dysrhythmia. The atrium fires at such a rapid rate that there is a block at the AV node, so that only every second, every third, or every fourth impulse reaches the ventricles. The ventricular response may be regular or irregular. Atrial flutter is a dangerous dysrhythmia in that ineffective atrial contraction may cause mural clots to form in the atria and consequently break loose, forming pulmonary or cerebral emboli. Atrial flutter may be seen in coronary artery disease, rheumatic heart disease, pulmonary embolism, and chronic obstructive pulmonary disease.

■ **THERAPEUTIC INTERVENTIONS**

Reduce the ventricular rate with digitalis, verapamil, or propranolol. Then administer quinidine or procainamide to convert or prevent the arrhythmia. (See Figure 5-29 on p. 99.) If the patient is symptomatic, use synchronous cardioversion. (See Figure 5-28 on p. 98.)

Atrial fibrillation

Rate	Atrial rate 400 to 800 beats/minute; ventricular rate varies
Rhythm	Ventricular rhythm *always* irregularly irregular
P waves	Irregular, rapid; "fib waves" replace P waves
QRS complexes	Present, normal duration usually
P/QRS relationship	Indistinguishable P waves; irregular ventricular response
PR interval	Indistinguishable

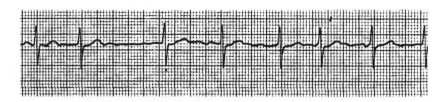

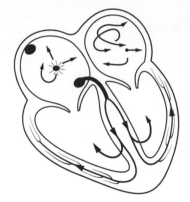

Random reentry circuits within atria; variable degree of block in AV node

■ **SIGNIFICANCE**

Multiple atrial pacemakers fire chaotically in rapid succession. The atria quiver and never firmly contract. The ventricles react in a sporadic fashion. Because of poor atrial emptying there is danger of mural clot formation and embolism. Cardiac output drops 15% to 20% because of lack of atrial kick. Atrial fibrillation is said to be uncontrolled if the ventricular rate is faster than 100 beats/minute. This dysrhythmia is frequently seen in the presence of coronary artery disease, pericarditis, congestive heart failure, rheumatic heart disease, hypertension, pulmonary embolus, hyperthyroidism, and digitalis toxicity.

■ **THERAPEUTIC INTERVENTIONS**

Check the ventricular response, both on the monitor and by checking apical pulse. Check the patient's blood pressure. If the patient is severely symptomatic (syncope, altered level of consciousness, deteriorating vital signs, and chest pain), administer synchronous cardioversion. (See Figure 5-28 on p. 98.) If the patient has been on digitalis therapy, obtain a serum digoxin level before cardioversion. If the patient has not been on digitalis therapy before the onset of this dysrhythmia, he or she may be treated with digitalis or quinidine following a successful synchronous cardioversion. If the patient is stable with atrial fibrillation, rate control is achieved with digitalis, beta blockers, and calcium channel blockers. Chemical conversion can be accomplished with quinidine, procainamide, and verapamil, or with newer agents such as flecainide, propafenone, sotalol, or amiodarone. Warfarin is used to prevent systemic thromboembolism. A new surgical technique called the Maze procedure is being used to abolish atrial fibrillation. (See Figure 5-29 on p. 99.)

Dysrhythmias Originating in the AV Junction

Junctional rhythm

Rate	Usually 40 to 60 beats/minute
Rhythm	Regular
P waves	May appear inverted or may not be present
QRS complexes	Present; normal duration
P/QRS relationship	P wave may appear inverted before or after the QRS complex or may be hidden in QRS
PR interval	Less than 0.12 second when P wave is present preceding QRS

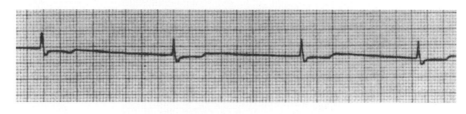

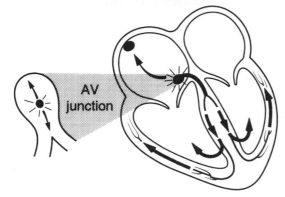

Impulse originates
in AV junction

■ **SIGNIFICANCE**

Usually when higher pacemakers fail, the AV junction takes over as the pacemaker of the heart. It is an unreliable pacemaker.

■ **THERAPEUTIC INTERVENTIONS**

If the patient has been on digitalis therapy, withhold digitalis and obtain a serum digoxin level to check for digitalis toxicity. There is no specific therapy for this dysrhythmia. If the patient becomes symptomatic (syncope, altered level of consciousness, and chest pain) as a result of the slow heart rate, give atropine sulfate. If the atropine is unsuccessful, transcutaneous pacing is indicated. (See Figure 5-27 on p. 97.)

Premature junctional complex (PJC)

Rate	Usually normal or bradycardic depending on the underlying rhythm
Rhythm	Irregular due to premature complex
P waves	May appear inverted or may not be present
QRS complexes	Present; normal duration
P/QRS relationship	P waves may appear inverted before or after the QRS complex or may be hidden in QRS; entire P/QRS complex is early
PR interval	Less than 0.12 second when P wave is seen in premature beat

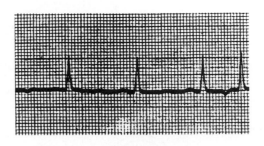

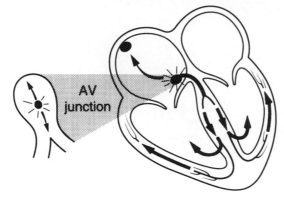

Junctional origin
of abnormal impulse

■ **SIGNIFICANCE**

The AV junction is the pacemaker. The dysrhythmia is usually seen in digitalis toxicity, ischemia, hypoxia, electrolyte imbalances, and congestive heart failure.

■ **THERAPEUTIC INTERVENTIONS**

If the patient is on digitalis therapy, withhold digitalis and obtain a serum digoxin level. Observe closely. Pharmacologic therapy may include quinidine or procainamide if the patient is symptomatic. Alcohol, caffeine, and nicotine should be withheld from the patient's daily routine.

Junctional tachycardia

Rate	60 to 180 beats/minute; 60 to 100 beats/minute is often called accelerated junctional rhythm
Rhythm	Regular
P waves	May appear inverted or may not be present
QRS complexes	Present; normal duration
P/QRS relationship	P waves may appear inverted before or after the QRS complex or may be hidden in QRS
PR interval	Less than 0.12 second when P wave is present

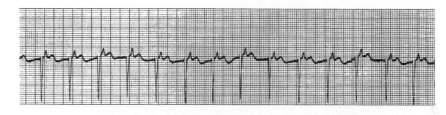

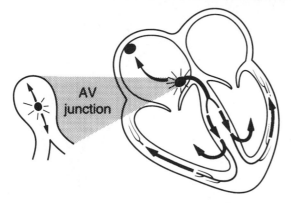

Ectopic focus in AV junction
beats regularly at rate of
60 -180 / minute

■ **SIGNIFICANCE**

A junctional focus takes over as the heart's pacemaker. Junctional tachycardia has the same causes as PJCs.

■ **THERAPEUTIC INTERVENTIONS**

Check vital signs. If the patient is on digitalis therapy, withhold digitalis and obtain a serum digoxin level. In the presence of hemodynamic instability, digitalis binding antibody may be administered. Usually no other treatment is necessary.

Wandering pacemaker

Rate	Usually 50 to 100 beats/minute
Rhythm	Usually regular or slightly irregular
P waves	Present; configuration varies
QRS complexes	Present; normal duration
P/QRS relationship	P wave precedes most QRSs, though it may disappear
PR interval	Normal

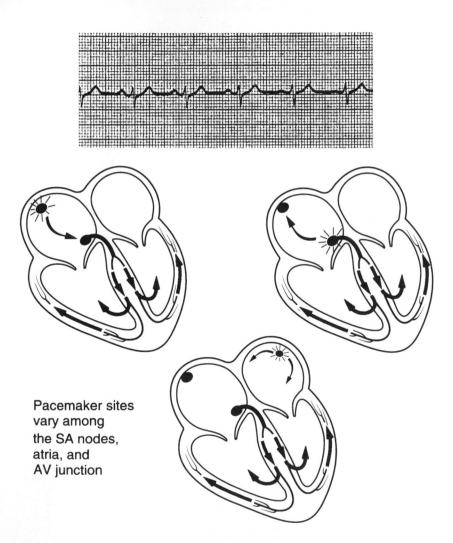

Pacemaker sites
vary among
the SA nodes,
atria, and
AV junction

■ **SIGNIFICANCE**

There is competition between two or more supraventricular foci in the SA node, atria, or AV junction, for control of the rhythm. Either the SA node is suppressed or other lower foci become excited and take over the pacemaker function of the heart.

■ **THERAPEUTIC INTERVENTIONS**

Treatment is usually unnecessary. If the patient is receiving digitalis, it may be wise to withhold the digitalis and obtain a serum digoxin level.

Paroxysmal supraventricular tachycardia (PSVT, reentry tachycardia)

Rate	100 to 280 beats/minute
Rhythm	Regular; sudden start and stop
P wave	Often buried in or distorting QRS; may be before QRS
QRS complexes	Present; usually normal duration though may be wide
P/QRS relationship	P wave for each QRS, or none seen
PR interval	Short or none

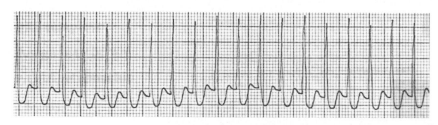

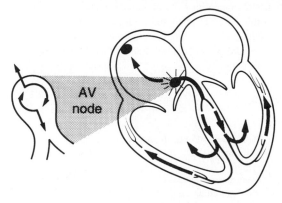

AV junction or atrium originates impulse

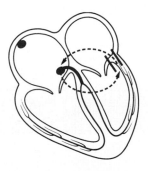

Circus movement between
AV node and accessory pathway

■ SIGNIFICANCE

Most frequently the rhythm is a reentry tachycardia occurring within the AV node. PSVT can also be caused by circus movement between the AV node and an accessory pathway. Least frequently, the tachycardia originates within the atria. PSVT can occur in a normal heart, or in association with hypoxia, ischemia, electrolyte imbalances, stretch of the myocardium as in congestive heart failure, rheumatic heart disease, acute pericarditis, myocardial infarction, mitral valve prolapse, or with preexcitation such as Wolff-Parkinson-White syndrome. Nonparoxysmal atrial tachycardia is caused by digitalis toxicity. Physical signs in the patient are dyspnea, angina, diaphoresis, fatigue, anxiety, dizziness, and polyuria.

■ THERAPEUTIC INTERVENTIONS

Record the rhythm in multiple leads before treatment so that the mechanism of the arrhythmia can be determined. AV nodal reentry tachycardia is usually benign and self-limiting or easily terminated with vagal maneuvers, e.g., carotid sinus pressure, gagging, Valsalva maneuver, facial immersion in cold water, or coughing. Since this arrhythmia is usually initiated with a PAC, advise the patient to avoid excess caffeine, nicotine, and stress. If the patient is symptomatic with the PSVT, vagal maneuvers or drugs such as adenosine (first line), verapamil, digoxin, beta blockers, and diltiazen are used. If this is unsuccessful, cardiovert. (See Figures 5-28 and 5-29 on pp. 98 and 99.)

If the patient is digitalis toxic, discontinue the digitalis preparation and correct any hypokalemia. Antiarrhythmic medications used in this case are phenytoin, lidocaine, and magnesium IV. If the patient is hemodynamically compromised, administer digitalis binding antibody.

Newer approaches being used are permanent ablation of the AV node by radiofrequency current, and surgical interruption of the accessory pathway.

Atrioventricular Blocks

First-degree AV block

Rate	Usually 60 to 100 beats/minute
Rhythm	Usually regular
P waves	Present
QRS complexes	Present; normal duration
P/QRS relationship	P wave preceding each QRS complex
PR interval	Greater than 0.20 seconds, consistent

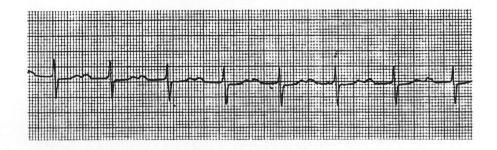

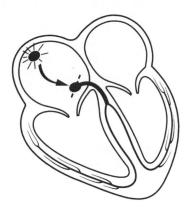

SA node originates impulse;
conduction delay at AV node

■ **SIGNIFICANCE**

The SA node initiates an impulse that is delayed through the AV node. This may be caused by anoxia, ischemia of the myocardium, AV node malfunction, edema following open heart surgery, myocarditis, thyrotoxicosis, rheumatic fever, and certain drugs, including digitalis, clonidine, and tricyclic antidepressants.

■ **THERAPEUTIC INTERVENTIONS**

Treatment for first-degree AV block is not necessary without symptoms. If symptomatic, treat the underlying cause. If the patient is on digitalis therapy, withhold digitalis and obtain a serum digoxin level. Observe the patient for a higher degree of block. If the patient becomes symptomatic (syncope, altered level of consciousness, chest pain), administer atropine. If atropine administration is unsuccessful, prepare for pacemaker placement.

Second-degree AV block—type I (Mobitz, type I or Wenckebach phenomenon)

Rate	Usually normal
Rhythm	Grouped beats
P waves	One preceding each QRS complex except for regular dropped ventricular complex at intervals
QRS complexes	Cyclic missed conduction; when QRS complex is present, it is of normal duration
P/QRS relationship	P wave before each QRS complex except for regular dropped ventricular complex at intervals
PR interval	Lengthens with each cycle until one QRS complex is dropped, then repeats

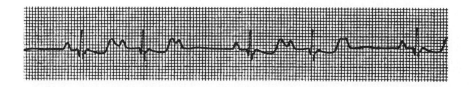

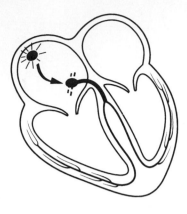

SA node originates impulse;
progressive conduction delay
at AV node

■ **SIGNIFICANCE**

Each atrial impulse takes longer to travel through the AV node, until a beat is finally dropped, and the entire cycle repeats itself. Although its cause is not well understood, this dysrhythmia is transient and commonly seen following inferior wall myocardial infarction or any other disorder that affects conduction through the AV node or the bundle of His. This includes myocarditis; open heart surgery; and medications such as digoxin, prorandol, or verapamil.

■ **THERAPEUTIC INTERVENTIONS**

Treatment is usually unnecessary without symptoms. Investigate cause and withhold digoxin. Observe for progression of the AV block. If perfusion is impaired or serious dysrhythmias result from bradycardia, consider atropine and then a transcutaneous pacemaker. (See Figure 5-27 on p. 97.)

Second-degree AV block—type II (Mobitz, type II)

Rate	Atrial rate usually 60 to 100 beats/minute; ventricular rate usually slow
Rhythm	Atrial regular/ventricular irregular
P waves	Two or more for every QRS complex
QRS complexes	Normal or prolonged duration when present
P/QRS relationship	Two or more nonconducted impulses appearing as P waves without QRS complexes following
PR interval	Normal or delayed on the conducted beat, but remains the same throughout the dysrhythmia

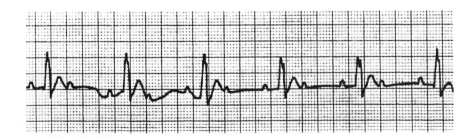

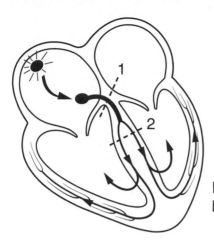

Partial intermittent block in
bundle of His or bundle branches

■ **SIGNIFICANCE**

One or more atrial impulses are not conducted through the AV node to the ventricles. This is usually the result of an inferior or anterior wall myocardial infarction, but may also be caused by anoxia, digitalis toxicity, edema following open heart surgery, or hyperkalemia.

■ **THERAPEUTIC INTERVENTIONS**

If the QRS is of normal duration, administer atropine. When this is ineffective or the QRS is wide, pacing is the treatment of choice. If the patient is on digitalis therapy, withhold digitalis and obtain a serum digoxin level. If hyperkalemia is the cause of the dysrhythmia, administer sodium polystrene sulfonate (Kayexalate) enema. Always administer supplemental oxygen. (See Figure 5-27 on p. 97.) Consider dopamine, epinephrine, and isoproterenol.

Complete AV block—third-degree heart block

Rate	Atrial rate 60 to 100 beats/minute; ventricular rate usually less than 60 beats/minute
Rhythm	Regular
P waves	Occur regularly
QRS complexes	Slow; narrow or wide (>0.12 second)
P/QRS relationship	Completely independent of each other
PR interval	Inconsistent

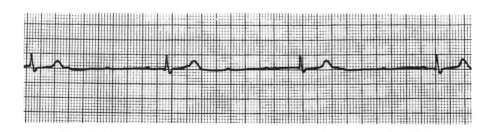

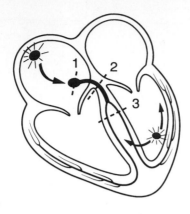

Complete block at AV node, bundle of His, or bundle branches; may have junctional or ventricular independent pacemaker

■ **SIGNIFICANCE**

In this dysrhythmia there is no conduction of the SA node impulse through the AV node. The AV junction or ventricle begins to initiate its own impulse; the atria and ventricles beat independently of each other. Causes may include digitalis toxicity, diaphragmatic or anterior myocardial infarction, myocarditis, or accidental injury during open heart surgery.

■ **THERAPEUTIC INTERVENTIONS**

If the patient is on digitalis therapy, withhold digitalis and obtain a digoxin level. Observe the ventricular rate closely. If the ventricular rate is slow, the patient will most likely be symptomatic (syncope, altered level of consciousness, and chest pain), and cardiac failure may soon result. Therapeutic intervention is the placement of a pacemaker. Be prepared to perform both basic and advanced life support. (See Figure 5-27 on p. 97.)

Junctional Escape Rhythm

Rate	May or may not be normal
Rhythm	P waves regular; QRS complexes regular
P waves	Vary; may be sinus, atrial, or junctional
QRS complexes	Normal duration or wide
P/QRS relationship	Varies; usually no relationship
PR interval	Inconsistent

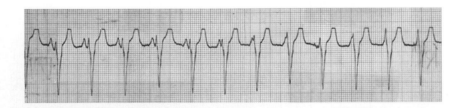

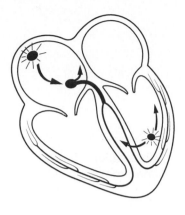

Junctional or ventricular focus
beating faster than sinus node

■ SIGNIFICANCE

The AV junction pacemaker accelerates to a rate exceeding that of the underlying sinus rate. There is independent beating of the atria and ventricles, but no heart block is present. This dysrhythmia is seen in acute inferior myocardial infarction and digitalis toxicity.

■ THERAPEUTIC INTERVENTIONS

Most often the patient is asymptomatic, and pacemaker therapy is not warranted. Direct therapy at the underlying cause. Digoxin and serum potassium levels should be checked.

Dysrhythmias Originating in the Ventricles

Premature ventricular complex (premature ectopic beat or extrasystole, PVC, PVB, VPD)

Rate	Usually 60 to 100 beats/minute
Rhythm	Irregular due to early beats
P waves	Present with each sinus beat; do not precede PVCs
QRS complexes	Sinus-initiated QRS complex normal; QRS of PVC wide and bizarre, greater than 0.12 second; full compensatory pause; usually has T wave of opposite polarity
P/QRS relationship	P wave before each QRS complex in normal sinus beats; no P wave preceding PVC
PR interval	Normal in sinus beat; none in PVC

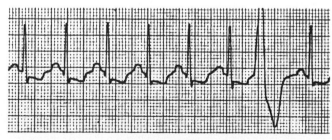

Single PVC

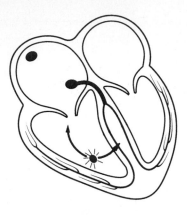

Ventricular origin of
abnormal impulse

■ **SIGNIFICANCE**

PVCs are indicative of an irritable ventricle. PVCs come from an impulse initiated by a ventricular cell. They may occur as a result of hypoxia, hypovolemia, ischemia, infarction, hypertrophy, hypokalemia, acidosis, or the use of alcohol, nicotine, caffeine, or many other drugs. PVCs may originate from the same focus (unifocal PVCs) or from various foci (multifocal PVCs). Multifocal PVCs are of different configurations. PVCs may occur in repetitious patterns. If they occur every other beat, the condition is called bigeminy. If they occur every third beat, it is called trigeminy. If they occur in a pair, they are called a couplet. If three occur together, they are called a triplet. A series of three or more consecutive PVCs is commonly known as ventricular tachycardia.

■ **THERAPEUTIC INTERVENTIONS**

If the cause of the PVCs is known, treat the cause. If the patient is hypoxic, administer oxygen. If the patient is hypokalemic, give potassium. If the patient is hypovolemic, initiate volume replacement. Usually isolated PVCs are not treated except for the first 4 hours after a myocardial infarction. There is little conclusive evidence that PVCs adversely affect survival and that treatment enhances survival. Treatment is lidocaine in the form of an IV bolus followed by additional boluses and an IV drip. Other drugs that may be administered are atropine (if the PVCs are related to a slow heart rate), procainamide, quinidine, phenytoin, bretylium, or propranolol.

Ventricular tachycardia (V tach or VT)

Rate	100 to 250 beats/minute
Rhythm	Regular
P waves	Not seen
QRS complexes	Wide and bizarre
P/QRS relationship	None
PR interval	None

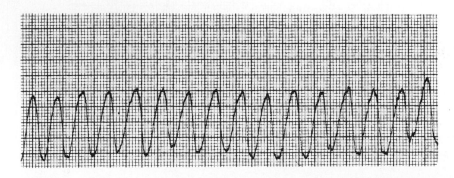

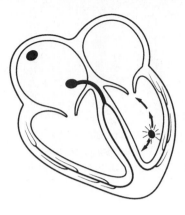

One ventricular pacemaker
fires rapidly

■ **SIGNIFICANCE**

This rhythm is actually several consecutive PVCs. It is rare in patients without underlying heart disease. The patient's hemodynamic response is based on the lack of atrial kick and the ventricular rate. Craney found that cardiac patients with a VT rate of 130 to 270 became dizzy, and loss of consciousness occurred beginning at a VT rate of 200.[3] Nonsustained VT (lasting less than 30 seconds) may not be treated unless the person is symptomatic or has underlying heart disease. Sustained VT is more often seen in those with prior myocardial infarction, chronic coronary artery disease, or dilated cardiomyopathy. Polymorphic VT (torsades de pointes) is often seen with drugs that prolong the QT interval, such as quinidine. If fast VT does not dissipate itself, it will deteriorate to ventricular fibrillation.

■ **THERAPEUTIC INTERVENTIONS**

Monomorphic VT at a rate faster than 150 beats per minute is treated in an emergency with synchronized cardioversion at 100, 200, 300, then 360 joules (J). Pulseless VT is treated as ventricular fibrillation. If the patient is stable, antiarrhythmic IV drugs such as lidocaine, procainamide, and bretylium are used. Polymorphic VT is treated by stopping the offending drug and giving IV potassium or IV magnesium. If this is not successful, use overdrive pacing or an IV isoproterenol drip. Oral antiarrhythmic drugs include quinidine, procainamide, flecainide, mexiletine, and amiodarone. An automatic implantable cardioverter defibrillator may be used when VT has resulted in cardiac arrest. If the site of the VT can be determined during electrophysiologic study, ablation or surgical subendocardial resection may be performed. (See Figures 5-24, 5-28, and 5-29 on pp. 94, 98, and 99.)

Ventricular fibrillation (VF)

Rate	Rapid, disorganized
Rhythm	Irregular
P waves	Not seen
QRS complexes	Extremely bizarre, wide patterns, appearing like baseline oscillations
P/QRS relationship	None
PR interval	None

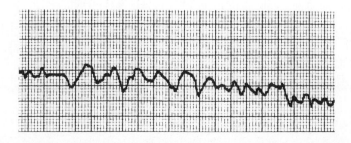

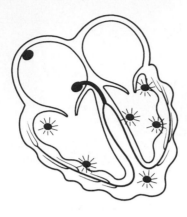

Ventricular ectopic
sites firing so fast
that quivering results

■ **SIGNIFICANCE**

This rhythm produces essentially no cardiac output; death will result if it is allowed to persist for more than 4 to 6 minutes. It is often initiated by ventricular tachycardia. Its most frequent cause is coronary artery disease.

■ **THERAPEUTIC INTERVENTIONS**

Begin basic and advanced cardiac life support immediately. The sooner defibrillation is performed, the greater the chance of success. Defibrillate three times at 200, 200 to 300 and 360 J, respectively. Administer 100% oxygen under positive pressure; administer epinephrine IV and repeat every 3 to 5 minutes. Allow the drug to circulate for 30 to 60 seconds and then reevaluate the patient's rhythm. If fibrillation continues, defibrillate at 360 J. If this is unsuccessful, the following treatments may be tried: (1) lidocaine, (2) bretylium, (3) magnesium sulfate, (4) procainamide, and in some cases (5) sodium bicarbonate. After each dose of medication, defibrillate with 360 J. If resuscitation is successful, the underlying cause of the arrest must be corrected. (See Figure 5-24 on p. 94.) Patients who survive at least one episode of cardiac arrest may receive an automatic implantable cardioverter defibrillator.

Idioventricular rhythm

Rate	20 to 40 beats/minute
Rhythm	Regular or irregular
P waves	None
QRS complexes	Wide and bizarre
P/QRS relationship	None
PR interval	None

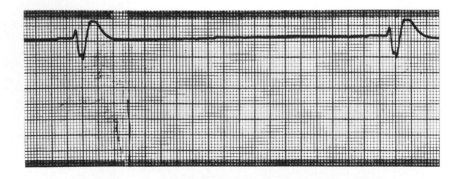

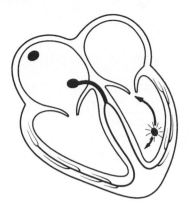

Ventricular focus originates
beat at very slow rate

■ **SIGNIFICANCE**

This dysrhythmia is associated with a poor prognosis; it probably indicates a large myocardial infarction with concurrent loss of a large amount of ventricular mass.

■ **THERAPEUTIC INTERVENTIONS**

Begin basic and advanced cardiac life support immediately. Intubate and give 100% oxygen under positive pressure. Administer epinephrine and atropine. (See Figure 5-25 on p. 95.)

Accelerated idioventricular rhythm

Rate	40 to 120 beats/minute
Rhythm	Regular
P waves	None
QRS complexes	Wide and bizarre
P/QRS relationship	None
PR interval	None

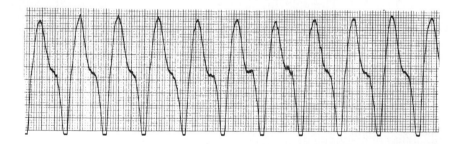

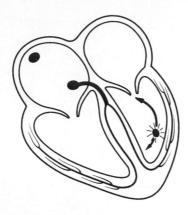

Ventricular focus originates beat
at rate of 40-120 / minute

■ **SIGNIFICANCE**

This arrhythmia is seen during reperfusion with thrombolytic therapy for coronary occlusion. It can also reflect myocardial necrosis.

■ **THERAPEUTIC INTERVENTIONS**

Often no drug intervention is needed. Keep the patient flat in bed and provide fluids until the arrhythmia disappears.

Asystole (ventricular standstill)

Rate	None
Rhythm	None
P waves	May or may not appear
P/QRS relationship	None
PR interval	None

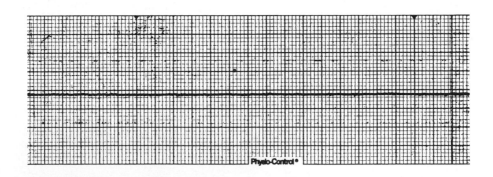

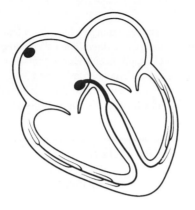

No impulses
from the heart

■ **SIGNIFICANCE**

Asystole often implies that the patient has been in cardiopulmonary arrest for a prolonged period; mortality is high (greater than 95%).

■ **THERAPEUTIC INTERVENTIONS**

Begin basic and advanced life support immediately. Intubate and give 100% oxygen under positive pressure. Administer epinephrine and atropine. Consider sodium bicarbonate administration. Confirm asystole by switching to another lead because occasionally ventricular fibrillation may appear as a flat line. Shocking asystole may eliminate return of spontaneous heart beats. Transcutaneous pacing may be effective only if asystole is of short duration. Consider termination of resuscitation efforts because this is a "terminal" rhythm. (See Figure 5-26 on p. 96.)

Pulseless electrical activity

Pulseless electrical activity (PEA) is a phenomenon in which some type of electrical activity other than VT or VF is present but there is not a palpable pulse. This group of dysrhythmias includes:

Electromechanical dissociation (EMD)
Pseudo-EMD
Idioventricular rhythms
Ventricular escape rhythms
Bradyasystolic rhythms
Post-defibrillation idioventricular rhythms

■ **SIGNIFICANCE**

Cardiac output is so low or nonexistent that the patient is essentially in cardiac arrest. Death almost always follows PEA, although there is survival from certain causes if recognized and treated early in the process. Causes include:

Hypovolemia
Hypoxia
Cardiac tamponade
Tension pneumothorax
Hypothermia
Massive pulmonary embolism
Drug overdoses, such as tricyclics, digitalis, beta blockers, calcium channel blockers
Hyperkalemia
Acidosis
Massive acute myocardial infarction

■ **THERAPEUTIC INTERVENTIONS**

Initiate CPR, intubate, and administer positive pressure breathing right away. Identify the cause and apply specific interventions. For example, give volume expanders in hypovolemia. With suspected cardiac tamponade, perform pericardiocentesis. In tension pneumothorax, apply needle decompression. Proper airway management and aggressive hyperventilation should be pursued since hypoventilation and hypoxemia are frequent causes of PEA. Medications used in PEA include epinephrine IV every 3 to 5 minutes and atropine. Sodium bicarbonate may be useful in hyperkalemia and acidosis, and with tricyclic antidepressant overdose. (See Figure 5-25 on p. 95.)

ADVANCED LIFE SUPPORT TECHNIQUES

Administration of Medications in Cardiac Arrest

The ideal route for drug administration during cardiopulmonary resuscitation is IV through a central vein located above the diaphragm. But often it is easier to place a peripheral IV line, and CPR does not have to be stopped to do so. When drugs are given peripherally compared to the central route, peak drug levels are lower and circulation time is increased. To speed up drug delivery to the central circulation, peripheral catheters should be large bore and placed proximally (e.g., antecubital). Any medication administered through a peripheral catheter should be given rapidly and flushed afterward with 20 to 30 ml of solution. Then elevate the extremity.

If insertion of an IV line is delayed, one may wish to consider administering medication via the endotracheal route. This route is particularly beneficial for children, in whom much time may be consumed attempting to find an IV route.

The lungs absorb medication rapidly, and the entire cardiac circulation passes through them, making the absorption of medication by the cardiovascular system rapid. It is interesting to note that the onset of action of atropine, epinephrine, and lidocaine given intratracheally to animals in cardiopulmonary arrest was 70% to 80% more rapid than the onset with IV drugs.

The following medications are readily absorbed via the intratracheal route:

Atropine	Isoproterenol
Bretylium	Lidocaine
Diazepam	Naloxone (Narcan)
Epinephrine (Adrenalin)	

The following medications should *not* be given via the intratracheal route:
Sodium bicarbonate; because of alkalinity and volume
Norepinephrine (Levophed); causes tissue necrosis and sloughing
Calcium chloride; causes tissue necrosis and sloughing

■ **PROCEDURE FOR INTRATRACHEAL ADMINISTRATION OF MEDICATIONS**

1. Advance a long, 35-μm, small-bore catheter beyond the end of the endotracheal tube.
2. Stop chest compressions.
3. Administer through the catheter 2 to 2½ times the recommended adult IV dose of the medication.
4. Follow with a 10-ml normal saline flush down the catheter.
5. Give four or five ventilations with the bag-valve device to distribute the medication.
6. Resume chest compressions.

The intraosseous route is an excellent alternative when IV access is not readily available, particularly in the pediatric patient. Although the intraosseous dose would be the same as the IV dose, some evidence suggests that higher intraosseous doses might be necessary, especially when epinephrine is administered.

Medication drips should be mixed in normal saline rather than D_5W. Hyperglycemia may lead to a worse neurologic outcome and increased mortality in the arrest victim. Supplemental administration of glucose should be reserved for documented hypoglycemia.

Carotid Sinus Massage

Carotid sinus massage is the procedure usually chosen before pharmacologic or electric therapies for cardioversion of PSVT. The procedure is performed to place pressure on the carotid bodies located in the carotid arteries. This pressure activates the autonomic nervous system, causing vagal nerve stimulation. As a result, conduction is slowed and the reentry circuit is interrupted, stopping the tachycardia.

■ **PROCEDURE**
1. Place the patient in a supine or Trendelenburg position with the neck extended.
2. Administer oxygen via nasal cannula at 4 to 6 L/min.
3. Initiate IV D_5W TKO. Atropine and lidocaine should be available.
4. Monitor the patient's ECG continuously.
5. Auscultate the carotids for the presence of bruits (murmurs); do not perform the massage if bruits are present.
6. Turn the patient's head to the left side. On the patient's right side, locate the carotid sinus by palpating the carotid artery just below the angle of the jaw (Figure 5-17).
7. Press the carotid artery between the fingers and the lateral processes of the vertebrae.
8. Apply pressure firmly in a small, circular motion, backward and medially.
9. Pressure should last no more than 5 seconds (less if a rhythm change is seen).
10. Carotid sinus massage may be repeated if it is unsuccessful the first time.

■ **SPECIAL NOTES**
Warn the patient that the procedure is uncomfortable.
Have a crash cart and transcutaneous pacemaker standing by during the procedure.
Stop the procedure if there is a rhythm change.
Never massage both sides at once.
Successful conversion is often preceded by short periods of asystole, followed by a few PVCs before normal sinus rhythm resumes.
If the procedure is successful, continue to monitor the patient.

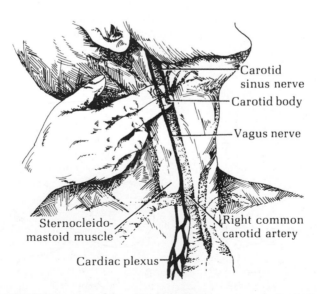

FIGURE 5-17. Location of the carotid sinus body.
(From Conover MB: *Understanding electrocardiography*, ed 7, St Louis, 1996, Mosby.)

■ **COMPLICATIONS**
  Dysrhythmias (ventricular tachycardia, ventricular fibrillation, asystole)
  Cerebral occlusion (CVA)
  Transient ischemia attack
■ **OTHER VAGAL MANEUVERS**
  Valsalva maneuver
  Facial immersion in cold water
  Digital rectal massage
  Gagging
  Coughing
  Breath holding
  Gag reflex stimulation

Precordial Thump ("Thumpversion")

Although the precordial thump may occasionally convert a patient out of VT or VF, the maneuver appears more likely to have no effect, or to exacerbate the rhythm (i.e., precipitate a pulseless rhythm or asystole). This is because the emergency rescuer has no control over when in the cardiac cycle the low-energy wave (approximately 4 J) will be delivered with the thump. Aggravation of the rhythm is likely if the thump is delivered during the vulnerable period (T wave).

Grauer and Cavallaro[4] recommend that the thump be used in "no-lose" situations. They generally reserve use of the thump for treatment of rhythms without a pulse (pulseless VT or VF), since there is nothing to lose from treatment of such rhythms. But in VT with a pulse, where there is "too much to lose," it is better to use synchronized countershock. It is also acceptable to avoid use of the thump in pulseless VT or VF when a defibrillator is close by. (See Figure 5-24 on p. 94.)

In acute onset asystole, rhythmic precordial thumps can produce a QRS complex and associated myocardial contraction until pacing is initiated.

■ **PROCEDURE** (Figure 5-18)
  1. Locate the mid portion of the sternum, halfway between the suprasternal notch and the costal angle.
  2. Make a fist with the dominant hand.
  3. Deliver one blow with the fleshy part of the fist to the mid-sternum from 18 to 12 inches above the chest.
  4. Check for return of pulse and continue with resuscitation as needed.

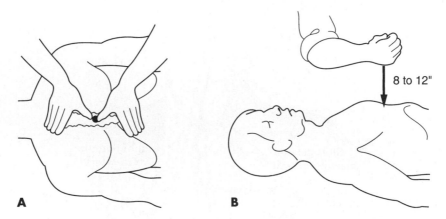

A   **B**

FIGURE 5-18. **A,** Finding correct location. **B,** Performance of precordial thump.
(From Persons CB: *Critical care procedures and protocols,* Philadelphia, 1987, Lippincott.)

Remember to never deliver more than one precordial thump, and do not delay other resuscitation techniques for the thump. The precordial thump is not used with children.

Defibrillation

The sooner defibrillation is delivered to a patient with pulseless ventricular tachycardia or ventricular fibrillation, the greater the chance of recovery. Without this intervention, death will ensue. Defibrillation depolarizes a critical mass of the myocardium so that the SA node or other intrinsic pacemaker can regain control.

On discovering a patient in pulseless ventricular tachycardia or ventricular fibrillation, the rescuer should defibrillate immediately three times if necessary. If unsuccessful, it is essential to begin basic and advanced life support techniques and medications before further defibrillation attempts. (See Figure 5-24 on p. 94.)

In addition to the manual mode, defibrillators are now available in automatic and semiautomatic designs, so rescuers can be more easily trained to defibrillate. It is essential to know how to operate the defibrillators in your work setting quickly and efficiently. Users should follow checklists each shift to ascertain that there is no malfunction of defibrillators. A more thorough evaluation by biomedical personnel is warranted every 3 to 6 months.

External defibrillation can be performed with the usual hand-held paddles or the newer "hands-off" disposable electrodes. Paddles and electrodes are available in adult and pediatric sizes. As soon as the adult paddles/electrodes fit onto a child's chest with good skin contact (usually over 1 year of age or 10 kg), they should be used, because transthoracic impedance is less and defibrillation more successful. Anterior-lateral paddle/electrode placement is commonly used (Figure 5-19), though anterior-posterior placement is an acceptable alternative (Figure 5-20). Paddles/electrodes should be placed 5 inches away from an internal pacemaker generator and never over nitroglycerin ointment/patches or EKG electrodes/wires. If the patient has an automatic implantable cardioverter defibrillator (ICD), the internal pads on the epicardium may deflect the energy when the paddles are in their usual location. Side-to-side location of the paddles/electrodes may be successful in this circumstance.

Remember that transthoracic impedance is lower with rapid, successive shocks, so initial shocks in the adult are stacked: 200, then 200 to 300, and finally 360 J without pulse checks in between. Initially, 2 J/kg are used with children followed by 4 J/kg.

Disposable defibrillation electrodes are pregelled with conductive medium. When using paddles, always apply a conductive medium to them, even in an emergency. This conductive medium decreases transthoracic

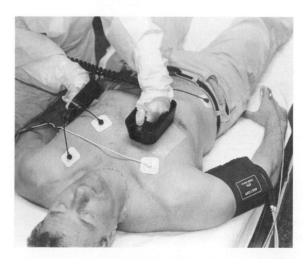

FIGURE 5-19. Anterior-lateral paddle placement for defibrillation.
(Courtesy Emilie Goudey, Lenox, Mass.)

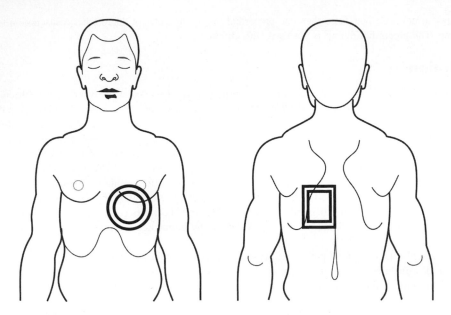

FIGURE 5-20. Anterior-posterior disposable defibrillation electrode placement.
(From Zoll PD: *1200 pacemaker/defibrillator operator's guide*, Woburn, Mass, 1992, Zoll Medical Corporation.)

impedance and prevents skin burns. Commercially available paste or disposable pregelled pads may be used with the paddles. *Never* use alcohol-soaked pads because alcohol will ignite. Make sure that the paste is not smeared between the paddles on the chest, or arcing of the current may occur. There should be enough paste on the paddles to cover them completely, but never so much that the paste slides down onto the rescuer's hand, creating an electrical hazard.

Before defibrillation remove temporary transvenous pacing wires from the generator so its internal circuitry is not damaged. Always check permanent pacemaker function after defibrillation. Do not delay CPR or external defibrillation when an ICD is in place; proceed with the usual emergency protocols. If the ICD discharges when the caregiver's hands are on the patient, a small amount of current may be felt, but it is not dangerous.

■ **EXTERNAL DEFIBRILLATION PROCEDURE**
1. Verify loss of consciousness and absence of pulse and respirations.
2. Turn the machine on.
3. Check that the "synchronous/defibrillate" switch is in the defibrillate mode.
4. Select the desired energy level.
5. If paddles are used, apply a conductive medium to their surfaces.
6. Apply the disposable electrodes or hard paddles to the patient's unclothed chest in the desired location.
7. Confirm the dysrhythmia of ventricular tachycardia or fibrillation on the monitor scope.
8. If paddles are used, apply 25 pounds of pressure to them to decrease transthoracic impedance.
9. Charge the machine.
10. Observe closely and state aloud, "All clear." This means no person should be touching the patient, the bed, or any equipment attached to the patient.
11. Discharge the defibrillator by pressing the discharge buttons simultaneously.
12. Quickly interpret the rhythm on the monitor scope and proceed with the second shock if needed.

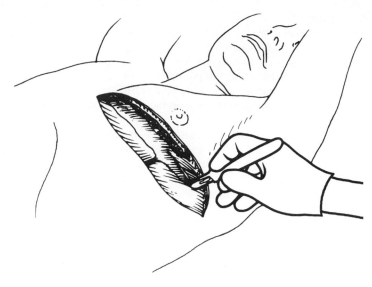

FIGURE 5-21. Emergency thoracotomy incision.
(From Wasserberger J et al: Emergency department thoracotomy, *Emer Med Clin North Am* 7(1):104, 1989.)

Emergency Thoracotomy/Open Chest Massage/Internal Defibrillation

Thoracotomy and open chest massage (direct cardiac massage) or cross-clamping of the aorta may be required in cases of penetrating wounds to the heart, repeat pericardial tamponade not relieved by pericardiocentesis, tension pneumothorax, crush injuries to the chest, or any other incident for which ready access to the intrathoracic cavity is needed. Other examples include patients in arrest with chest wall deformities such as those found in patients with COPD and barrel chest.

■ **EQUIPMENT**

Gloves, masks, goggle, gowns	Sterile towels or drapes
Scalpel and blade	Suture material
Rib retractor	Vascular clamps
Forceps needle holder	Good lighting
Scissors	Povidone-iodine
Suction	
Defibrillator with internal paddles	
4 × 4 inch gauze soaked in saline	

■ **PROCEDURE (PERFORMED BY A PHYSICIAN)**
1. Place patient in supine position.
2. Ensure that patient is being ventilated.
3. Ensure placement of two large-bore IV lines.
4. Cleanse skin rapidly with povidone-iodine.
5. Apply simple skin draping.
6. Make a curvilinear incision 2 to 3 cm lateral to the left sternal border, extending to the midaxillary line in the fourth or fifth intercostal space (Figure 5-21).
7. Spread the ribs and retract the lungs.
8. Introduce a gloved hand into the chest cavity.
9. Open the pericardial sac if necessary.

10. Massage the heart gently.
11. Perform internal defibrillation if needed (see below).
12. Determine if there is volume in the heart.
13. Determine if cross-clamping of the aorta is required.
14. Determine if there is an injury and repair it if possible.
15. It may be necessary to cross-clamp the aorta if bleeding is massive.
16. Once the procedure has been accomplished, transport the patient to the operating suite for irrigation, repair, closure, and chest tube placement.

Thoracotomy is of limited usefulness in medically caused cardiopulmonary arrest. Studies have shown improved survival when the chest is opened early during resuscitation efforts. Thoracotomy should only be performed by a trained physician.

■ **INTERNAL DEFIBRILLATION PROCEDURE**
1. Replace the external paddles of the defibrillator with internal paddles.
2. Turn the machine on.
3. Ensure that the "synchronous/defibrillate" switch is in the defibrillate mode.
4. Use sterile saline-soaked sponges as conductive medium; place them on the surfaces of the electrodes.
5. Select the dosage level (usually 10 to 20 J in an adult).
6. Place one paddle over the apex of the left ventricle and the other over the base of the right ventricle.
7. Charge the machine.
8. Ensure that all personnel are standing clear of the victim, the bed, and the electrical equipment.
9. Press the discharge buttons and discharge the current.
10. Quickly interpret the rhythm and assess pulses and breathing status; if these are not acceptable, resume internal massage and continue ventilation.

Cardioversion (Synchronous Electrical Countershock)

Synchronous cardioversion is the delivery of a countershock to the chest wall timed to coincide with the QRS. In this way, the shock is not delivered on the T wave, when it could initiate ventricular fibrillation. Synchronized cardioversion is used when a fast tachycardia is accompanied by signs and symptoms of intolerance. These dysrhythmias include ventricular tachycardia, paroxysmal supraventricular tachycardia, atrial fibrillation, and atrial flutter. If a patient has a wide-complex tachycardia of unknown etiology with hemodynamic instability, it should be treated as if it is ventricular tachycardia. Synchronized cardioversion is immediately indicated. (See Figures 5-28 and 5-29 on pp. 98-99.)

Synchronized cardioversion can be an elective procedure for the conversion of atrial fibrillation and flutter when pharmacologic means have not worked. In the presence of digitalis toxicity, cardioversion should not be performed.

The patient in ventricular tachycardia who is pulseless, unconscious, hypotensive, or in pulmonary edema should receive unsynchronized shocks. This avoids any delay when attempting synchronization, since defibrillators may have difficulty differentiating the QRS from a T wave at a very fast rate.

This procedure should only be undertaken by adequately trained personnel who will not only be able to perform the procedure, but who will be able to manage any emergency situation that may result from the cardioversion.

■ **NONEMERGENCY PROCEDURE**
1. Explain the procedure to the patient.
2. Obtain written consent from the patient.
3. Give anticoagulation therapy for several weeks before the procedure.
4. Withhold digitalis for 24 to 72 hours before the procedure; a safe digitalis level in atrial fibrillation may be a toxic level in normal sinus rhythm.
5. Give the patient nothing by mouth (NPO) for 12 hours before the procedure to prevent emesis and aspiration.

6. Determine the serum potassium level; hypokalemia predisposes the patient to ventricular fibrillation.
7. Ask the patient to void.
8. If the patient wears dentures, remove them.
9. Continue at No. 4 of emergency procedure.

■ **EMERGENCY PROCEDURE**

1. Give a brief explanation of the procedure to the patient and/or the family.
2. Obtain consent from the patient or family if possible.
3. If the patient wears dentures, remove them.
4. Keep the room very quiet and dim (usually less sedation will be required).
5. Have a crash cart, transcutaneous pacemaker, and inhalation equipment standing by.
6. Give D_5W IV TKO with an 18-gauge or larger cannula.
7. Have midazolam (Versed) or diazepam (Valium) ready in bolus form; administer it slowly by IV push at small increments until the patient is no longer awake and alert.
8. Ensure that the patient is disconnected from all other electric equipment and oxygen.
9. Turn on the defibrillator unit.
10. Apply ECG electrodes to the patient away from the defibrillator paddle sites. Select a lead with a tall R wave.
11. Obtain a precardioversion 12-lead ECG and have it read by a physician; mark the strip with name, date, and time.
12. Turn on "synchronous" button and verify sensing of the QRS.
13. Set the energy level to 100 J.
14. Run an ECG strip throughout the procedure.
15. If hard paddles are used, cover the surfaces with conductive medium. (*Never* use alcohol-soaked pads— they will explode!)
16. Place the paddles or disposable defibrillation electrodes just to the right of the sternum in the second or third intercostal space and in the fifth intercostal space at the anterior axillary line.
17. Charge the machine.
18. Push down on the paddles with 25 pounds of pressure.
19. Quickly double-check the room to ensure that all personnel are standing clear of the patient, bed, and equipment. Announce, "All clear."
20. Press the discharge buttons simultaneously and hold them until the shock is delivered.
21. Observe the patient closely for respiratory rate and observe the ECG for the resulting rhythm.
22. If the procedure is unsuccessful, repeat it using 200, 300, then 360 J.
23. If the procedure is successful, run a postcardioversion ECG and mark the strip with date, name, and time.

■ **CARE OF PATIENT AFTER CARDIOVERSION**

1. Check the vital signs every 15 minutes for 1 hour, then every 30 minutes for 2 hours, then every 2 hours.
2. Monitor the cardiac rhythm and document any dysrhythmias.
3. Tend to burns that may have been produced by paddles.
4. Keep the patient under observation for 24 hours.
5. If there are no problems, the patient may be discharged.

■ **EARLY COMPLICATIONS**

Asystole	Ventricular tachycardia or fibrillation
Junctional rhythm	Embolization
Premature ventricular contractions	

■ **LATE COMPLICATIONS**

Reversion to atrial fibrillation or atrial flutter
Embolization

Pacemakers

A pacemaker is a technical system for providing low-energy electrical stimulation to the myocardium, which will result in depolarization of the heart. Temporary pacing is instituted in patients with hemodynamically unstable bradycardia (i.e., those with hypotension, change in mental status, myocardial ischemia, or pulmonary edema). Pacing is also used in bradycardic situations accompanied by PVCs if pharmacologic means have not increased the heart rate and eliminated these PVCs. The danger here is that the PVCs, if untreated, may lead to ventricular tachycardia or ventricular fibrillation. (See Figure 5-27 on p. 97.) In asystole, pacing is not usually successful if a long period of hypoperfusion has existed because the heart is then unable to respond to the pacing stimuli. If pacing is to be used successfully in the cardiac arrest victim, it should be started early. (See Figure 5-26 on p. 96.) Finally, pacing may be used to "overdrive" atrial and ventricular tachyarrhythmias. If the pacing is instituted for a few seconds at a rate faster than the tachycardia and then abruptly stopped, the heart's normal (and slower) pacemaker may take over. This overdrive pacing technique should be done only by skilled practitioners with a defibrillator nearby since it may accelerate the rate or trigger ventricular fibrillation.

Standby temporary pacing may be used in the following circumstances:

Stable bradycardias, when it is suspected that the patient may become unstable in the near future

Acute myocardial infarction

Symptomatic sinus node dysfunction

Second-degree heart block, type II

Third-degree heart block

Newly acquired left bundle branch block, right bundle branch block, alternating bundle branch block, or bifascicular block

Components of a pacemaker system

■ **GENERATOR**

The generator houses the electronic circuitry that directs the pacing rate, current released, sensing of the patient's own underlying beats, and timing. In addition it contains the power source or battery.

■ **ELECTRODES**

The contact point with the myocardium (or chest wall) from which the energy is discharged is called the electrode.

■ **LEAD WIRE**

The insulated lead wire connects the generator to the electrodes. It carries the electrical stimulus to the heart and relays information about the patient's own beats back to the generator.

Mode of pacing—demand versus fixed rate

Many pacemakers are set to the demand mode, in which they fire when needed. A sensing circuit looks for the patient's own underlying beats. If the patient's rate falls below a preset rate, the pacemaker fires. Occasionally pacemakers may be set to fire at a fixed rate no matter what the patient's own heart is doing. The problem with this mode of pacing is that the paced beats may compete with the patient's own beats. There is a remote possibility that the pacemaker may fire on the patient's own T wave, causing ventricular tachycardia or fibrillation. In asystole, the fastest way to initiate temporary pacing may be in the fixed rate mode.

Types of pacemaker systems
Temporary transcutaneous (external)

Many of the newer defibrillators also have the ability to perform transcutaneous pacing. Disposable electrodes are placed anterior and posterior on the chest. The caregiver dials the appropriate settings and initiates pacing through the chest wall. See the procedure below. Because the skeletal muscle contraction is painful to the patient, IV sedation or analgesia is given. Electrical capture is usually obtained at 40 to 100 mA. Patients who require greater amounts of energy to capture the ventricle are those with large hearts, increased anterior-posterior chest size, large chest muscle mass, large pleural effusion, and pericardial tamponade. This system is

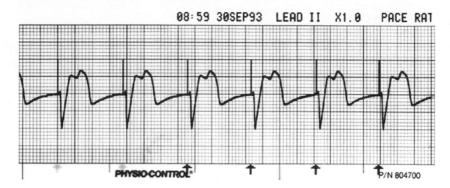

FIGURE 5-22. Ventricular capture with a transcutaneous pacemaker.

used in emergencies until the patient is stabilized, and then consideration is given to placement of a temporary transvenous catheter when the personnel and equipment are available. It is also used when pacing is needed for only a short duration, such as a bradycardia resulting from a medication side effect or overdose.

■ **PROCEDURE FOR TRANSCUTANEOUS PACING**
1. Administer an IV analgesic/sedative medication.
2. Prepare the patient's skin for electrode application. The skin should be clean and dry. Clip the hair to promote electrode adherence, though shaving may be necessary in an emergency.
3. Attach the pacing electrodes to the pacing cable. Affix the pacing electrodes to the patient so that they "sandwich the heart." The anterior electrode is located at a left V2 or V3 position and the posterior electrode under the scapula to the left of the spine.
4. Attach the ECG electrodes to the ECG cable and apply to the patient's skin in the designated locations. These ECG electrodes must always be in place if demand pacing is used, so that the patient's own beats can be sensed.
5. Turn on the defibrillator/external pacing unit.
6. Select the pacing mode (usually demand) and the pacing rate (usually 60 to 100 beats per minute).
7. Ensure that the machine is sensing the patient's own ECG complexes.
8. If the patient is awake, activate the pacemaker at the lowest current setting. Increase the mA until ventricular electrical capture occurs. Electrical capture is verified by a pacing spike followed by a wide QRS and a tall broad T wave in the opposite direction (Figure 5-22).
9. Increase the mA by 5% to 10% to ensure consistent capture.
10. If the patient is unconscious, initiate pacing with the mA up to maximum. Confirm electrical capture and decrease the mA until only that which is necessary for capture is used.
11. Verify mechanical capture by checking for a pulse and blood pressure. *Caution:* Assess the pulse in the right femoral artery, for a carotid artery pulse may be difficult to detect due to the muscle contraction with pacing. Measure blood pressure in the right arm because falsely elevated pressures are found in the left arm during transcutaneous pacing.

■ **PROBLEMS ENCOUNTERED WITH TRANSCUTANEOUS PACING**
   Patient discomfort
Tell the patient in advance that he will feel a "thumping" sensation in his chest.
Give the patient adequate IV analgesia/sedation before initiating pacing.
Do not place the pacing electrodes over the nipple, cuts or abrasions, ECG electrodes, nitroglycerin patches or ointment, alcohol or acetone skin prep.
Place the pacing electrode under the breast of the female patient rather than over breast tissue.
Use only the amount of current necessary to capture the ventricle.
Change the pacing electrodes every 24 hours.

Lack of electrical capture

Increase the mA.

Check for adequate adherence to the patient's skin. The posterior electrode may have slid out of position because of diaphoresis.

Check that all the cable connections are intact.

Change position of the pacing electrodes. Alternate positions are side-to side and anterior-lateral.

Correct any underlying acidosis and hypoxia that could be keeping the myocardium from responding to the electrical stimulus.

Inability to sense the patient's underlying rhythm

Increase the size of the ECG pattern on the monitor.

Select a different lead.

Check for adherence of the ECG electrodes.

Change the position of the ECG electrodes to achieve different leads.

■ **ADVANTAGES**

It can be done with minimal training by a variety of caregivers.

It is quickly and simply initiated.

The procedure is noninvasive and thus low risk.

It is especially useful in patients with bleeding disorders, a compromised immune system, or who are receiving thrombolytic therapy.

It allows more controlled insertion of a transvenous wire.

It is less costly than other types of pacing.

■ **DISADVANTAGES**

It is uncomfortable for the patient.

Temporary transvenous

In the transvenous approach a pacing catheter is threaded through a major vein such as the brachial, internal jugular, subclavian, or femoral, so that the electrodes are in contact with the endocardium of the right ventricle at the apex. The catheter may have a small balloon at its tip to help float it into position. Its location is then tracked by ECG recordings taken from the end of the pacing wire. The catheter may also be a stiffer type that is inserted under the guidance of fluoroscopy. This pacing wire is then connected to an external generator. Dials on the face of this generator are manipulated by the caregiver to control pacing rate, energy output, and sensing of the patient's own heart beats (Figure 5-23). If pacing wires are placed in the atria and ventricles (dual chamber pacing), the AV interval is also set on the generator.

■ **ADVANTAGES**

It performs reliably once in place.

The patient experiences minimal discomfort during use.

■ **DISADVANTAGES**

It must be inserted by a physician.

Placement is time-consuming.

CPR must be interrupted during placement.

Fluoroscopy is sometimes required.

20% develop complications (e.g., pneumothorax, pericardial tamponade, infection, bleeding, thrombus formation).

The amount of energy it takes to capture the ventricle increases over time.

Its direct pathway to the heart presents a microshock hazard to the patient.

Temporary transthoracic

This emergency method of passing a needle directly through the chest wall until contact is made with the myocardium has been abandoned recently. Problems with this technique were a high risk of complications (e.g., pneumothorax, hemothorax, hemopericardium), delay in chest compressions, and poor reliability of pacing.

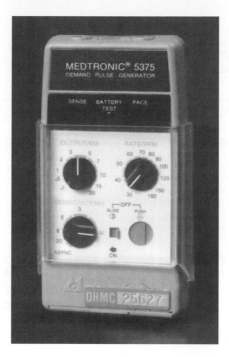

FIGURE 5-23. A temporary transvenous pacemaker generator.

Permanent

In a permanent pacing system all the components are placed internally during an elective surgical procedure. Electrodes are put in contact with the endocardium of the right ventricle and/or atrium via a transvenous approach, or rarely the electrodes are screwed into the epicardium. The generator is usually located subclavicular, though it may be in the abdominal area. Settings are changed in the generator by placing a handheld programmer over the chest wall. Most patients are now followed in a pacemaker clinic in which their ECG is sent via telephone from their home to a technician or nurse who checks the function of their pacemaker. Permanent pacemakers are now being incorporated into automatic implantable cardioverter defibrillators to pace patients out of their tachyarrhythmias or to provide back-up pacing when asystole or bradycardia occurs after defibrillation.

ADVANCED LIFE SUPPORT ALGORITHMS FOR ADULTS

The American Heart Association released new advanced cardiac life support algorithms in November, 1992[5] (Figures 5-24 to 5-29). It is suggested that these algorithms be used as educational tools rather than as dictums of emergency care. They are designed to provide a basic plan of care and are not meant to be followed blindly. Some patients may require care not outlined in or varied from that in the algorithms. When clinically appropriate, flexibility is accepted and encouraged. Also, they emphasize: Treat the patient, not the monitor. Adequate airway, ventilation, oxygenation, chest compressions, and defibrillation are more important than administration of medications and take precedence over initiating an intravenous line or injecting agents.

Text continued on page 108.

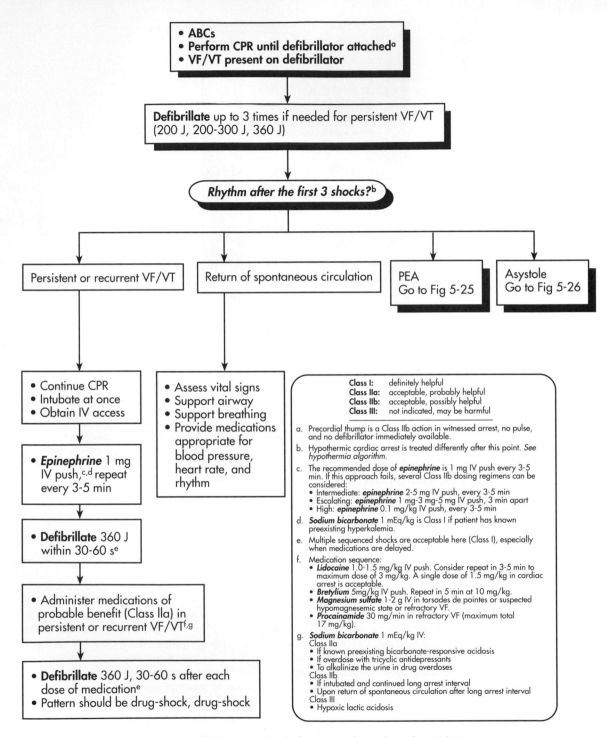

- ABCs
- Perform CPR until defibrillator attached[a]
- VF/VT present on defibrillator

Defibrillate up to 3 times if needed for persistent VF/VT (200 J, 200-300 J, 360 J)

Rhythm after the first 3 shocks?[b]

| Persistent or recurrent VF/VT | Return of spontaneous circulation | PEA Go to Fig 5-25 | Asystole Go to Fig 5-26 |

- Continue CPR
- Intubate at once
- Obtain IV access

- *Epinephrine* 1 mg IV push,[c,d] repeat every 3-5 min

- **Defibrillate** 360 J within 30-60 s[e]

- Administer medications of probable benefit (Class IIa) in persistent or recurrent VF/VT[f,g]

- **Defibrillate** 360 J, 30-60 s after each dose of medication[e]
- Pattern should be drug-shock, drug-shock

- Assess vital signs
- Support airway
- Support breathing
- Provide medications appropriate for blood pressure, heart rate, and rhythm

Class I: definitely helpful
Class IIa: acceptable, probably helpful
Class IIb: acceptable, possibly helpful
Class III: not indicated, may be harmful

a. Precordial thump is a Class IIb action in witnessed arrest, no pulse, and no defibrillator immediately available.

b. Hypothermic cardiac arrest is treated differently after this point. *See hypothermia algorithm.*

c. The recommended dose of *epinephrine* is 1 mg IV push every 3-5 min. If this approach fails, several Class IIb dosing regimens can be considered:
   - Intermediate: *epinephrine* 2-5 mg IV push, every 3-5 min
   - Escalating: *epinephrine* 1 mg-3 mg-5 mg IV push, 3 min apart
   - High: *epinephrine* 0.1 mg/kg IV push, every 3-5 min

d. *Sodium bicarbonate* 1 mEq/kg is Class I if patient has known preexisting hyperkalemia.

e. Multiple sequenced shocks are acceptable here (Class I), especially when medications are delayed.

f. Medication sequence:
   - *Lidocaine* 1.0-1.5 mg/kg IV push. Consider repeat in 3-5 min to maximum dose of 3 mg/kg. A single dose of 1.5 mg/kg in cardiac arrest is acceptable.
   - *Bretylium* 5mg/kg IV push. Repeat in 5 min at 10 mg/kg.
   - *Magnesium sulfate* 1-2 g IV in torsades de pointes or suspected hypomagnesemic state or refractory VF.
   - *Procainamide* 30 mg/min in refractory VF (maximum total 17 mg/kg).

g. *Sodium bicarbonate* 1 mEq/kg IV:
   Class IIa
   - If known preexisting bicarbonate-responsive acidosis
   - If overdose with tricyclic antidepressants
   - To alkalinize the urine in drug overdoses
   Class IIb
   - If intubated and continued long arrest interval
   - Upon return of spontaneous circulation after long arrest interval
   Class III
   - Hypoxic lactic acidosis

FIGURE 5-24. Algorithm for ventricular fibrillation and pulseless ventricular tachycardia (VF/VT).
(From American Heart Association: *Advanced cardiac life support,* Dallas, 1997, The Association.)

Includes
- Electromechanical dissociation (EMD)
- Pseudo-EMD
- Idioventricular rhythms
- Ventricular escape rhythms
- Bradyasystolic rhythms
- Postdefibrillation idioventricular rhythms

- Continue CPR
- Intubate at once
- Obtain IV access

- Assess blood flow using Doppler ultrasound, end-tidal CO_2, echocardiography, or arterial line

Consider possible causes
(Parentheses = possible therapies and treatments)

- Hypovolemia (volume infusion)
- Hypoxia (ventilation)
- Cardiac tamponade (pericardiocentesis)
- Tension pneumothorax (needle decompression)
- Hypothermia (see hypothermia algorithm)
- Massive pulmonary embolism (surgery, *thrombolytics*)

- Drug overdoses such as tricyclics, digitalis, β–blockers, calcium channel blockers
- Hyperkalemia[a]
- Acidosis[b]
- Massive acute myocardial infarction

- *Epinephrine* 1 mg IV push,[a,c] repeat every 3-5 min

- If absolute bradycardia (<60 BPM) or relative bradycardia, give *atropine* 1 mg IV
- Repeat every 3-5 min to a total of 0.03-0.04 mg/kg[d]

Class I: definitely helpful
Class IIa: acceptable, probably helpful
Class IIb: acceptable, possibly helpful
Class III: not indicated, may be harmful

a. *Sodium bicarbonate* 1 mEq/kg is Class I if patient has known preexisting hyperkalemia.
b. *Sodium bicarbonate* 1 mEq/kg:
   Class IIa
   - If known preexisting bicarbonate-responsive acidosis
   - If overdose with tricyclic antidepressants
   - To alkalinize the urine in drug overdoses
   Class IIb
   - If intubated and continued long arrest interval
   - Upon return of spontaneous circulation after long arrest interval
   Class III
   - Hypoxic lactic acidosis
c. The recommended dose of *epinephrine* is 1 mg IV push every 3-5 min. If this approach fails, several Class IIb dosing regimens can be considered:
   - Intermediate: *epinephrine* 2-5 mg IV push, every 3-5 min
   - Escalating: *epinephrine* 1 mg-3 mg-5 mg IV push, 3 min apart
   - High: *epinephrine* 0.1 mg/kg IV push, every 3-5 min
d. The shorter *atropine* dosing interval (3 min) is possibly helpful in cardiac arrest (Class IIb).

FIGURE 5-25. Algorithm for pulseless electrical activity (PEA) or electromechanical dissociation (EMD).
(From American Heart Association: *Advanced cardiac life support,* Dallas, 1997, The Association.)

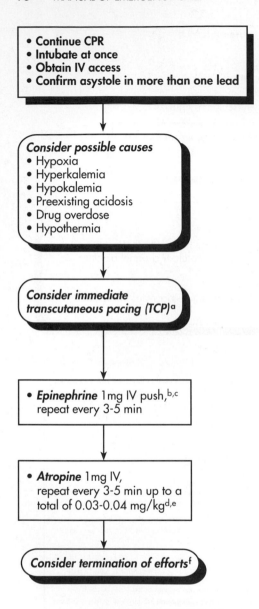

Class I: definitely helpful
Class IIa: acceptable, probably helpful
Class IIb: acceptable, possibly helpful
Class III: not indicated, may be harmful

a. TCP is a Class IIb intervention. Lack of success may be due to delays in pacing. To be effective TCP must be performed early, simultaneously with drugs. Evidence does not support routine use of TCP for asystole.

b. The recommended dose of *epinephrine* is 1mg IV push every 3-5 min. If this approach fails, several Class IIb dosing regimens can be considered:
   • Intermediate: *epinephrine* 2-5 mg IV push, every 3-5 min
   • Escalating: *epinephrine* 1 mg-3 mg-5 mg IV push, 3 min apart
   • High: *epinephrine* 0.1 mg/kg IV push, every 3-5 min

c. *Sodium bicarbonate* 1 mEq/kg is Class I if patient has known preexisting hyperkalemia.

d. The shorter *atropine* dosing interval (3 min) is Class IIb in asystolic arrest.

e. *Sodium bicarbonate* 1 mEq/kg:
   Class IIa
   • If known preexisting bicarbonate-responsive acidosis
   • If overdose with tricyclic antidepressants
   • To alkalinize the urine in drug overdoses
   Class IIb
   • If intubated and continued long arrest interval
   • Upon return of spontaneous circulation after long arrest interval
   Class III
   • Hypoxic lactic acidosis

f. If patient remains in asystole or other agonal rhythm after successful intubation and initial medications and no reversible causes are identified, consider termination of resuscitative efforts by a physician. Consider interval since arrest.

FIGURE 5-26. Asystole treatment algorithm.
(From American Heart Association: *Advanced cardiac life support*, Dallas, 1997, The Association.)

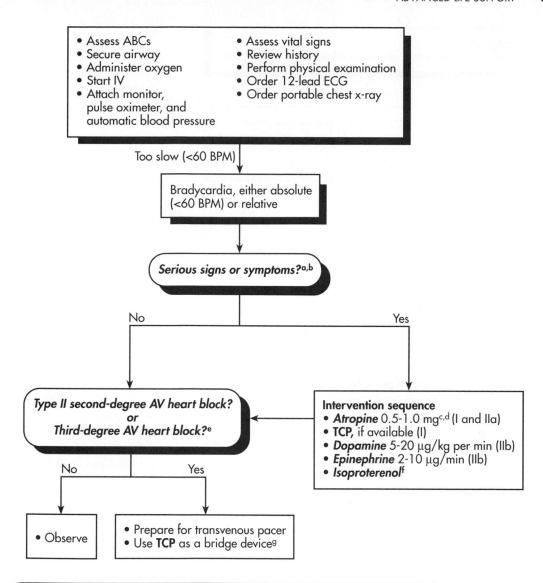

FIGURE 5-27. Bradycardia algorithm (with the patient not in cardiac arrest).

(From American Heart Association: *Advanced cardiac life support*, Dallas, 1997, The Association.)

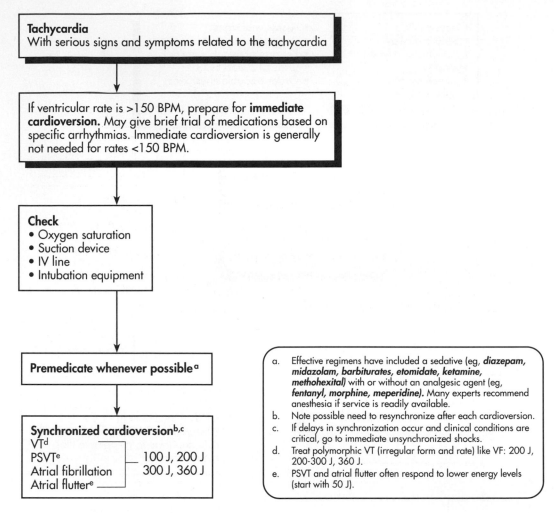

FIGURE 5-28. Electrical cardioversion algorithm (with the patient not in cardiac arrest).
(From American Heart Association: *Advanced cardiac life support,* Dallas, 1997, The Association.)

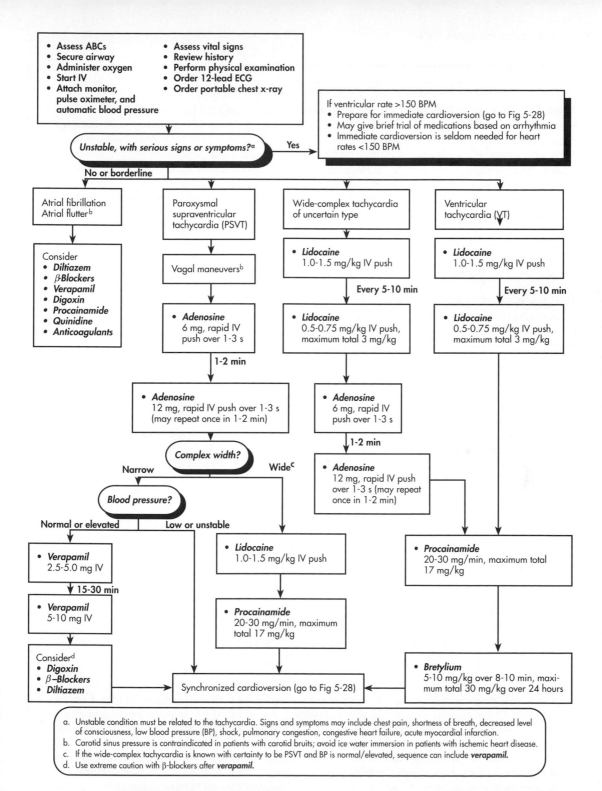

- Assess ABCs
- Secure airway
- Administer oxygen
- Start IV
- Attach monitor, pulse oximeter, and automatic blood pressure

- Assess vital signs
- Review history
- Perform physical examination
- Order 12-lead ECG
- Order portable chest x-ray

If ventricular rate >150 BPM
- Prepare for immediate cardioversion (go to Fig 5-28)
- May give brief trial of medications based on arrhythmia
- Immediate cardioversion is seldom needed for heart rates <150 BPM

Unstable, with serious signs or symptoms?[a]   **Yes**

No or borderline

Atrial fibrillation
Atrial flutter[b]

Consider
- *Diltiazem*
- *β-Blockers*
- *Verapamil*
- *Digoxin*
- *Procainamide*
- *Quinidine*
- *Anticoagulants*

Paroxysmal supraventricular tachycardia (PSVT)

Vagal maneuvers[b]

- *Adenosine*
  6 mg, rapid IV
  push over 1-3 s

1-2 min

- *Adenosine*
  12 mg, rapid IV push over 1-3 s
  (may repeat once in 1-2 min)

Wide-complex tachycardia of uncertain type

- *Lidocaine*
  1.0-1.5 mg/kg IV push

Every 5-10 min

- *Lidocaine*
  0.5-0.75 mg/kg IV push, maximum total 3 mg/kg

- *Adenosine*
  6 mg, rapid IV push over 1-3 s

1-2 min

- *Adenosine*
  12 mg, rapid IV push over 1-3 s (may repeat once in 1-2 min)

Ventricular tachycardia (VT)

- *Lidocaine*
  1.0-1.5 mg/kg IV push

Every 5-10 min

- *Lidocaine*
  0.5-0.75 mg/kg IV push, maximum total 3 mg/kg

Complex width?   **Narrow**   **Wide[c]**

Blood pressure?

Normal or elevated   **Low or unstable**

- *Verapamil*
  2.5-5.0 mg IV

15-30 min

- *Verapamil*
  5-10 mg IV

Consider[d]
- *Digoxin*
- *β–Blockers*
- *Diltiazem*

- *Lidocaine*
  1.0-1.5 mg/kg IV push

- *Procainamide*
  20-30 mg/min, maximum total 17 mg/kg

- *Procainamide*
  20-30 mg/min, maximum total 17 mg/kg

Synchronized cardioversion (go to Fig 5-28)

- *Bretylium*
  5-10 mg/kg over 8-10 min, maximum total 30 mg/kg over 24 hours

a. Unstable condition must be related to the tachycardia. Signs and symptoms may include chest pain, shortness of breath, decreased level of consciousness, low blood pressure (BP), shock, pulmonary congestion, congestive heart failure, acute myocardial infarction.
b. Carotid sinus pressure is contraindicated in patients with carotid bruits; avoid ice water immersion in patients with ischemic heart disease.
c. If the wide-complex tachycardia is known with certainty to be PSVT and BP is normal/elevated, sequence can include *verapamil.*
d. Use extreme caution with β-blockers after *verapamil.*

FIGURE 5-29. Tachycardia algorithm.

(From American Heart Association: *Advanced cardiac life support,* Dallas, 1997, The Association.)

BOX 5-1   Advanced Life Support Drugs and Electrical Therapy (Adult)

Adenosine: 3 mg/mL in 2mL vial (total = 6 mg) *Indications* •First drug for narrow-complex PSVT. •May be used diagnostically (after lidocaine) in wide-complex tachycardias of uncertain type. *Precautions* •Transient side effects include flushing, chest pain or tightness, brief periods of asystole or bradycardia, ventricular ectopy. •Less effective in patients taking theophyllines; avoid in patients receiving dipyridamole. *Adult Dosage IV rapid push:* (1) Place patient in mild reverse Trendelenburg position before administration of drug. (2) Initial bolus of 6 mg given *rapidly* over 1 to 3 seconds followed by normal saline bolus of 20 mL; then elevate the extremity. (3) Repeat dose of 12 mg in 1 to 2 minutes if needed. (4) A third dose of 12 mg may be given in 1 to 2 minutes if needed. *Injection Technique* (1) Record rhythm strip during administration. (2) Draw up adenosine dose and flush in two separate syringes. (3) Attach both syringes to the IV injection port closest to patient. (4) Clamp IV tubing above injection port. (5) Push IV adenosine as *quickly* as possible (1 to 3 seconds). (6) While maintaining pressure on adenosine plunger, push normal saline flush *as rapidly as possible* after adenosine. (7) Unclamp IV tubing.

Aminophylline: 25 mg/mL in 10 mL vial (total = 250 mg); 50 mg/mL in 10 mL vial (total = 500 mg) *Indications* •Third-line agent for acute pulmonary edema. *Precautions* •May cause VT or other tachyarrhythmias. •Watch for toxicity in patients with congestive heart failure. •Avoid in PSVT and acute ischemic heart disease. •Do not mix with other drugs. *Adult Dosage IV Loading Dose and Infusion:* (1) 5 mg/kg given over 30 to 45 minutes. (2) Never exceed 500 mg loading dose. (3) Follow with infusion of 0.5 to 0.7 mg/kg per hour.

Amrinone: 5 mg/mL in 20 mL vial (total = 100 mg) *Indications* •Severe congestive heart failure refractory to diuretics, vasodilators, and conventional inotropic agents. *Precautions* •Do not mix with dextrose solutions or other drugs. •May cause tachyarrhythmias, hypotension, or thrombocytopenia. •Can increase myocardial ischemia. *Adult Dosage IV Loading Dose and Infusion:* (1) 0.75 mg/kg, given over 10 to 15 minutes. (2) Follow by infusion of 5 to 15 μg/kg per minute titrated to clinical effect. (3) Optimal use requires hemodynamic monitoring.

Atropine sulfate: 0.1 mg/mL in 10 mL preloaded syringe (total = 1 mg) can be given via endotracheal tube. *Indications* •First drug for symptomatic bradycardia (Class IIa). •Second drug (after epinephrine) for asystole or bradycardic pulseless electrical activity (Class IIb). *Precautions* •Use with caution in presence of myocardial ischemia and hypoxia. •Increases myocardial oxygen demand. •Avoid in hypothermia. •Seldom effective for infranodal (type II) AV block and new third-degree block with wide QRS complexes (Class IIb). (In these patients may cause paradoxical slowing. Be prepared to pace or give catecholamines.) *Adult Dosage Asystole or Pulseless Electrical Activity:* (1) 1 mg IV push. (2) Repeat every 3 to 5 minutes (if asystole persists) to a maximum dose of 0.03 to 0.04 mg/kg. *Bradycardia:* (1) 0.5 to 1.0 mg IV every 3 to 5 minutes as needed; not to exceed total dose of 0.03 to 0.04 mg/kg. (2) Use shorter dosing interval (3 minutes) and higher doses (0.04 mg/kg) in severe clinical conditions. *Endotracheal Administration:* 2 to 3 mg diluted in 10 mL normal saline.

β-Blockers, *Metoprolol:* 1 mg/mL in 5 mL vial (total = 5 mg); *Atenolol:* 0.5 mg/mL in 10 mL ampule (total = 5 mg); *Propranolol:* 1 mg/mL in 1 mg ampule; 4 mg/mL in 5 mL vial (total = 20 mg); *Esmolol:* 10 mg/mL in 10 mL ampule (total = 100 mg); *Labetalol:* 5 mg/mL in 20 mL ampules. *Indications* •To convert to normal sinus rhythm or to slow ventricular response (or both) in supraventricular tachyarrhythmias (PSVT, atrial fibrillation, or atrial flutter). β-Blockers are second-line agents after adenosine, diltiazem, or digoxin. •To reduce myocardial ischemia and damage in AMI patients with elevated heart rates, blood pressure, or both. •For emergency antihypertensive therapy for hemorrhagic and acute ischemic stroke. *Precautions* •Concurrent IV administration with IV calcium channel blocking agents like verapamil

BOX 5-1   Advanced Life Support Drugs and Electrical Therapy (Adult)—cont'd

or diltiazem can cause severe hypotension. •Avoid in bronchospastic diseases, cardiac failure, or severe abnormalities in cardiac conduction. •Monitor cardiac and pulmonary status during administration. •May cause myocardial depression. **Adult Dosage** *Metoprolol:* •5 mg slow IV at 5-minute intervals to a total of 15 mg. *Atenolol:* (1) 5 mg slow IV (over 5 minutes). (2) Wait 10 minutes, then give second dose of 5 mg slow IV (over 5 minutes). (3) In 10 minutes, if tolerated well, may start 50 mg PO; then give 50 mg PO twice a day. *Propranolol:* (1) 1 to 3 mg slow IV. Do not exceed 1 mg/min. (2) Repeat after 2 minutes if necessary. *Esmolol:* (1) 0.5 mg/kg over 1 minute, followed by continuous infusion at 0.05 mg/kg per minute. (2) Titrate to effect. Esmolol has a short half-life (<10 minutes). *Labetalol:* 10 mg labetalol IV push over 1 to 2 minutes. May repeat or double labetalol every 10 minutes to a maximum dose of 150 mg, *or* give initial dose as a bolus, then start labetalol infusion 2 to 8 μg/min.

Bretylium: 50 mg/mL in 10 mL prefilled syringe (total = 500 mg); 50 mg/mL in 10 mL vial (total = 500 mg) **Indications** •Cardiac arrest from VF/VT after defibrillation, epinephrine, lidocaine (Class IIa). •Refractory/recurrent VT after full doses of lidocaine (Class IIa). •Class IIa as first antiarrhythmic for hypothermic VF. **Precautions** •Side effects include hypotension, nausea, and vomiting. **Adult Dosage** *Cardiac arrest* (1) 5 mg/kg IV bolus. May give 10 mg/kg in 5 minutes if needed. (2) One 500-mg ampule IV bolus with a second dose of two 500-mg ampules in 5 minutes is acceptable. *Stable VT* (1) 5 to 10 mg/kg IV over 8 to 10 minutes; wait 10 to 30 minutes before next dose. (2) Maximum total dose, 30 mg/kg over 24 hours. (3) Maintenance infusion: 1 to 2 mg/min.

Calcium chloride: 100 mg/mL in 10 mL vial (total = 1 g; a 10% solution) **Indications** •Known or suspected hyperkalemia (e.g., renal failure). •Hypocalcemia (e.g., after multiple blood transfusions). •As an antidote for toxic effects (hypotension and arrhythmias) from calcium channel blocker overdose. •Used prophylactically before IV calcium channel blockers to prevent hypotension. **Precautions** •Do not use routinely in cardiac arrest. •Do not mix with sodium bicarbonate. **Adult Dosage** *IV Slow Push:* (1) 8 to 16 mg/kg (usually 5 to 10 mL) IV for hyperkalemia and calcium channel blocker overdose. (2) 2 to 4 mg/kg (usually 2 mL) IV for prophylactic pretreatment before IV calcium channel blockers.

Cardioversion (synchronized): (1) Administered via remote defibrillation electrodes or hand-held paddles from a defibrillator/monitor. (2) Place defibrillator/monitor in synchronized (sync) mode. (3) Sync mode delivers energy just after the R wave. **Indications** •All tachycardias (rate > 150 beats/min) with serious signs and symptoms related to the tachycardia. •May give brief trial of medications based on specific arrhythmias. **Precautions** •In critical conditions, go to immediate unsynchronized shocks. •Urgent cardioversion is generally not needed if heart rate is 150 beats/min or less. •Reactivation of sync mode is usually required after each cardioversion. •Prepare to defibrillate immediately if cardioversion causes VF. •Synchronized cardioversion cannot be performed unless the patient is connected to monitor leads; lead select switch must be on lead I, II, or III and not on "paddles." **Adult Dosage** *Technique:* (1) Premedicate whenever possible. (2) Engage sync mode. (3) Look for sync markers on the R wave. (4) "Clear" the patient before each shock. (5) Deliver shocks in the following sequence: 100 J, 200 J, 300 J, 360 J. Use this sequence for each of the following: VT†, PSVT‡, atrial flutter‡, atrial fibrillation. †Treat polymorphic VT (irregular form and rate) with same currents used for VF: 200 J, 200 to 300 J, 360 J. ‡PSVT and atrial flutter often respond to lower energy levels; start with 50 J. •Press "charge" button, "clear" the patient, and press both "shock" buttons simultaneously.

Defibrillation: (1) Use conventional monitor/defibrillator. (2) Use automated or shock advisory defibrillator. (3) Administer shocks via remote adhesive electrodes or hand-held paddles. **Indications** •First interventions for VF or pulseless VT (Class I). **Precautions** •Always "clear" the patient before discharging a

Continued

BOX 5-1   Advanced Life Support Drugs and Electrical Therapy (Adult)—cont'd

defibrillation shock. •Do not delay defibrillation for VF/VT. •Asystole should not be routinely shocked. •Treat VF/VT in hypothermic cardiac arrest with up to 3 shocks. Repeat shocks for VF/VT only after core temperature rises above 30°C. •If patient in VF/VT has an automatic implantable cardioverter defibrillator (AICD), perform external defibrillation per ACLS guidelines. If AICD is delivering shocks, wait 30 to 60 seconds for completion of cycle. •If patient has implanted pacemaker, place paddles and pads several inches from the pacing generator. *Adult Dosage Adult Defibrillation Energy Levels:* (1) 200 J, first shock. (2) 200 to 300 J, second shock. (3) 360 J, third shock. (4) If these shocks fail to convert VF/VT, continue at 360 J for future shocks. (5) If VF recurs, shock again at the last successful energy level. (6) Biphasic devices shock at lower energy levels (approximately 150 J). In some clinical settings, initial and repeated shocks at these lower energy levels are acceptable.

Digibind (digoxin-specific antibody therapy): 40 mg vial (each vial binds about 0.6 mg digoxin). *Indications* Digoxin toxicity with the following: •Uncontrolled life-threatening arrhythmias. •Shock or congestive heart failure. •Hyperkalemia (potassium level > 5.0 mEq/L). •Steady-state serum levels above 10 to 15 mg/mL. *Precautions* •Serum digoxin levels rise after digibind therapy and should not be used to guide continuing therapy. *Adult Dosage Chronic intoxication:* 3 to 5 vials may be effective. *Acute Overdose:* (1) IV dose varies according to amount of digoxin ingested. (2) Average dose is 10 vials (400 mg); may require up to 20 vials (800 mg). (3) See package insert for details.

Digoxin: 0.25 mg/mL or 0.1 mg/mL supplied in 1 or 2 mL ampule (totals = 0.1 to 0.5 mg). *Indications* •To slow ventricular response in atrial fibrillation or atrial flutter. •Third-line choice for PSVT (after vagal maneuvers, adenosine, diltiazem, verapamil). *Precautions* •Toxic effects are common and are frequently associated with serious arrhythmias. •Avoid electrical cardioversion if patient is receiving digoxin unless condition is life threatening; use lower current settings (10-20J). *Adult Dosage IV Infusion* (1) Loading doses of 10 to 15 μg/kg lean body weight provide therapeutic effect with minimum risk of toxic effects. (2) Maintenance dose is affected by body size and renal function.

Diltiazem: 5 mg/mL in 5 or 10 mL vials (total = 25 or 50 mg). *Indications* •To control ventricular rate in atrial fibrillation and atrial flutter. •Use after adenosine to treat refractory PSVT in patients with narrow QRS complex and adequate blood pressure. •As an alternative, use verapamil. *Precautions* •Do not use calcium channel blockers for wide-QRS tachycardias of uncertain origin. •Avoid calcium channel blockers in patients with Wolff-Parkinson-White syndrome plus rapid atrial fibrillation or flutter, in patients with sick sinus syndrome, or in patients with AV block without a pacemaker. •Expect blood pressure drop resulting from peripheral vasodilation (greater drop with verapamil than with diltiazem). •Avoid in patients receiving oral β-blockers. •Concurrent IV administration with IV β-blockers can cause severe hypotension. *Adult Dosage Acute Rate Control:* (1) 15 to 20 mg (0.25 mg/kg) IV over 2 minutes. (2) May repeat in 15 minutes at 20 to 25 mg (0.35 mg/kg) over 2 minutes. *Maintenance infusion:* 5 to 15 mg/hour, titrated to heart rate.

Dobutamine: 12.5 mg/mL in 20 mL vial (total = 250 mg). *IV infusion:* Dilute 250 mg (20 mL) in 250 mL normal saline or D_5W. *Indications* •Consider for pump problems (congestive heart failure, pulmonary congestion) with systolic blood pressure of 70 to 100 mm Hg and no signs of shock. *Precautions* •Avoid when systolic blood pressure <100 mm Hg and signs of shock are present. •May cause tachyarrhythmias, fluctuations in blood pressure, headache, and nausea. *Adult Dosage IV Infusion:* (1) Usual infusion rate is 2 to 20 μg/kg per minute. (2) Titrate so heart rate does not increase by more than 10% of baseline. (3) Hemodynamic monitoring is recommended for optimal use.

BOX 5-1   Advanced Life Support Drugs and Electrical Therapy (Adult)—cont'd

Dopamine: 40 mg/mL in 5 mL ampule (total = 200 mg); 160 mg/mL in 5 mL ampule (total = 800 mg); *IV infusion:* Mix 400 to 800 mg in 250 mL normal saline, lactated Ringer's solution, or D_5W. ***Indications*** •Second drug for symptomatic bradycardia (after atropine). •Use for hypotension (systolic blood pressure ≤ 70 to 100 mm Hg) with signs and symptoms of shock. ***Precautions*** •May use in patients with hypovolemia but only after volume replacement. •Use with caution in cardiogenic shock with accompanying congestive heart failure. •May cause tachyarrhythmias, excessive vasoconstriction. ***Adult Dosage*** *Continuous infusions (titrate to patient response) Low Dose:* 1 to 5 μg/kg per minute ("renal doses"). *Moderate Dose:* 5 to 10 μg/kg per minute ("cardiac doses"). *High Dose:* 10 to 20 μg/kg per minute ("vasopressor doses").

Epinephrine: 1 mg/10 mL in preloaded 10 mL syringe (total = 1 mg); 1 mg/mL in glass 1 mL ampule (total = 1 mg); 1 mg/mL in multi-dose 30 mL vial (total = 30 mg). ***Indications*** •*Cardiac arrest:* VF, pulseless VT, asystole, pulseless electrical activity (Class I). •*Symptomatic bradycardia:* After atropine, dopamine, and transcutaneous pacing (Class IIb). •*Anaphylaxis, severe allergic reactions:* Combine with large fluid volumes, corticosteroids, antihistamines. ***Precautions*** •Raising blood pressure and increasing heart rate may cause myocardial ischemia, angina, and increased myocardial oxygen demand. ***Adult Dosage*** *Cardiac arrest* (1) First dose: 1 mg IV push; may repeat every 3 to 5 minutes. (2) Alternative regimens for second dose (Class IIb) (a) Intermediate: 2 to 5 mg IV push, every 3 to 5 minutes. (b) Escalating: 1 mg, 3 mg, 5 mg IV push, each dose 3 minutes apart. (c) High: 0.1 mg/kg IV push, every 3 to 5 minutes. (3) Endotracheal Route 2.0 to 2.5 mg diluted in 10 mL normal saline. *Profound Bradycardia:* 2 to 10 μg/min infusion (add 1 mg of 1:1000 to 500 mL normal saline; infuse at 1 to 5 mL/min).

Flumazenil: 0.1 mg/mL in 5 and 10 mL vials (totals = 0.5 to 1.0 mg). ***Indications*** •Reverse respiratory depression and sedative effects of benzodiazepines. ***Precautions*** •Effects may not outlast effect of benzodiazepines. •Monitor for later respiratory depression. •Do not use in suspected tricyclic overdose. •Do not use in seizure-prone patients. •Do not use in unknown drug overdose. ***Adult Dosage*** *First Dose,* 0.2 mg IV over 15 seconds. *Second Dose,* 0.3 mg IV over 30 seconds. If no adequate response, give third dose. *Third Dose,* 0.5 mg IV given over 30 seconds. If no adequate response, repeat once every minute until adequate response or until a total of 3 mg is given.

Furosemide: 10 mg/mL in 2, 4, and 10 mL ampules or vials (totals = 20 mg, 40 mg, and 100 mg). ***Indications*** •For adjuvant therapy of acute pulmonary edema in patients with systolic blood pressure > 90 to 100 mm Hg (without signs and symptoms of shock). •Hypertensive emergencies. •Increased intracranial pressure. ***Precautions*** •Dehydration, hypovolemia, hypotension, hypokalemia, or other electrolyte imbalance may occur. ***Adult Dosage*** *IV Infusion* (1) 0.5 to 1.0 mg/kg given over 1 to 2 minutes. (2) If no response, double dose to 2.0 mg/kg, slowly over 1 to 2 minutes.

Glucagon: Powdered in 1 and 10 mg vials. Reconstitute with provided solution. ***Indications*** •Adjuvant treatment of toxic effects of calcium channel blocker or β-blocker. ***Precautions*** •Do not mix with saline. •May cause vomiting, hyperglycemia. ***Adult Dosage*** *IV infusion* 1 to 5 mg over 2 to 5 minutes.

Heparin: 0.5 to 1.0 mL ampules, vials, and prefilled syringes; 1, 2, 5, and 30 mL multidose vials; concentrations range from 1000 to 40,000 IU/mL. ***Indications*** •Adjuvant therapy in AMI. •Begin heparin with alteplase. ***Precautions*** •Same contraindications as for thrombolytic therapy, as follows: (a) active bleeding (b) recent intracranial, intraspinal, or eye surgery (c) severe hypertension (d) bleeding disorders (e) gastrointestinal bleeding. •Doses and laboratory targets appropriate when used with thrombolytic therapy. •Heparin reversal if necessary. *Protamine* 25 mg IV infusion over 10 minutes or longer. (Calculate dose as

Continued

BOX 5-1   Advanced Life Support Drugs and Electrical Therapy (Adult)—cont'd

1 mg protamine per 100 IU of heparin remaining in the patient; heparin plasma half-life is 60 minutes.) *Adult Dosage IV infusion* (1) Initial bolus 80 IU/kg. (2) Continue 18 IU/kg per hour (round to the nearest 50 IU). (3) Adjust to maintain activated partial thromboplastin time (aPTT) 1.5 to 2.0 times the control values. (4) Target range for aPTT after first 24 hours is between 60 and 85 seconds (may vary with laboratory). (5) Check aPTT at 6, 12, 18, and 24 hours. (6) If aPTT <60 seconds at 24 hours, repeat bolus with 20 IU/kg heparin; increase infusion by 3 IU/kg per hour; recheck aPTT in 2 hours.

Isoproterenol: 1 mg/mL in 1 mL vial. *IV infusion:* Mix 1 mg in 250 mL normal saline, lactated Ringer's solution, or D_5W. **Indications** •Refractory torsades de pointes unresponsive to magnesium sulfate. •*Temporary* control of bradycardia in heart transplant patients. •Class IIb at low doses for symptomatic bradycardia. **Precautions** •Do not use for treatment of cardiac arrest. •Increases myocardial oxygen requirements, which may increase myocardial ischemia. Do not give with epinephrine; can cause VF/VT. **Adult Dosage** *IV infusion* (1) Infuse at 2 to 10 µg/min. (2) Titrate to adequate heart rate. (3) In torsades de pointes titrate to increase heart rate until VT is suppressed.

Lidocaine: 20 mg/mL in preloaded 5 mL syringe (total = 100 mg); 10 mg/mL in 5 mL vial (total = 50 mg), can be given via endotracheal tube. **Indications** •Cardiac arrest from VF/VT (Class IIa). •Stable VT, wide-complex tachycardias of uncertain type, wide-complex PSVT (Class I). **Precautions** •*Prophylactic* use in AMI patients is *not* recommended. •Reduce maintenance dose (not loading dose) in presence of impaired liver function or left ventricular dysfunction. **Adult Dosage** *Cardiac Arrest From VF/VT* (1) Initial dose: 1.0 to 1.5 mg/kg IV. (2) For refractory VF may repeat 1.0 to 1.5 mg/kg IV in 3 to 5 minutes; maximum total dose, 3 mg/kg. (3) A single dose of 1.5 mg/kg IV in cardiac arrest is acceptable. (4) Endotracheal administration: 2 to 4 mg/kg. *Perfusing Arrhythmia* For stable VT, wide-complex tachycardia of uncertain type, significant ectopy, use as follows: (a) 1.0 to 1.5 mg/kg IV push. (b) Repeat 0.5 to 0.75 mg/kg every 5 to 10 minutes; maximum total dose, 3 mg/kg. *Maintenance infusion* 2 to 4 mg/min (30 to 50 µg/kg per minute).

Magnesium sulfate: 2 and 10 mL ampules of 50% $MgSO_4$ (total = 1 g and 5 g); 10 mL in preloaded syringe (total = 5 g/10 mL). **Indications** •Cardiac arrest associated with torsades de pointes or suspected hypomagnesemic state. •Refractory VF (after lidocaine and bretylium). •Torsades de pointes with a pulse. •Life-threatening ventricular arrhythmias due to digitalis toxicity, tricyclic overdose. •Consider prophylactic administration in hospitalized patients with AMI (Class IIa). **Precautions** •Occasional fall in blood pressure with rapid administration. •Use with caution if renal failure is present. **Adult Dosage** *Cardiac arrest* 1 to 2 g (2 to 4 mL of a 50% solution) diluted in 10 mL of D_5W IV push. *Acute Myocardial Infarction* (1) Loading dose of 1 to 2 g, mixed in 50 to 100 mL of D_5W, over 5 to 60 minutes IV. (2) Follow with 0.5 to 1.0 g/hour IV for up to 24 hours. *Torsades de pointes* (1) Loading dose of 1 to 2 g mixed in 50 to 100 mL of D_5W, over 5 to 60 minutes IV. (2) Follow with 1 to 4 g/hour IV (titrate dose to control the torsades).

Mannitol: 150, 250, and 1000 mL IV containers (strengths: 5%, 10%, 15%, 20%, and 25%). **Indications** •Increased intracranial pressure in management of neurologic emergencies. **Precautions** •Monitor fluid status and osmolarity (not to exceed 310 mOsm/kg). •Caution in renal failure because fluid overload may result. **Adult Dosage** *IV Infusions* (1) Administer 0.5 to 1.0 g/kg over 5 to 10 minutes. (2) Additional doses of 0.25 to 2 g/kg can be given every 4 to 6 hours as needed. (3) Use in conjunction with mild hyperventilation.

BOX 5-1   Advanced Life Support Drugs and Electrical Therapy (Adult)—cont'd

Morphine sulfate: 2 to 10 mg/mL in 1 mL syringes. ***Indications*** •Chest pain and anxiety associated with AMI or cardiac ischemia. •Acute cardiogenic pulmonary edema (if blood pressure is adequate). ***Precautions*** •Administer slowly and titrate to effect. •May compromise respiration; therefore use with caution in the compromised respiratory state of acute pulmonary edema. •Causes hypotension in volume-depleted patients. •Reverse, if needed, with naloxone (0.4 to 2.0 mg IV). ***Adult Dosage*** *IV infusion* 1 to 3 mg IV (over 1 to 5 minutes) every 5 to 30 minutes.

Naloxone hydrochloride: 0.4 and 1 mg vials, ampules, and syringes. ***Indications*** •Respiratory and neurologic depression due to narcotic intoxication. ***Precautions*** •May cause narcotic withdrawal. •Effects may not outlast effects of narcotics. •Monitor for later respiratory depression. •Rare anaphylactic reactions have been reported. ***Adult Dosage*** *IV infusion* (1) 0.4 to 2.0 mg every 2 minutes. (2) Use higher doses for complete narcotic reversal. (3) Can administer up to 10 mg over short period (<30 minutes).

Nitroglycerin: *Parenteral* Ampules: 5 mg in 10 mL, 8 mg in 10 mL, 10 mg in 10 mL; Vials: 25 mg in 5 mL, 50 mg in 10 mL, 100 mg in 10 mL; *Sublingual tablets:* 0.3 and 0.4 mg; Aerosol spray: 0.4 mg per dose. ***Indications*** •Chest pain of suspected cardiac origin. •Unstable angina. •Complications of AMI, including congestive heart failure, left ventricular failure. •Hypertensive crisis or urgency with chest pain. ***Precautions*** •With evidence of AMI, limit systolic blood pressure drop to 10% if patient is normotensive, 30% drop if hypertensive, and avoid drop below 90 mm Hg. •Do not mix with other drugs. •Patient should sit or lie down when receiving this medication. •Do not shake aerosol spray because this affects metered dose. ***Adult Dosage*** *IV infusion* (1) Infuse at 10 to 20 μg/min. (2) Route of choice for emergencies. (3) Use appropriate IV sets provided by pharmaceutic companies. (4) Titrate to effect. *Sublingual route* 0.3 to 0.4 mg; repeat every 5 minutes. *Aerosol spray* Spray for 0.5 to 1.0 second at 5-minute intervals.

Norepinephrine: (1) 1 mg/mL in 4 mL ampule. (2) Mix 4 mg in 250 mL of D_5W or 5% dextrose in normal saline. (3) Avoid dilution in normal saline alone. ***Indications*** •For severe cardiogenic shock and hemodynamically significant hypotension (systolic blood pressure < 70 mm Hg). •This is an agent of last resort for management of ischemic heart disease and shock. ***Precautions*** •Increases myocardial oxygen requirements because it raises blood pressure and heart rate. •May induce arrhythmias. Use with caution in patients with acute ischemia; monitor cardiac output. •Extravasation causes tissue necrosis. ***Adult Dosage*** *IV infusion* (only route) 0.5 to 1.0 μg/min titrated to improve blood pressure (up to 30 μg/min).

Oxygen: Delivered from portable tanks or installed, wall-mounted sources through delivery devices. ***Indications*** •Any suspected cardiopulmonary emergency, especially (but *not* limited to) complaints of shortness of breath and suspected ischemic chest pain. •NOTE: Pulse oximetry provides a useful method to "dose" oxygen; aim to keep oxygen saturation level above 96%. ***Precautions*** •Observe closely when using with pulmonary patients known to be dependent on hypoxic respiratory drive (very rare situation). •Pulse oximetry inaccurate in low cardiac output states or with vasoconstriction. ***Adult Dosage***

DEVICE	FLOW RATE	O$_2$ (%)
Nasal prongs	1-6 L/min	24-44
Venturi mask	4-8 L/min	24-40
Partial rebreather mask	6-10 L/min	35-60
Bag-valve mask	15 L/min	up to 100

Continued

BOX 5-1   Advanced Life Support Drugs and Electrical Therapy (Adult)—cont'd

Procainamide: 100 mg/mL in 10 mL vial (total = 1 g); 500 mg/mL in 2 mL vial (total = 1 g). ***Indications*** •Recurrent VT not controlled by lidocaine. •Refractory PSVT. •Refractory VF/pulseless VT. •Stable wide-complex tachycardia of unknown origin. •Atrial fibrillation with rapid rate in Wolff-Parkinson-White syndrome. ***Precautions*** •If cardiac or renal dysfunction is present, reduce maximum total dose to 12 mg/kg and maintenance infusion to 1 to 2 mg/min. •Proarrhythmic, especially in setting of AMI, hypokalemia, or hypomagnesemia. ***Adult Dosage*** *Cardiac arrest* (1) 30 mg/min IV infusion (maximum total dose, 17 mg/kg). (2) In refractory VF/VT, 100 mg IV push doses given every 5 minutes are acceptable. *Other indications* 20 to 30 mg/min IV infusion until one of the following occurs: (a) Arrhythmia suppression (b) Hypotension (c) QRS widens by more than 50% (d) Total dose of 17 mg/kg is given. *Maintenance infusion* 1 to 4 mg/min.

Sodium bicarbonate: 50 mL preloaded syringe (8.4% sodium bicarbonate provides 50 mEq/50mL). ***Indications*** Specific indications for bicarbonate use are as follows: •Class I if known preexisting hyperkalemia. •Class II if known preexisting bicarbonate-responsive acidosis (e.g., diabetic ketoacidosis); tricyclic antidepressant overdose; to alkalinize the urine in aspirin or other overdose. •Class IIb if prolonged resuscitation with effective ventilation; upon return of spontaneous circulation after long arrest interval. •Class III (not useful or effective) in hypoxic lactic acidosis or hypercarbic acidosis (e.g., cardiac arrest and CPR without intubation). ***Precautions*** •Adequate ventilation and CPR, not bicarbonate, are the major "buffer agents" in cardiac arrest. •Not recommended for routine use in cardiac arrest patients. ***Adult Dosage*** *IV infusion* (1) 1 mEq/kg IV bolus. (2) Repeat half this dose every 10 minutes thereafter. (3) If rapidly available, use arterial blood gas analysis to guide bicarbonate therapy (calculated base deficits or bicarbonate concentration). *Blood Gas Interpretation Rules* (1) Rule 1: An acute change in $Paco_2$ of 1 mm Hg is associated with an increase or decrease in pH of 0.008 U (relative to normal $Paco_2$ of 40 mm Hg and normal pH of 7.4). (2) Rule 2: A pH change of 0.01 U is the result of a base change of 0.67 mEq/L. (3) Rule 3: The total body bicarbonate deficit equals the base deficit (mEq/L) times the patient's weight (in kg) times 0.3. Complete buffer correction is seldom indicated. Use one fourth to one half the calculated dose.

Sodium nitroprusside: 10 mg/mL in 5 mL vial (total = 50 mg); mix 50 or 100 mg in 250 mL D_5W only. ***Indications*** •Hypertensive crisis. •To reduce afterload in heart failure and acute pulmonary edema. •To reduce afterload in acute mitral or aortic valve regurgitation. ***Precautions*** •Light sensitive; therefore, wrap drug reservoir in aluminum foil. •May cause hypotension, thiocyanate toxicity, and CO_2 retention. •Other side effects include headaches, nausea, vomiting, and abdominal cramps. ***Adult Dosage*** *IV infusion* (1) Begin at 0.10 μg/kg per minute and titrate upward every 3 to 5 minutes to desired effect (up to 5.0 μg/kg per minute). (2) Use with an infusion pump; use hemodynamic monitoring for optimal safety. (3) Action occurs within 1 to 2 minutes. (4) Cover drug reservoir and tubing with opaque material.

Thrombolytic agents: *Alteplase,* recombinant (Activase), tissue plasminogen activator (TPA). 50 and 100 mg vials reconstituted with sterile water to 1 mg/mL; for all four agents, use two peripheral IV lines, *one line exclusively for thrombolytic administration; Anistreplase* (Eminase); anisoylated plasminogen streptokinase activator complex (APSAC)—reconstitute 30 units in 50 mL sterile water or D_5W; *Reteplase,* recombinant (Retavase) 10-unit vials reconstituted with sterile water to 1 Ug/mL; *Streptokinase* (Streptase)-reconstitute to 1 mg/mL. ***Indications*** *For AMI in Adults* •ST elevation (1 mm or more in at least two contiguous leads) or new or presumably new BBB; strongly suspicious for injury. •In context of signs and symptoms of AMI. •Time from onset of symptoms <12 hours. *For Acute Ischemic Stroke (Alteplase is the only thrombolytic agent approved for acute ischemic stroke.)* •Sudden onset of focal neurologic deficits or alterations in consciousness (e.g., language abnormality, motor arm, facial droop). •Absence of intracerebral or subarachnoid hemorrhage or mass effect on CT scan. •Absence of variable or rapidly improving neurologic deficits. •Alteplase can be started in <3 hours from symptom onset. ***Precau-***

BOX 5-1   Advanced Life Support Drugs and Electrical Therapy (Adult)—cont'd

tions *Specific exclusion criteria* •Active internal bleeding (except menses) within 21 days. •History of cerebrovascular, intracranial, or intraspinal event within 3 months (stroke, arteriovenous malformation, neoplasm, aneurysm, recent trauma, recent surgery). •Major surgery or serious trauma within 14 days. •Aortic dissection. •Severe, uncontrolled hypertension. •Known bleeding disorders. •Prolonged CPR with evidence of thoracic trauma. •Lumbar puncture within 7 days. •Recent arterial puncture at noncompressible site. •During the first 24 hours of thrombolytic therapy for ischemic stroke, do not administer aspirin or heparin. *Adjuvant Therapy for AMI* •160 to 325 mg aspirin chewed as soon as possible. •Begin heparin immediately and continue for 48 hours if alteplase or retavase is used. ***Adult Dosage*** *Alteplase, recombinant (TPA),* recommended total dose is based on patient's weight. For AMI the total dose should not exceed 100 mg; for acute ischemic stroke the total dose should not exceed 90 mg. Note that there are two approved dose regimens for AMI patients, and a *different* regimen for acute ischemic stroke. *For AMI* (1) Accelerated infusion (1.5 hours) (a) Give 15 mg IV bolus. (b) Then 0.75 mg/kg over next 30 minutes (do not exceed 50 mg). (c) then 0.50 mg/kg over next 60 minutes (do not exceed 35 mg). (2) 3-hour infusion (a) give 60 mg in first hour (initial 6 to 10 mg is given as a bolus). (b) then 20 mg/hour for 2 additional hours. *For Acute Ischemic Stroke* (1) give 0.9 mg/kg (maximum 90 mg) infused over 60 minutes. (2) give 10% of the total dose as an initial IV bolus over 1 minute. (3) give the remaining 90% over the next 60 minutes. *Anistreplase (APSAC)* 30 IU IV over 2 to 5 minutes. *Reteplase, recombinant* (1) give first 10-unit IV bolus over 2 minutes. (2) 30 minutes later give second 10-unit IV bolus over 2 minutes. (Give NS flush before and after each bolus). *Streptokinase* 1.5 million IU in a 1-hour infusion.

Verapamil: 2.5 mg/mL in 2, 4, and 5 mL vials (totals = 5, 10, and 12.5 mg) ***Indications*** •Drug of second choice (after adenosine) to terminate PSVT with narrow QRS complex and adequate blood pressure. ***Precautions*** •Do not use calcium channel blockers for wide-QRS tachycardias of uncertain origin. •Avoid calcium channel blockers in patients with Wolff-Parkinson-White syndrome and atrial fibrillation, sick sinus syndrome, or second- or third-degree AV block without pacemaker. •Expect blood pressure drop caused by peripheral vasodilation. IV calcium can restore blood pressure, and some experts recommend prophylactic calcium administration before giving calcium channel blockers. •Concurrent IV administration with IV β-blockers may produce severe hypotension. •Use with extreme caution for patients receiving oral β-blockers. ***Adult Dosage*** *IV infusion* (1) 2.5 to 5.0 mg IV bolus over 1 to 2 minutes. (2) Second dose: 50 to 10 mg, if needed, in 15 to 30 minutes. Maximum dose, 30 mg. (3) Alternative: 5 mg bolus every 15 minutes to total dose of 30 mg. (4) Older patients: Administer over 3 minutes.

Transcutaneous Pacing: External pacemakers have either *fixed* rates (nondemand or asynchronous mode) or *demand* rates (range: 30 to 180 beats/min). Current outputs range from 0 to 200 mA. ***Indications*** •Class I for hemodynamically unstable bradycardia (e.g., blood pressure changes, altered mental status, angina, pulmonary edema). •Class I for pacing readiness in setting of AMI, as follows: (a) Symptomatic sinus node dysfunction. (b) Type II second-degree heart block. (c) Third-degree heart block. (d) New left, right, or alternating bundle branch block or bifascicular block. •Class IIa for bradycardia with escape rhythms. •Class IIa for overdrive pacing of tachycardias refractory to drug therapy or electrical cardioversion. •Class IIb for bradyasystolic cardiac arrest. Not routinely recommended. If used, use early. ***Precautions*** •Contraindicated in severe hypothermia or prolonged bradyasystolic cardiac arrest. •Conscious patients may require analgesia for discomfort. •Avoid using carotid pulse to confirm mechanical capture. Electrical stimulation causes muscular jerking that may mimic carotid pulse. ***Adult Dosage*** *Technique* (1) Place pacing electrodes on chest per package instructions. (2) Turn the pacer *on*. (3) Set demand rate to approximately 80 beats/min. (4) Set current (mA) output as follows: (a) *Bradycardia:* increase milliamperes from minimum setting until capture is achieved (characterized by a widening QRS and a broad T wave after each pacer spike). (b) *Asystole:* Begin at full output (mA) and decrease if capture is achieved.

TABLE 5-2 Drugs Used in Pediatric Advanced Life Support

DRUGS	DOSAGE (PEDIATRIC)	REMARKS
Adenosine	0.1-0.2 mg/kg	Rapid IV bolus
Atropine sulfate	0.02 mg/kg	Minimum dose: 0.1 mg Maximum single dose: 0.5 mg in child. 1.0 mg in adolescent
Bretylium	5 mg/kg; may be increased to 10 mg/kg	Rapid IV
Dopamine hydrochloride	2-20 μg/kg per min	α-Adrenergic action dominates at ≥15-20 μg/kg per min
Dobutamine hydrochloride	2-20 μg/kg per min	Titrate to desired effect.
Epinephrine for bradycardia	IV/IO: 0.01 mg/kg (1:10,000, 0.1 ml/kg) ET: 0.1 mg/kg (1:1000, 0.1 ml/kg)	Be aware of total dose of preservative administered (if preservatives are present in epinephrine presentation) when high doses are used.
Epinephrine for asystolic or pulseless arrest	*First dose:* IV/IO: 0.01 mg/kg (1:10,000, 0.1 ml/kg ET: 0.1 mg/kg (1:1000, 0.1 ml/kg IV/IO doses as high as 0.2 mg/kg of 1:1000 may be effective. *Subsequent doses:* IV/IO/ET: 0.1 mg/kg (1:1000, 0.1 ml/kg) • Repeat every 3-5 min. IV/IO doses as high as 0.2 mg/kg of 1:1000 may be effective.	Be aware of total dose of preservative administered (if preservatives are present in epinephrine preparation) when high doses are used.
Epinephrine infusion	Initial at 0.1 μg/kg per min Higher infusion dose used if asystole present	Titrate to desired effect (0.1-1.0 μg/kg per min).
Lidocaine	1 mg/kg	Rapid IV push
Lidocaine infusion	20-50 μg/kg per min	
Sodium bicarbonate	1 mEq/kg per dose	Infuse slowly and only if ventilation is adequate.

(Modified from American Heart Association: *1997-99 Handbook of emergency cardiovascular care for healthcare providers,* Dallas, 1999, American Heart Association.)

Therapeutic interventions in the algorithms are classified as follows:

CLASS	THERAPEUTIC INTERVENTION
I	Usually indicated and always acceptable; considered safe and effective.
IIa	Available evidence suggests it is probably useful and effective.
IIb	May be helpful and is probably not harmful, but not well established by evidence.
III	Inappropriate without supporting data, and possibly harmful.

Within the flow diagrams themselves are the Class I recommendations. The footnotes in these algorithms present Class IIa, IIb, and III recommendations. Box 5-1 and Table 5-2 show adult and pediatric medications recommended for use when delivering advanced life support.

REFERENCES

1. American Heart Association: *Advanced cardiac life support,* Dallas, 1997, American Heart Association.
2. Benumof JL: Management of the difficult adult airway, *Anesthesiology* 75:1087, 1991.
3. Craney J et al: *What is the relationship between ventricular tachycardia rate and hemodynamic compromise?* Presented at the American Association of Critical Care Nurses National Critical Care Nursing Research Conference, May 12, 1991, Boston, Mass.
4. Grauer K, Cavallaro D: *ACLS certification preparation,* St Louis, 1993, Mosby Lifeline.
5. American Heart Association: Guidelines for cardiopulmonary resuscitation and emergency cardiac care, *JAMA* 268:2171, 1992.

SUGGESTED READINGS

ACC, AHA: Task force report: guidelines for the early management of patients with acute myocardial infarction, *J Am Coll Cardiol* 16: 249, 1990.

Aehlert B: *ACLS quick review study guide,* St Louis, 1994, Mosby.

Lezon K: Code blue: defibrillate, *Nurs 98* 28(4): 58-60, 1998.

Martin DR: Initial countershock in the treatment of asystole, *Resuscitation* 26: 62, 1993.

Neumar RW, Ward KR: Cardiopulmonary arrest. In Rosen P, Barkin R, editors: Emergency Medicine, St Louis, 1998, Mosby.

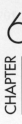

CHAPTER 6

Intravenous Therapy

Jessie M. Moore

INTRAVENOUS LINES

An intravenous (IV) line is initiated so that fluids, medications, blood, and blood products can be placed into the vascular circulation. To initiate an IV line, one should have general familiarity with the vasculature of the access site. When determining where to start the line, consider the urgency of the situation—urgency may take priority over the best long-term site location. In the emergency situation, where IV access is critical, the IV is often started in the most accessible site.

TYPES OF INTRAVENOUS SOLUTIONS

Dextrose Intravenous Solutions

Available in various concentrations, and in combination with other solutions; is the main way of providing calories in fluid administration. Dextrose 5% in water (D5%W) contains 5 grams of glucose per 100 ml, and is considered an isotonic solution. Dextrose 10% and greater are hypertonic solutions. The 5% and 10% solutions may be given peripherally; higher than 10% concentrations are given through central veins, with the exception of Dextrose 50%, given slowly through peripheral veins.[1]

■ **USES**
Keep open (TKO) IV lines, nonelectrolyte hydration, calorie replacement.

■ **PRECAUTIONS**
Should not be used in the same IV line with blood, as it causes damage to red blood cells. May affect the stability of admixtures (ampicillin, phenytoin); check compatibility. May increase intracranial pressure in head injuries.[2]

Sodium Containing Intravenous Solutions

Available in hypotonic solution (0.45% NS, containing 77 mEq each of sodium and chloride), isotonic solutions (0.9% NS, containing 154 mEq each of sodium and chloride), and in hypertonic solutions (greater than 0.9% NS).

■ **USES**
Restoration of water and salt loss in hypovolemic shock and dehydration, administration with blood products, medication administration, and in metabolic alkalosis.

■ **PRECAUTIONS**
Use caution in any condition involving sodium retention. Large infusions can lead to hypokalemia, acidosis, circulatory overload, or hypernatremia.

Multiple Electrolyte Solutions

Ringer's Injection: An isotonic solution containing sodium, potassium, calcium, and chloride in approximate plasma concentrations.

Lactated Ringer's: Isotonic solution as above, with lactate added as a buffer.

■ **USES**

Replacement of extracellular fluid losses, volume expansion in severe shock and cardiac arrest.

■ **PRECAUTIONS**

Excess quantities may cause overhydration, electrolyte excess (particularly sodium), and metabolic alkalosis (Lactated Ringer's). Use caution in patients with cardiac or renal disorders. Lactated Ringer's is contraindicated in patients with hepatic disorders.

Alkalizing Solutions

■ **SODIUM BICARBONATE**

Solutions containing 5 to 10% sodium bicarbonate may be used to treat metabolic acidosis, severe hyperkalemia, and to alkalinize urine and enhance excretion of acid toxins (i.e., salicylate, lithium).[1,3]

■ **PRECAUTIONS**

Extravasation may cause tissue necrosis and/or sloughing. Excess administration may cause metabolic acidosis, hypokalemia, and hypocalcemia.

DELIVERY SYSTEMS

Glass vs. Plastic Containers

Plastic bags are the modern standard for IV solutions, with the exception of solutions that are incompatible with some properties of plastics (fat emulsions, insulin, nitroglycerin, lorazepam).[1] Glass bottles must be vented for air to replace the fluid in the bottle and allow free flow of the solution. Use of vented IV administration sets is the most common method used.

Plastic bags do not require venting and adapt easily to rapid infusion devices such as pressure infusion sleeves. Bags are susceptible to puncture when opening or adding admixtures, and should be discarded if any leakage is detected.

Intravenous Administration Sets

Primary administration set: main tubing carrying fluid to the IV site; can be gravity tubing, infusion pump tubing or microbore syringe pump tubing.

Secondary administration set: used to administer medication of additional fluid; may be intermittent or continuous. Should have built-in safety device; that is, recessed needle in rigid cap, or blunt plastic cannula device, to reduce risk of accidental disconnection and needle injury.

Metered volume chamber set: Small volume chamber between the solutions container and an administration set. Allows more accurate control of volume infused, commonly used in pediatric and neonatal patient therapy.

Primary Y tubing and blood administration sets: used for infusion of blood products, have larger internal tubing diameter, larger drop factor than standard tubing, and screen filters for removal of byproducts of stored blood.

Nitroglycerin administration set: some studies have indicated that nitroglycerin adheres to PVC tubing to varying degrees. These sets are made with non PVC material, causing minimal loss of the drug during administration. They are, however, more expensive, and because nitroglycerin administration is titrated to clinical effect, many clinicians elect to use standard sets. Tubing changes will cause potential fluctuations in actual drug delivery until the saturation point of the tubing is reached.

Infusion pump sets: device specific; may or may not require special tubing to infuse correctly; follow manufacturer's instructions. *Always* use roller clamp devices when pumps are not operational to prevent accidental infusion of the fluid.

Flow Control Devices

Back check valves: prevent retrograde flow of solutions to the primary fluid container.

Flash balls: latex rubber cone located at the patient connection of a primary infusion set. Formerly a common feature on administration sets, most have been replaced with a resealable latex port. Flash balls should never be used to improve blood flow or restore patency because microemboli may be dislodged.[1]

Patient-controlled anesthesia (PCA) pumps: can deliver continuous or on-demand doses of analgesic; generally have a lock-out feature on rate control to prevent tampering.

Heparin or saline locks: peripheral IV cannulas without tubing attached. The distal end of the cannula is plugged. The purpose of this lock is to have ready access to a vein should the need arise or to have brief access to a vein should an intravenous medication be given. The cannula should be filled with a heparinized saline or normal saline solution (per institution policy), so that it will not clot while it is not in use.

Drop factors

The drop factor is the number of drops delivered by a given tubing that equal 1 ml. It is essential to rate adjustment calculations. There are two common distinctive types.

Macrodrip   Regular size, commonly 10, 12, 15, or 20 drops/ml; must be used for rapid fluid administration.
Microdrip   Most commonly 60 drops/ml; used for pediatric fluid administration, medication drips, and in volume restricted patients.

Flow rate determination

IV rates are commonly ordered in ml/hr. The following formula helps to determine the drops/min.

$$\frac{\text{Drop factor (drops/ml)}}{\text{minutes/hour(60)}} \times \text{ml/hr (ordered)} = \text{drops/min}$$

Example: An IV is ordered to infuse at 150 ml/hr using a macrodrip tubing with a drop factor of 15 drops/ml.

$$\frac{15 \text{ drops/ml}}{60 \text{ min/hr.}} \times 150 \text{ ml/hr} = \text{desired drops/min}$$

Answer: 37.5 or 38 drops/min (when determining drops per minute, always round to a whole number).

INTRAVENOUS CATHETERS AND CANNULAS

Peripheral Intravenous Devices

Winged needles: also known as a scalp vein or "butterfly"; a stainless steel needle with two winglike plastic projections mounted where the needle meets the catheter to facilitate placement and anchoring. Recommended for 1 to 4 hours of use.

Over-the-needle catheter: a tapered catheter fitted over the needle; the needle is used to puncture the skin and vein, the catheter is advanced over the needle, and the needle is removed from the patient. Some versions have winged protrusions to improve handling and securing of the devices.

Through-the-needle catheter: steel or plastic needle makes the venipuncture, then the softer plastic catheter is advanced through the needle. Previously, the needle remained on the device, secured by an outer plastic clip; newer versions use splittable needles, which are removed and leave only the softer catheter attached to the patient.

Plain plastic catheter: used when cutdown intravenous lines are placed; threaded into vein through an open sterile procedure.

Dual lumen peripheral catheter: has two totally separate infusion channels, allowing infusion of solutions not compatible through the same site. The total lumen size of the catheter is larger and necessitates a larger vessel site choice.

Catheter Size and Length

Recommendations for cannula size selection:[1]

SIZE	CLINICAL APPLICATION
14-18 g	Trauma, surgery, blood
20 g	Continuous or intermittent infusion, blood
22 g	Intermittent or general infusion, children, and elderly
24 g	Fragile veins for intermittent or general infusions

Length of plastic catheter commonly ranges from ⅝ to 2 inches, but may be up to 12 inches. Catheters that are threaded 3 to 10 inches are considered midarm or midline catheters. Peripherally inserted central catheters (PICC) are inserted peripherally, but terminate in the superior vena cava and are considered central lines.

Fluid administration rate is limited by the diameter and length of tubing and catheter; the rule of thumb for rapid volume infusion is a large-bore (16 gauge or greater), short catheter (1¼ inch commonly used).

Color coding of catheter hubs is not universal in the medical device industry, therefore it is essential that all IV sites be labeled with the size of catheter placed. Most catheters are made of variations of plastic; new material features include reduced thrombogenesis, minimized vein trauma, and reduced complications. Some materials expand and increase in size once in the vessel.[1]

Central Venous Catheters

Nontunneled catheters or PICC lines (peripherally inserted central catheters): inserted by specially trained nurses; tip lies in superior vena cava, used for several weeks to months.

Percutaneously inserted devices: central lines inserted by direct skin puncture; then the subclavian or internal jugular vessel is cannulated with a central venous catheter; can be single or multiple lumen.

Tunneled catheters: silicone cuffed catheters placed surgically in central vessels and tunneled under the skin to an exit point located to facilitate self-care and maintenance. Examples include Hickman, Broviac, RAAF, and Groshong catheters; may be single or multiple lumen.

Implanted ports: single- or double-lumen device placed surgically under the skin with the terminal in the central vena cava. Implantable ports are easily palpable under the skin, with a dense latex or silicone septum overlying a reservoir. The septum can withstand 1000 to 2000 needle sticks. A noncoring needle, called a Huber needle, must be used to access the device. This needle deflects the entry through the septum, rather than coring it (Figures 6-1 and 6-2).

Alternative Access Devices

Dialysis access devices
Dialysis access sites have traditionally not been used for routine intravenous therapy needs. However, new silicone type dialysis type catheters are now being used for intermittent therapy in some practice settings. Dialysis shunts should be accessed only by trained personnel.

Intraosseous needle
Steel needle inserted into the bone, can carry both fluid and medication directly into the vascular system. Can be used in adults, more commonly used in children. Size: 18 g. recommended for children, 15-16 g. needle for adults.

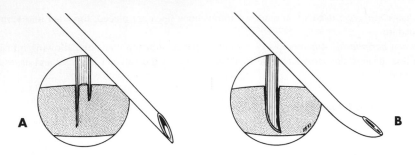

FIGURE 6-1. Huber tipped needle. **A,** Hypodermic needle. **B,** Noncoring needle.
(From Bard Access Systems, Salt Lake City, Utah.)

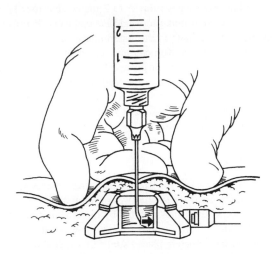

FIGURE 6-2. Cross section of an implanted port.
(From Bard Access Systems, Salt Lake City, Utah.)

INSERTION PROCEDURES

Peripheral Site Selection

The choice of an IV site depends on:
Purpose of the IV line and length of time the IV will be in place
Clinical condition of the patient
Age and size of the patient
Condition of the vein

General Principles

Avoid use of an extremity with arteriovenous fistula or graft, an affected extremity of a stroke patient, or an affected arm of a postmastectomy patient. Access of these sites in emergency situations is sometimes necessary; follow institution policy and monitor the site more closely for swelling if use is required.

Avoid use of lower extremities because of the increased risk of thrombophlebitis. Exception: children under walking age.

The most distal site on the extremity should be selected. If reinsertion of a previous IV is indicated, the new site should be proximal to the discontinued site.

Recommended veins on the adult patient are the metacarpal (dorsal hand), cephalic (radial aspect of the forearm), basilic (ulnar aspect of the arm), and median (ulnar aspect and antecubital fossa). The antecubital fossa veins are at greater risk for mechanical phlebitis and infection, and should not be the preferred site except in extreme emergency situations.[1]

The external jugular vein is often overlooked. It is large and easy to cannulate, and can accommodate a very large-bore catheter. It should be considered as an IV site in cardiopulmonary arrest and multiple trauma, especially when large volume fluid resuscitation is required.

Site Preparation

1. Apply a tourniquet 4 to 6 inches above the proposed site on an extremity.
2. Keep the tourniquet in place for no more than 5 minutes or just until the vein dilates. If the vein does not dilate enough for cannulation, rub the vein or tap lightly; hold the limb in a dependent position; apply heat with a hot pack or warm towel, or have the patient open and close the fist.
3. The recommended cleansing procedure is to apply 70% isopropyl alcohol for a minimum of 30 seconds, allow to air dry, and apply a povidine iodine (betadine) or chlorhexidrine gluconate (Hibiclens) to the site. All site preps should be applied with friction, working outward from the insertion site.[1]
4. The routine use of 1% lidocaine before catheter insertion is NOT recommended.[1]

Peripheral Venipuncture Technique

1. Always use standard precautions for body fluids when initiating intravenous lines.
2. Stabilize the vein by applying traction to the side of the insertion site.
3. The depth of the vein in the subcutaneous tissue will determine the angle used to enter the skin (10 degree to 30 degree angle).
4. Puncture the skin and the vein with the bevel of the needle facing upward.
5. Advance the needle slowly.
6. Check for a blood return ("flashback"), advance the catheter $\frac{1}{16}$ inch, pull the stylet back slightly, and advance the catheter into the vein.
7. Remove the tourniquet.
8. Remove the stylet and connect the IV administration set and begin flow.
9. If difficulty occurs in threading the catheter, initiating the flow of IV fluid may help "float" the catheter into the vein.
10. Do *not* reinsert the stylet into the catheter; catheter fragmentation and embolism can occur!
11. Place a small dab of antimicrobial ointment at the puncture site (per institution policy).
12. Secure the hub of the cannula to prevent movement of the catheter.
13. Site dressings of gauze or transparent semipermeable membranes may be use to cover and protect the insertion site (per institutional policy).
14. Make a loop with the IV tubing and secure it.
15. Label the IV site (type, gauge, time, date, and initials).
16. All sharps should be safely disposed of using proper safety techniques.

INTRAVENOUS THERAPY IN PEDIATRIC PATIENTS

Site Considerations

The IV sites of choice in an infant or small child are the dorsum of the hand, the dorsum of the foot, and the scalp (in an infant). In the newborn, the umbilical vein should not be overlooked. Be sure to anchor an IV extra securely in an infant or small child because movement may dislodge it.

Tips for Intravenous Insertion in Pediatric Patients[1,4]

1. Rubber bands or ⅜ inch penrose drains may be used as tourniquets.
2. Position the young child in a passive restraint such as a papoose board before beginning the procedure.
3. A flashlight placed beneath the extremity helps illuminate tissue surrounding the vein and outlines the targeted vein.
4. Insert the needle with bevel *down,* to prevent puncture of the back wall.
5. Spasms can occur in small veins; stop advancing the catheter and place a warm compress over the vein. Resume advancing the catheter when the spasm stops.
6. Use a syringe with normal saline to "float" the catheter into the vein once the stylet is removed. This prevents clotting in the catheter and also confirms correct placement even when a significant blood return was not detected.
7. Padded tongue blades can function as arm boards for hand sites; these may be placed prior to insertion if desired.

INTRAVENOUS THERAPY IN OLDER ADULT PATIENTS

Site selection

Dorsal hand sites are less desirable; loss of subcutaneous fat and thinning of the skin can lead to mechanical inflammation and infiltration.

Tips for intravenous insertion in older adult patients[1,4]

1. Side lighting is more effective in visualizing vein shadows below the skin. Bright overhead light may cause a "washout" effect on visualization of the vein.
2. Tourniquet use: if the vein is visible and already distended, do not use the tourniquet, as excessive distension of the vein may cause vein damage or rupture on insertion. If veins are not distended, allow a few moments longer after placing the tourniquet, as venous return is slower in the elderly patient.
3. Avoid using sclerosed, hard veins, as the wall of the vessel may be thickened, leaving a narrow or occluded lumen.
4. Avoid valves, or decrease the gauge size to thread the catheter through the valve.
5. Veins tend to roll because of decreased subcutaneous tissue mass. To immobilize, find the vessel's axis, place the thumb directly along the axis, 2 to 3 inches below the intended site, and the index finger above the insertion site.
6. Use of subcutaneous lidocaine before IV insertion may cause subcutaneous tissue swelling and other complications in the elderly person.
7. Light tapping may enhance vein dilation; slapping may cause vessel rupture.
8. In fragile veins, preflush the catheter with normal saline before attempting access; the preflushed catheter will show blood return more quickly.
9. Maintain stabilization of the skin while using the one-handed technique to advance the catheter.
10. To float the catheter into tortuous veins: release the tourniquet, remove the stylet, connect the IV and slowly infuse the fluid while gently advancing the catheter.

PATIENT EDUCATION

Inform the patient and family of the rationale for therapy.

Explain any special requirements related to positioning, intake and output measurement, and potential adverse reactions.

Complications

Hematoma
Infiltration
Phlebitis
   bacterial, mechanical, or chemical
Thrombosis
Catheter fragmentation and embolism
Extravasation
Cellulitis
Fluid overload
Sepsis

Preventive Measures

Avoid areas of flexion for IV sites.

Use strict aseptic techniques.

Use the smallest gauge catheter that is appropriate.

Use large veins to provide greater hemodilution when administering irritating medications.

Securely tape catheters to prevent excessive movement at the site entry.

Avoid the use of lower extremities.

Inspect catheters for defects before use.

Never reinsert a stylet into an over-the-needle catheter.

Assess the patient's circulatory and pulmonary status before and during intravenous therapy.

VENOUS CUTDOWN

A venous cutdown is a minor surgical procedure that is used if a peripheral IV site cannot be located or if a large volume of fluid is to be administered over a short period of time. A cutdown is usually done on the basilic vein (just above the elbow) or the saphenous vein (above the ankle). The saphenous vein is usually chosen when a cutdown is performed on a child (Figure 6-3).

■ **EQUIPMENT**

Surgical gloves
Surgical mask
Scalpel handle and blades (11- or 15-gauge)
Vascular scissors
Suture scissors
Lidocaine (1% or 2%)
Suture material
Forceps
4 × 4-inch gauze squares
Sterile towels
Catheter (may use infant-feeding tube or IV connecting tubing)
Antiseptic solution
Hemostats

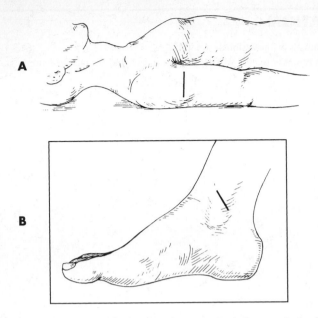

FIGURE 6-3. Common sites of venous cutdown. **A,** Cephalic vein. **B,** Saphenous vein.

Syringe and needle (25-gauge)
Antibiotic ointment
IV setup
Tape
Small vein retractor

■ **PROCEDURE (USUALLY PERFORMED BY A PHYSICIAN)** (Figure 6-4)
  1. Prepare the extremity with antiseptic solution.
  2. Drape the limb.
  3. Apply a local anesthetic.
  4. Make a transverse incision.
  5. Dissect the tissue down to the vein.
  6. Lift the vein.
  7. Nick the vein with a scalpel.
  8. Insert the cannula.
  9. Secure the cannula with a suture.
 10. Suture the wound around the cannula.
 11. Apply antibiotic ointment.
 12. Tape the cannula in place.
 13. Label the IV site (gauge and type of cannula, date, time, caregiver's initials).

CENTRAL VEIN CANNULATION

Catheterization of the subclavian vein (Figure 6-5) is used to provide volume and to enable measurement of the central venous pressure. Catheterization of the internal jugular vein is used to provide large volumes over a short period of time. It should be remembered that catheterizing these sites carries a risk of pneumothorax. They should only be used in urgent situations.

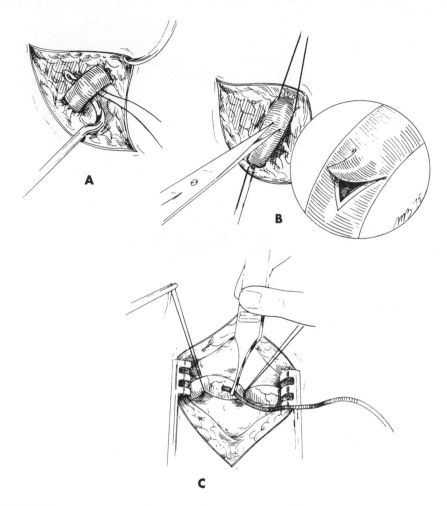

FIGURE 6-4. Venous cutdown. **A,** Isolating the vein. **B,** Cutting the vein. **C,** Inserting the cannula.

Subclavian Vein

This vein is located in the neck between the median and middle thirds of the clavicle and the sternal notch.

1. Place the patient in Trendelenburg's position to increase the size of the vein and decrease the possibility of air embolism.
2. Place a rolled towel between the patient's shoulder blades to provide a better angle.
3. Prepare the neck and upper chest with an antiseptic solution.
4. Anesthetize the area with 1% lidocaine at the inferior edge of the clavicle where the medial and middle thirds join.
5. Insert a 14-gauge or larger cannula (with a syringe on the end to avoid air embolism), aiming toward the suprasternal notch and keeping the cannula just under the clavicle.
6. Aspirate as the needle is advancing; if nonpulsating blood is drawn, the vein has been cannulated.
7. Advance the catheter through the needle; do not pull back on the catheter because it may be sheared off.
8. When the catheter is in place, withdraw the needle.

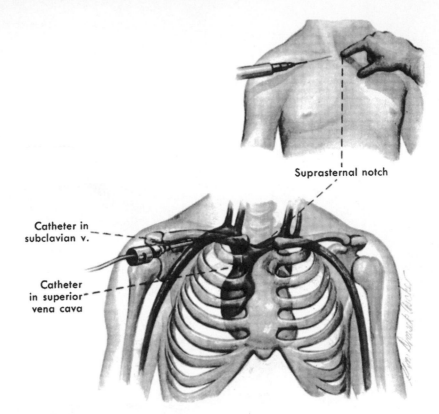

FIGURE 6-5. Technique of percutaneous intraclavicular subclavian catheterization. Needle, inserted under midclavicle and aimed in three dimensions at top of posterior aspect of sternal manubrium (indicated by fingertip in suprasternal notch), lies in a plane parallel with frontal plane of patient and will enter anterior wall of subclavian vein.
(From *Needle and cannula techniques,* Chicago, 1971, Abbott Laboratories.)

9. Clip on the catheter guard so that the needle will not shear off the catheter.
10. Suture the catheter and guard in place.
11. Apply antibiotic ointment to the puncture site.
12. Apply a dry sterile dressing.
13. Apply a waterproof dressing.
14. Label the cannulation site.

Internal Jugular Vein

1. Place the patient in Trendelenburg's position to increase the size of the vein and decrease the possibility of air embolism.
2. Place a rolled towel between the shoulder blades to provide a better angle.
3. Prepare the neck and upper chest with an antiseptic solution.
4. Drape the neck and upper chest area.
5. Anesthetize the area with 1% lidocaine at the junction of the middle and lower thirds of the anterior border of the sternocleidomastoid muscle.
6. Insert a 14-gauge or larger cannula (with a syringe on the end to avoid air embolism) close behind the sternocleidomastoid muscle, aiming toward the space formed by the clavicular and sternal heads.
7. Aspirate as the needle is advancing; if nonpulsating blood is drawn, the vein has been cannulated.

8. Advance the catheter through the needle; do not pull back on the catheter because it may be sheared off.
9. When the catheter is in place, withdraw the needle carefully.
10. Clip the catheter guard so that the needle will not shear the catheter.
11. Suture the catheter and guard in place.
12. Apply antibiotic ointment to the puncture site.
13. Apply a dry sterile dressing.
14. Apply a waterproof dressing.
15. Label the cannulation site.

CENTRAL VENOUS PRESSURE

The central venous pressure (CVP) is a measurement of the right-sided pressures of the heart, blood volume, effectiveness of the heart as a pump, and vascular tone.

■ **PROCEDURE USING A SUBCLAVIAN INTRAVENOUS LINE**
1. Place the patient in a supine (flat) position.
2. Measure at the midaxillary line (5 cm from the top of the chest) in the fourth intercostal space at the level of the right atrium.
3. Place the manometer zero-reading at this point.
4. Fill the manometer from the attached IV solution (do not let it overflow).
5. Turn the stopcock on the IV line open to the patient and the manometer. The fluid level will fall and fluctuate (decreasing on inspiration and increasing on expiration).
6. When the fluid level appears stable, note where the top of the fluid column reaches.
7. Record this reading as the CVP.
8. Adjust the stopcock to close the manometer and open the IV line to the patient (make sure to readjust the IV solution drip rate).

The normal range of CVP is 4 to 10 cm of water pressure. A value greater than 10 cm may indicate tamponade, right heart failure, fluid overload, pulmonary edema, tension pneumothorax, or hemothorax. A value below 4 cm may indicate hypovolemia, vasodilation, dehydration, septic shock, or drug-induced shock.

INTRAOSSEOUS INFUSIONS

An intraosseous infusion is the administration of IV fluids and drugs directly into the bone marrow. It is best performed on children under the age of 2 when they are in:
• Cardiopulmonary arrest
• Hypovolemic shock
• Status epilepticus

It may also be performed in any other condition where the administration of fluid or medication is critical to the child's survival and the establishment of an IV is difficult.

Locate the anterior medial surface of the tibia, 2 cm below the tibial tuberosity (Figure 6-6). Other sites that may be used are the distal anterior femur, the medial malleolus, and the iliac crest.

Prepare the area with Betadine. Using a metal biopsy needle, such as an Illinois Sternal Bone Marrow Needle (Figure 6-7) or a Jamsheedy needle, advance the needle through the skin, fascia, and bony cortex with a back-and-forth boring motion. The needle is angled away from the joint space to avoid the growth plate. It is apparent that the needle is in the bone marrow when there is a popping sensation followed by a sudden absence of resistance, when the needle can stand upright without manual support, and when fluid flows freely through the needle. Aspirate, using a syringe. If bone marrow is returned, the needle has been placed correctly.

Once the needle is in place, tape it and infuse solutions and/or medications.

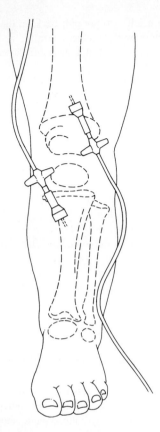

FIGURE 6-6. Recommended sites for an intraosseous infusion.

ACCESSING VENOUS ACCESS DEVICES

Various procedures in accessing VADs are used throughout the country; however, it can be reasonably assumed that the fundamental requirement for successful VAD maintenance is strict adherence to established protocols. Below are basic steps utilized during accessing for blood sampling.

Nontunneled and Tunneled Catheters

1. Good hand washing and aseptic technique are essential in preparing to access the device.
2. Sterile gloves should always be worn.
3. Gather needed equipment before access.
   Laboratory tubes/test requisition
   Heparinized saline (10 U/ml)
   Alcohol wipes
   Two 10-cc syringes, one filled with saline
   18-gauge needles
   Syringes large enough to draw required amount of blood
   Sterile Luer-Lock caps

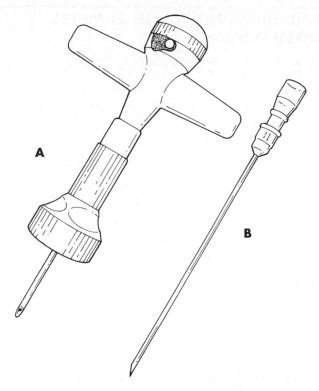

FIGURE 6-7. **A,** A 16-gauge disposable Illinois Sternal Bone Marrow Aspiration Needle. **B,** A 3-inch, 18-gauge B-D spinal needle.
(From ®Becton, Dickinson and Co., Rutherford, NJ.)

4. Prepare sterile barrier/place equipment on barrier.
5. Turn off any infusions/dual or triple lumen; clamp catheters that will not be used for blood sampling.
6. Clamp catheter to be used and remove Luer-Lock cap from catheter hub.
7. Attach 10-cc syringe to hub; withdraw 6 ml of blood for discard/clamp catheter.
8. Attach syringe large enough to accommodate blood needed for samples and withdraw that amount. Remember to draw samples for blood cultures first. Blood needed for clotting studies should not be drawn from heparinized catheters.
9. Clamp catheter, remove collection syringe, inject blood samples into appropriate laboratory tubes.
10. Flush catheter with 10 cc N/S, then reattach to infusion. If dual-lumen or triple-lumen catheter, unclamp other catheters and restart those infusions.
11. If catheter is to be capped, flush with heparinized saline (10 U/ml), wipe hub with alcohol wipe, then cap with sterile Luer-Lock cap and tape for added security.

NOTE: Groshong catheters do *not* require heparin flush.

12. Label blood sample tubes and send to laboratory.

ACCESSING AND DRAWING BLOOD SAMPLES FROM IMPLANTED PORTS

1. Have the patient lie supine or in semi-Fowler's position.
2. Wash hands thoroughly.
3. Palpate site to locate the port and septum; examine the site for signs and symptoms of infection.
4. Cleanse the site with povidone/iodine swabs; start at center and cleanse outward in a circular motion.
5. Make a small wheal above injection site with 1% lidocaine if patient desires.
6. Place needed equipment on sterile barrier.
    10-cc syringe filled with N/S
    18-gauge needle
    90 degree Huber needle
    Sterile gloves
7. Prime Huber needle with N/S.
8. Cannulate the port with the Huber needle; push the needle through the skin and septum until the bottom of the port is felt.
9. Check for correct placement by flushing with remaining saline in syringe; a correctly accessed port will flush easily without pain or swelling (infiltration).
10. Apply antimicrobial ointment to site.
11. Stabilize needle by placing 2 × 2-inch gauze pads under wings of needle and tape.
12. Clamp tubing and remove syringe.
13. Hook up to infusion tubing and tape connections. If no infusion is ordered, cap with sterile Luer-Lock cap after heparin flush.

Blood Sampling from Implanted Port

1. If access is required, follow above procedure.
2. If access has been achieved, gather necessary equipment
    Alcohol wipes
    Two 10-cc syringes, one filled with saline
    One heparinized saline
    Blood collection tubes/requisitions/labels
    Syringe of appropriate size to draw required amount of blood
3. Wear sterile gloves.
4. Stop infusion and clamp the short extension tubing attached to the Huber needle hub.
5. If no infusion, ensure that tubing is clamped and remove Luer-Lock cap.
6. Attach 10-cc syringe, unclamp tubing, withdraw 6 cc of blood.
7. Clamp tubing, disconnect this syringe, and discard it.
8. Attach collection syringe, unclamp tubing, and slowly and steadily withdraw required amount of blood. Do not draw clotting studies from heparinized catheters.
9. Clamp tubing, disconnect syringe.
10. Flush Huber needle with 10 cc N/S and reconnect to infusion.
11. If no infusion, flush with heparinized saline (10 U/ml) then cap with sterile Luer-Lock cap.
12. Inject laboratory specimen tubes with blood, label and send to lab.

COMPLICATIONS INVOLVING VENOUS ACCESS DEVICES

1. **Infection** may occur at exit site, port pocket along catheter tunnel, or as septicemia.
2. **Obstruction:** Withdrawal occlusion—occurs when hospital personnel are unable to withdraw blood samples; fluid can still be infused unless there is intraluminal occlusion of the catheter.
    Intraluminal obstruction—occurs when blood cannot be withdrawn nor can fluids be infused.

- Most commonly caused by clot formation or precipitation of drugs.
- May require gentle instillation of thrombolytic agent (usually urokinase), always ordered by a physician.
3. **Extravasation:** Leakage from a vein or catheter into subcutaneous tissue. Symptoms are pain, swelling, erythema.
   Certain drugs can cause tissue necrosis.
   - Greatest risk is with implantable ports, usually secondary to dislodgment of Huber needle.
4. **Damaged catheters:** Only tunneled catheters can be repaired if damaged in the external portion.

DISCONTINUATION OF INTRAVENOUS THERAPY

Peripheral catheters should be removed immediately if signs of infiltration or phlebitis are observed. Always use standard precautions for body fluid exposure, and remove the catheter smoothly and steadily. Apply pressure to the insertion site with dry sterile gauze until bleeding stops. Note catheter integrity, and document actions and any abnormal findings.

Central Catheter Removal

1. Place patient in a supine position with head of bed flat.
2. Clip and remove any sutures.
3. Instruct the patient to perform a Valsalva maneuver.
4. Remove the catheter with a steady gently pulling motion.
5. Apply pressure to the insertion site with a sterile gauze until the bleeding stops.
6. Apply a sterile occlusive dressing over the insertion site, per institution policy.
7. Visually inspect the catheter.
8. Document actions and any abnormal findings.

Indwelling venous access devices should be removed only by personnel trained in the procedure.

REFERENCES

1. Terry J: *Intravenous therapy: clinical principles and practice,* Philadelphia, 1995, Saunders.
2. Cardona VD et al: *Trauma nursing: from resuscitation through rehabilitation,* ed 2, Philadelphia, 1994, Saunders.
3. Proehl JA et al: *Emergency nursing: a physiologic and clinical perspective,* ed 2, Philadelphia, 1995, Saunders.
4. Weinstein SM: *Plumer's principles and practice of intravenous therapy,* ed 6, Philadelphia, 1997, Lippincott.

Laboratory Specimens

Nancy M. Bonalumi

Collection and analysis of laboratory specimens is an important component of emergency nursing care. The information provided from laboratory results supports the caregiver in developing a diagnosis and treatment plan for the patient.

Proper collection technique impacts the reliability of test results; thus competency in the sampling method is crucial. The information found in this chapter will assist nurses in obtaining specimens correctly and understanding the significance of specific test results.

DRAWING BLOOD FOR BLOOD GAS MEASUREMENT

Selection of Site

Choose the radial, brachial, or femoral artery (Figure 7-1).
Avoid limbs that demonstrate poor circulation.
Avoid limbs where hematomas are present.
If the radial artery is selected, check for the presence of a positive Allen test.

Suggested Equipment

Nonsterile examination gloves
Container of crushed ice (plastic bag or emesis basin is fine)
Rubber or cork stopper or commercial blood gas cap
5-ml glass syringe or specially treated plastic syringe
Two 22-gauge, 1.5-inch needles
Two alcohol swabs
Sodium heparin, 0.5 ml (1000 U/ml)
One small dry gauze pad
Gummed label for syringe
Laboratory requisition slip with the following information: Concentration of oxygen patient is receiving and by what route (Fio_2) and patient's rectal temperature at the time the specimen is collected (both parameters affect calculation of values).

Drawing the Specimen

1. Explain the procedure to the patient.
2. Draw up 0.5 ml heparin into a *glass* or specially treated plastic syringe.
3. Flush the syringe with heparin (expel all air bubbles).
4. Replace the needle.
5. Select the puncture site.

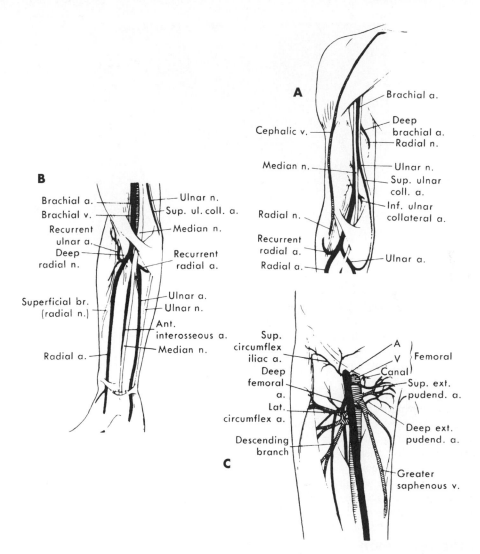

FIGURE 7-1. **A,** Brachial artery, a continuation of axillary artery. *Advantages:* Easy to locate, not much arterial spasm, and easy to immobilize. *Disadvantages:* Radial and medial nerves in close proximity, making venous sampling possible. **B,** Radial artery extends from neck of radius to median side of styloid process. *Advantages:* No close proximity to veins; thus venous sampling is unlikely. *Disadvantages:* Puncture may produce spasm and artery is very small. **C,** Femoral artery branches from abdominal aorta and branches to superficial epigastric, superficial circumflex iliac, external pudendal, deep femoral, and descending genicular arteries. *Advantages:* Easily accessible. *Disadvantages:* May have large amount of interstitial bleeding before it is noticed. Close proximity to vein makes venous sampling possible.
(From Budassi SA: An emergency nurse's guide to drawing arterial blood gases, *JEN* 3(2):24, 1977.)

6. Straighten the limb of the selected puncture site and position it on a firm surface.
7. Apply gloves.
8. Palpate the artery: assess the pulse and position of the artery.
9. Cleanse area over the puncture site with an alcohol swab (be sure to use plenty of friction and allow the alcohol to dry before the actual puncture).
10. Immobilize the artery between two fingers (be careful not to contaminate the puncture site).

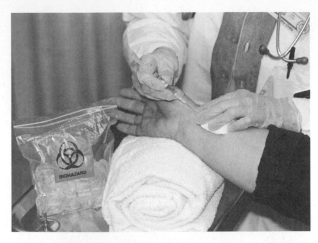

FIGURE 7-2. Puncture of radial artery.
(Courtesy Emilie Goudey, Lenox, Mass.)

11. Penetrate both the skin and the artery at a 45- to 90-degree angle, holding the syringe like a pencil (Figure 7-2).
12. If the syringe begins to fill and the plunger begins to move spontaneously, this is usually an indication that the needle is in the artery.
13. If the syringe does not begin to fill spontaneously, withdraw the needle slightly (it may have gone all the way through the artery).
14. If systolic blood pressure is less than 100 mm Hg, the syringe may not fill spontaneously, and it may be necessary to manually withdraw the plunger (e.g., during CPR).
15. If the blood sample is not bright red or is bluish in color, this may indicate that the specimen is venous—make another attempt at an arterial specimen.
16. Obtain 3 to 5 ml of arterial blood (some laboratories will accept less for analysis).
17. Withdraw the needle quickly.
18. Apply direct pressure with dry gauze.
19. Maintain pressure for 5 minutes (make certain to time it on your watch or the wall clock—it is difficult to estimate 5 minutes).

Care of the Specimen

1. Expel all air bubbles from the sample.
2. Stick the needle into a cork or rubber stopper or remove the needle and cap the syringe.
3. Place the gummed label (containing patient's name and hospital number) on the syringe.
4. Place the syringe into the container of ice.
5. Send the specimen to the laboratory immediately along with the completed laboratory request form. (If the specimen is being sent to a small laboratory, it frequently is helpful to call the laboratory before obtaining the arterial specimen so that the blood gas analyzer can be calibrated before the specimen arrives in the laboratory.)

Aftercare

Ensure that pressure is maintained over the puncture site for at least 5 minutes (sandbags will not do—use fingers!).

Do not use dressings or bandages that interfere with visualization of the puncture site. Patients with blood dys-

	pH	CARBONIC ACID	BICARBONATE
ACIDOSIS	Low	Increase	Decrease
ALKALOSIS	High	Decrease	Increase

Acid-base balance is normally maintained by three different body systems: the respiratory system, the renal system, and the buffer system.

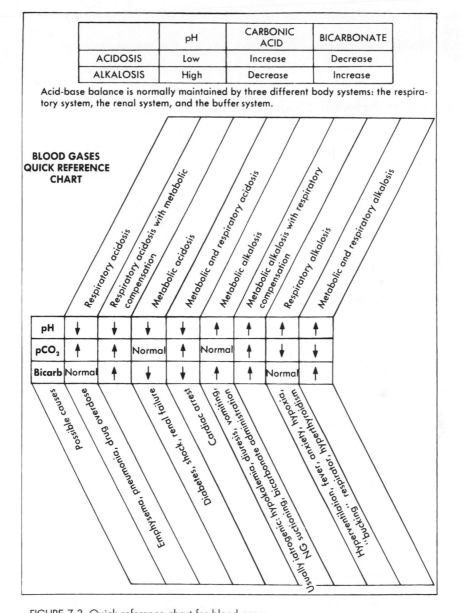

FIGURE 7-3. Quick reference chart for blood gases.
(From Budassi SA: An emergency nurse's guide to drawing arterial blood gases, *JEN* 3(2):24, 1977.)

crasias or those who are anticoagulated may require a longer period of pressure to ensure that bleeding has ceased.

Observe the puncture site for at least 1 minute following removal of manual pressure for formation of a hematoma.

Reassess pulse.

Interpretation of Arterial Blood Gas Values

Notice the pH value: 7.35 to 7.45 = normal; above 7.45 = alkalosis; below 7.35 = acidosis.

Notice the bicarbonate level: 22 to 26 mEq = normal; above 26 mEq = metabolic alkalosis; below 22 mEq = metabolic acidosis.

Notice the Pco_2 value: 35 to 40 mm Hg = normal; above 45 mm Hg = respiratory acidosis; below 35 mm Hg = respiratory alkalosis.

Make an acid-base "diagnosis" on the basis of these criteria. Consider the effect of compensatory mechanisms on blood gas values. Even when the values are abnormal, they may not all fit the criteria. The variance is caused by the compensatory action—see the examples in Figure 7-3.

THE COLLECTION OF LABORATORY SPECIMENS

The Collection of Blood

Most patients have blood samples collected at some time during their emergency department visit. These blood values may be used to establish a baseline, identify trends, or diagnose a particular condition. Always explain to the patient that blood is going to be drawn for some test. If the patient asks the reason for the tests, try to explain. The patient should be lying or sitting while the specimen is being collected.

Selection of the site

Usually the median cephalic vein, located in the antecubital fossa, is used for the collection of blood. You may use any other peripheral site that is readily accessible. If an IV line must also be initiated, consider establishing the IV line and withdrawing a blood sample from that line before connecting the IV solution. This will save the patient an additional puncture and may save time.

Methods to find a vein

Apply a tourniquet and leave it in place for no longer than 5 minutes.

Lower the extremity, causing the site from which the specimen is to be collected to be dependent.

Apply warm soaks to the area.

Have the patient open and close his or her hand.

Use good direct lighting.

Feel for a vein with the fingers; sometimes good large veins are a bit deeper and cannot be visualized, but can be palpated.

In an absolute emergency situation, when a site for drawing blood cannot be located, the specimen may be drawn from the femoral vein. This site is not routinely recommended because of the increased incidence of infection and/or embolism.

Procedure

Once the site has been identified, cleanse it with an antiseptic solution such as alcohol or an iodine-based solution (be sure to check to see if the patient is allergic to any of these preparations). Avoid using alcohol if you are drawing an ethanol level.

NOTE: Use nonsterile examination gloves during procedure.

Palpate the site above the proposed needle entry point; do not touch the actual site.

Have the patient open and close a fist to allow for venous filling.

Stabilize the vein with a thumb.

Draw the skin taut below the site to prevent the vein from moving during puncture.

Insert the needle at a 30-degree angle with the bevel facing up.

If using a Vacutainer, insert the laboratory tube at this point.

If using the needle-and-syringe technique, begin to pull back on the plunger of the syringe at this point.

Once the correct amount of blood has been collected, release the tourniquet.

Place a dry, sterile 2 × 2-inch gauze square over the needle insertion site and withdraw the needle.

Place a slight amount of pressure over the puncture site.

Place specimens into the correct laboratory tubes if the needle-and-syringe technique was used.

Do not force blood with pressure through the needle and into the laboratory tube.

Be sure to agitate carefully any tube that contains any type of preservative or chemical to allow for its dissemination.

Label all tubes carefully with the patient's name, hospital number, the date, and the caregiver's initials.

Do not have the patient bend the arm at the elbow to decrease bleeding; instead, have the patient elevate the arm.

Blood Sampling from Implanted Ports

Procedure

1. Gather equipment
   Alcohol swab
   Povidone-iodine swabsticks (3)
   Sterile gloves
   1 empty 5 cc Luer-Lock syringe
   1-5 cc syringe filled with 3 cc of sterile saline
   1-3 cc syringe filled with 3 cc of heparin solution 1:100 units (unless specified otherwise by physician)
   Empty 10 cc Luer-Lock syringe with 20 g, 1-inch needles
   Blood tubes
   Noncoring (Huber) straight point 22 g 1-inch needle
   Vacutainer needle/sleeve (optional)
2. Wash hands
3. Explain procedure to patient and assist to a comfortable position.
4. Palpate the implant site to locate the device septum.
5. Cleanse site vigorously with alcohol for one (1) minute.
6. Cleanse site with povidone-iodine swabstick three (3) times, using a circular motion and moving from the center outward to a 2-inch radius. Allow to dry for three (3) minutes.
7. Attach a 5 cc Luer-Lock syringe to a 20 g, 1-inch noncoring (Huber) needle. A standard straight needle must never be used to puncture the septum.
8. Apply sterile gloves.
9. Stabilize the implant device under the skin using the thumb and forefinger of the nondominant hand.
10. Hold syringe with noncoring (Huber) needle perpendicular to injection site.
11. Puncture the skin and device's rubber septum until needle reaches needle stop.
12. Grasp and stabilize needle against needle stop. The needle must be held securely against the needle stop below the rubber septum to avoid injection of solution into the subcutaneous tissue. Never use an angular motion or twist the needle and syringe once in the septum. This action will tear the septum and may create a leakage path.
13. Withdraw 5 cc of blood and discard sample and syringe.
14. Attach a new 10 cc syringe and withdraw the necessary amount of blood for the laboratory tests ordered.

If more than 10 cc of blood is required, remove and connect another 10 cc syringe for removal of additional blood.

15. Attach the 5 cc syringe filled with sterile saline.
16. Fill the necessary blood tubes.
17. Aspirate for blood return and inject the sterile saline steadily into the device.
18. While continuing to stabilize the port with sterile hand:
   a. Remove needle from 3 cc syringe containing heparin solution.
   b. Remove 5 cc syringe from noncoring (Huber) needle and attach heparin-filled syringe.
   c. Aspirate for blood return and inject heparin solution.
19. Remove syringe and needle while maintaining stability of the port.
20. Examine the injection site carefully and apply Band-Aid if necessary.

Point of Care Testing

Point of care testing is a method to rapid screen for critical laboratory values, performed by a hand-held or stationary analyzer, usually located at or near the patient's bedside. Because of the rapid turn around time for results (less than 5 minutes for most tests), this method of obtaining selected laboratory studies is becoming increasingly popular. I-STAT® is one example of this technology, offering electrolyte (sodium, potassium, and chloride), blood urea nitrogen (BUN), glucose, Ca + (ionized calcium), pH, $PaCO_2$, PaO_2 and hematocrit values through direct measurement and HCO_3 (bicarbonate), TCO_2 (total carbon dioxide) Base excess, SaO_2 (oxygen saturation) anion gap and hemoglobin values via calculated methodologies.

The benefits of point of care testing include precise, accurate laboratory-quality results within minutes, ease of use, and immediate access to patient results at equal or lower laboratory costs than traditional laboratory methods.

Procedure

1. Obtain venous blood sample.
2. Apply 2 to 3 drops whole blood to test cartridge.
3. Insert cartridge into analyzer.
4. Results will be displayed when test is completed.

LABORATORY ANALYSIS

The laboratory data base is an essential component in the assessment of patients in the emergency department. Expensive at best, laboratory tests should not be ordered indiscriminately, but should follow an interview and examination process that indicates the appropriate testing requirements for each patient.

A number of laboratory tests are frequently used within the emergency setting. In some departments it is a nursing responsibility to order routine tests when their need is established, whereas in other departments such

TABLE 7-1   Tubes for Drawing Blood

TUBE	PRESERVATIVE OR ANTICOAGULANT	TEST
Red top	None	Serologies, chemistry panels, routine chemistries
Lavender top	Ethylenediaminetetraacetate (EDTA)	Hematology, lipoprotein electrophoresis, acid phosphatase
Blue top	Sodium citrate (0.5 g)	Coagulation studies
Gray top	Sodium fluoride	Blood glucose, blood alcohol, drug screens and tests that will not be evaluated soon
Green top	Sodium heparin	Special procedures

Modified from Sheehy SB, Barber JM: *Emergency nursing: principles and practice,* ed 2, St Louis, 1985, Mosby.

orders are carried out by the physician on duty. In either case, a working knowledge of the common tests and the types of containers used to collect test specimens is necessary for the nurse involved (Table 7-1).

Specific Tests

Table 7-2 provides a quick overview of commonly ordered laboratory tests and corresponding normal lab values for each test.

Complete blood count

A complete blood count (CBC) is a routine hematologic screening test on serum; it includes hemoglobin, hematocrit, total red blood cell (RBC) count, white blood cell count and differential, and mean corpuscular cell volume (MCV), mean cell hemoglobin concentration (MCHC), and mean cell hemoglobin (MCH). Elements of this test may on occasion be ordered separately, which will lower the cost to the patient. Five milliliters of venous blood is generally required.

Urinalysis

A urinalysis should always be a clean-catch or catheter specimen collected in a sterile, dry container and examined within 30 minutes if unrefrigerated. The standard examination includes appearance, pH, specific gravity, glucose and ketones, protein semiquantitation, and microscopic examination of the sediment for casts, crystals, RBCs, and bacteria.

Blood glucose

Venous blood for glucose levels should be obtained as a clot specimen in a patient whom you suspect has an abnormality in glucose metabolism. Collect the specimen before starting intravenous solution infusions or administering dextrose. Two to three milliliters is necessary to perform the test. Record the conditions under which the blood was drawn—that is, whether the patient was fasting, approximate time of last meal, and so on.

Blood urea nitrogen

The BUN test measures the amount of circulating urea in the blood, which is the end product of protein metabolism and is normally excreted in the urine. An elevation of the BUN may indicate renal failure, renal hypoperfusion, or obstructive uropathy. A 1-ml amount of venous blood is required to perform the test.

Serum electrolytes

The venous specimen should be withdrawn from a vein and collected in a specimen container in as atraumatic a procedure as possible to avoid hemolysis, which results in a false elevation of the serum potassium. Electrolytes include potassium, chlorides, and carbon dioxide content. Although each of these elements can be tested individually, the implications of the result may change depending on the values of the other electrolytes in concert with one another.

Serum creatinine

The serum creatinine test evaluates renal functions by measuring creatinine, a waste product that is found in skeletal muscle and is usually filtered by the renal glomerulus. The serum creatinine may be elevated in acute renal failure. A 3-ml amount of venous blood is needed to perform the test.

Cardiac enzymes

The presence of specific cardiac enzymes assists in the diagnosis of acute myocardial infarction. Laboratory studies include creatinine kinase, creatinine kinase-myocardial band (CK-MB), myoglobin and troponin-T. A 5-ml volume of venous blood is required for this test.

TABLE 7-2   Normal Laboratory Values for Commonly Ordered Laboratory Tests

Serum chemistry
Bilirubin (Bili)
    Total   0.3–1.5 mg/dL
    Direct   0–0.2 mg/dL
Creatinine (Creat)
    Female   0.6–1.1 mg/dL
    Male   0.8–1.3 mg/dL
Urea nitrogen (BUN)   8–23 mg/dL
Glucose-fasting (Gluc)   65–110 mg/dL
Electrolytes (Lytes)
    Potassium (K^+)   3.8–5.0 mEq/L
    Chlorides (Cl)   95–103 mEq/L
    Carbon dioxide (CO_2)   24–30 mM
    Sodium (Na)   136–142 mEq/L

Arterial blood gases

    pH   7.35–7.45
    Po_2 80–105 mm Hg
    Pco_2 35–45 mm Hg

Serum enzymes

Amylase   15–90 U/L
Creatinine phosphokinase (CPK)   25–145 mU/ml
Lactic dehydrogenase (LDH)   110–250 mU/ml
Alanine amino transaminase (SGPT)   5–35 mU/L
Aspartate amino transaminase (SGOT)   10–40 mU/ml

Hematology
Coagulation
Bleeding time   <8 minutes
Partial thromboplastin time (PTT)   24–36 seconds
Prothrombin time (PT)   70%–100%
Thrombin time   11.9–18.5 seconds
Hematocrit
    Female   37%–47%
    Male   42%–52%
Hemoglobin
    Female   12.0–16.0 g/dL
    Male   14.0–18.0 g/dL
Erythrocytes
    Female $4.2–5.4 \times 10^6$ cu mm
    Male $4.6–6.2 \times 10^6$ cu mm
Sedimentation rate
    Female   up to 20 mm/hr
    Male   up to 9 mm/hr
Leukocytes $4.8–10.8 \times 10^3$ cu mm
Platelets $150–400 \times 10^3$ cu mm
Urinalysis
    Color   yellow
    pH   4.6–8
    Specific gravity   1.001–1.035
    Glucose   Ø

Toxic screen

A toxic screen may be ordered specific to a certain drug or as a screen for sedatives, hypnotics, and narcotics. It measures the exact amount of circulating drug per volume of plasma. This is a very expensive test and takes a long time to run. Most facilities send the specimen out to a bioanalysis laboratory, but this delays receipt of the results because of transit time. A 5-ml amount of venous blood is required to perform this test.

Serum drug level

A serum drug level is generally ordered specific to a drug such as digoxin. It measures the concentration of drug in the blood at the time the level is drawn. The test requires 2 to 5 ml of venous blood.

Serum amylase

Serum amylase is generally evaluated in patients with upper abdominal pain. The test measures the amount of circulating amylase, which is a digestive enzyme for carbohydrates and is elevated most notably in acute pancreatitis. This test requires 3 ml of venous blood.

Arterial blood gases

Arterial blood gases are analyzed from arterial specimens collected in heparinized tubes or syringes. Elements include serum pH, P_{CO_2}, P_{O_2}, and bicarbonate levels. Results help determine the acid-base status of the internal environment and the degree of oxygenation of the tissues. Most test results include the percentage of oxygen saturation of the red blood cells. The minimal specimen required is 3 ml, which is collected under aseptic conditions.

White blood count and differential

A white blood count (WBC) and differential may be ordered instead of a CBC when an infection is suspected. However, both these elements must be ordered and evaluated together, since the WBC may not be elevated even in severe infections, whereas the differential will. Mild to moderate leukocytosis may indicate an infectious process that is bacterial in origin. The differential is an evaluation of the different types of leukocytes that are found in the serum: neutrophils (56% of the total), eosinophils (2.7%), basophils (0.3%), and lymphocytes (34%). Neutrophils are also called "polys," or polymorphonucleocytes, and "segs," or segmented cells. Monocytes are nongranular leukocytes and may be seen in chronic inflammatory conditions in small numbers. Bands are new neutrophils that are formed in response to overwhelming bacterial invasion that taxes the older neutrophil population. Such a condition is referred to as a *shift to the left*. The WBC and differential are collected in a clot tube devoid of preservatives or anticoagulants. To perform the test, 3 to 5 ml venous blood is needed.

Coagulation studies

Various elements of the coagulation series evaluate the different stages of clotting. The studies include protime, partial thromboplastin time, platelet count, Lee white clotting time, and prothrombin consumption time.

Prothrombin time

This test identifies defects in stage 3 of coagulation. A calcium-binding anticoagulant is added to the patient's serum, and the time between addition of this element and the formation of a fibrin clot is measured.

Partial thromboplastin time

This test identifies defects in stage 2 of coagulation. It measures factors XII, XI, X, IX, VIII, V, II, and I. The test measures the clotting time of plasma when elements of the clotting process are added to calcium-free and platelet-poor plasma in a predetermined sequence.

Prothrombin consumption time (PCT)

This test measures prothrombin utilization time. It identifies defects in stage 1 and 2 of coagulation and is also used to elevate coagulation of blood.

Platelet count

This test identifies the number of platelets in a peripheral smear and confirms defects in stage 1 of coagulation.

Lee-White clotting time

This test measures the time it takes for a fibrin clot to form in venous blood and identifies defects in stage 4 of coagulation.

BLOOD SAMPLING IN PEDIATRIC PATIENTS

Specimens may be obtained by finger-stick, heel-stick, or regular venipuncture technique, depending on the amount of the specimen required. If using conventional venipuncture technique, the appropriate size needle for collection would be between 19 or 23 gauge. Pediatric-size vacuum tubes are available in 3- and 5-ml sizes.

Finger-Stick/Heel-Stick Technique

Cleanse the site.
Apply a small sterile dressing at the completion of the procedure.

BLOOD FOR BLOOD CULTURES

Particular care must be taken when obtaining specimens for blood culture.
1. Separate containers are required for specimens for aerobic, anaerobic, and fungal cultures.
2. The stopper of a culture medium container must be cleansed using betadine followed by dry wiping or air drying.
3. It is recommended that the caregiver wear sterile gloves when obtaining the specimen to avoid contamination of the puncture site.
4. The site must also be prepared in the same way as the culture medium stopper.
5. The needle must be changed each time a culture medium is inoculated.
6. The ratio of blood to medium should be 1:10.
7. The laboratory slip is labeled with the patient's name, hospital number, date, time, and body temperature, and any antibiotics the patient is taking are listed.
8. The culture medium container is labeled with the patient's name, the hospital number, date, time, and caregiver's initials; also include the patient's hospital/emergency department number.

SPINAL FLUID

Usually three to five specimens are sent to the laboratory following a spinal tap.
1. Number the tubes serially during collection.
2. If only one tube is collected, this tube should be sent to the microbiology section of the laboratory for division of the specimen under aseptic conditions following examination for necessary cultures.
3. Transport specimens to the laboratory immediately following collection; do not allow these specimens to sit in the department for prolonged periods.

URINE SPECIMENS

All urine specimens collected in the emergency department should be obtained by at least a midstream clean catch. On occasion it will be necessary to obtain a urine specimen by catheterization of the bladder.
1. Use sterile containers.
2. If the physician orders a urinalysis, split the urine and save a specimen (refrigerated) in case a culture and sensitivity test is ordered later.
3. Do not allow specimens to remain at room temperature for more than 30 minutes.

PERCUTANEOUS FLUID OR WOUND DRAINAGE SPECIMENS

Fluids from body cavities or wounds should be collected in a sterile syringe and then transferred to a sterile test tube or bottle. Be sure that specimens collected for anaerobic testing are free of air bubbles before being sent to the lab. If the patient is taking any medication, be sure to indicate what it is on the laboratory slip.

EMESIS AND GASTRIC LAVAGE MATERIAL

If the specimen is to be collected from gastric lavage, be sure to send the sample from the initial aspirate. If it is known or suspected what the ingested substance is or if there is an unusual smell about the patient, be sure to indicate this on the laboratory slip—it may aid in identification of toxic material.

STOOL SPECIMENS

If stool is to be sent to the laboratory for culture, it should be warm and newly evacuated. It should be sent to the laboratory in a sterile container. If the specimen is obtained by rectal swabbing, be sure that there is particulate matter on the swab. *Do not add saline or any other liquid to the specimen because this may destroy certain parasites.*

THROAT SWABS AND SPUTUM SPECIMENS

A throat culture is usually obtained via the oropharyngeal route using a long, sterile, cotton-tipped swab. The swab should then be placed in a sterile culture tube and transported to the laboratory as soon as possible.

Sputum can be collected directly into a dry, sterile container. The specimen should come from deep within the tracheobronchial tree. Saliva is not an acceptable sputum specimen. The specimen should be taken to the laboratory immediately. If the patient cannot cough or is unconscious, it may be necessary to obtain a specimen by suctioning the tracheobronchial tree.

SUGGESTED READINGS

Carrol P: Clarifying the CBC, *RN* 60: 29-34, 1997.
Carroll P: Lab reports: only as good as the sample, *RN* 60(9):26-28, 1997.
Frizzell J: Avoiding lab test pitfalls, *AJN* 98(2): 34-38, 1998.
Hutsko GM, Jones JB, Danielson L: Using point-of-care testing to speed patient care: one emergency department's experience, *J Emerg Nurs* 21(5):408-412, 1995.
Mattox D, Gorski L: Implanted venous access ports, *Home Health Focus* 1(8):6-7, 1995.
Sheehy SB: *Emergency nursing: principles and practice,* ed 4, St Louis, 1997, Mosby.
Sheehy SB, Jimmerson CL: *Manual of clinical trauma care: the first hour,* ed 3, St Louis, 1999, Mosby.
Werman HA, Brown CG: White blood cell and differential counts, *Emerg Med Clin North Am* 4(1): 41, 1986.

CHAPTER 8

Basic Legal Issues for Emergency Nurses

Genell Lee

A skilled emergency nurse will have a basic understanding of legal principles that have an impact on the delivery of emergency care.

CONSENT

The first major legal principle of concern to emergency nurses, and the patients for whom they provide care, is consent. The integrity of the individual and the individual's right to privacy requires consent for treatment, invasive procedures, surgical intervention, and release of any medical information about the patient's condition. Informed consent requires disclosure of information about the risks and benefits of treatment or procedures. The patient can then decide whether to consent. In emergency situations, state law generally allows for implied consent. The state, through its laws, can provide that the patient would, if he could, consent in emergencies. Although policies may require that a family member sign if the emergency department patient is unable to sign a consent, the law typically requires that two physicians certify that an emergency exists and consent for the patient.

Age of the Patient

One of the first components of consent is the age of the individual patient. The age at which a person can consent to medical treatment is governed by state law. Often, the age for medical consent is less than the legal age of majority (or the time when the law distinguishes between being a minor and an adult). Although hospital policy may dictate that a parent or guardian sign for a minor, the law generally recognizes that a minor of a certain age has the legal authority to decide on medical treatment. State law may allow a younger age of consent for certain situations. For example, a minor with a sexually transmitted disease, suspected HIV, or pregnancy-related complaints, can often consent to treatment at a very young age. Emancipated minors are another possible exception. Emancipated minors provide their own support, live on their own, and may have court documents showing the removal of legal age restrictions.

Competency of Patient

Also of concern are those patients who are not legally competent to consent. An individual declared incompetent by a court will have a guardian appointed to decide what is in the patient's best interest, including consent for treatment. A patient with a diminished capacity to comprehend issues surrounding consent may pose a dilemma. For instance, a patient who ingests drugs or alcohol may not fully comprehend consent issues. When a person with some diminished capacity attempts to refuse treatment, the emergency nurse may find little help from policies, procedures, or even the law. A description and evaluation of the patient's behavior and degree of understanding of risks are very important.

A patient with the legal capacity to *consent* to treatment also has the legal right to *refuse* treatment or withdraw consent. In the emergency department, patients may refuse treatment at different intervals in their care. Patients who leave without being seen (LWBS), against medical advice (AMA), or walk out of the emergency department without telling anyone, decide to withdraw consent for treatment for reasons often known only to them. Patients with a diminished capacity resulting from ingestion of alcohol and drugs often demand to leave the emergency department AMA. If the patient does not understand, and verbalize, the risks associated with leaving the ED, signing an AMA form is very little legal protection.

Patients with mental illness can also pose difficult issues related to consent. Psychiatric patients retain the right to consent and to refuse treatment. One exception is the patient who expresses suicidal or homicidal ideation. Assessment of the dangerousness of the patient, to self or others, is imperative before allowing a mentally ill patient to sign an AMA form. State law governs the ability to hold mentally ill patients who are evaluated to be a suicidal or homicidal risk.

Managed care delivery systems often request, or may require, immediate notification when a patient covered by a plan presents to the ED. Confusion sometimes exists regarding who should notify the managed care plan, what to tell them, and what to do with the answer. Recognizing that the managed care plan can only provide authorization for *payment,* not *treatment,* is imperative for the emergency nurse, and others in the ED. Consent for treatment rests with the patient.

Finally, consent is required for the release of the patient's medical information. Although no federal law protects a patient's medical record information, state laws typically do provide a measure of privacy. Certainly patients have an expectation that their most personal information—illnesses, injuries, and treatments—will be kept private unless consent is given for its release. The privacy surrounds all their information, not only the information included in the record. Conflict can often arise in the emergency department when a minor, of legal age to consent, refuses to inform a parent about diagnosis and treatment. The emergency nurse often feels torn and becomes embroiled in the conflict. The duty is to the patient and the emergency nurse must always keep that focus.

Special consideration is given those patients undergoing treatment for alcohol, drug abuse, or mental illness. Again, the hallmark of consent is that the patient decides whether to provide or deny consent or release information to other persons. Box 8-1 provides an outline of consent issues.

Reportable Conditions/Situations

Although consent remains with the patient or the patient's legal representative, sometimes the state legislature decides that the state will override the patient's right to consent for the release of medical information. Most states require the reporting of violent crime to the appropriate law enforcement agency. Thus, patients with gunshot wounds, stab wounds, burns, or injuries sustained in a motor vehicle crash may not be allowed, by state law, to refuse or in any way eliminate the hospital's legal responsibility to notify law enforcement.

Similarly, the state has an interest in protecting those in vulnerable situations who cannot protect themselves. Most states require the reporting of child or elder abuse and neglect to the proper authorities. Reporting to a law enforcement agency for a criminal investigation, or a state agency for protective services, is a matter of state law.

The state also has an interest that often overrides the individual's right to privacy in containing communicable disease. Reporting of emergency department patients seen and treated for a communicable disease is also a matter of state law. Reporting generally occurs to a local health department or other entity responsible for the public health and welfare. The types of communicable diseases that may require reporting include, but are not limited to, tuberculosis, HIV, gonorrhea, bacterial meningitis, and syphilis. The list can be extensive and state law should be consulted.

Public health hazards, such as rabies, may require the reporting of a potential source. A patient with dog or other animal bites is often a reportable condition. Firecracker or fireworks injuries, particularly in minors, may be a public health hazard that needs reporting to the proper authorities.

BOX 8-1   Common Consent Questions and Answers

Q: How old is the patient?

A: Minors have special rules. Consider:
1. Age
2. Type of problem (pregnancy-related, sexually transmitted disease, and so forth may have additional special rules).
3. Emancipated or married or parent

Q: Is consent given for treatment and special procedures?

A:
1. Informed: patient understands risks and benefits of treatment or procedure.
2. Implied: in an emergency, the patient, unable to consent, would likely want to be treated. May require written physician certification.
3. Managed care: "precertification" is consent for payment, *not* treatment.

Q: Is the patient impaired in any way that might affect the ability to consent?

A:
1. Age (see minors above)
2. Mental illness that reflects inability to understand risks and benefits of treatment or procedure (note that mental illness alone does not indicate an inability to consent).
3. Chemical impairment: drugs, alcohol, hypoxia.
4. Legally declared incompetent: if so, consent generally is given by guardian designated by an appropriate court.
5. Language barrier.
6. Illness, such as dementia or Alzheimer's, that may affect comprehension.

Q: Has the patient refused or withdrawn consent?

A:
1. Patient left without being seen (LWBS).
2. AMA: ensure patient understands the risks of refusing or withdrawing consent.
3. Advanced directive in place for either specific situations or appointment of alternative decisionmaker (health care proxy).

Q: Has the patient consented to release of private, confidential medical information?

A:
1. Signed release of information.
2. Special protections exist for:
   a. Psychiatric treatment
   b. Alcohol or drug treatment
   c. HIV status
   d. Sexually transmitted diseases
3. May precipitate conflict when minor involved (parent wants information and minor refuses).

Q: Does the law mandate reporting regardless of patient's consent?

A: Examples of reportable conditions (check state law for further clarification):
1. Child abuse or neglect
2. Elder abuse or neglect
3. Certain injuries:
   a. Gunshot wounds
   b. Stab wounds
   c. Physical assault
   d. Sexual assault
   e. Domestic violence
   f. Dog bites
4. Communicable diseases:
   a. Tuberculosis
   b. Rubella
   c. Bacterial meningitis
   d. HIV (some states)
5. Other situations:
   a. Death in emergency department
   b. Suicide (some states require reporting of attempted suicide)
   c. Seizures or episode of unconsciousness while driving or operating a motor vehicle
   d. Motor vehicle crash producing injury

PSYCHIATRIC PATIENTS

Patients with mental illness are of special concern in the emergency department. Patients expressing suicidal or homicidal ideation should receive a psychiatric evaluation. In patients impaired by drugs or alcohol, a proper evaluation is often difficult. Whether or not a psychiatric patient may be held involuntarily is a matter governed by state law.

The use of restraints or seclusion in psychiatric patients may not be directly covered by state law. However, other laws may be applicable. Issues of battery (for example, touching a patient without his consent) and false imprisonment (for example, restricting a patient's movement to a definite area) may be a concern. However, proper documentation of the patient's words and behavior can prove, if needed, the underlying safety rationale for restraint or seclusion.

FORENSIC ISSUES

Patients who present to the emergency department in the custody of law enforcement personnel retain their right to consent to treatment. If law enforcement personnel request that the emergency nurse collect evidence for legal purposes, such as blood or urine for detection of alcohol or drugs, a specific policy should exist to address the nurse's role. Conflict may occur if the patient refuses and law enforcement personnel insist. State law typically addresses the collection of specimens from patients who are in the custody of law enforcement personnel.

Other types of evidence collection that may occur in the emergency department include obtaining evidence from victims of sexual assault, photographs of injuries, and collection of clothing from victims of violent crime. State law may also require the reporting of certain types of cases to the local coroner or medical examiner.

EMERGENCY MEDICAL TREATMENT AND ACTIVE LABOR ACT

The Emergency Medical Treatment and Active Labor Act (EMTALA) is a federal law passed by Congress to prevent hospitals from transferring emergency patients, particularly those who are unstable, because of their inability to pay. Media reports of patients, either in active labor or an unstable condition, transferred to hospitals for financial reasons generated Congressional hearings and resulted in the legislation. A summary of the highlights of EMTALA is outlined in Box 8-2.

NURSING PRACTICE

The scope of practice for licensed nurses is determined by each state's nurse practice act. The state's designated regulatory body, typically a board of nursing, publishes regulations governing licensure, practice activities, continuing education, and disciplinary procedures. Each licensed nurse should be aware of the scope of practice outlined by his or her respective board of nursing. A physician's order to perform a procedure that is beyond the scope of nursing practice can have significant consequences for the nurse who performs the activity.

In the ever-changing healthcare delivery system, hospitals may replace licensed nurses with unlicensed personnel as a cost-saving measure. Generally, the licensed nurse is required to supervise the unlicensed staff member. Pitfalls can occur in this arrangement. Delegation of activities that should only be performed by licensed nurses to an unlicensed staff member may result in disciplinary action against the licensed nurse.

Any policy or position statements published by the board of nursing regarding delegation to unlicensed personnel should be carefully reviewed before job descriptions and policies and procedures are implemented. If unlicensed personnel are performing nursing functions, the nursing board's position statement is likely to address that issue. The National Council of State Boards of Nursing, Inc., www.ncsbn.org/, makes its position paper on delegation available on the Internet.

BOX 8-2   EMTALA Highlights

1. *All individuals . . .*
2. *Presenting to the emergency department:* on hospital property, including hospital-owned ambulance. Is not restricted to ED entrance or system.
3. *Entitled to an appropriate medical screening examination:*
   a. What is appropriate is not defined in the law.
   b. Should be addressed in the hospital's medical staff bylaws and by the governing body.
   c. Do not differentiate between patients based on financial status (beware treating managed care patients differently).
4. *To determine the existence of an emergency medical condition:*
   a. Threat to life or limb; *or*
   b. Severe pain; *or*
   c. Active labor.
5. *Resources of hospital used, including ancillary services and on-call physicians, to determine the existence of an emergency medical condition.*
6. *Hospitals with specialized capabilities must accept transfers if capacity to treat* (for example, sufficient resources available: personnel, equipment, beds).
7. Transfers require:
   a. *Consent of patient or patient representative;*
   b. *Accepting physician;*
   c. *Accepting facility;*
   d. *Appropriate vehicle* (mode):
   e. *Appropriate equipment;*
   f. *Qualified personnel* (be knowledgeable about scope of practice of transferring personnel to determine if personnel are qualified to transport patient);
   g. *Records must accompany patient.*

From EMTALA Highlights from the Emergency Medical Treatment and Active Labor Act, 42 U.S.C.A. § 1395dd (Supp. 1995).

SUMMARY

The emergency nurse practices in a complex environment that is a microcosm of a complex society. Fear of litigation cannot override the responsibility to provide safe, competent nursing care to patients seeking emergency care. An understanding of the basic legal concepts encountered on a daily basis can reduce the fear of litigation and provide protection in the event litigation occurs.

SUGGESTED READINGS

Brent NJ: *Nurses and the law: a guide to principles and application,* Philadelphia, 1997, WB Saunders.

Derse AR: Legal and ethical issues in the emergency department, *Emerg Med Clin North Am* 13: 213, 1995.

Fackler ML, Riddick L: *Clinicians' inadequate descriptions of gunshot wounds obstruct justice: clinical journals refuse to expose the problem: proceedings American Academy of Forensic Sciences, II,* Colorado Springs, Colo, 1996, McCormick-Armstrong.

George GE, Quatrone JD, Goldstone M: The duty to document—what are the limits?, *J Emerg Nurs* 23(5): 467-469, 1997.

George GE, Quatrone JD, Goldstone M: Slip and fall cases: beware, *J Emerg Nurs* 23(6): 633-634, 1997.

Lee G: Legal and regulatory constructs. in ENA: *Sheehy's emergency nursing: principles and practice,* ed 4, St Louis, 1998, Mosby.

Legal handbook: ways to improve and safeguard your practice, *Nurs 97* 27(6): 32, 1997.

Morrison A: Incorrect restraint use: deadly protection, *Nurs 97* 27(6): 32, 1997.

Rozovsky FA: *Consent to treatment,* ed 2, Boston, 1995, Little, Brown.

Southard P: Legal issues, In *Emergency nurses association core curriculum,* ed 4, Philadelphia, 1994, WB Saunders.

CHAPTER 9

Shock and Hemodynamic Monitoring

Ingrid B. Mroz ■ Lisa B. McCabe

Shock is a complex syndrome that develops because of inadequate or inappropriate tissue perfusion or an inability of tissues to utilize available oxygen and nutrients, leading to cellular hypoxia and a buildup of toxic metabolites, which results in tissue damage and organ dysfunction. Three main components responsible for supplying the cells with nutrients and oxygen are the:

Heart, which functions as a pump

Blood, fluid which serves as the transporter

Vascular system, which provides the transportation network.

If radical changes occur in any of these areas, shock may rapidly ensue.

CLASSIFICATION OF SHOCK

Hypovolemic

Critical loss of intravascular volume that may be caused by trauma; hemorrhage from other causes (GI bleeding or a ruptured ectopic pregnancy); severe burns; or dehydration resulting from diarrhea, polyuria, profuse diaphoresis, emesis, or excessive nasogastric suctioning.

Cardiogenic

Inefficiency of the heart as a pump; occurs in myocardial infarction, cardiac tamponade, pulmonary embolus, myocarditis, or cardiomyopathies.

Distributive

Maldistribution of blood volume because of changes in vascular resistance and permeability.

1. *Septic* An overwhelming infection that causes an endotoxin release that results in vasodilation and decreased tissue perfusion.
2. *Anaphylactic* A severe allergic reaction that results in histamine release, increased capillary permeability, and dilation of the arterioles and venules.
3. *Neurogenic* Massive dilation of arterioles and venules caused by loss of sympathetic tone.

Obstructive

Obstruction to the outflow of blood from the heart caused by massive pulmonary embolism, pericardial tamponade, tension pneumothorax, or severe aortic stenosis.

The first hour of therapeutic intervention for shock is usually the most important. Management can be difficult, and the mortality rate is high. To choose the appropriate therapeutic intervention, it is vital to determine if the cause is a volume deficit problem, a pump failure problem, or a vascular dilation problem.

Despite the initiating etiology of shock, the final common pathway for all categories of shock is inadequate oxygen delivery at the cellular level. The immediate end-points of therapy for all categories of shock are to restore and maintain adequate delivery of oxygen and nutrients by preventing or reversing anaerobic metabolism.

It is, however, important to note that the most important factor in the success of early treatment is the experience of the medical and nursing staff,[1] for early recognition of decreased oxygen delivery and prompt initiation of therapy to restore tissue perfusion and oxygenation is critical to improving patient outcome.

PATHOPHYSIOLOGY OF SHOCK

Understanding the basic pathophysiology of shock is an essential component toward further appreciation of the clinical presentation and progression seen with each category of shock.

Regardless of the etiologic event, the primary pathophysiologic outcome in shock consists of hypoperfusion, which results in tissue hypoxia, acidosis, and end organ dysfunction.[2]

Rice[3] describes the shock state as having the potential for progressing through four stages:

Initial stage
Compensatory stage
Progressive stage
Refractory stage

Speed of progression and clinical manifestations seen with each stage will vary with each patient. The following pathophysiologic mechanisms are described according to each stage of shock:

Initial Stage

- Decrease in cardiac output
- Decrease in tissue perfusion
- Decrease in aerobic metabolism
- Increase in anaerobic metabolism
- Increase in lactic acid production

Compensatory Stage

- Decrease in cardiac output
- Activation of compensatory mechanisms

Compensatory mechanisms in shock

The activation of compensatory mechanisms occurs in an attempt to preserve vital organ function. The four most prominent mechanisms are discussed below.

■ SYMPATHETIC NERVOUS SYSTEM

When the sympathetic nervous system is activated following trauma, epinephrine is released. Epinephrine causes an increase in heart rate. Cardiac output and blood pressure increase, resulting in peripheral vasoconstriction.

■ RENIN-ANGIOTENSIN MECHANISM

When renal perfusion is decreased, the renin-angiotensin mechanism is activated. When renin is released, it causes the release of angiotensin I and angiotensin II. This effect causes the release of aldosterone into the system. Aldosterone causes increased sodium reabsorption at the renal tubule level. As sodium is reabsorbed, fluid is also reabsorbed. This fluid is then shunted into the venous system, resulting in increased intravascular volume, increased blood return to the right side of the heart, increased cardiac output, and increased blood pressure. Aldosterone may be a factor in decreased urinary output.

■ **RELEASE OF ANTIDIURETIC HORMONE**

In hypovolemic states, the anterior pituitary gland releases antidiuretic hormone (ADH). ADH causes the reabsorption of water at the renal collecting duct level. The water is shunted into the venous system, where it causes an increased intravascular volume, increased blood return to the right side of the heart, increased cardiac output, decreased urine output, and increased blood pressure. Like aldosterone, ADH release may also be a factor in decreased urinary output.

■ **INTRACELLULAR FLUID SHIFT**

Fluid shifts from intracellular spaces to intravascular spaces, causing increased vascular volume, increased blood return to the right side of the heart, increased cardiac output, and increased blood pressure. Because of the "cellular dehydration," the patient, if awake, will complain of being thirsty.

Progressive Stage

- Inadequacy or failure of compensatory mechanisms
- Hypoperfusion of vital organs
- Decrease in cardiac output
- Decrease in blood pressure
- Decrease in myocardial oxygen supply
- Decrease in myocardial function
- Increase in capillary permeability

Refractory Stage (Irreversible)

- Multiple system organ failure
- Profound hypoperfusion
- Severe hypoxemia
- Renal shutdown
- Intractable circulatory failure

Throughout the four stages of shock, five main organ systems are affected.

EFFECT OF SHOCK ON THE FIVE VITAL ORGANS

Heart

Decreased coronary artery perfusion causes decreased function of the heart muscle as a pump; stroke volume and blood pressure decrease.

Brain

If oxygen and nutrient supplies are inadequate, brain function diminishes and unconsciousness ensues.

Lungs

As the partial pressure of oxygen decreases because of decreased blood volume or blood pressure, gas exchange does not take place at the capillary membrane level.

Liver

Glycogen stores are depleted by an excess of circulating epinephrine; metabolic acids that are normally detoxified in the liver cause acidosis.

Kidneys

A drop in cardiac output causes a decrease in blood flow through the kidneys; decreased urinary output and renal failure result.

TYPES OF SHOCK

Hypovolemic Shock

Hypovolemia is the most common cause of shock, resulting from a loss of blood, plasma, or fluid and electrolytes. The most common cause of hypovolemic shock is trauma that produces ruptured internal organs, lacerations, disrupted vasculature, long bone fractures, or pelvic fractures. Hypovolemic shock may also result from other conditions that result in fluid volume loss, such as a massive crush injury, severe burn injury, gastrointestinal bleed, ruptured aortic aneurysm, aortic dissection, ruptured ectopic pregnancy, peritonitis, intestinal obstruction, severe diarrhea, severe nausea and vomiting, or severe diaphoresis.

In general, the easiest way to discuss hypovolemic shock is in terms of blood loss resulting from trauma. The degree of shock depends on the following:
- Amount of blood lost
- Rate of blood loss
- Age of the patient
- Patient's overall physical condition
- Patient's ability to mobilize compensatory mechanisms

The blood volume of an adult (expressed in milliliters) is equal to 70% or 80% of *ideal* body weight in kilograms. A child contains 80 to 90 ml/kg of body weight.[4] The diagnosis of hypovolemic shock is made by clinical observation, physical examination, laboratory analysis, arterial pressure, central venous pressure (CVP), and pulmonary capillary occlusive pressure (PaOP) measurements. The initial goal in the treatment of hypovolemic shock is identifying and treating the cause while restoring volume by rapid infusion of fluids.

Classification of hypovolemic shock

Four classes of hypovolemic shock have been described[4]:

Class I: Less than 15% blood loss

■ SIGNS AND SYMPTOMS
- Mild tachycardia

■ THERAPEUTIC INTERVENTIONS
- Control bleeding
- Replace primary fluid losses

Class II: 15% to 30% blood loss

■ SIGNS AND SYMPTOMS
- Tachycardia
- Mild decrease in pulse pressure
- Mild increase in diastolic pressure
- Mild increase in respiratory rate
- Mildly cool skin

■ **THERAPEUTIC INTERVENTIONS**
- Manage airway.
- Administer oxygen.
- Administer IV fluids.
- Control bleeding if possible.
- Consider surgery.

Class III: 30% to 40% blood loss

■ **SIGNS AND SYMPTOMS**
- Airway difficulties possible
- Tachypnea
- Tachycardia
- Hypotension
- Restlessness, anxiety, or decreased level of consciousness
- Cool, clammy skin
- Cool extremities
- Delayed capillary refill
- Decreased urinary output
- Decreased CVP and PaOP

■ **THERAPEUTIC INTERVENTIONS**
- Manage airway.
- Administer oxygen.
- Administer IV fluids.
- Administer crystalloids and blood products.

NOTE: Replace blood loss with crystalloids at a rate of 3 L of crystalloids to 1 L of blood loss.

- Consider autotransfusion.
- Control bleeding, if possible.
- Prepare patient for diagnostic studies and/or surgery.

Class IV: Greater than 40% blood loss

■ **SIGNS AND SYMPTOMS**
- Decreased level of consciousness
- Tachycardia
- Hypotension
- Narrowed pulse pressure
- Tachypnea
- Cool, clammy skin
- Delayed capillary refill
- Decreased urinary output
- CVP less than 5 mm H_2O
- PaOP less than 4 mm H_2O

■ **THERAPEUTIC INTERVENTIONS**
- Manage airway.
- Administer oxygen.
- Administer IV fluids.
- Give blood products as soon as possible.
- Control bleeding, if possible.
- Consider emergency surgical intervention.

Distributive Shock

Distributive shock occurs when there is an abnormal distribution of intravascular volume because of a decrease in vascular resistance. Categories of distributive shock include septic, anaphylactic, and neurogenic shock.

Septic shock

Septic shock is usually caused by an overwhelming gram-negative infection that results in vasodilation and decreased tissue perfusion. It may also be caused by immune system suppression, invasion of organs by toxic substances, or the failure of the immune system to react to bacteria. It is important to remember that blood volume in septic shock is essentially normal. The infection may come from a source such as an indwelling urinary catheter or a severe burn injury, or it may occur as a postpartum complication. Mortality from septic shock is high—30% to 50%.[5] Death from septic shock is more common in the very young and the very old.

The usual cause of the infection is a gram-negative bacillus such as *Escherichia coli, Pseudomonas, Aerugionsa, Klebsiella pneumoniae, Proteus, Salmonella,* or *Bacteroides.* It is occasionally caused by gram-positive cocci such as *Streptococcus pneumoniae, Staphylococcus aureus,* and *Staphylococcus epidemidus.* On rare occasions, fungi, viruses, or yeast are causative agents. Bacteria enter the vascular system and cause the release of endotoxins into the circulation. This causes fluid leaks into the interstitial spaces, increased vascular permeability and vasodilation, and hypotension.

■ **SIGNS AND SYMPTOMS**
- Decreased blood pressure or normal blood pressure with widened pulse pressure
- Decreased cardiac output
- Tachycardia
- Hyperventilation
- Hypocapnia
- Hyperpyrexia
- Chills/tremors/rigors
- Pink, warm, dry skin
- Petechiae
- Decreased level of consciousness
- Metabolic acidosis
- Nausea and vomiting
- Diarrhea
- Positive cultures

Initially, the presentation of septic shock is that of a hypodynamic state.[6] The initial response is arterial and venous vasodilation that results in decreased preload and decreased systemic vascular resistance ultimately causing hypotension. Shock may later progress to a hypodynamic state. In hypodynamic shock the cardiac output falls as a consequence of decreased intravascular volume and myocardial depression leading to decreased cellular perfusion. This causes a stagnation of blood and resultant anaerobic metabolism and acidosis.

■ **THERAPEUTIC INTERVENTIONS**
- High-flow oxygen
- IV fluids
- Antibiotics (be sure to obtain cultures first)
- Inotropic agents and vasodilators for alpha-adrenergic effects
- Dopamine (Intropin)
- Dobutamine (Dobutrex)
- Naloxone (Narcan): considered investigational
- Corticosteroids (controversial)
- Heparin (controversial)
- Surgical intervention

Anaphylactic shock

Anaphylactic shock is an antigen/antibody reaction that occurs when a sensitized person is exposed to an antigen that is characterized by acute changes in vascular permeability and bronchial hyperactivity. It develops rapidly (usually within 20 minutes following exposure)[6] and may be caused by medications (e.g., antibiotics, such as penicillin), contrast media, sera, insect bites and stings, or ingestion of foodstuffs. When the antigen/antibody reaction occurs, a histamine release causes arterioles, venules, and capillaries to dilate. When the capillaries dilate, capillary permeability increases and intravascular fluid leaks into the interstitial spaces. This causes a form of relative hypovolemia and shock.

■ **SIGNS AND SYMPTOMS**
- Respiratory difficulty:
    Stridor
    Airway obstruction
    Bronchospasm
    Wheezing
- Hypotension
- Tachycardia
- Dysrhythmias
- Urticaria/angioneurotic edema
- Pruritus
- Warm skin
- Cardiopulmonary arrest

■ **THERAPEUTIC INTERVENTIONS**
- ABCs
- High-flow oxygen
- IV fluids
- Epinephrine 0.1 to 0.5 ml of a 1:10,000 solution by slow IV push (may be repeated in 5 to 15 minutes if necessary). Propranolol (Inderal) should be available in the event persistent hypertension and tachycardia occur.
- Aminophylline for bronchospasm
- Beta-agonist aerosol (e.g., metaproterenol) for bronchospasm
- Antihistamines: (e.g., diphenhydramine) to decrease circulating histamines
- Steroids to reduce inflammatory response

Neurogenic shock

Neurogenic shock is caused by a decrease of sympathetic tone. This results in a dilation of arterioles and venules, which causes relative hypotension. Neurogenic shock may result from deep general anesthesia, spinal anesthesia, spinal cord injury, or severe brainstem injury at the level of the medulla. It is usually a diagnosis of exclusion when all other causes of shock are ruled out.

■ **SIGNS AND SYMPTOMS**
- Decreased blood pressure
- Rapid, shallow respirations or no respirations
- Bradycardia
- Paraplegia or quadriplegia
- Cool, clammy skin above the level of the lesion
- Priapism
- History of recent spinal anesthesia
- History of recent head trauma

■ **THERAPEUTIC INTERVENTIONS**
- ABCs
- Supine position
- IV fluids with crystalloids

- IV vasopressors for alpha-agonist effects
- Dopamine
- Phenylephrine
- Cervical spine protection

Cardiogenic Shock

Cardiogenic shock (seen with a 35% to 70% destruction of the left ventricular myocardium) is defined as a low cardiac output state with hypotension and signs of inadequate tissue perfusion.[7] Characterized as primary cardiac pump failure, it may be seen in the setting of acute myocardial infarction, myocardial contusion, myocardial rupture, myocarditis, cardiomyopathies, dysrhythmias, or pericardial tamponade. Pump failure is the inability of the heart to produce an adequate cardiac output. When myocardial infarction occurs, part of the myocardium becomes dysfunctional. If the infarct is large (usually involving more than 40% of the ventricle),[8] cardiac output decreases. When cardiac output decreases, blood pressure also decreases and tissue perfusion becomes inadequate, causing shock.

Therapeutic interventions are aimed at improving cardiac output, increasing tissue perfusion, and limiting myocardial damage.

■ SIGNS AND SYMPTOMS

- Signs of myocardial infarction (chest pain, nausea and vomiting, syncope)
- ECG changes indicative of myocardial infarction
- Cardiac dysrhythmias
- Elevated cardiac isoenzymes
- Shallow, rapid respirations
- Hypoxemia
- Decreased peripheral pulses
- Decreased blood pressure (if blood pressure increases, it does so at the expense of myocardial ischemia)
- Decreased cardiac output/cardiac index
- Elevated pulmonary artery occlusive pressure (greater than 18 mm Hg)
- Decreased level of consciousness (or anxiety or restlessness)
- Pale, cool, clammy skin
- Oliguria (less than 0.5 to 1 ml/kg/hour)
- Metabolic acidosis

■ THERAPEUTIC INTERVENTIONS

Aimed at optimizing preload, afterload, and contractility (See section on hemodynamic monitoring.)

- Correcting preload
  Low preload:
    Decreased CVP
    Decreased PaOP
    Decreased PAD
      Administer fluids
  High preload:
    Elevated CVP
    Elevated PAOP
    Elevated PAD
      Administer diuretics, venodilation (nitroglycerin)
- Correcting afterload
  Low afterload:
    Decreased blood pressure
    Decreased SVR
      Administer dopamine

High afterload:
>   Increased blood pressure
>   Elevated SVR
>   Administer sodium nitroprusside, dobutamine
- Correcting contractility (inotropy):
    Low cardiac output
>   Administer dobutamine, epinephrine, and dopamine (if afterload within normal limits)
- Intraaortic balloon pump (IABP) to increase cardiac output, oxygen delivery, and blood flow to the coronary arteries and to decrease myocardial oxygen consumption
- High-flow oxygen and/or therapeutic intubation
- Antiarrhythmic agents

Obstructive Shock

Obstructive shock occurs as a result of an obstruction to the outflow of blood from the heart or from an increased resistance to ventricular filling (diastole). Massive pulmonary contusion, coarctation of the aorta, or aortic stenosis may cause an obstruction of outflow of blood, whereas pericardial tamponade or tension pneumothorax may result in increased resistance to ventricular filling.[9] Regardless of the causes, the end result is a decrease in cardiac output and inadequate tissue perfusion.

Pulmonary embolism

■ **SIGNS AND SYMPTOMS (WILL VARY ACCORDING TO CAUSE)**
- Dyspnea
- Tachypnea
- Chest pain
- Anxiety
- Hypoxemia

■ **THERAPEUTIC INTERVENTIONS (WILL VARY ACCORDING TO CAUSE)**
- Oxygen
- System anticoagulation
- IV access

Coarctation of aorta

■ **SIGNS AND SYMPTOMS (WILL VARY ACCORDING TO CAUSE)**
- Systemic hypertension (upper extremities)
- Lower blood pressure in lower extremities

■ **THERAPEUTIC INTERVENTIONS (WILL VARY ACCORDING TO CAUSE)**
- IV access
- Oxygen
- Prepare patient for cardiac catheterization, aortogram and/or operating room

Aortic stenosis

■ **SIGNS AND SYMPTOMS (WILL VARY ACCORDING TO CAUSE)**
- Chest pain
- Dyspnea
- Cyanosis
- Syncope
- Hypoxemia
- Cough
- Mental status changes

■ **THERAPEUTIC INTERVENTIONS (WILL VARY ACCORDING TO CAUSE)**
- IV access
- Supportive treatment of symptoms
- Prepare patient for cardiac catheterization or operating room (valve replacement)
- Oxygen

Pericardial tamponade

■ **SIGNS AND SYMPTOMS (WILL VARY ACCORDING TO CAUSE)**
- Elevated CVP
- Cyanosis
- Distended neck veins
- Decreased CO
- Decreased blood pressure
- Muffled heart sounds

■ **THERAPEUTIC INTERVENTIONS (WILL VARY ACCORDING TO CAUSE)**
- IV access
- Oxygen
- Pericardiocentesis/pericardial window

Tension pneumothorax

■ **SIGNS AND SYMPTOMS (WILL VARY ACCORDING TO CAUSE)**
- Decreased CVP
- Decreased CO
- Decreased blood pressure
- Hypoxemia
- Severe shortness of breath
- Jugular vein distension
- Tracheal deviation
- Mediastinal shift

■ **THERAPEUTIC INTERVENTIONS (WILL VARY ACCORDING TO CAUSE)**
- IV access
- Oxygen
- Needle thoracostomy
- Chest tube placement

FLUID REPLACEMENT

One of the most important therapeutic interventions for a patient in shock is to gain vascular access so that fluids and blood products can be administered to replace volume and to increase preload and cardiac output to improve oxygen delivery. The number of intravenous accesses required depends on the severity of shock.

Sites

Choose sites that can accommodate large-bore cannulas for rapid fluid volume replacement. In the emergency setting, when time is critical, choose sites that are easily accessible and easy to cannulate.

Peripheral

External jugular vein
Antecubital (fossa) vein
Saphenous vein
Femoral vein

Central

Internal jugular vein
Subclavian vein

CAUTION: Caution should be exercised in using subclavian or jugular veins for treatment of hypovolemic shock, since the great veins are usually collapsed, increasing the possibility of complications such as hemothorax or pneumothorax.[10]

Surgical cutdown

Brachial vein
Femoral vein
Saphenous vein

Intraosseous

Intraosseous infusion is a temporary method to obtain intravascular access in children when other vascular sites are not readily available. A rigid needle is placed through the bone cortex into the medullary cavity. The anterior medial aspect of the tibia is the preferred site. Positioning the needle 1 to 3 cm below the proximal tibial tuberosity is preferred, although any site along the tibia may be used. The midanterior distal one-third of the femur, iliac crest, humerus, and sternum are other sites that may be considered (depending on the patient's age). Intraosseous access should be replaced with conventional intravenous access as soon as possible.

Size of Cannula

Use the largest-gauge, shortest-length cannula possible. Whenever possible, in the adult patient, use a 16-gauge or larger cannula, so that both IV fluids and blood products can be infused. If a surgical cutdown is performed, attempt to cannulate the vein with a catheter 8 French or larger.

Type of Tubing

Use standard *macrodrip* tubing (do not use *microdrip*) or other larger commercially available tubing. Inline manual pumping devices may be used to facilitate rapid fluid flow. Avoid IV extension tubing and standard stopcocks whenever possible during the resuscitation phase of fluid replacement. The increased length of tubing causes an increase in the coefficient of friction and slows the flow rate and delivery rate of the fluid. The inner diameter of standard stopcocks will slow flow rate.

CAUTION: Use only high-flow stopcocks.

IV Adjuncts

A rapid infusion device or pressure cuff used on an IV bag significantly increases the rate of fluid delivery. If warming devices are used, be sure that the product chosen does not slow fluid flow rate.

Temperature of Fluids

Ideally, fluids should be warmed to 39° to 41° C. Rapidly infused fluids that are room temperature or colder may cause hypothermia. Commercially available fluid warmers may be used to warm fluids and blood. IV fluids may also be warmed by placing bags of IV fluids near the defrosting unit in prehospital vehicles, placing chemical heat packs on IV bags, coiling IV tubing through basins of warm water, and heating IV bags in a microwave. Whichever method is chosen, fluid temperatures must never exceed 41° C.

CAUTION: Remember, blood and blood products *cannot* and *should not* be microwaved.

Types of Fluids

The choice of replacement fluid for resuscitation of shock depends on the type and severity of shock. Crystalloid solutions are usually the solutions of choice in early phases of shock and in the resuscitation phases of trauma. There continues to be considerable controversy in selecting the correct fluid to resuscitate patients in moderate to severe shock. At this time, there is evidence to support the opinion that crystalloids and colloids probably have equal effects, if the amount administered yields the same hemodynamic end points.[10] The American College of Surgeons Committee on Trauma (ACSCOT) recommends the following fluid replacement schedule:[4]

> 15% to 30% blood loss—crystalloid solutions
> >30% to 40% blood loss—crystalloid solutions and blood products

When administering crystalloids, remember that they should replace blood volume loss on a 3:1 ratio.

Crystalloids

Crystalloid solutions used to increase intravascular volume in shock contain electrolytes in isotonic or hypertonic concentrations. Crystalloids are readily available and relatively inexpensive options for volume replacement without risks of disease transmission or allergic reaction.

■ ISOTONIC SOLUTIONS

Isotonic solutions have a concentration that is similar to the normal concentration of extracellular fluid.
- 0.9% sodium chloride
- Lactated Ringer's injection
- Ringer's solution

CAUTION: Administration of large amounts of normal saline may cause hyperchloremia, hypernatremia, and acidosis.

CAUTION: Administration of large amounts of lactated Ringer's solution may elevate lactate level in patients who may be in lactic acidosis.

■ HYPERTONIC SOLUTIONS

Hypertonic solutions have a concentration greater than extracellular fluid. Administration of hypertonic solutions draws interstitial and intracellular fluid into the intravascular space.
- 3% sodium chloride
- 5% sodium chloride
- 7.5% sodium chloride

Hypertonic solutions are being used experimentally in prehospital care and in some institutions.

CAUTION: *May* lead to hypernatremia, hyperchloremia, metabolic acidosis, and hyperosmolarity.

NOTE: Consider administering hypertonic solutions via infusion pump. The most frequently recommended crystalloid solutions are Ringer's lactate solution and 0.9% sodium chloride solution.

Colloids

Colloids are efficient volume expanders that do not diffuse easily across normal capillary membranes and increase plasma oncotic pressure.

Blood/blood components

In major hypovolemic situations consider the administration of whole blood or packed cells. The amount of blood to request for type and cross-match depends on local protocol. In general, in instances of major trauma, blood should be typed and cross-matched for at least four units, with instructions to the blood bank to keep two units ahead of demand.

If a patient has received 3 to 4 L of crystalloid solution without improvement and/or stabilization of vital signs, the need for blood products becomes evident.

Fresh whole blood. This is the ideal solution; it contains red blood cells (and hemoglobin), plasma, and clotting factors. Potential complications associated with administration of fresh whole blood include volume overload, infusion of excess potassium and sodium, and infusion of anticoagulant.

Packed red blood cells. This is whole blood in which plasma has been extracted. Because plasma contains factors that may cause transfusion reactions and transmit infectious diseases, the risks of these are greatly reduced when using packed cells. In addition to reducing these risks, the amount of citrate, phosphate, free potassium, and debris is less than that contained in whole blood. Packed red blood cells improve the oxygen-carrying capacity of the blood while preventing fluid overload.

Problems inherent with the administration of large amounts of packed cells involve bleeding disorders, as a result of platelets and clotting factors that are minimally functional. The patient must be observed very closely for abnormal bleeding.

O negative packed red blood cells. When blood is required immediately without time for type and cross-match for type-specific matching, O negative packed cells should be given. O negative type blood can be universally accepted. When large amounts of O negative blood have been administered, there may be a reaction later when type-specific or type and cross-matched blood is given.

Type-specific, uncross-matched red blood cells. Type-specific uncross-matched cells may be given, if one can wait 15 to 20 minutes for the processing of type-specific, uncross-matched blood. Type-specific blood is preferable to O negative blood.

Type-specific, cross-matched red blood cells. Processing of type-specific and cross-matched red cells may take 30 minutes to 1 hour. Type-specific and cross-matched red blood cells are the most preferable type because risk of transfusion reactions are lower. However, in the resuscitation phase of shock, one may not have the luxury of waiting an hour for type and cross-matched red blood cells.

Albumin

Human serum albumin (5%) is a volume expander derived from the plasma utilized to increase or maintain oncotic pressure. Human serum albumin does not contain blood group antibodies. The shelflife of albumin is 3 to 5 years.

CAUTION: Albumin and Plasmanate are not recommended for use in trauma resuscitation, as they may increase bleeding from raw, abraded surfaces, they infuse slowly, they may cause an error in the type and cross-match process for blood, and they are relatively expensive.

CAUTION: In many shock states the capillary membranes may allow diffusion of colloids from the intravascular space into the interstitium.

■ STROMA-FREE HEMOGLOBIN

This material is hemoglobin that has been extracted from current or outdated red blood cells. The advantages are that it has no incompatibility factors and a great affinity for oxygen. The disadvantages are its 2-hour to 4-hour half-life and the fact that its affinity for oxygen is so great that oxygen does not release easily. There are also indications that stroma-free hemoglobin causes increased coagulation problems. At the present time, stroma-free hemoglobin is under clinical investigation.

Plasma substitutes

Currently available plasma substitutes include hetastarch, low-molecular-weight dextran, and high-molecular-weight dextran. Advantages of plasma substitutes include the following: readily available, can be administered without delay associated with typing and cross-matching blood, and do not transmit hepatitis or HIV. Plasma substitutes do not contain plasma proteins, clotting factors, or improve oxygen transport.

■ **DEXTRAN**

Dextran is a polysaccharide prepared from sucrose. Low-molecular-weight (dextran 40) and high-molecular-weight (dextran 70) dextrans are volume expander alternatives that improve intravascular volume for approximately 24 hours.[10] When administered in large doses, dextran can alter coagulation and result in prolongation of bleeding times as well as impairing platelet function.

■ **HYDROXYETHYL (HETASTARCH)**

Hetastarch is a synthetic compound with an indefinite shelf-life. Hetastarch has similar volume expansion characteristics as 5% albumin, but Hetastarch may last up to 36 hours, and is less expensive than 5% albumin.

CAUTION: Limit total volume to 1500 ml/day.

■ **PERFLUOROCHEMICAL EMULSIONS (PERFLUOROCARBON)**

Perfluorocarbon is a synthetic product that is known to effectively load and unload oxygen. The question of long-term effects still remains. Perfluorocarbon is currently under investigation and not generally available for clinical use.

Massive Transfusion Considerations

If a patient has received more than 50% of his or her blood volume over a 3-hour period, observe the patient for the following conditions.

Hypothermia

Unwarmed blood may lead to hypothermia. Hypothermic conditions shift the oxyhemoglobin curve to the left. Cold blood products have a higher viscosity and therefore infuse at a slower flow rate.

Hyperkalemia

When red blood cells hemolyze, potassium is released. As some red blood cell hemolysis is inevitable, one must carefully monitor the patient's serum electrolytes, especially potassium, and treat resulting findings appropriately. If hyperkalemia does occur, it is usually transient, and as the patient stabilizes, this condition usually corrects itself.

Hypocalcemia

Banked blood contains citrate. Citrate binds free calcium. If citrated whole blood is administered at greater than 100 ml/min, give 10 ml of a 10% solution of calcium chloride with each 10 U of whole blood.[4]

Acidosis

Banked blood has a pH of 7.1. Multiple transfusions of banked blood may lead to acidosis. Monitor arterial blood gases for acidosis and ECG for dysrhythmias that are induced by acidosis.

Alkalosis

Although initially acidosis is a concern, eventually the citrate contained in banked blood is converted to bicarbonate in the liver. Monitor the patient's arterial blood gases for alkalosis.

Coagulopathies

Loss of clotting factors in most banked blood results in prolonged coagulation times and coagulation disorders: consumptive coagulopathy, dilutional coagulopathy, impaired production of clotting factors, and platelet dysfunction. One should carefully monitor the patient's prothrombin time, partial thromboplastin time, and platelet count, and watch for any excessive bleeding. Administer 1 U of fresh frozen plasma for 10 U of whole blood given.

Debris

Banked blood often contains debris. Although it is not known if this debris is harmful, it is recommended that a 160-mm micropore filter be used during massive transfusions.[4]

Autotransfusion

Autotransfusion is a procedure in which blood is collected, filtered, anticoagulated, and then reperfused into the same patient. Autotransfusion is most commonly used as a therapy for hypovolemic shock.

When there is a massive blood loss into the thoracic cavity and banked blood is not readily available, autotransfusion should be considered. In the emergency setting, autotransfusion should be used in patients who have suffered chest trauma with accompanying hypotension or in patients requiring an open thoracotomy where blood loss is expected to be 500 cc or more. Blood from sources other than the thorax are considered contaminated and should not be used.

Most autotransfusion systems (ATS) use a closed-chest drainage system designed with access to the collection chamber for retransfusion. Blood that has been drained into the collection chamber to be used for autotransfusion should be retransfused within 6 hours of initiating collection.[12]

The use of anticoagulant in autotransfusion continues to be controversial. It has been recommended that addition of anticoagulant may be more appropriate in patients with large volume blood loss than in patients whose blood loss is slow and gradual.[13]

Advantages

- Readily available
- No time delay for lab type and cross-match
- No risk of transfusion reaction
- Fresh whole blood, intact clotting factors, platelets, red blood cells
- No risk of communicable disease transmission

Disadvantages

- Increase in free plasma hemoglobin as a consequence of hemolysis
- Potential for coagulopathies
- Potential for air embolism
- Potential for microembolization of fat and/or microaggregates

Contraindications

- Blood greater than 4 hours old
- Large clots
- Known coagulopathy
- Enteric contamination
- Malignant neoplasms
- Pericardial, mediastinal, or systemic infections
- Poor liver or renal function

Consider obtaining the following baseline lab values before initiating autotransfusion:

Complete blood count (CBC)	Split products of fibrinogen
Hemoglobin	BUN and creatinine
Hematocrit	Serum potassium
PT and PTT	Serum calcium
Platelets	Arterial blood gases
Thrombin time	Urinalysis
Plasma fibrinogen	

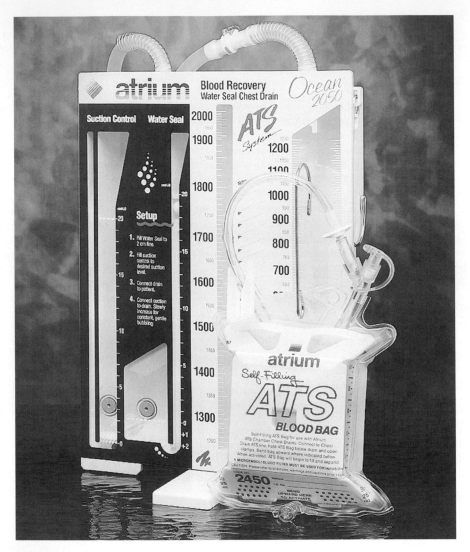

FIGURE 9-1. Atrium Autotransfusion System (ATS) (closed chest drainage).
(From Atrium Medical Corp., Hollis, NH.)

Procedure: Collection Using the Atrium Autotransfusion System

See Figure 9-1.

1. Fill water seal to 2 cm.
2. Fill suction control chamber to ordered suction pressure.
3. Assure ATS access line is clamped.
4. Connect patient.
5. Apply regulated suction until gentle bubbling occurs.
6. Closely monitor blood volume outputs in collection chamber.
7. When 500 cc of blood volume has drained into the collection chamber, clamp the ATS blood bag clamp.
8. Remove spike port cap.

9. Insert ATS bag spike into ATS access line using a firm twisting motion.
10. Place bag below closed chest drainage system.
11. Open ATS access line and blood bag clamps.
12. Gently bend ATS bag upward where indicated to initiate blood transfer.
13. Once blood evacuation is complete, clamp ATS access line and blood bag clamps.
14. Disconnect blood bag from ATS access line.

Reinfusion

1. Prime a microemboli blood filter and IV blood tubing with 0.9% sodium chloride solution.
2. Spike ATS blood bag with primed microemboli filter and blood tubing.
3. Hang ATS blood bag.
4. Open filtered air vent on top of ATS blood bag.
5. Open IV clamp to complete priming and assure all air has been evacuated.
6. Attach to patient IV access.
7. Begin infusion.

CAUTION: If using a pressure infusor, close the filtered air vent.

Maximum infusor pressure is 150 mm Hg.
Do not infuse entire blood volume in ATS blood bag through blood filter and IV tubing—air emboli can result.
Record chest drainage.
Record amount of autotransfused blood.
Document type and amount of anticoagulant used.
Observe the patient for:
    Excessive bleeding
    Hypothermia
    Air embolism
    Fat embolism

HEMODYNAMIC MONITORING

Successful management of shock, regardless of the classification, may be optimized by the use of hemodynamic monitoring. Hemodynamic status can be assessed through noninvasive methods (noninvasive BP, orthostatic vital signs, urine output, and evaluation of mental status) or with the use of invasive methods (pulmonary artery catheters, central venous catheters and arterial catheters.)

Invasive hemodynamic monitoring provides continuous physiologic data about the cardiovascular system. The information provided by this technology is a valuable adjunct to other assessment data.

Controversies currently exist surrounding the use of invasive hemodynamic monitoring.

Evidence suggests that data alone obtained from invasive hemodynamic monitoring cannot predict outcome and/or improve survival. Intelligent use of the data can guide the practitioner toward successful use of volume and pharmacological agents for patients in shock.[14]

Noninvasive Monitoring

- Blood pressure
- Postural vital signs

■ **POSTURAL VITAL SIGNS**

Postural vital signs should be assessed in all patients with (1) evidence of significant fluid loss through bleeding, vomiting, diarrhea, perspiration, or wound drainage; (2) unexplained tachycardia; (3) hypotension without tachycardia; (4) history or suspicion of chronic or concealed bleeding; or (5) blunt abdominal or chest trauma.

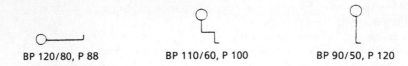

BP 120/80, P 88   BP 110/60, P 100   BP 90/50, P 120

FIGURE 9-2. Charting postural vital signs.
(From Bookman LB, Simoneau JK: Postural vital signs, *JEN* 3:43, 1977.)

Contraindications. Postural vital signs are not indicated if other injuries or the patient's general condition preclude safe administration of the test.

Rationale for the test. When a patient assumes a vertical position, gravity tends to cause sequestration (pooling) of blood in the capacitance vessels of the legs and trunk. Normally, individuals adapt readily to this postural change through rapid vasoconstriction of the vessels in which the blood tends to pool. This adjustment is not possible for the volume-depleted patient whose vasoconstrictor potential has already been maximally used.

Interpreting results. Postural changes (from lying to sitting or standing) that result in a *decrease* of 20 mm Hg or more in the systolic or diastolic blood pressure or an *increase* of 20 beats or more per minute in the pulse rate is a *positive* test result. The patient should be considered *hypovolemic* until proved otherwise.

CAUTION: The patient may experience weakness, dizziness, visual disturbances, or fainting during the test. These symptoms are promptly eliminated in most instances when the patient lies down again. Be certain to protect the patient during the assessment of postural vital signs to prevent injuries.

Procedure

1. With the patient supine, take and record the blood pressure and pulse as a baseline against which changes of both measures taken after position changes can be evaluated.
2. Have the patient sit up to a 90-degree position, and again record the blood pressure and pulse.
3. Have the patient stand, if possible, and again record the blood pressure and pulse. If significant changes occur, or if the patient's symptoms become acute during the sitting portion of the test, eliminate the third step and consider the results of the sitting portion positive.

Correct charting of the results is done in the following manner (Figure 9-2):

Invasive Monitoring

- Arterial pressure
- Central venous pressure (CVP)
- Pulmonary artery pressure (systolic [PAS] and diastolic [PAD])
- Pulmonary artery occlusive pressure ("wedge pressure" PaOP)
- Cardiac output/index (C0/C1)
- Systemic vascular resistance (SVR)

Definitions

The following terms are commonly used while caring for the patient requiring hemodynamic monitoring:

preload   The volume of blood filling the ventricles during diastole. Central venous pressure (CVP) reflects right ventricular (RV) preload. Pulmonary artery diastolic (PAD) and pulmonary artery occlusive/wedge (PaOP) reflect left ventricular preload.[15]

afterload   The resistance the ventricles must work against during systole to eject its volume. Pulmonary vascular resistance (PVR) reflects RV afterload. Systemic vascular resistance (SVR) reflects left ventricular (LV) afterload.

contractility   The force with which the heart muscle contracts.

Arterial Pressure Monitoring

Invasive arterial pressure monitoring provides direct measurement of arterial systolic and diastolic blood pressure. In addition, the presence of an arterial catheter allows for blood sampling for determination of arterial blood gas values and other laboratory studies.

Arterial pressure monitoring is achieved through cannulation of an artery either percutaneously or via surgical cutdown. The arterial vessels most commonly used are the radial and femoral arteries. The brachial artery may be used for short-term monitoring. The artery is cannulated using sterile technique and the cannula is attached to a pressurized system that provides a continuous infusion (3 cc/hr) of heparinized saline to maintain patency of the system.

Patient preparation

Before insertion of the arterial catheter, an Allen's test should be performed. An Allen's test assesses the ability of the ulnar artery to maintain perfusion if the radial artery is cannulated (Figure 9-3).

Equipment needed:

Sterile drapes

Sterile gloves

Betadine solution/ointment

1% lidocaine for infiltration

TB or 3-cc syringe

20 gauge 1½ inch Intracath

Heparinized saline (1000 U/500 cc N/S)

Pressure tubing/transducer

Monitor with pressure measurement capability

Pressure bag

Transducer holder

Benzoin

Tape

Bandages

2 × 2s

Interpreting results

■ WAVEFORM ANALYSIS

The arterial pressure consists of two phases: systole and diastole. Arterial systole signifies opening of the aortic valve with subsequent rapid ejection of blood into the aorta. Following this ejection, there is runoff of blood from the proximal aorta to the peripheral arteries. On the arterial waveform (Figure 9-4), this event is displayed as a sharp rise in pressure followed by a fall in pressure. As the pressure decreases, the aortic valve quickly closes, resulting in a small elevation in arterial pressure on the downslope. This is termed the *dicrotic notch*. Diastole occurs following closure of the aortic valve and continues until the next systole.[16]

Mean arterial pressure (MAP) is the average arterial pressure during systole and diastole. MAP is influenced by cardiac output or the volume of blood in the arterial system and the elasticity or resistance of the arteries (SVR).[17]

The formula for calculating MAP is:

$$Pd + \frac{Ps - Pd}{3}$$

where

Pd = diastolic pressure

Ps = systolic pressure.

Normal values

Systolic pressure (SBP) = 110 to 120 mm Hg

Diastolic pressure (DBP) = 70 to 80 mm Hg

Mean arterial pressure (MAP) = 70 to 105 mm Hg[18]

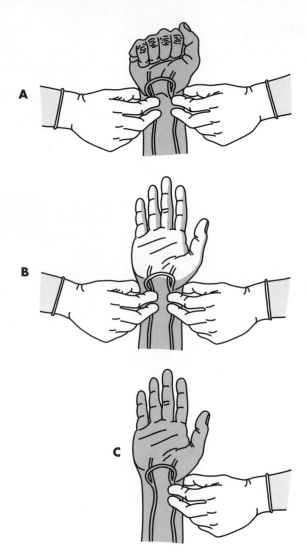

FIGURE 9-3. Assessing for Allen's Signs. **A,** Occlude both arteries with firm pressure. **B,** Raise arm to blanch hand. **C,** Release ulnar artery for return of color to hand.

(From Sheehy SB: *Emergency nursing: principles and practice,* ed 3, St Louis, 1992, Mosby.)

Potential complications

An invasive monitoring device has potential complications inherent in its use. Complications seen with invasive arterial monitoring may include:
- Thrombosis/emboli
- Infection/sepsis
- Neurovascular compromise/distal ischemia
- Bleeding
- Coagulopathy (secondary to heparin)

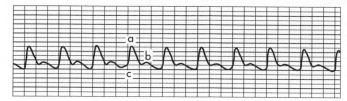

FIGURE 9-4. Arterial waveform. **A,** Systole. **B,** Dicrotic notch. **C,** Diastole.

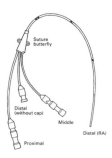

FIGURE 9-5. Central venous catheter.
(From Abbott Laboratories, Mountain View, Calif.)

■ **THERAPEUTIC INTERVENTIONS**
- Frequent neurovascular assessments of extremity
- Meticulous site care
- Immobilization of extremity
- Frequent assessment for site bleeding/oozing

Central venous pressure monitoring

Central venous pressure (CVP) monitoring provides information about:
- Pressure in the great veins
- Blood volume
- Right ventricular function
- Central venous return[19]

Catheter placement for pressure measurement can be performed percutaneously or via surgical cutdown. Veins commonly used for cannulation include internal and external jugular and subclavian veins and, less frequently, the antecubital veins.

Central venous catheters are manufactured with single, double, or triple lumens. CVP can also be measured via a pulmonary artery catheter (Figure 9-5.)

The decision to place a single-lumen or multilumen central line is determined by the actual or anticipated venous access needs of the patient. Considerations to help make the decision include:
- Need for CVP monitoring
- Need for frequent blood sampling
- Amount and frequency of medication administration
- Need for blood/blood product administration
- Need for maintenance fluid/nutritional support
- Patient's current vascular access

Recommendations exist regarding the use of the various ports of multilumen catheters:

The distal port (16-gauge/brown*) should be used for pressure monitoring, administration of blood products, and general access, since it is within close proximity to the right atrium.

The middle port (18-gauge/blue*) may be used for general access.

*Color and gauge may vary with manufacturer.

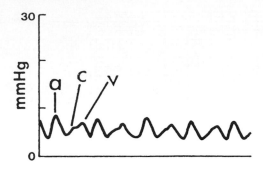

FIGURE 9-6. Central venous pressure waveform with identified **a, c,** and **v** waves.
(From Abbott Laboratories, Mountain View, Calif.)

The proximal port (18-gauge/white*) is recommended for blood sampling and general access.
All ports of these catheters should be flushed with 2.5 mL of heparin (100 U/ml) following intermittent use.[14]

CVP can be measured using pressurized systems and a transducer (*see* Arterial Pressure Monitoring) or a water manometer.

Central pressures obtained from pressurized systems are measured in mm Hg. Those values obtained from a water manometer are measured in cm H_2O.

Normal values:

2 to 6 mm Hg

2 to 8 cm H_2O

To convert mm Hg to cm H_2O, multiply mm Hg $\times$ 1.36.[17] All central venous pressure measurements are mean pressures.

Patient preparation and equipment: *See* Pulmonary Artery Pressure Monitoring.

Interpreting results: Central venous pressure waveform analysis

The CVP waveform consists of three positive waves: **a, c,** and **v** followed by **x, x_1,** and **y** descent or negative waves. The **a** wave signifies atrial systole and is immediately followed by the **x** descent, which reflects atrial relaxation. The **c** wave signifies closure of the tricuspid valve and may have a distinct appearance, may appear as a notch on the **a** wave, or may be absent. The **v** wave signifies right atrial filling, which occurs concomitantly during right ventricular (RV) systole. During RV systole, the closed leaflets of the tricuspid valve bulge into the right atrium. The **y** descent following the **v** wave represents opening of the tricuspid valve and RV filling (Figure 9-6).[16]

Central veins are influenced by the intrathoracic pressure changes that occur during the respiratory cycle. During spontaneous respiration (inspiration), negative pressure within the intrathoracic space causes the CVP to drop. Pressures rise during spontaneous expiration. The opposite phenomenon occurs with mechanically delivered breaths.

The pressure that is delivered with mechanically controlled breaths results in positive pressure within the intrathoracic space during both the inspiratory and expiratory phases of controlled ventilation.[20] During inspiration and to a lesser degree during expiration, the CVP will rise.

To minimize the influence that these changing pressures have on the waveform, CVP should be measured at end expiration, whether the patient is breathing spontaneously or with mechanical ventilation.[16] Intrathoracic pressures at end expiration are relatively constant and allow for a more stable pressure waveform (Figures 9-7 and 9-8).[21]

*Color and gauge may vary with manufacturer.

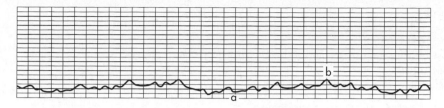

FIGURE 9-7. Central venous pressure waveform during spontaneous respirations. **A,** Inspiration. **B,** End expiration.

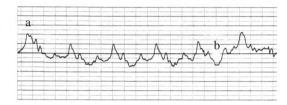

FIGURE 9-8. Central venous pressure waveform during mechanical ventilation. **A,** Inspiration. **B,** End expiration.

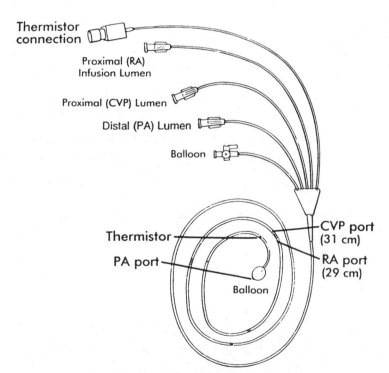

FIGURE 9-9. Pulmonary artery thermodilution catheter.

Potential complications

- Pneumothorax (related to insertion)
- Hemothorax (related to insertion)
- Vessel thrombosis/occlusion
- Bleeding
- Infection/sepsis

- Air embolus
- Neurovascular compromise (at an antecubital site)

■ **THERAPEUTIC INTERVENTIONS**

Frequent neurovascular assessment of extremity (if indicated)

Meticulous site care

Maintenance of a closed system

Pulmonary artery pressure monitoring

Pulmonary artery (PA) pressure monitoring provides direct measurement of pressure within the pulmonary artery. Monitoring is achieved through percutaneous cannulation of a central vein. Central veins commonly used include internal and external jugular and subclavian veins. Femoral and antecubital veins may be used if necessary. Use of a PA catheter allows for direct monitoring of PA pressures (systolic, diastolic, and mean) and central venous pressure and indirect measurement of left ventricular function (PA occlusive/wedge pressure [PaOP]) (Figure 9-9). Other hemodynamic values that may be obtained using the PA catheter include:

- Cardiac output/index
- Systemic vascular resistance
- SvO_2 (mixed venous oxygen saturation)*

Patient preparation

The patient is prepared for any central vein catheterization using aseptic technique. The patient is placed in the Trendelenburg position to allow for venous distention. The skin is prepped with povidone/iodine solution, and the area is draped with sterile towels. The site is infiltrated with 1% lidocaine before cannulation to provide local anesthesia. A percutaneous sheath introducer is inserted first; this allows for immediate vascular access via the side port. Before the PA catheter insertion, the nurse connects and primes all ports of the catheter with a heparinized flush solution. If a fiberoptic catheter is used, the nurse should perform a preinsertion calibration via the oximetric computer/monitor. The PA catheter is advanced into position via the diaphragm of the introducer. It is advanced into the right atrium (RA), right ventricle (RV), and then the PA (Figure 9-10). Continuous cardiac monitoring is required during and after the procedure. During placement of the PA catheter, the role of the nurse may include:

- Observing for cardiac dysrhythmias (PVCs, V-tach)
- Administering lidocaine IVP if indicated (1 mg/kg)
- Observing waveforms and recording pressures (RA, RV, PA systolic and diastolic, PaOP)
- Inflating and deflating the catheter balloon according to physician direction

After the catheter is successfully inserted, a portable chest x-ray is taken to confirm catheter placement and to check for pneumothorax.

PaOP measurements should not be performed by nursing staff until chest x-ray film confirmation and physician approval are obtained. Pulmonary infarction may occur if the catheter tip is too far advanced into the pulmonary vasculature.

*Using a fiberoptic pulmonary catheter.

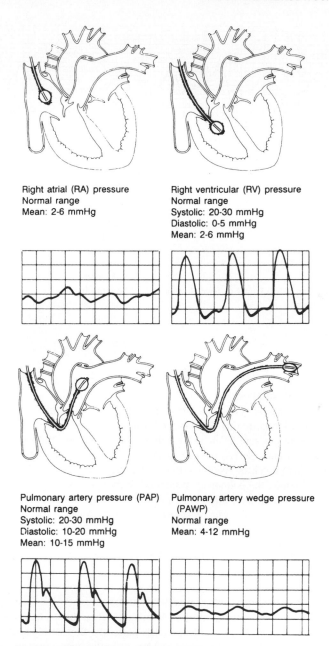

Right atrial (RA) pressure
Normal range
Mean: 2-6 mmHg

Right ventricular (RV) pressure
Normal range
Systolic: 20-30 mmHg
Diastolic: 0-5 mmHg
Mean: 2-6 mmHg

Pulmonary artery pressure (PAP)
Normal range
Systolic: 20-30 mmHg
Diastolic: 10-20 mmHg
Mean: 10-15 mmHg

Pulmonary artery wedge pressure
  (PAWP)
Normal range
Mean: 4-12 mmHg

FIGURE 9-10. Flow directed balloon-tipped catheter as it passes through the right side of the heart, wedging in a distal pulmonary artery with corresponding pressure waveforms and normal values.

(From Alspach JG: *AACN care curriculum for critical care nursing*, ed 4, Philadelphia, 1991, WB Saunders.)

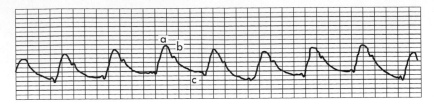

FIGURE 9-11. Pulmonary artery waveform. **A,** Systole. **B,** Dicrotic notch. **C,** Diastole.

Equipment needed:

Sterile drapes
Sterile gloves
Povidone/iodine solution/ointment
1% lidocaine for infiltration
3 cc syringe
Heparinized saline solution (1000 U/500 cc normal saline)
Pressure tubing/transducers
Pressure monitor
Cardiac output computer*

Percutaneous sheath
Introducer kit (8.5 FR)*
Pulmonary artery catheter (#7 French)*
Monitor/computer for SvO_2†
Lidocaine (100 mg Bristojet)
Pressure bag
Transducer holder
Benzoin
Tape
2 × 2s

Interpreting results

■ PULMONARY ARTERY WAVEFORM ANALYSIS

PA pressure consists of two phases: systole and diastole. Systole signifies opening of the pulmonic valve with subsequent rapid ejection of blood into the PA. On the PA waveform, this event is displayed as a sharp rise in pressure followed by a fall in pressure as the volume decreases. When pressures within the right ventricle become less than pressures within the PA, the pulmonic valve abruptly closes. This abrupt closure of the pulmonic valve produces a small notch on the downslope called the *dicrotic notch.* Diastole follows closure of the pulmonic valve. During diastole, the pulmonary system receives runoff blood flow. Further blood flow from the right ventricle does not occur until the next systole. Provided that there is no pulmonary or mitral valve disease, the PA diastolic value (end-diastolic pressure) corresponds closely to the left ventricular end-diastolic pressure (LVEDP)[15] (Figure 9-11).

Normal PA systolic pressure (same as RV systolic):   20 to 30 mm Hg
Normal PA end-diastolic pressure: 8 to 12 mm Hg

See Interpreting Results, Central Venous Pressure Monitoring.

■ PULMONARY ARTERY OCCLUSIVE/WEDGE PRESSURE WAVEFORM ANALYSIS

PaOP is obtained following balloon inflation of the PA catheter. When the PA catheter is positioned in a small branch of the pulmonary artery and balloon inflation takes place, the flow of blood to that segment of the vessel is occluded. PaOP reflects left atrial pressure and has a similar appearance to right atrial pressure (presence of **a, c,** and **v** waves). The **a** wave represents left atrial systole, the **c** wave, often difficult to observe, signifies closure of the mitral valve, and the **v** wave represents filling of the left atrium.[16]

Similar to a CVP reading, a PaOP (PAW) pressure is recorded as a mean value[16] (Figure 9-12).

Normal PaOP = 4 to 12 mm Hg

*Not required for CVP catheter placement.
†Only if fiberoptic PA catheter is used.

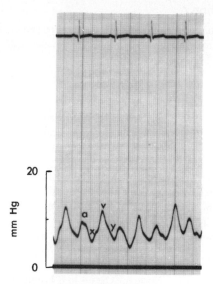

FIGURE 9-12. Normal pulmonary artery wedge (PAW) pressure waveform showing *a* and *v* waves and *x* and *y* descents. The mean of this PAW pressure is about 8 mm Hg.

(From Daily EK, Schroeder JS: *Techniques in bedside hemodynamic monitoring,* ed 4, St Louis, 1989, Mosby.)

Potential complications

Potential complications seen with pulmonary artery pressure monitoring include:
- Thrombosis/emboli
- Infection/sepsis
- Bleeding
- Coagulopathy (secondary to heparin)
- Pneumothorax
- Hemothorax
- Pulmonary infarction
- Air embolus
- Ventricular dysrhythmias
- Ventricular perforation
- Distal neurovascular compromise*

■ THERAPEUTIC INTERVENTIONS
- Meticulous site care
- Maintenance of a closed system
- Performing wedge pressures only when indicated
- Ongoing assessment of PA waveform
- Continuous cardiac monitoring
- Assuring that balloon is deflated after each wedge pressure is obtained
- Routine documentation of catheter position (in cm)

*Seen with femoral or peripheral sites.

Cardiac output determination

Cardiac output (CO) is the amount of blood ejected from the left ventricle per minute. CO is a product of stroke volume and heart rate. Stroke volume (SV) equals the amount of blood ejected by the left ventricle with each contraction.

$$CO = SV \times HR$$

where HR = heart rate.[17]

Using the PA catheter, cardiac output is measured via the thermodilution method. The thermodilution method is based on the theory of temperature change as an indicator of circulating blood volume. The thermistor port of the PA catheter, when attached to a cardiac output computer, provides an accurate measurement of blood temperature (core temp).

The nurse quickly injects a predetermined amount (usually 10 mL) of room temperature* D_5W through the proximal lumen of the PA catheter. This procedure is repeated three times. An average of the three values is obtained provided they are within an acceptable range of each other. Studies have shown an expected variance of 4% to 10% to occur between sequential measurements.[21]

The thermistor senses the temperature of the blood in the PA: the cardiac output computer calculates the cardiac output in liters per minute[15]:

$$Normal\ CO = 4\ to\ 8\ L/min$$

Cardiac index (CI) or the corrected CO according to body size and based on body surface area (BSA) is determined by[17]:

$$CI = CO/BSA$$
$$Normal\ CI = 2.5\ to\ 4.0\ L/min$$

Physiologic changes that may influence CO/CI include:
- Any changes in heart rate (affects diastolic filling time)
- Changes in preload (increased preload, increased CO; decreased preload, decreased CO)
- Extreme changes in afterload (decrease in CO)
- Venous constriction (increase in CO)
- Venous dilation (decrease in CO)
- Hypothermia (decreases in CO)

Systemic Vascular Resistance

Systemic vascular resistance represents the average resistance to blood flow within all vascular beds of the systemic circulation. SVR is a calculated value rather than a direct value. Pressure differences from either end of the circulatory system and measurements of blood flow determine SVR.[19]

$$SVR = \frac{MAP - CVP}{CO} \times 80$$
$$Normal\ values = 770\ to\ 1500\ dyne\ sec/cm$$

Any change in MAP, CVP, or CO will influence SVR.
   Conditions resulting in a decreased SVR:
- Neurogenic shock
- Hyperthermia
- Cardiogenic shock (uncompensated)

*Iced injectate may be indicated in the hypothermic patient to allow for an adequate temperature difference.

- Hypovolemia (uncompensated)

Conditions resulting in an elevated SVR:

- Hypothermia
- Hypovolemia (compensated)
- Low cardiac output (compensated)

Accuracy of Data

To ensure accuracy and reliability of the data obtained from any pressurized hemodynamic monitoring system, the following steps should take place before data collection:

1. Zero-calibrate the system to atmospheric air.
2. Leveling:
   - Phlebostatic axis or midchest (Figures 9-13 and 9-14)
   - Insertion site
3. Check all connections for tightness and proper alignment.
4. Check catheter for proper position.
5. Check extremity for proper position and alignment.
6. Determine dynamic response by performing a square wave test (Figure 9-15).

A "pole mount" system describes a system where the transducer is leveled to the phlebostatic axis or midchest position. There is recent evidence to suggest improved accuracy when leveling the transducer to the site of the catheter. This is called *patient mount*. The dynamic response represents a function of the entire monitoring system, which includes any component of the fluid path between the transducer and the catheter tip. This response measures the ability of the fluid-filled system to accurately reproduce pressure changes that occur in the cardiovascular system (waveforms). A good dynamic response reflects[22]:

- Accurate representation by the transducer due to a high natural frequency of the monitoring system
- The pressures within the patient's blood vessels
- Pressures within the heart chambers

The square wave test reflects the dynamic response of a hemodynamic system. This test is performed by activating the fast flush mechanism. The portion of the wave that is square is produced by the fast flush. Closure of the fast flush system produces the wave or oscillation after the square wave[22] (Figure 9-16).

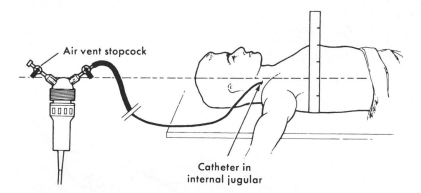

FIGURE 9-13. The patient's midchest position is measured, marked, and used as an anatomic reference point for placement of the transducer.

(From Daily EK, Schroeder JS: *Techniques is bedside hemodynamic monitoring*, ed 4, St Louis, 1989, Mosby.)

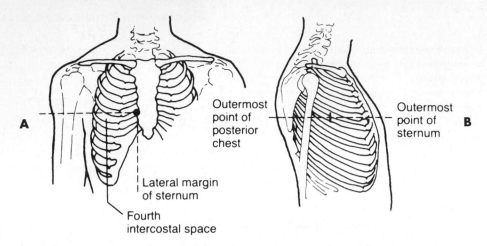

FIGURE 9-14. The phlebostatic axis. The crossing of two imaginary lines defines the assumed position of the monitoring catheter tip within the body (i.e., right atrial levels). **A,** A line that passes from the fourth intercostal space at the lateral margin of the sternum down the side of the body beneath the axilla. **B,** A line that runs horizontally at a part midway between the outermost position of the anterior and posterior surfaces of the chest.

(From Darovic G: *Hemodynamic monitoring, invasive and noninvasive clinical application*, Philadelphia, 1987, WB Saunders.)

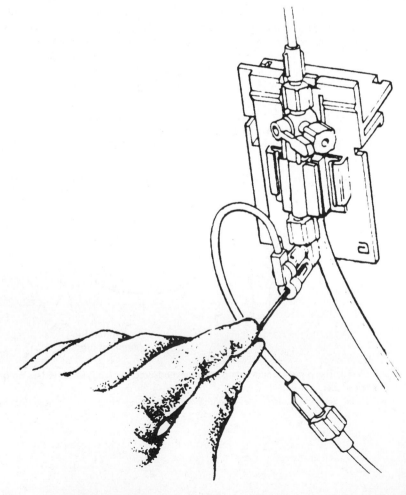

FIGURE 9-15. Method for performing a square wave test.

(From Abbott Laboratories, Mountain View, Calif.)

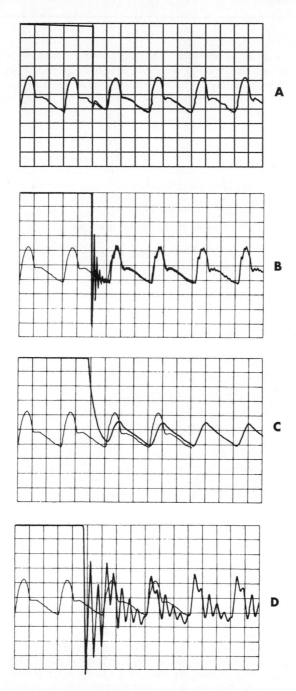

FIGURE 9-16. Assessing dynamic response. **A,** Optimally damped. The fast flush trace ends with small undershoot followed by an even smaller overshoot. **B,** Acceptable. The fast flush trace ending in rapid oscillations that subside before the next patient waveform indicates a high natural frequency system. Patient waveform distortion will be minimal despite underdamping. **C,** Overdamped. The fast flush trace slowly returns toward the next patient waveform without any sign of oscillation. **D,** Highly underdamped. The fast flush trace ends in a series of oscillations that persist into the next patient waveform. (From Abbott Laboratories, Mountain View, Calif.)

CONCLUSION

The clinical presentation of shock can occur for a variety of reasons. The common thread in all shock states is a reduction in tissue perfusion with a resultant imbalance of cellular oxygen supply and demand. Measures to optimize CO and oxygen delivery to improve tissue perfusion remain the hallmarks of treatment. Prompt diagnosis and treatment remain essential contributing factors in reducing the overall morbidity and mortality in shock states.

REFERENCES

1. Herckes R, Bihari DJ: Management of shock. In Tinker J, Zapol W, editors: *Care of the critically ill patient,* New York, 1992, Springer-Verlag.
2. Mouchawar A, Rosenthal M: A pathophysiological approach to the patient in shock. In Rosenthal M, editor: *Recent advances in critical care medicine: international anesthesiology clinics,* Boston, 1993, Little, Brown.
3. Rice V: Shock a clinical syndrome: an update. Part 2, The stages of shock, *Crit Care Nurs* 11(5):74, 1991.
4. American College of Surgeons' Committee on Trauma: *Advanced trauma life support instructor manual,* Chicago, 1997, the Committee.
5. Emergency Nurses Association: *Sheehy's emergency nursing: principles and practice,* ed 4, St Louis, 1998, Mosby.
6. Summers G: The clinical and hemodynamic presentation of the shock patient, *Crit Care Nurs Clin North Am* 2(2):161, 1990.
7. Houston M: Pathophysiology of shock, *Crit Care Nurs Clin North Am* 2(2):143, 1990.
8. Franaszek JB: Cardiogenic shock. In Rosen P et al, editors: *Emergency: emergency medicine,* ed 4, St Louis, 1997, Mosby.
9. Boyd J, Stanford G, Chernow B: The pathophysiology of shock. In Tinker J, Zapol W, editors: *Care of the critically ill patient,* New York, 1992, Springer-Verlag.
10. Trunkey DD, Salber PR, Mills J: Shock. In Saunders CE, Ho MT, editors: *Current emergency diagnosis and treatment,* Norwalk, Conn, 1992, Appleton & Lange.
11. Kuhn MM: Colloids versus crystalloids, *Critical Care Nurse* 11(5):37, 1991.
12. American Association of Blood Banks: *Standards for blood banks and transfusion services manual,* ed 18, Bethesda, Md, 1998, the Association.
13. Blansfield J: Emergency autotransfusion in hypovolemia, *Crit Care Nurs Clin North Am* 2(2):195, 1990.
14. Holder C, Alexander J: A new and improved guide to IV therapy, *AJN* 43, 1990.
15. Palmer D: Advanced hemodynamic assessment, *Dimens Crit Care Nurs* 1(3):139, 1982.
16. Daily E: *Techniques in bedside hemodynamic monitoring,* ed 5, St Louis, 1994, Mosby.
17. *American Association of Critical Care Nurses, core curriculum for critical care nursing,* ed 5, Philadelphia, 1998, Saunders.
18. Swearingen PL: *Manual of critical care: applying nursing diagnoses to adult critical illness,* St Louis, 1988, Mosby.
19. Darovic G: *Hemodynamic monitoring: invasive and noninvasive clinical application,* ed 2, Philadelphia, 1995, Saunders.
20. Thielen J: Air emboli: a potentially lethal complication of central venous lines, *Focus* 17(5):374, 1990.
21. Quaal S: Hemodynamic monitoring: a review of the literature, *Appl Nurs Res* 1(2):58, 1988.
22. Abbott Critical Care Systems: *Hemodynamic monitoring learning program,* Chicago, 1989, Abbott Laboratories, Hospital Product Division.

SUGGESTED READINGS

Ackerman MH, Evans NJ, Ecklund MM: Systemic inflammatory response syndrome, sepsis, and nutritional support, *Crit Care Nurs Clin North Am* 6:321, 1994.
Ackerman MH: The systemic inflammatory response, sepsis, and multiple organ dysfunction: new definitions for an old problem, *Crit Care Nurs Clin North Am* 6:243, 1994.
Cowley SR: The pathogenesis of septic shock, *Heart Lung* 25:124, 1996.
Fiddian-Green RG, Haglund U, Gutierrez G et al: Goals for the resuscitation of shock, *Crit Care Med* 21:S25, 1993.
Gattinoni L et al: A trial of goal oriented hemodynamic therapy in critically ill patients, *N Engl J Med* 333:1025, 1995.
Goodnough LT: Current red blood cell transfusion practices, *AACN Clin Issues* 7:212, 1996.
Kelly KM: Does increasing oxygen delivery improve outcome? Yes, *Crit Care Clin* 12:635, 1996.
Summers G: The clinical and hemodynamic presentation of the shock patient, *Crit Care Nurs Clin North Am* 2:161, 1990.
Tuchschmidt JA, Mecher CE: Predictors of outcome from critical illness: shock and cardiopulmonary resuscitation, *Crit Care Clin* 10:179, 1994.
Von Reuden KT, Dunham CM: Sequelae of massive fluid resuscitation in trauma patients, *Crit Care Nurs Clin North Am* 6:463, 1994.

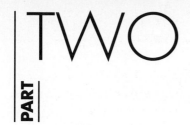

Medical Emergencies

Cardiac Emergencies

Diane Panton Lapsley

Chest pain can be the chief patient complaint in a variety of different but serious cardiac emergencies. Any time the heart is in jeopardy the caregiver must ascertain the problem and begin treating it without the luxury of lengthy assessments or in-depth history taking. This chapter presents the essential elements of cardiac assessment in the emergency setting. It then outlines, by point of origination, various cardiac conditions that can produce chest pain and the corresponding emergency treatments. Common noncardiac conditions that produce chest pain are also listed. Finally, congestive heart failure, a common cardiac emergency, is discussed. This chapter is not designed to be a definitive course in cardiac care, but rather provides rapid detection methods and initial treatment options for suspected cardiac problems.

ASSESSMENT OF CHEST PAIN

Determine vital signs, skin vital signs (color, temperature, and moistness), pulse oximetry and/or arterial blood gas (ABG).
Examine a rhythm strip (lead II or MCL) for the presence of dysrhythmias.
Further examine the chief complaint and obtain a brief history.
Use the PQRST mnemonic to assist in gathering facts about the pain.

P = Provokes

What provokes the pain? What makes it better? What makes it worse?

Q = Quality

What does it feel like? Is it sharp? Dull? Burning? Stabbing? Crushing? (Try to let the patient describe it before offering choices.)

R = Radiates

Where does the pain radiate? Is it in one place? Does it go to any other place?

S = Severity

How severe is the pain? On a scale of 1 to 10, with 1 being the least pain and 10 being the worst, what rating would you give the pain? (Watch for nonverbal clues with this question. A patient may be writhing in pain and tell you the pain is a 2, or a patient may sit there very calmly and quietly and tell you the pain is a 10.)

T = Time

When did it start? How long did it last?

Other Useful Data to Collect

Find out if the patient has a history (or a family history) of heart disease, lung disease, stroke, or hypertension.

Ask if the patient is taking any medications. (Use words such as "heart pills" or "water pills" if necessary.)

Ask if it hurts to take a deep breath.

Find out what the patient was doing when the pain began.

Ask if the patient has ever had this pain before.

Ask if it is different this time.

Check the patient for level of consciousness.

Check the patient's pupils for equality, reaction to light, and accommodation. (Remember that 10% of the population has unequal pupils.)

Examine the jugular veins for distension.

Check the trachea to see that it is in a midline position.

Inquire as to a recent history of trauma.

In these early phases of myocardial infarction, it is essential to pay particular attention to the relief of pain and the prevention of dysrhythmias.

ELECTROCARDIOGRAPH MONITORING

Monitoring on a four-lead monitoring system (with an automatic lead switch button) is shown in Figure 10-1.

When monitoring on a three-lead ECG monitor (without an automatic lead switch button), the best lead placement to use is Lead II or MCL_1. Leads II and MCL_1 are the best leads to monitor for dysrhythmias.

Standard 12-Lead Electrocardiograph

The standard 12-lead ECG (Figures 10-2 and 10-3) takes 12 views of the heart's electrical activity and records it on standardized ECG paper or in the computer system.

Before beginning:

1. Check to be sure that all leads are placed correctly.
   a. "Green and white on the right, Christmas trees (red and green) below the knees" is a helpful memory aid.
   b. Ensure that there is a conduction medium between the electrodes and the patient.
   c. Avoid placing the electrodes over large muscle masses.
   d. Remove excess hair if necessary to ensure good skin contact. (You may need to rub the skin with an alcohol pad to remove excess dry skin or hair particles.)
2. Ensure that lead wires are not touching anything metal (this will cause 60-cycle interference).
3. If 60-cycle interference occurs, check for the following:
   a. Loose leads
   b. Leads and wires against metal
   c. Other electrical machines that could be unplugged
4. If the patient will be transferred to a coronary care or intensive care unit where an ECG will be done each day, mark the chest where chest leads are placed to ensure that the leads will have the same placement each time the ECG is recorded.
5. Attempt to maintain the patient's modesty. Explain what you are doing.
6. Record the patient's name, the date, and the time the ECG was taken directly on the ECG strip.
7. Interpret the strip or relay it to the appropriate individual for interpretation.

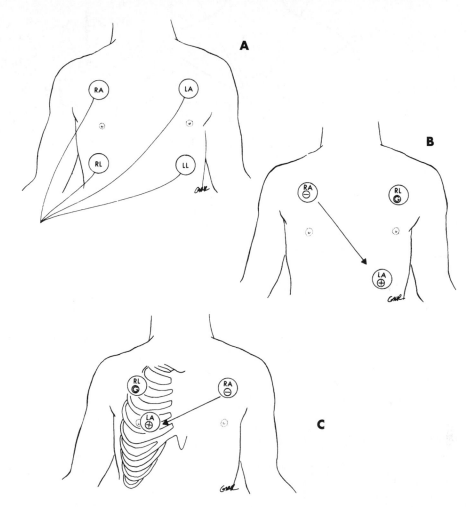

FIGURE 10-1. Lead placement for four-lead monitoring system (with automatic lead switch button). **A,** Monitoring on three-lead system (without automatic lead switch button). **B,** Lead II. **C,** Lead MCL$_1$.

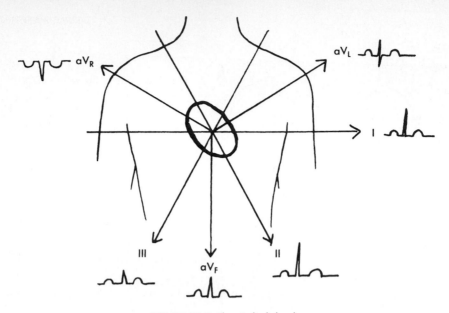

FIGURE 10-2. The six limb leads.

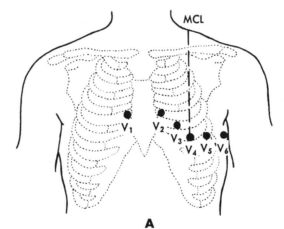

A

FIGURE 10-3. Electrode positions of the precordial leads. **A,** V_1, fourth intercostal space at right sternal border; V_2, fourth intercostal space at left sternal border; V_3, halfway between V_2 and V_4; fifth intercostal space at midclavicular line; V_5, anterior axillary line directly lateral to V_4, V_6, midaxillary line directly lateral to V_5. **B,** Precordial reference figure. Leads V_1 and V_2 are called right-sided precordial leads; leads V_3 and V_4, midprecordial leads; and leads V_5 and V_6, left-sided precordial leads.

(Modified from Andreoli K et al: *Comprehensive cardiac care: a text for nurses, physicians, and other health practitioners,* ed 6, St Louis, 1987, Mosby.)

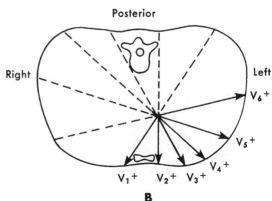

B

Interpretation

When current flows toward a lead (arrowheads, positive electrode), an upward ECG deflection occurs. When current flows away from a lead (arrowhead, positive electrode), a downward deflection of the ECG occurs. When current flows perpendicular to a lead (arrowhead, positive electrode), diphasic deflection of the ECG occurs.

When examining a 12-lead ECG, examine each of the 12 leads individually and note any of the following:

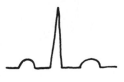

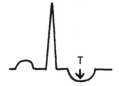

Normal

Ischemia
   T wave inversion
   (intramural eschemia)
   Decreased blood supply
   ST Segment depression
   (subendocardial ischemia)

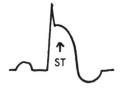

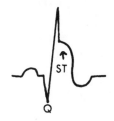

Injury
   Acute or
   recent; the
   more elevated
   the ST segment,
   the more recent
   the injury

Infarct
   Significant Q wave
   greater than 0.04 seconds
   wide and greater than
   25% of the associated
   R wave
   Indicates myocardial
   necrosis

The leads directly recording the area of infarct will demonstrate changes. An anterior wall myocardial infarction appears in leads V_2, V_3, V_4.

Limb leads

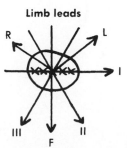

Chest leads

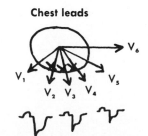

An inferior wall myocardial infarction appears in leads II, III, and V_F.

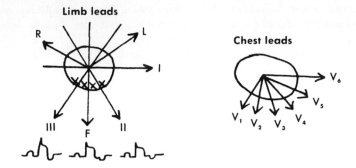

A lateral wall myocardial infarction appears in leads I, aV_L, V_5, and V_6.

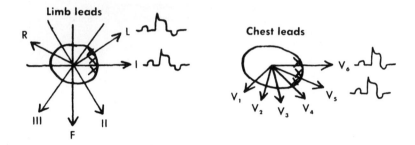

A posterior wall myocardial infarction appears in leads V_1 and V_2. The first **r** wave is tall, there is a depressed ST segment, and there is an elevated **t** wave.

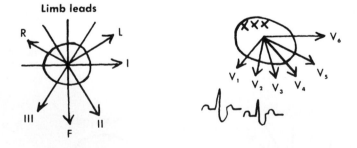

Plotting a simple axis

An axis is a graphic representation of the main vector in the heart.

■ **EQUIPMENT**

12-lead ECG

Graph paper

Ruler

Writing instrument

■ **PROCEDURE**

1. Draw leads I and aV$_F$ lines on graph paper.

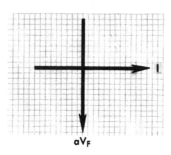

2. Examine lead I of the ECG.
   a. Determine if it is positive or negative.
   b. Determine by how much.

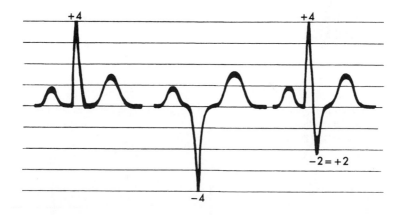

3. Plot the positive inflection or negative deflection on the graph paper by drawing a perpendicular line.
   a. Positive goes *toward* the lead.
   b. Negative goes *away from* the lead.

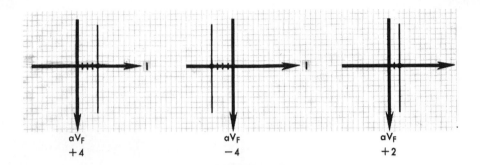

4. Examine lead aV_F of the ECG.
   a. Determine if it is positive or negative.
   b. Determine by how much.

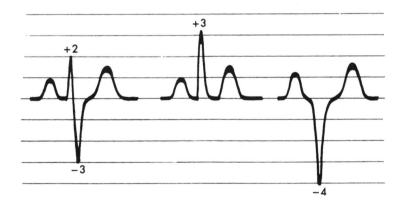

5. Plot the positive inflection or negative deflection on the graph paper by drawing a perpendicular line.
   a. Positive goes *toward* the lead.
   b. Negative goes *away from* the lead.

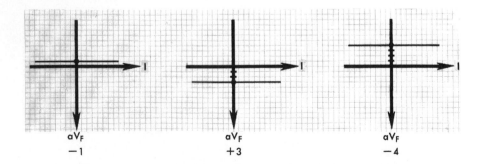

6. The intersection of the plots of leads I and aV_F is the axis.

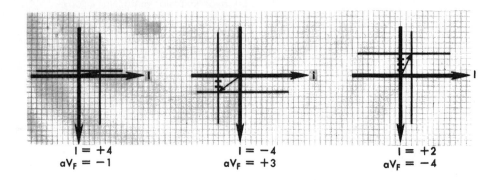

$$I = +4$$
$$aV_F = -1$$

$$I = -4$$
$$aV_F = +3$$

$$I = +2$$
$$aV_F = -4$$

7. Superimpose a protractor compass over the graph paper to determine the exact degree of axis or estimate the degree of axis by quadrants.

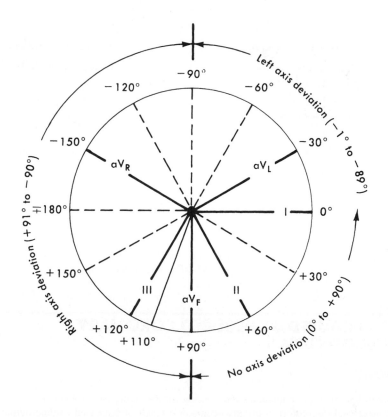

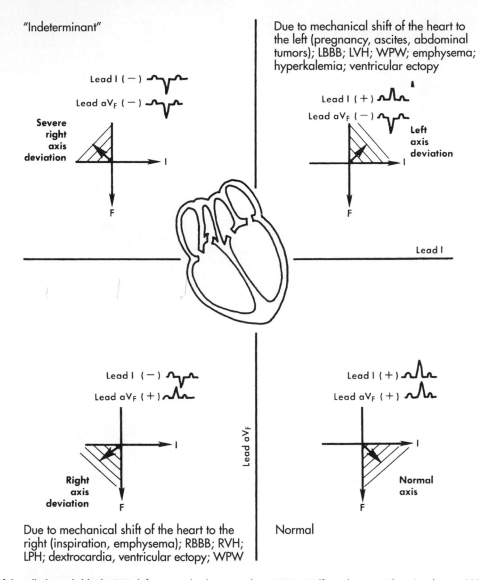

"Indeterminant"

Lead I (−)

Lead aV$_F$ (−)

Severe
right
axis
deviation

Due to mechanical shift of the heart to
the left (pregnancy, ascites, abdominal
tumors); LBBB; LVH; WPW; emphysema;
hyperkalemia; ventricular ectopy

Lead I (+)

Lead aV$_F$ (−)

Left
axis
deviation

Lead I

Lead I (−)

Lead aV$_F$ (+)

Right
axis
deviation

Lead I (+)

Lead aV$_F$ (+)

Normal
axis

Lead aV$_F$

Due to mechanical shift of the heart to the
right (inspiration, emphysema); RBBB; RVH;
LPH; dextrocardia, ventricular ectopy; WPW

Normal

LBBB, left bundle branch block; LVH, left ventricular hypertrophy; WPW, Wolfe-Parkinson White Syndrome; RBBB, right
bundle branch block; RVH, right ventricular hypertrophy; LPH, left posterior hemiblock.

CHEST PAIN CAUSED BY REDUCED CORONARY ARTERY BLOOD FLOW

Angina Pectoris

When the myocardium becomes anoxic, a condition known as angina pectoris occurs.

Described as retrosternal discomfort, it usually occurs as a result of increased cardiac output and increased
oxygen demand with an underlying diseased coronary artery system.

TABLE 10-1   Differential Diagnosis of Angina

	STABLE ANGINA	UNSTABLE ("PREINFARCTION") ANGINA
Location of pain	Substernal; may radiate to jaws and neck and down arms and back	Substernal; may radiate to jaws and neck and down arms and back
Duration of pain	1 to 15 minutes	5 minutes, occurring more frequently
Characteristic of pain	Ache, squeezing, choking, heavy; burning	Same as stable angina, but more intense
Other symptoms	None, usually	Diaphoresis; weakness
Pain worsened by	Exercise; activity; eating; cold weather; reclining	Exercise; activity; eating; cold weather, reclining
Pain relieved by	Rest; nitroglycerin; isosorbide (Isordil)	Nitroglycerin
ECG findings	Transient ST depression; disappears with pain relief	ST segment depression; often T-wave inversion; but ECG may be normal

Most angina is caused by a partial occlusion of the coronary arteries, usually because of atherosclerosis.

It can also be caused by arterial spasms, emboli, or a dissecting aortic aneurysm.

Is not usually sharply localized.

Refer to Table 10-1 for a differential diagnosis of angina.

stable (typical)   The pain that occurs is predictable and follows events such as exercise, heavy work, or strain.

unstable (preinfarction)   Attacks are prolonged and more severe and occur more frequently. May occur at rest.

Prinzmetal's (variant)   The pain occurs while the patient is at rest or with exercise (unpredictable). During the attack the ST segment may be elevated. The pain may be intense and prolonged, and not quickly relieved with nitroglycerin. Treatment includes nitrates, calcium channel blockers, and low-dose aspirin. Consider PTCA if there is a fixed lesion, or consider CABG if multivessel disease is present.

Myocardial Infarction

Myocardial infarction (MI) is a localized ischemic necrosis of an area of the myocardium caused by a narrowing of one or more of the coronary arteries. The narrowing may be caused by a thrombus, spasm, or hemorrhage. The size and location of the infarction depend on the location of the block in the coronary artery (Table 10-2).

Clinical findings in myocardial infarction

Pain of sudden onset that lasts from several minutes to several days. It is usually localized in the substernal area and radiates up into the jaw or down into the arm. It also may have an atypical presentation, such as a toothache or other painful sensation.

Frequently described as crushing, sharp, or burning, or as a pressure, tightness, or choking.

Nausea and vomiting.

Blood pressure is usually decreased.

Increased pulse.

Edema caused by decreased cardiac output and increased venous pressure.

Heart sounds will vary depending on the physiologic status of the myocardium.

Therapeutic interventions
Medications

■ **NITROGLYCERIN**
   Sublingual
   Administer an initial dose of nitroglycerin 0.4 mg or 1/150 g.
   Monitor blood pressure before and after nitroglycerin administration.
   Do not administer nitroglycerin unless systolic blood pressure is above 100 mm Hg.

TABLE 10-2 Coronary Arteries in Myocardial Infarction

RIGHT CORONARY ARTERY

LEFT CORONARY ARTERY

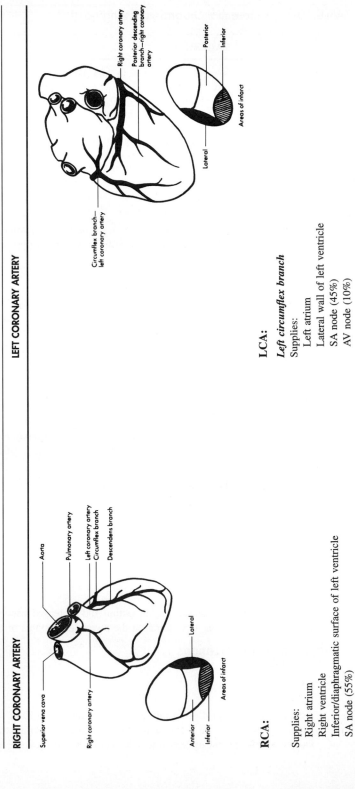

RCA:

Supplies:
Right atrium
Right ventricle
Inferior/diaphragmatic surface of left ventricle
SA node (55%)
AV node (90%)
Bundle of His

LCA:

Left circumflex branch
Supplies:
Left atrium
Lateral wall of left ventricle
SA node (45%)
AV node (10%)
Posterior/inferior division of left bundle

Block causes:
Infarction of posterior or inferior wall of left ventricle
Right ventricle infarction
In inferior myocardial infarction (leads II, III, aV_F) anticipate second-degree heart block, Mobitz type I block (Wenckebach)

Block causes:
Lateral wall infarction
Posterior wall infarction (near base)
In lateral wall MI, ECG changes seen in leads I, AV_L, V_{5-6}

Left anterior descending branch
Supplies:
Anterior wall of left ventricle
Interventricular septum
Bundle of His
Right bundle
Posterior/inferior division of left bundle
Apex of left ventricle
Block causes:
Infarction of anterior wall of left ventricle
Effect on papillary muscle (which attaches to mitral valve)
In anterior myocardial infarction (leads V_2, V_3, V_4) anticipate second-degree heart block, Mobitz type II block or third-degree block

If the initial dose is not effective, administer an additional tablet (again, ensuring that the patient's systolic pressure is greater than 100 mm Hg). A third dose can be given if needed and tolerated.

Intravenous

Administer a bolus of 12.5 to 25 mcg followed by an infusion of 10 to 20 mcg/min and increase by 5 to 10 mcg/min every 5 to 10 min until pain is relieved, systolic blood pressure drops to less than 90 mmHg, or heart rate increases to over 110 bpm. Maximum IV dose is 200 mcg/min. Side effects of nitroglycerin include hypotension with tachycardia and ischemia, and headache. Avoid giving nitroglycerin to patients with right ventricular infarction. Use caution when giving nitroglycerin and heparin together as it may inhibit heparin, which may require larger doses of heparin for recommended aPTT. The heparin may need to be adjusted when nitroglycerin is discontinued.

■ BETA BLOCKER THERAPY

Beta blocker therapy has been shown to reduce mortality and morbidity after AMI. It reduces the incidence of ventricular fibrillation, decreases myocardial oxygen demand by decreasing heart rate, systemic arterial pressure and myocardial contractility. Reinfarction and recurrent ischemia are decreased. Beta-blocking agents are contraindicated in patients with heart rates less than 60 bpm, systolic blood pressure less than 100 mmHg, moderate to severe left ventricular failure, heart block, severe COPD, or asthma. Side effects include AV block, excess bradycardia, and hypotension. Common beta-blocking agents include:

Esmolol: administer a 500 mcg/Kg/min bolus followed by 50 to 250 mcg/Kg/min. Bolus and administration doses may be repeated.

Metoprolol: administer 5 mg IV bolus over 2 min times 3 doses. Oral doses range from 50 to 100 mg bid.

Propranolol: administer 0.033 mg/Kg IV bolus over 2 min times 3 doses every 5 min. Oral dose is 20-80 mg qid.

Atenolol: administer 5 mg IV over 5 min times 2 doses. Oral dose is 100 mg qd.

■ OXYGEN

Administer via nasal prongs to prevent hypoxemia.

■ ASPIRIN

Administer 160 to 325 mg chewed for rapid absorption. The antiplatelet activity of aspirin has been shown to decrease mortality after AMI. Do not give to patients who are hypersensitive to salicylates or who have active ulcer disease.

■ ANGIOTENSIN CONVERTING ENZYME (ACE) INHIBITORS

ACE inhibitors are useful for large or anterior wall MI, heart failure without hypotension, and patients with prior MI. Common agents are enalapril, captopril, and lisinopril.

■ MORPHINE SULFATE

Morphine sulfate is the drug of choice for chest pain of myocardial origin. Besides relieving pain as a narcotic-analgesic, morphine sulfate reduces preload and decreases myocardial oxygen demand.

Administer slowly intravenously at a dosage of 2 to 10 mg, titrated to effect.

Do not give if systolic blood pressure is below 90 mm Hg.

If hypotension should occur, elevate the patient's legs to facilitate venous return to the central circulation, as for nitroglycerin-induced hypotension.

If there is respiratory depression, administer naloxone hydrochloride (Narcan) 0.8 mg IV. Naloxone acts rapidly to reverse the effects of morphine sulfate.

The presence of chronic obstructive pulmonary disease is a relative contraindication to the use of morphine sulfate.

■ ANTIDYSRHYTHMICS

Consider antidysrhythmics only for life-threatening or severely symptomatic dysrhythmias.

Lidocaine: administer an IV bolus of 1 to 1.5 mg/Kg, additional bolus of 0.5 to 0.75 mg/Kg every 5 to 10 min up to 3 mg/Kg. A maintenance infusion of 1 to 4 mg/min may follow.

Thrombolytic therapy

A pharmacologic agent is administered to dissolve thrombi that typically form at the site of atherosclerotic lesion.

■ **GOALS**

Prevention of myocardial necrosis

Reduction of myocardial ischemia

Limitation of myocardial infarct size

Improvement of left ventricular function

■ **INDICATIONS**

Acute chest pain indicative of MI within 6 hours of onset.

ECG evidence of ST-segment elevation or new left bundle branch block

■ **CONTRAINDICATIONS**

Previous hemorrhagic stroke, aortic dissection, active internal bleeding.

Known intracranial bleed

Other stroke or cerebrovascular event within 1 year

Types of agents

Streptokinase, anisoylated plasminogen activator complex (APSAC), tissue plasminogen activator (t-PA), and recombinant tissue plasminogen activator (rt-PA).

Method of administration: Intravenous

NOTE: Heparin therapy is initiated concurrently with t-PA or rt-PA to prevent rethrombosis.

Streptokinase: 1.5 million units IV over 60 min

APSAC: 30 units IV over 2 to 5 min

t-PA: Standard dose is 10 mg IV push over 1 to 2 min followed by a 50 mg infusion over 1 hour, then 20 mg infusion over 1 hour, then another 20 mg infusion over 1 hour. A total of 100 mg is infused over 3 hours.

Accelerated dose by weight: 15 mg IV bolus over 1 to 2 min, followed by 0.75 mg/kg IV infusion over 30 min (maximum of 50 mg), then followed by 0.50 mg/kg IV infusion over 60 min (maximum of 35 mg).

rt-PA: Accelerated dose is 15 mg bolus IV over 1-2 min, followed by an infusion of 50 mg over 30 min then 35 mg over 60 min.

■ **COMPLICATIONS**

Bleeding

Reocclusion/reinfarction

Allergic reaction with SK, APSAC

Reperfusion dysrhythmias

Hematoma at insertion site

Hypotension

Primary percutaneous transluminal coronary angioplasty (PTCA)

Primary percutaneous transluminal coronary angioplasty (PTCA) is a nonsurgical method of revascularizing myocardial tissue. Under sterile conditions in a catheterization lab, a steerable catheter is threaded into the coronary artery through a femoral artery sheath and positioned at the site of the coronary stenosis. The plaque is flattened against the artery wall (i.e., PTCA) or removed altogether (i.e., PDCA).

■ **GOALS**

Prevention of myocardial necrosis

Reduction of myocardial ischemia

Limitation of myocardial infarct size

Improvement of left ventricular function

CHEST PAIN ORIGINATING FROM THE PERICARDIUM

Acute Pericarditis

Acute pericarditis is an inflammation of the pericardial sac and can occur as a result of the following conditions:

Idiopathic—following viral or febrile illness. Etiology may not be able to be established.
Infection—viral, bacterial, or fungal in origin
Connective tissue disease
Malignancy—breast, lung, and other tumors can metastasize to the pericardium
Uremia
Drug induced
Postmyocardial infarction (Dressler's syndrome)
Postpericardiotomy

■ SIGNS AND SYMPTOMS

Severe chest pain that increases with respirations or activity
Fever and chills
Diaphoresis
Dyspnea
Tachycardia or other dysrhythmias
Pericardial friction rub (increased when patient leans forward)
Malaise
ST segment elevation of 1 to 3 mm in all ECG leads except aV_R and V_1
Decreased blood pressure (if effusion has occurred)

■ THERAPEUTIC INTERVENTIONS

Treatment of underlying etiology
Chest x-ray film—may assist in establishing etiology
Oxygen
Sedation
Rest
Antibiotics
Analgesia (salicylates)
Nonsteroidal antiinflammatories
Corticosteroids
Pericardiectomy for constrictive pericarditis

Cardiac Tamponade

Cardiac tamponade is a condition in which blood leaks into the pericardial sac. It may be caused by:

Infection
Neoplasm
Open heart surgery
Cardiac catheterization
Dissecting aortic aneurysm
Trauma—most common cause

The compression of the heart caused by the increased fluid in the pericardial sac prevents adequate venous return from the systemic circulation. This produces a critical decrease in cardiac output.

■ SIGNS AND SYMPTOMS

The speed and severity in which signs and symptoms develop depend on the rate of fluid accumulation, pericardial compliance, and intravascular volume. An initial but temporary hypertensive state can exist as decreased cardiac output causes a compensatory vasoconstriction and an increase in peripheral vascular resistance. The patient may develop profound shock with as little as 150 to 200 ml of blood into the pericardial sac. Other signs and symptoms include:

Tachycardia
Elevated CVP (greater than 15 mm Hg)
Decreased blood pressure
Distended neck veins ⎫
Distant heart sounds ⎬ Beck's Triad*
Decreased arterial pressure ⎭
Decreased systolic blood pressure
Narrow pulse pressure
Weak, thready pulse
Cyanosis
Increased respiratory rate
Dyspnea
Paradoxical pulse (see below)
Restlessness
Loss of apical cardiac impulse
Shock
Widening cardiac silhouette on chest x-ray film

Paradoxical pulse

Paradoxical pulse is found in one third of patients experiencing acute pericardial tamponade. It will be noted by an abnormal fall of more than 10 mm Hg in systolic blood pressure during inspiration.

■ **PROCEDURE**
1. Apply a blood pressure cuff to the patient's arm.
2. Inflate the cuff to a level above systolic pressure.
3. Deflate the cuff slowly until the first systolic sound is heard. During normal inspiration the systolic sound will disappear.
4. Deflate the cuff until all systolic sounds can be heard during both inspiration and expiration.
5. Note the point at which all systolic sounds can be heard.
6. The difference in millimeters of mercury between the pressure at which the systolic sound disappears during inspiration and the pressure at which all systolic sounds can be heard is called a paradox.

NOTE: A paradox of more than 10 mm Hg indicates a paradoxical pulse.

■ **THERAPEUTIC INTERVENTIONS**
CVP monitoring
Oxygen
Volume expansion using normal saline, plasma, dextran, blood, or vasoconstriction using vasopressors
Pericardiocentesis (see below)

Pericardiocentesis

See Figure 10-4.

■ **EQUIPMENT**
21-gauge spinal needle (at least 6 inches long)
50-ml syringe
Fluoroscopy (Procedure should ideally be done in cardiac catheterization lab)
Echocardiography

*These 3 symptomatic findings (i.e., decreased blood pressure, distended neck veins, and distant heart sounds) are known in combination as Beck's Triad.

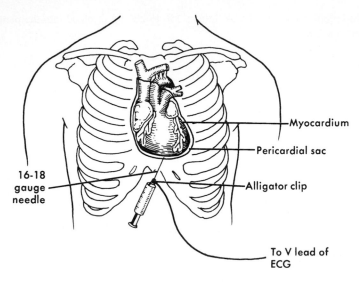

FIGURE 10-4. Pericardiocentesis.

Alligator clips (sterile)
Kelly clamp
3-channel ECG machine
Defibrillator
Three-way stopcock (metal)
Local anesthetic agent
Antiseptic solution
Gloves
Sterile drapes

■ **PROCEDURE**
1. Position the patient supine with trunk elevated 45 degrees.
2. Prepare the patient's chest at the left inferior costal margin and the xiphoid.
3. Administer a local anesthetic to the area.
4. Attach the limb leads to the patient's extremities and to the V5 and V6 precordial leads.
5. Attach one end of an alligator clip to the hub of the 16-gauge needle and the other end of the clip to the V lead of the ECG machine.
6. Attach the needle to the syringe via the three-way stopcock.
7. Run the ECG machine on the V-lead setting.
8. Advance the needle in a subxiphoid approach between the left inferior costal margin and the xiphoid at a 30- to 45-degree angle to the body, advancing toward the tip of the right scapula.
9. Gently aspirate the syringe as the needle is advanced; if blood returns and there is no ST-segment elevation on the ECG, the needle has probably entered the pericardial sac. If an ST-segment elevation appears on the ECG, the needle has pierced the epicardium. If this occurs, withdraw the needle slowly until the ST segment returns to normal. If the needle has gone all the way through to the myocardium, a pulsation will be felt up through the needle and the syringe.
10. Once blood is being withdrawn from the pericardial sac, attach a Kelly clamp to the needle at the level of the skin to avoid accidental advancement of the needle.

NOTE: Blood withdrawn from the pericardial sac should not clot because it has been defibrinated in the sac. Also, samples should be placed in sterile tubes for lab analysis.

■ **COMPLICATIONS**
  Laceration of a coronary artery
  Laceration of the lung or liver
  Laceration of the ventricle
  Cardiac dysrhythmias
  Increased tamponade

CHEST PAIN OF AORTIC ORIGIN

Aortic Dissection

Aortic dissection affects twice as many men as women, especially between the ages of 50 and 70. It is frequently seen in conjunction with arteriosclerotic heart disease and hypertension. Other causes of dissection are trauma and Marfan's syndrome, which occur primarily in the young (Figure 10-5).

An aortic dissection is a tear in the intimal layer of the aorta that allows blood to leak between the intimal and medial layers. There are three types of aortic dissection.

Type I

Dissection of the descending aorta to and beyond the aortic arch (occurs in two thirds of cases).

Type II

Dissection of the ascending aorta alone.

Type III

Dissection from beyond the left subclavian artery.

Dissection may cause occlusion of major vessels that branch off from the aorta, such as the myocardial, cerebral, mesenteric, and renal vessels. Rupture of the dissection may have two results: (1) rupture into the pericardial sac causing pericardial tamponade and (2) rupture into the chest cavity causing exsanguination.

■ **SIGNS AND SYMPTOMS**
  Chest pain—described as sudden, excruciating or tearing; anteroposterior in nature (may be confused with myocardial infarction, back pain, pericarditis, or peptic ulcer). Occurs in 90% of cases.

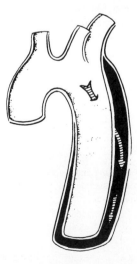

FIGURE 10-5. A dissecting aortic aneurysm.

Dyspnea
Orthopnea
Diaphoresis
Pallor
Apprehension
Syncope
Tachycardia
Absence of major arterial pulses *unilaterally*
Blood pressure differences between arms (in a thoracic aortic dissection)
Hypertension
Pulse at the sternoclavicular joint
Murmur of aortic insufficiency (in type II)
Hemiplegia or paraplegia
Shock
Widened mediastinum

■ **THERAPEUTIC INTERVENTIONS**

NOTE: The aim is to prevent rupture.

High Fowler's position
Oxygen
IV D$_5$W TKO
Nitroprusside to keep systolic blood pressure at 100 to 120 mm Hg
Propranolol
Much support and reassurance
Preparation for surgery—emergent if systolic blood pressure drops below 100 mm Hg

CHEST PAIN OF OTHER ORIGINS

Hyperventilation

Hyperventilation is one of the most common conditions. It may occur as a result of anxiety, or it may be caused by a disease process such as salicylate overdose, myocardial infarction, or intracerebral bleeding. Pay close attention to associated signs and symptoms that may lead to the discovery of an underlying disorder. Avoid "tunnel vision" and keep your mind open to all possibilities for the cause. Hyperventilation may be a response to a disease process that, when treated with the traditional breathing into a paper bag, could cause serious complications. Medical illness *must be ruled out* before assuming that the hyperventilation is caused by anxiety or an hysterical response.

■ **CAUSES**

Anxiety
Pregnancy
Fever from any cause
Trauma
Pain
Liver disease
Pulmonary embolus
Stress
Diabetic ketoacidosis
High altitude
Thyrotoxicosis

Pulmonary hypertension
Pulmonary edema
Smoke inhalation
Anemia
Intracerebral bleeding and increased intracranial pressure
Central nervous system lesion
Fibrosis of lung tissue
Exercise
Fatigue

No matter what the cause of hyperventilation, it is accompanied by a fall in Pco_2 (hypocapnia), which causes constriction of cerebral vasculature, respiratory alkalosis, and symptoms of tetany. Pco_2 may drop to as low as 15 mm Hg.

■ **SIGNS AND SYMPTOMS**

Anxiety or panicky appearance
Shortness of breath
Tingling of fingers and toes
Periorbital numbness
Carpopedal spasm
Syncope
Confusion

■ **THERAPEUTIC INTERVENTIONS**

Therapeutic intervention for hyperventilation syndrome *should only* be undertaken *after* medical disease and trauma have been ruled out as the cause of the hyperventilation.

Speak with the patient; make the patient aware of what is going on.

Have the patient talk. (It is difficult to hyperventilate while talking.)

Act in a calm, reassuring manner; never be demanding or demeaning.

Demonstrate proper breathing for the patient and say, "Breathe as I am breathing."

Once the patient seems to be aware of what is going on, have the patient watch a clock with a second hand and breathe once every 5 seconds.

If none of these seems to be working, have the patient rebreathe into a paper bag (carbon dioxide rebreathing).

Always remember to look for underlying causes of hyperventilation other than anxiety or hysteria.

OTHER CAUSES OF CHEST PAIN

See Table 10-3 for differential diagnosis.
Hiatal hernia
Gastric or peptic ulcer
Pancreatitis
Esophageal spasm
Pulmonary embolus
Pneumonia
Pleurisy
Trauma
Degenerative disk disease
Costochondritis (Tietze's syndrome)
Herpes Zoster syndrome
Thoracic outlet

TABLE 10-3   Differential Diagnosis of Chest Pain

CAUSE	ONSET OF PAIN	CHARACTERISTIC OF PAIN	LOCATION OF PAIN
Acute myocardial infarction	Sudden onset; lasts more than 30 minutes to 1 hour	Pressure, burning, aching, tightness, choking	Across chest; may radiate to jaws and neck and down arms and back
Angina	Sudden onset; lasts only few minutes	Aches, squeezing, choking, heaviness, burning	Substernal; may radiate to jaws and neck and down arms and back
Dissecting aortic aneurysm	Sudden onset	Excruciating, tearing	Center of chest; radiates into back; may radiate to abdomen
Pericarditis	Sudden onset or may be variable	Sharp, knifelike	Retrosternal; may radiate up neck and down left arm
Pneumothorax	Sudden onset	Tearing, pleuritic	Lateral side of chest
Pulmonary embolus	Sudden onset	Crushing (but not always)	Lateral side of chest
Hiatal hernia	Sudden onset	Sharp, severe	Lower chest; upper abdomen
Gastrointestinal disturbance or cholecystitis	Sudden onset	Gripping, burning	Lower substernal area, upper abdomen
Degenerative disk (cervical or thoracic spine) disease	Sudden onset	Sharp, severe	Substernal; may radiate to neck, jaw, arms, and shoulders
Degenerative or inflammatory lesions of shoulder, ribs, scalenus anterior	Sudden onset	Sharp, severe	Substernal; radiates to shoulder
Hyperventilation	Sudden onset	Vague	Vague

HISTORY	PAIN WORSENED BY	PAIN RELIEVED BY	OTHER
Age 40 to 70 years; may or may not have history of angina	Movement, anxiety	Nothing; no movement, stillness, position, or breath holding; only relieved by medication (morphine sulfate)	Shortness of breath, diaphoresis, weakness, anxiety
May have history of angina; circumstances precipitating; pain characteristic; response to nitroglycerin	Lying down, eating, effort, cold weather, smoking, stress, anger, worry, hunger	Rest, nitroglycerin	Unstable angina occurs even at rest
Nothing specific, except that pain is usually worse at onset		Nothing	Blood pressure difference between right and left arms, murmur of aortic regurgitation
Short history of upper respiratory infection or fever	Deep breathing, trunk movement, maybe swallowing	Sitting up, leaning forward	Friction rub, paradoxic pulse over 10 mm Hg.
None	Breathing	Nothing	Dyspnea, increased pulse, decreased breath sounds, deviated trachea
Sometimes phlebitis Deep vein thrombosis Recent surgery	Breathing	Not breathing	Cyanosis, dyspnea, profound anxiety, hypoxemia, cough with hemoptysis
May have none	Heavy meal, bending, lying down	Bland diet, walking, antacids, semi-Fowler's position	
May have none	Eating, lying down	Antacids	
May have none	Movement of neck or spine, lifting, straining	Rest, decreased movement	Pain usually on outer aspect of arm, thumb, or index finger
May have none	Movement of arm or shoulder	Elevation and arm support to shoulder postural exercises	
Hyperventilation, anxiety, stress, emotional upset	Increased respiratory rate	Slowing of respiratory rate	Be *sure* hyperventilation is from nonmedical cause!

CONGESTIVE HEART FAILURE

Congestive heart failure (CHF) is a symptom complex in which the heart can no longer produce sufficient cardiac output, at normal filling pressure, to meet metabolic demands. CHF may be seen as an individual entity or in conjunction with pulmonary edema, angina, or MI.

Onset of symptoms may be sudden (acute pulmonary edema) or gradual (chronic CHF). Symptoms are associated with abnormalities in systolic or diastolic function and are accompanied by congestion. Causes of congestive heart failure include

Hypertension—systemic or pulmonary
Fluid overload
Increased intracranial pressure
Myocardial infarction with failure (most common of CHF)
Valvular heart disease
Coronary artery disease
Cardiomyopathy
Dysrhythmias
Tachycardia (more than 180 beats/minute)
Bradycardia (less than 30 beats/minute)
Fever from any cause
Hyperthyroidism
Postpneumothorax
Adult respiratory distress syndrome (ARDS)
Oxygen toxicity
Uremic pneumonia
Intracranial tumors
Drugs such as methotrexate, busulfan, hexamethonium, and nitrofurantoin
Acquired immunodeficiency syndrome (AIDS)
Infective endocarditis
Viral myocarditis
Anemia
Pericardial disease
Pulmonary embolus

■ **SIGNS AND SYMPTOMS**
Exercise intolerance
Dyspnea on exertion
Weakness
Dependent edema
Distended neck veins
Hepatomegaly
Bilateral rales
Increased circulation time
Weight gain

■ **MONITORING PARAMETERS**

Vital signs

Cardiac monitor

Auscultation of the lungs

Auscultation of the heart

Observation of neck veins

Observation for peripheral edema

Obtaining a history and performing a brief physical examination

Pulse oximetry/arterial blood gas

Chest x-ray film, echocardiogram

CBC, lytes, BUN, CR

Cardiac enzymes

■ **THERAPEUTIC INTERVENTIONS**

Acute

High flow oxygen—may require intubation

Morphine sulfate—venous dilation decreases preload; sedation relieves anxiety and depression of respiratory center reduces hyperventilation

Diuretics—reduces preload. Rapid-acting loop diuretics; if no clinical response within 15 to 30 minutes, repeat dose

Aminophylline—used if bronchospasm present not relieved by oxygen, morphine, and diuretics

Dopamine or dobutamine to increase contractile force with systolic dysfunction

Rotating tourniquets

IV D_5W at TKO

Sodium nitroprusside for vasodilation

Chronic

Oxygen therapy

Digitalis therapy—used in presence of reduced left ventricular ejection fraction

Weight loss if overweight

Risk factor reduction (smoking, high cholesterol, alcohol abuse)

Exercise program

Diuretics

Low-sodium diet

Angiotensin-Converting Enzyme (ACE) Inhibitors—systemic vasodilation reduces afterload:

Captopril

Enalapril

Lisinopril

SUGGESTED READINGS

ACC/AHA Guidelines for the management of patients with acute myocardial infarction: a report of the American College of Cardiology/American Heart Association Task Force on Practice Guidelines, *J Am Coll Cardiol,* 28(5):1328-1428, 1996.

Casey K et al: Myocardial infarction: review of clinical trails and treatment strategies, *Crit Care Nurs* 18(2): 39-52, 1998.

Hayes DD: Bradycardia: keeping the current flowing, *Nurs 97* 27(6): 50-56, 1997.

Riegel B, Thomason T, Carlson B: Nursing care of patients with acute myocardial infarction: results of a national survey, *Crit Care Nurs* 17(5): 23-33, 1997.

Sayre MR, Gibler WB: New approaches to ruling out acute ischemic coronary syndrome in the emergency department, *Ann Emerg Med* 27(1): 75-78, 1996.

Sims JM: Premature ventricular contractions, *Nurs 97* 27(8): 43-44, 1997.

Yealy DM, Delbridge TR: Dysrhythmias. In Rosen P, Barkin R, editors: *Emerg Med,* St Louis, 1998, Mosby.

CHAPTER 11

Pulmonary Emergencies

Anne P. Manton

GENERAL ASSESSMENT

Severe dyspnea is a common chief complaint in the emergency setting. Questions to ask to assist with a diagnosis include:

- When did this begin?
- What brought it on? What were you doing when it started?
- Did it come on gradually or suddenly?
- Is it difficult to get air out?
- Has this ever happened before?
- Is it extremely difficult to breathe?
- Do you have pain?
- Do you have a cough?
- Do you have difficulty swallowing?
- Have you ever had lung disease? Heart disease? Asthma? High blood pressure?
- Do you smoke?
- Are you taking any medications? For your heart? For retained water?
- Do you have difficulty walking up stairs?

Other assessment parameters in the patient with a pulmonary disorder are:

Ensure ABCs.

Auscultate lungs (remember, noisy breathing is obstructed breathing).

Check level of consciousness.

Check skin vital signs (color, temperature, and moistness).

Check character of respirations.

Check for use of accessory muscles.

Check oxygen saturation (pulse oximetry).

Check for paradoxical chest movement.

PULMONARY EMBOLUS

Pulmonary embolus is one of the most difficult diagnoses to make because it is often confused with myocardial infarction, pneumothorax, and other conditions involving chest pain. It is not a disease, but rather a complication of a disease. Pulmonary embolus is caused by a free-flowing thrombus from the venous system of the legs, pelvis, or right side of the heart.

The thrombus lodges in a branch of the pulmonary artery, causing partial or total occlusion and sometimes infarction. An embolus may consist of clotted blood, fat, air, or amniotic fluid. Septic emboli from blood-borne bacteria and tumor emboli from intravascular metastases also occur.

■ **CAUSES**

Trauma

Long-bone fractures

Surgery (especially abdominal or pelvic)

Obesity

Decreased peripheral circulation

Congestive heart failure with myocardial infarction

Thrombophlebitis

Cardiac disease

Atrial fibrillation

Prolonged immobilization

Acute infections

Blood dyscrasias

Amniotic fluid emboli (in childbirth)

Air emboli (from scuba diving or poor IV technique)

Oral contraceptives

Neoplasms

■ **PREVENTION**

Frequent ambulation on long trips

Avoiding long periods of standing

Early postoperative ambulation

Adequate hydration

Elastic stockings (or intermittent pressure boots) for those on bed rest

Range of motion exercises for those on bed rest

Good IV technique

Careful management and movement of severely traumatized patients

Prophylactic anticoagulants for high-risk patients

■ **SIGNS AND SYMPTOMS**

There may be absolutely no prodromal signs or symptoms preceding a terminal event. When signs and symptoms do appear, they may be vague. The following is a list of some of the more common signs and symptoms:

Shortness of breath

Tachypnea

Tachycardia

Cough

Hemoptysis

Angina-like chest pain (or pleuritic chest pain)

Pallor or cyanosis

Crackles or wheezing on auscultation

Anxiety

Occasionally decreased blood pressure

Change in mental status

Accentuation of pulmonic heart sounds

Signs of right-sided heart failure, including distended neck veins

Right bundle branch block with right axis deviation, peaked T waves in limb leads, and depressed T waves in the right precordial leads (V_1, V_2, and V_3)

■ **DIAGNOSTIC TESTS**

Posteroanterior and lateral chest x-ray films

Ventilation/perfusion scan

Pulmonary angiography

■ **THERAPEUTIC INTERVENTIONS**

Monitor and maintain ABCs

Oxygen at high flow rate

Initiate and maintain vascular access

Monitor ABGs and oxygen saturation

Analgesia (usually meperidine—avoid morphine)

Bronchodilators

Treatment of dysrhythmias

Heparin (5000 U bolus, then 1000 U per hour continuous infusion); monitor clotting times carefully

Thrombolytic therapy (TPA, urokinase)

Much reassurance

When 60% of the pulmonary vasculature is blocked, cardiac function is compromised. If a large pulmonary embolus lodges in the main, right, or left pulmonary artery, sudden death may occur.

SPONTANEOUS PNEUMOTHORAX

Whenever air enters the pleural space, a loss of negative pressure results, thereby causing collapse of the lung (partially or totally) on the affected side. Spontaneous pneumothorax may occur in the absence of trauma. It occurs most often in young persons (16 to 26 years old) and is more commonly associated with males than females. The usual cause is a ruptured congenital bleb or a bulla that has developed from chronic obstructive pulmonary disease. Other causes of spontaneous pneumothorax include:

Too great mechanical ventilation pressures

Rupture of a cyst

Abscess

Fungal disease

Cancer

Tuberculosis

Trauma

Chest compression in cardiopulmonary resuscitation

Tracheostomy complication

Subclavian puncture complication

■ **SIGNS AND SYMPTOMS**

The signs and symptoms of spontaneous pneumothorax may be minimal. Classic signs and symptoms are usually associated with pneumothorax of 40% or greater.

Dyspnea

Tachypnea

Cough

Cyanosis

Sudden onset of pleuritic chest pain

Agitation

Decreased breath sounds

Severe signs and symptoms of tension pneumothorax include:

Decreased motion of chest wall

Mediastinal shift

Distended neck veins

Deviated trachea

Tympany on percussion

Shock

The definitive diagnosis of pneumothorax is made by chest x-ray examination. If symptoms are severe, however, do not delay therapeutic intervention until a chest x-ray film is available.

■ **THERAPEUTIC INTERVENTIONS**

Therapy is aimed toward reexpansion of the collapsed lung.

Oxygen
Analgesia
Needle placement in the anterior chest wall or chest tube
Initiate and maintain vascular access
Monitor ABGs and oxygen saturation
Bed rest in high Fowler's position
Much reassurance

PLEURAL EFFUSION

Abnormal collections of pleural fluid in the pleural space result in an effusion. Effusions take up space in the thoracic cavity, thus reducing lung volumes. Pleural effusions may be classified as transudative or exudative. Transudative effusions are caused by systemic factors. Exudative effusions, in which fluid movement is facilitated out of capillaries and into pleural space, results from increased capillary permeability.

■ **CAUSES**

TRANSUDATIVE	EXUDATIVE
CHF	Infectious diseases
Cirrhosis	Neoplastic diseases
Pericardial disease	Collagen vascular diseases (systemic lupus erythematosus,
Pulmonary	rheumatoid pleuritis)
embolus	Postabdominal surgery
Peritoneal dialysis	Trauma

■ **SIGNS AND SYMPTOMS**

Dull, aching chest pain
Dullness to percussion (affected area)
Decreased breath sounds over affected area
Decreased chest movement
Egophony (near top of fluid line)
Pleural friction rub
Dyspnea
Cough
Local or referred pleuritic pain
Signs and symptoms of congestive heart failure, infection, or pleural effusion
Chest x-ray film—two views: effusion will appear as a homogeneously dense opaque area. Fluid will often shift with change in body position.

■ **THERAPEUTIC INTERVENTIONS**

Thoracentesis
Oxygen
Analgesia
Subsequent treatment based on underlying cause

PNEUMONIA

Pneumonia results from a bacterial, viral, mycoplasmal, or fungal infection. The patient will often have a history of recent upper respiratory tract infection, otitis media, or conjunctivitis before the onset of pneumonia. However, the patient could have no known medical problems before pneumonia is manifest. It frequently appears in very young or very old persons who are debilitated in some way.

Pneumonia is classified according to the organism that causes it and according to its location (bronchial or lobar). Some of the more common predisposing factors for pneumonia are:

Debilitation
Underlying cardiovascular disorder
Underlying pulmonary disorder
Air pollution
Prolonged immobility
Tracheal intubation
Smoking
Diabetes mellitus
Steroids
Immunosuppression
Aspiration (frequently seen in alcohol or drug abusers or persons with head injury)
Foreign body

■ SIGNS AND SYMPTOMS

Bacterial pneumonia

Dyspnea
Sudden onset
Chills
Fever 39.4° to 40° C (103° to 104° F)
Toxicity
Productive cough and purulent sputum
Chest pain (may be referred diaphragmatically and be mistaken for a gastrointestinal disorder)
Diaphoresis
Tachypnea
Nausea and vomiting
Cyanosis
Rales
Recent otitis media
Recent conjunctivitis
Apprehension
Abdominal distension

Nonbacterial pneumonia

Same symptoms as bacterial pneumonia
Insidious onset
Preceded by upper respiratory infection
Myalgia
Headache
May have seasonal pattern
Cough may be nonproductive

■ THERAPEUTIC INTERVENTIONS

Oxygen
Bed rest in high Fowler's position
Monitor ABGs and oxygen saturation
Hydration
Antibiotic therapy appropriate to the causative organism
Expectorants
Bronchodilators as needed
If aspiration pneumonia, evaluate swallowing

■ **COMPLICATIONS**

Rupture of pneumatocele producing pneumothorax

Empyema

Therapeutic intervention for both of these complications is placement of a chest tube.

PULMONARY EDEMA

The key to survival in pulmonary edema is prompt recognition and rapid therapeutic intervention. Pulmonary failure is also known as backward failure or circulatory overload. It is most often a result of backward pressure into the left side of the heart and lungs. This transmits an increased pressure into the pulmonary capillaries and produces a leak of fluid from the capillaries into the alveoli (Box 11-1). Normally the fluid content of the lungs is about 20% of their total volume. In acute pulmonary edema, the fluid content of the lungs can rise as high as 1000% of normal.

Pulmonary edema is a symptom complex, not a diagnosis. Several diseases may produce pulmonary edema:

Myocardial infarction (with left ventricular failure)

Aortic insufficiency

Aortic stenosis

Mitral stenosis

Myocarditis

Amyloidosis

Drug toxicity

Cardiomyopathy

Hypertension

Coronary artery disease

Dysrhythmias (tachycardias > 180 beats per minute and bradycardias <30 beats per minute)

Hyperthermia

Hyperthyroidism

Exercise

Severe congestive heart failure

Adult respiratory distress syndrome

Heroin overdose

Inhalation of pulmonary irritants

BOX 11-1   Mechanism of Pulmonary Edema of Cardiac Origin

Left ventricular failure
↓
Increased pressure in left ventricle
↓
Increased pressure in pulmonary venous system
↓
Loss of plasma oncotic pressure
↓
Leak of fluid into interstitial tissue
↓
Reflex spasm of airways (cardiac asthma) and pulmonary alveoli
↓
Pulmonary edema and interference with gas exchange
↓
Decreased Po_2 and acidosis

Pulmonary embolism
High altitude
Neurogenic causes
Volume overload
Anemia
Uremia
Disseminated intravascular coagulation (DIC)
Near-drowning
Renal impairment
Lymphatic obstruction
Bacteremic sepsis
Beriberi
General anesthesia

■ **SIGNS AND SYMPTOMS**

Shortness of breath
Chest tightness
Cough
Cyanosis (central and peripheral)
Rales, rhonchi, wheezing
Distended neck veins
Pink, frothy sputum
Peripheral edema
Tachycardia
Paroxysmal nocturnal dyspnea (PND) or orthopnea
Cheyne-Stokes respirations
S_3 gallop and decreased heart sounds

■ **THERAPEUTIC INTERVENTIONS**

The following therapeutic interventions will alter circulatory and ventilatory dynamics but may not alter the underlying disease process. Once the patient is out of a life-threatening condition, status must be reevaluated to determine proper therapeutic intervention for the condition that caused the pulmonary edema.

Monitor and maintain ABCs
Place the patient in high Fowler's position with legs dependent.
Administer high-flow oxygen to treat hypoxia.
Place patient on a cardiac monitor.
Monitor for dysrhythmias
Monitor ABGs and oxygen saturation
Initiate an IV line for the administration of medications.
Administer morphine sulfate
Administer nitroglycerin to cause venous pooling and dilated vasculature that produces a decreased venous return to the right heart, provided that blood pressure is in an acceptable range.
Give furosemide or other diuretics to reduce intravascular volume.
Place a Foley catheter to monitor urine output.
Give reassurance. These patients experience feelings of suffocation and doom. They need much verbal support and touch communication.

HIGH-ALTITUDE PULMONARY EDEMA

High-altitude pulmonary edema (HAPE) usually occurs in patients who have made a very rapid ascent to altitudes above 10,000 feet over sea level and have engaged in heavy physical activity for the first 3 days at that altitude. It can occur much sooner in patients with underlying pulmonary or cardiac disease. Symptoms may begin to occur from 6 to 36 hours after a change of altitude. HAPE can also occur in patients who normally live at high altitudes but go to sea level for 2 or more weeks and then return to high altitudes. It may be seen in patients with no history of cardiac or pulmonary disease who have marked hypertension. Therapeutic intervention is return to a lower altitude, oxygen therapy, and bed rest.

ASTHMA

Asthma is reversible airway disease where there is an obstruction of air flow caused by one or more of the following ("the three Ss"):

Spasm

Swelling

Secretions

These produce bronchospasm, hypoxia, and epinephrine release (fight or flight response). Asthma may occur at any age and may be the result of:

Allergies to foods (e.g., shellfish, chocolate) or inhalants (e.g., pollen, rubber latex proteins, mold, animal dander)

Hyperirritability or hyperresponsiveness of the tracheobronchial tree to inhalants such as chemicals, dust, gases, or insecticides

Emotional factors

Exercise

Cold weather

Smoking

Allergies

Cardiogenic causes

Nasal polyps

Mechanical obstructions (such as tumors)

Respiratory infections

Air pollutants

Sinusitis

Medications

Food additives

REMEMBER: All that wheezes is not asthma; all that is asthma does not necessarily wheeze. Asthma may be manifested by repetitive coughing.

■ SIGNS AND SYMPTOMS

Wheezing (most commonly expiratory, but may also be inspiratory). *Remember that in severe bronchospasm there may be no wheezing, as there may be no air movement.*

Dyspnea

Cough

Tachycardia

Hypertension

Mild cyanosis

Use of accessory muscles of respiration

Chest tightness

"Anxiety" or restlessness because of epinephrine release and/or air hunger

Pulsus paradoxus of >12 mmHg

Tachypnea

Hyperresonance or percussion

Possible history of asthma

■ THERAPEUTIC INTERVENTIONS

Bed rest in high Fowler's position

Oxygen with humidification

Monitor ABGs and oxygen saturation

Administer bronchodilators or metered dose inhaler

Initiate and maintain vascular access

Monitor for dysrhythmias

Corticosteroids

Fluid and electrolyte replacement—ensure good hydration

Much verbal reassurance

STATUS ASTHMATICUS

Status asthmaticus is severe asthma that does not respond to therapy. The diagnosis is usually made through the patient's history.

■ **SIGNS AND SYMPTOMS**

Signs and symptoms are the same as asthma but more severe and prolonged.

Dyspnea (usually increases gradually over a few days)

Chest tightness

Tachycardia

Nonproductive cough

Wheezing on inspiration and expiration (if bronchospasm is severe there may be no wheezing because there may be no air movement)

Extreme anxiety

Acid-base imbalance hypoxemia

Increased work of breathing

Jugular vein distension

Sitting forward, using accessory muscles of respiration

Mild cyanosis

Distended neck veins in expiration

■ **THERAPEUTIC INTERVENTIONS**

Arterial blood gas determinations

Humidified oxygen

Bronchodilators by inhalation

IV fluid hydration

Intubation if severe

Corticosteroids

Antacids

Expectorants

Accurate recording of intake and output

BRONCHITIS

Bronchitis is a syndrome in which there is a frequent and productive cough. The cause of bronchitis is believed to be chronic irritation of the bronchial mucosa by such things as smoking, air pollution, or chronic inhalation of irritant substances. Acute bronchitis may be seen with or shortly after upper respiratory infection.

■ **SIGNS AND SYMPTOMS**

Dyspnea

Productive cough that worsens in the evenings or when there is damp weather

May have fever if acute

Prolonged expiratory phase

Rhonchi

■ **THERAPEUTIC INTERVENTIONS**

Removing the cause (the source of the irritation)

Rest

Relaxation
Bronchodilators
Expectorants
Antibiotics
Fluids (at least 4 liters per day by mouth)
Position to facilitate breathing
Postural drainage, if indicated
Monitor ABGs and oxygen saturation
Oxygen, if indicated (use with caution in COPD)

CHRONIC OBSTRUCTIVE PULMONARY DISEASE

Chronic obstructive pulmonary disease (COPD) is a process in which there is a loss of elasticity in the lung tissue and destruction of the alveolar walls. The patient with COPD will have much difficulty exhaling and will have difficulty with gas exchange. The specific cause of COPD is not known, but smoking appears to contribute to it (90% of COPD patients have a history of heavy smoking—more than 1 pack per day). Other causative factors may include pollution, industrial inhalants such as silicon, and tuberculosis.

■ **SIGNS AND SYMPTOMS**
Patient states that he or she has emphysema
Severe dyspnea that increases over a number of days
Cyanosis (especially of the lips, nailbeds, and earlobes)
Orthopnea
Clubbing of fingers
Faint breath sounds, wheezes, or rales
Prolonged expiratory phase of respiration
Hyperresonance on percussion
Pursed-lip breathing
Use of accessory muscles of respiration
Subclavicular and tracheal drawing-in on inspiration
Productive cough
History of smoking
Barrel chest

■ **THERAPEUTIC INTERVENTIONS**
Bed rest in high Fowler's position
Initiate and maintain vascular access
Monitor ABGs and oxygen saturation
Monitor for cardiac dysrhythmias
May need aggressive ventilator support
Bronchodilators; first line of defense is beta-agonists by inhalation (reduce standard nebulized dose 25 to 50% in patients with known cardiac disease)
Oxygen at 2 L/min; observe the patient carefully; do not hesitate to give oxygen if the patient is hypoxic; the most severe life-threatening problem for these patients is hypoxemia
Adequate hydration

SMOKE INHALATION

The inhalation of smoke and other noxious fumes usually occurs during a fire in an enclosed space. Severe pulmonary damage, such as chemical pneumonitis or asphyxia caused by increased levels of carboxyhemoglobin, may result. The burning of synthetic materials produces noxious chemicals that produce additional problems in the respiratory tract (Table 11-1).

TABLE 11-1   Toxic Products of Combustion

MATERIAL	USE	MAJOR TOXIC CHEMICAL PRODUCTS OF COMBUSTION
Polyvinyl chloride	Wall and floor covering, telephone cable insulation	Hydrogen chloride (P), phosgene (P), carbon monoxide
Polyurethane foam	Upholstery	Isocyanates, (toluene-2,4-diisocyanate) (P), hydrogen cyanide
Lacquered wood veneer, wallpaper	Wall covering	Acetaldehyde (P), formaldehyde (P), oxides of nitrogen (P), acetic acid
Acrylic	Light diffusers	Acrolein (P)
Nylon	Carpet	Hydrogen cyanide, ammonia (P)
Acrilan	Carpet	Hydrogen cyanide, acrolein (P)
Polystyrene	Miscellaneous	Styrene, carbon monoxide

From Genovesi MG et al: Toxic products of combustion, *Chest* 71:441, 1977.
P, pulmonary irritant.

When caring for the victim of smoke inhalation, ask a few questions:
- How long were you exposed?
- Were you in a confined space?
- What type of material burned?
- How much of the material burned?

The primary manifestation of smoke inhalation is pulmonary edema. This may not appear for 24 to 48 hours.

■ **SIGNS AND SYMPTOMS**

Mild irritation of the upper airways or burning pain in the throat or chest
Singed nasal hairs
Hypoxia
Oral mucosal burns, redness, or blistering
Facial burns
Sputum that contains carbon
Rales
Rhonchi
Wheezes
Dyspnea
Restlessness or agitation
Cough
Hoarseness
Other signs of pulmonary edema (usually appear hours later)

■ **THERAPEUTIC INTERVENTIONS**

ABCs
Humidified oxygen
Initiate and maintain vascular access
Monitor arterial blood gas values and oxygen saturation
Carboxyhemoglobin levels
Coughing, chest physical therapy, suctioning
Admission and observation for 24 to 48 hours
Endotracheal intubation, cricothyrotomy, or tracheostomy if indicated
Bronchodilators
Nasogastric tube
Steroids

CARBON MONOXIDE POISONING

Carbon monoxide is a colorless, odorless gas formed by the burning of organic matter. Inhalation of CO can lead to tissue hypoxia. CO has a 200 to 250 times greater affinity for hemoglobin than does oxygen. In the bloodstream CO displaces oxygen from the hemoglobin molecule thus decreasing oxygen content. CO also shifts the oxyhemoglobin dissociation curve to the left. This impairs the ability of hemoglobin to release oxygen molecules and may cause tissue injury. The brain and heart are most sensitive to CO poisoning.

■ **SIGNS AND SYMPTOMS**
   Carboxyhemoglobin levels 20% to 40%
   Headache
   Dizziness
   Hypotension
   Changes in mental status
   Nausea and vomiting
   Angina (with preexisting heart disease)
   Levels greater than 40%
   Dysrhythmias
   Seizures
   Coma

■ **THERAPEUTIC INTERVENTIONS**
Maintain ABCs
Monitor cardiac rhythm
High-flow oxygen
Intubation
Hyperbaric oxygen therapy

ADULT RESPIRATORY DISTRESS SYNDROME

Adult respiratory distress syndrome (ARDS) (otherwise known as shock lung, pulmonary contusion, congestive atelectasis, posttraumatic lung, and traumatic wet lung) is a pulmonary insult caused by a sudden congestion and atelectasis with hyaline membrane formation resulting from loss of surfactant and build-up of mucus along the alveoli. It is a syndrome of acute progressive failure caused by a variety of insults, such as:
Cardiopulmonary bypass
Infection/sepsis
Pulmonary edema
Inhaled toxins
Hemorrhagic shock
Massive transfusions
Lung contusion
Pancreatitis
Near-drowning
Overly aggressive fluid resuscitation
Emboli
Aspiration
Overdose
Eclampsia
Disseminated intravascular coagulation
Initially the lungs appear normal. Then there is progressive atelectasis, increased interstitial and alveolar edema, and marked ventilation-perfusion abnormalities that result in progressive hypoxemia and difficulty in breathing as lung compliance decreases.

■ SIGNS AND SYMPTOMS
Dyspnea
Tachypnea
Tachycardia
Cyanosis
Hypoxemia
Anxiety/restlessness
Hypocapnea
Pulmonary hemorrhage
Hypotension

■ THERAPEUTIC INTERVENTIONS
Monitor and maintain ABCs
Intubation—endotracheal or tracheostomy
Ventilation with volume-cycled ventilator and positive-end expiratory pressure (PEEP)
Initiate and maintain vascular access
Dehydration with diuretics and fluid restriction
Medication, possibly with steroids to enhance surfactant production; perhaps heparin
Suction

Benefits of PEEP
Prevents the collapse of alveoli.
Increases functional residual capacity.
Improves VQ relationship.
Combats pulmonary edema.
Enhances Fio_2

Dangers of PEEP
Oxygen toxicity
Fluid overload
Decreased cardiac output
Possible pneumothorax (especially in patients with chronic obstructive pulmonary disease)
Infection
If PEEP fails, hyperbaric oxygenation may be used if a chamber is readily available, or one may elect to use a bypass oxygenator as a last effort.

NEAR-DROWNING

Drowning or near-drowning occurs when an individual cannot stay afloat because of fatigue, lack of skill as a swimmer, panic, an acute medical incident while in the water (for example, a myocardial infarction or a seizure), being traumatized, or hyperventilating in preparation for a long-distance swim underwater. A near-drowning may also be a suicide attempt.

There are three categories of near-drowning and drowning:

dry drowning   Asphyxiation caused by decreased oxygen as a result of laryngotracheal spasm (prevents entrance of water as well as oxygen into trachea), causing cerebral anoxia, edema, and unconsciousness.

wet drowning   The victim makes a desperate respiratory effort, and the lungs fill with fluid rather than air.

secondary drowning   The recurrence of respiratory distress (usually in the form of pulmonary edema or aspiration pneumonia) that occurs following successful resuscitation from the initial near-drowning incident. It can occur anywhere from 1 hour to several days after the incident.

Seawater

Seawater is a hypertonic solution; fluid traverses into the alveoli because of an osmotic pull across the alveolar capillary membrane that results in pulmonary edema; it also causes hemoconcentration and hypovolemia.

Fresh water

Fresh water is a hypotonic solution; fluid traverses rapidly out of the alveoli into the blood by diffusion. Because the fresh water contains contaminants such as chlorine, algae, and mud, surfactant breakdown occurs and fluid begins to seep into the alveoli once again, resulting in pulmonary edema; it also causes hemodilution and hypervolemia.

■ **SIGNS AND SYMPTOMS**

History of immersion
Dyspnea that progresses
Wheezing
Rales
Rhonchi
Cough (sometimes with pink, frothy sputum)
Tachycardia
Cyanosis
Chest pain
Mental confusion
Seizure
Unconsciousness
Respiratory or cardiac arrest

■ **THERAPEUTIC INTERVENTIONS**

ABCs
Protection of cervical spine
Monitor ABGs and oxygen saturation
Monitor core body temperature
Warming, if needed
High-flow oxygen intubation if necessary
PEEP
Frequent suctioning
Elevating head of bed if C-spine cleared
Correction of acid-base imbalances
Antibiotics
Steroids
Isoproterenol or epinephrine for bronchospasm
Bronchodilators
Nasogastric tube
Central venous pressure line, arterial pressure line, or pulmonary capillary wedge pressure line to monitor fluid resuscitation
Admission for a minimum of 24 hours of observation

NOTE: Do not attempt to drain fluid from the lungs at the time of the incident, as this would waste time that could be used in the resuscitation effort.

This chapter reviews many of the common pulmonary conditions seen in the emergency department. Patients with these conditions often exhibit signs of air hunger and are usually extremely anxious. Rapid assessment, intervention, and reassurance are key to preventing life-threatening respiratory complications. Airway or breathing problems are often components of other medical emergencies such as multiple trauma or myocardial infarction, which are discussed in other chapters of this book.

SUGGESTED READINGS

Baum GL, Wolinsky E: *Textbook of pulmonary disease,* ed 5, Boston, 1994, Little, Brown.
Beyda DH: Childhood submersion injuries, *J Emerg Nurs* 24(2): 140-144, 1998.

Campolo S: Spontaneous pneumothorax, *Am J Nurs* 97(2):30, 1997.

Dobson ME, Ruben FL: The special challenge of pneumonia in the elderly, *J Resp Dis* 14(10):1145, 1993.

Fine MJ et al: A prediction rule to identify low-risk patients with community-acquired pneumonia, *N Engl J Med* 336:243, 1997.

Frakes MA: Asthma in the emergency department, *J Emerg Nurs* 23(5):429, 1997.

Glankler DM: Caring for the victim of near drowning, *Crit Care Nurs* 13:25, 1993.

Goldhaber SZ, Morpurgo M: Diagnosis, treatment and prevention of pulmonary embolism, *JAMA* 268(13):1727, 1992.

Goodwin SR, Boysen PE, Modell JH: Near-drowning—adults and children. In Ayres SM, Grenvik A, Holbrook PR et al, editors: *Textbook of critical care,* ed 3, Philadelphia, 1995, Saunders.

Grossman J: The evolution of inhaler technology, *J Asthma* 31:55, 1994.

Koller MH, Schuster DP: The acute respiratory distress syndrome, *N Engl J Med* 332:27, 1995.

Li JTC: Do peak flow meters lead to better asthma control? *J Resp Dis* 16(4):381, 1995.

Mathias S: Resurgence of tuberculosis: implications for emergency nurses, *J Emerg Nurs* 23(5):425, 1997.

Molitor L: A 55-year-old patient with chronic lung disease and intractable shortness of breath, *J Emerg Nurs* 24(2): 199-200, 1998.

Moser KM: Treating pulmonary embolism: who, what, and how? *J Resp Dis* 15(2):122, 1994.

O'Hanlon-Nichols T: Basic assessment series: the adult pulmonary system, *AJN* 98(2): 39-45, 1998.

Owen A: Respiratory assessment revisited, *Nurs 98* 28(4): 48-49, 1998.

Richman F: Asthma diagnosis and management: new severity classifications and therapy alternatives, *Clin Rev* 7(8):76, 1997.

Toogood J: Helping your patients make better use of MDIs and spacers, *J Resp Dis* 15(2):151, 1994.

Neurologic Emergencies

Kathy M. Dolan

Several types of neurologic emergencies bring a patient to the emergency department. Some of the more common ones are presented in this chapter.

HEADACHE

The chief complaint of a headache is a symptom of some underlying disorder and is not a diagnosis in itself. The diagnosis of headache is based on the patient's history.

- Is this the first headache?
- When did it start?
- Was there any trauma?
- Is there nausea or vomiting?
- Is there meningismus?
- Have there been any personality changes since the onset?
- Has there been any memory loss?
- Have there been any recent infections?
- Have there been any recent vision problems? Diplopia? Photophobia?
- Have there been any recent neurologic problems?
- Has blood pressure been elevated? For how long?
- Have there been any emotional problems?
- Is the patient currently taking any medications?
- Has the patient ever had any seizures? Recently?

Using the PQRST mnemonic, assess the pain:

P = Provokes: What makes the pain better? What makes it worse? Has the patient taken any medications for it?

Q = Quality: What does the pain feel like? Describe it.

R = Radiates: Where is the pain? Where does it go?

S = Severity: How severe is the pain? (This is not a particularly good index item for assessing headache because it is very subjective.)

T = Time: When did it start? When did it end? How long did it last?

Some common causes of headache:

Stress
Systemic illness
Intracranial hemorrhage
Intracranial tumor
Intracranial inflammations
Vascular problems
Temporal arteritis
Trauma

Migraine Headaches

■ **SIGNS AND SYMPTOMS**
Recurrent pain
Severe pain
Pulsatile pain
Motor and visual problems
Anorexia
Nausea and vomiting
Emotional irritability
Syncope
Diaphoresis
Photophobia/phonophobia
Gastrointestinal disturbances
May be preceded by "aura"
Possible family history of migraines

Cluster Headaches *(a form of migraine headache)*

■ **SIGNS AND SYMPTOMS**
Unilateral pain
Severe pain
Pain usually on one side of face or in one eye
Nasal congestion
Lacrimation
Ptosis
Diaphoresis
■ **THERAPEUTIC INTERVENTIONS**
Pain relief
    Usually with dihydroergotamine or sumatriptan
    Possibly with a narcotic analgesic
Nausea and vomiting relief
    With antiemetics
Anxiety relief
    With a sedative

Tension Headaches

Tension headaches usually occur in times of emotional distress. Pain is believed to be caused by contraction of the scalp and the muscles of the cervical area.
■ **SIGNS AND SYMPTOMS**
Dull headache (a tight, constricting feeling)
Bilateral pain (frontal or occipital)
■ **THERAPEUTIC INTERVENTIONS**
Mild analgesics
Identifying the cause of the pain and treating it

Traumatic Headaches

Local tissue damage from trauma may result in a headache, probably caused by muscle contractions and tension on the extracranial vasculature. Concussions and contusions are frequently followed by headaches. Intracerebral bleeds are usually accompanied by the complaint of a severe headache if the patient is conscious. For further information on intracranial bleeds, see Chapter 22.

Extracranial Headaches

There are many causes of extracranial headaches. These may include:
Glaucoma
Toothaches
Ear problems
Sinus congestion
These headaches are treated in accordance with their cause.

Temporal Arteritis

Temporal arteritis is a condition in which there is severe headache in one temporal area. The pain may also involve the neck or jaw area or both.
■ **SIGNS AND SYMPTOMS**
Severe headache
Patient is usually over 50 years old
Pain when temporal area is touched
Visual disturbances
History of polymyalgia rheumatica
■ **THERAPEUTIC INTERVENTIONS**
Steroids
Biopsy for definite diagnosis

HYPERTENSION

Hypertension is a product of cardiac output multiplied by peripheral vascular resistance. It can be benign or malignant (Table 12-1). A patient with a blood pressure of 160/90 or higher should be considered hypertensive. A diastolic blood pressure of greater than 130 mm HG is considered a hypertensive crisis. If hypertension is present with any of the following, the situation is considered an absolute emergency:
Cerebrovascular accident
Myocardial infarction
Grade III or IV retinopathy
Angina pectoris
Congestive heart failure
Renal insufficiency
Aortic dissection
The elevated blood pressure may be determined in the following ways:
On physical examination (especially with sustained abdominal bruit)

TABLE 12-1   Comparison of Benign and Malignant Hypertension

	BENIGN (GRADUAL PHASE)	MALIGNANT (ACCELERATED PHASE)
Duration	More than 10 years	Less than 2 years
Onset	Gradual; frequently asymptomatic	Sudden; symptomatic
Encephalopathy	Rarely	Often

In accordance with family history

By age (if the patient is less than 25 years old and has hypertension, it is probably caused by renal vascular disease)

By laboratory examination (urinalysis, BUN, creatinine, electrolytes, uric acid, calcium, lipids, and glucose)

By chest x-ray examination

By ECG

By intravenous pyelogram

Some patients will have an elevated blood pressure but no evidence of end-organ damage. This may be because the blood pressure increase is secondary to some other problems, such as:

Drug withdrawal (especially clonidine or propranolol)

Drug interactions (such as the combination of monoamine oxidase inhibitors and Chianti wine)

Direct drug effects (such as from amphetamines, tricyclics, or phencyclidine)

Pheochromocytoma

Head trauma

Guillain-Barré syndrome

Therapeutic intervention focuses on the underlying cause. Essential hypertension usually originates from the kidneys, adrenal glands, nervous system, coarctation of the aorta, or toxemia.

■ **SIGNS AND SYMPTOMS**

Headache

Epistaxis

Tinnitus

Syncope

■ **COMPLICATIONS** (TABLE 12-2)

Minor

Coronary hypertrophy

Left ventricular hypertrophy

Grade III retinopathy

Abnormal ECG or dysrhythmias

Conduction disturbances

Major

Cerebrovascular accident

Aortic dissection

TABLE 12-2   Complications of Hypertension

	I	II	III	IV
Fundi	Vascular spasms	Vascular sclerosis	Hemorrhage and/or exudates	Papilledema
Heart	Left ventricular hypertrophy	Congestive heart failure	Myocardial ischemia	Myocardial infarction
Vascular	Atherosclerosis	Aneurysm with or without rupture	Dissection of aneurysm	Rupture of aneurysm
Brain	Cerebrovascular insufficiency	Encephalopathy	Cerebral thrombosis	Intracranial or subarachnoid hemorrhage
Renal	Benign nephrosclerosis	Malignant nephrosclerosis	Impaired renal function; low specific gravity; proteinuria; hematuria	Elevated creatinine and BUN

Congestive heart failure
Renal insufficiency
Encephalopathy
Grade IV retinopathy
Myocardial infarction
Cerebral thrombosis
Peripheral vascular insufficiency
Sudden death

Hypertensive Encephalopathy

■ **SIGNS AND SYMPTOMS**
Fluctuating levels of consciousness or coma
Headaches
Seizures
Grade IV retinopathy

■ **THERAPEUTIC INTERVENTIONS**
Administration of an antihypertensive agent (Table 12-3)
Treatment of underlying condition

Hypertensive Cerebrovascular Syndromes (Transient Ischemic Attacks and Hemorrhages)

■ **SIGNS AND SYMPTOMS**
Headache
Decreased level of consciousness

■ **THERAPEUTIC INTERVENTIONS**
For intracerebral bleeding
Oxygen
Furosemide
Possible surgery
For cerebrovascular accident
Sodium nitroprusside

Toxemia

■ **SIGNS AND SYMPTOMS**
Elevated blood pressure
Peripheral edema
Proteinuria
Seizures
Decreased level of consciousness

■ **THERAPEUTIC INTERVENTIONS**
Immediate delivery (via induction of labor or cesarean section)
Diazoxide
Sodium nitroprusside
Magnesium sulfate for seizures

TABLE 12-3 Commonly Used Antihypertensive Medications

DRUG	COMMON BRAND NAME	DOSE (DAILY)	MAJOR ACTION	COMMON SIDE EFFECTS	UNIQUE PROBLEMS
Thiazide diuretics	Diuril, Hydrodiuril, Esidrix, Zaroxolyn	0.5-2 g 25-50 mg 25-100 mg 5-10 mg	Renal sodium and water increase by inhibition of Na reabsorption in distal tubule	Hypokalemia, decreased glomerular filtration rate, increased uric acid	Further compromise of impaired renal or hepatic functions, severe hyperglycemia
Furosemide	Lasix	40-200 mg	Inhibits Na reabsorption in ascending limb of Henle's loop	Fluid and electrolyte imbalance, hyperuricemia	Eighth nerve damage (rare)
Alpha-methyldopa	Aldomet	1-2 g	Central effect most profound	Sedation, postural hypotension, retention of sodium and water, impotence common	Positive direct Coombs' test (20%), hemolytic anemia, reversible liver damage, drug fever
Propranolol	Inderal	80-160 mg (may be much higher)	Beta-adrenergic blockade	Exacerbates congestive heart failure, exacerbates asthma, many central nervous system side effects (e.g., depression, hallucinations)	Masks signs and symptoms of hypoglycemia
Clonidine	Catapres	0.4-2 g	Many actions both peripheral and central (most important); causes stimulation of central centers that inhibit sympathetics	Dry mouth, sedation	Hyperirritability, marked rebound of hypertension with acute withdrawal
Hydralazine	Apresoline	100-200 mg/day, rarely more than 400 mg/day	Direct relaxation of smooth muscles, arteries much more than veins	Numerous effects including headaches, palpitations, dizziness, nasal congestion, flushing, peripheral neuropathy, myocardial, ischemia	Acute rheumatoid states (10%), lupus-like syndrome
Reserpine (rarely used)	Many preparations such as Serpasil	0.1-1.0 mg	Depletes catecholamine status leading to decreased peripheral resistance and cardiac output	Depression (do not use if patient is depressed), gastrointestinal upset	Extrapyramidal tract signs, gastrointestinal bleeding
Spironolactone	Aldactone	100 mg	Competitive antagonist of aldosterone in renal tubules	Hyperkalemia with or without other diuretics	Gynecomastia, masculinization, gastrointestinal upset

Generic	Brand	Dose	Mechanism of action	Side effects	Other effects
Triamterene	Dyrenium	200-300 mg	Direct action on tubular transport, not competitive antagonist of aldosterone	Hyperkalemia	Gastrointestinal symptoms, megaloblastic anemia (rare)
Prazosin	Minipress	3 mg to start, with first dose 1 mg only; may increase to 20 mg slowly	Alpha-adrenergic blocking agent at postsynaptic receptors	Postural hypotension; syncope, especially in salt-depleted patient (first dose phenomenon); palpitations, drowsiness, headache	Positive antinuclear factor ($\frac{1}{3}$ of patients)
Minoxidil	Loniten	10-40 mg	Vasodilation by direct relaxation of arteriolar smooth muscle	Fluid retention, reflex activation of sympathetic nervous system	Pericardial effusion
Guanethidine	Ismelin	25-50 mg	Inhibition of sympathetic nerves, inhibition of indirect activity of sympathetic amines (e.g., tyramine), presynaptic action caused by impaired release of neurotransmitter from peripheral adrenergic neurons	Postural hypotension (severe), weakness, fluid retention, precipitation of congestive heart failure	Hypertensive crisis (rare) with use in patients with pheochromocytoma or with sympathomimetics in "cold remedies"; in relation to tricyclics, guanethidine action is antagonized, and if tricyclics are withdrawn, profound hypotension may result if guanethidine is continued.
Labetalol	Normodyne	600 mg	Vasodilation by alpha$_1$ adrenoreceptor blockade; also beta blockade	Fatigue, dizziness Postural hypotension (uncommon) Bradycardia (uncommon) Contraindications: Asthma Heart failure Heart block Severe tachycardia	Hypertensive crisis possible if used when pheochromocytoma is present
Captopril	Capoten	75-450 mg	Competitive inhibition of angiotensin-I converting enzyme	Proteinuria Hypotension, especially when CHF is present Elevated BUN	Agranulocytosis

From Rosen P et al: *Emergency medicine*, ed 2, St Louis, 1987, Mosby.

Left Ventricular Failure

- ■ SIGNS AND SYMPTOMS
  Dyspnea
  Pink, frothy sputum
  Rales
  Bronchospasm
- ■ THERAPEUTIC INTERVENTIONS
  Oxygen
  Antihypertensive agent

Aortic Dissection

(See Chapter 10.)
- ■ SIGNS AND SYMPTOMS
  Chest pain that radiates to back
  Hypertension
  Blood pressure discrepancies between arms
  Pulse discrepancies between femoral areas
- ■ THERAPEUTIC INTERVENTIONS
  Sodium nitroprusside
  Beta blockade
  Surgery

Drug Overdose

- ■ THERAPEUTIC INTERVENTIONS
  Sodium nitroprusside

Drug Withdrawal

- ■ THERAPEUTIC INTERVENTIONS
  Clonidine—alpha and beta blockade
  Propranolol—bed rest, nitroglycerin

Pulmonary Edema

- ■ SIGNS AND SYMPTOMS
  Shortness of breath
  Possible chest tightness
  Anxiety
  Inability to lie flat
  Rales, rhonchi, wheezes
  Distended neck veins
  Pink, frothy sputum
- ■ THERAPEUTIC INTERVENTIONS
  Morphine sulfate
  Nitroglycerin
  Oxygen/positive pressure
  Furosemide
  Bed rest in high Fowler's position

Aminophylline
Monitor condition

MAO Inhibitors

■ THERAPEUTIC INTERVENTIONS
Phentolamine
Phenoxybenzamine

Glomerulonephritis

■ THERAPEUTIC INTERVENTIONS
Hydralazine
Diazoxide
Furosemide

Hyperthyroidism

■ THERAPEUTIC INTERVENTIONS
Alpha and beta blockade
Iodine
Propylthiouracil

SEIZURES

A seizure is a symptom, not a disease. It is a period of abnormal electrical activity in the brain. There are two classes of seizures:

Generalized, which include tonic-clonic and absence
Partial, which includes focal

Seizures may occur as a result of head trauma, tumor, vascular disorders, metabolic abnormalities, overdoses, or infections. It is important to obtain past history of seizures, information on what happened preceding the seizure, any history of recent trauma, and the patient's vital signs.

Generalized Seizures

Tonic-clonic (formerly Grand Mal)

In tonic-clonic seizure there is a sudden loss of organized muscle tone. This causes a severely decreased level of consciousness, extensor muscle spasms, apnea, and bilateral clonic movements. The patient fades into a postictal state in which there is muscle relaxation, deep breathing, and a depressed level of consciousness. The seizures may be idiopathic or may be caused by an easily identifiable condition, such as hypoxia.

■ THERAPEUTIC INTERVENTIONS
Protect airway patency, administer oxygen.
Protect patient from injury.
Administer naloxone 0.8 mg and dextrose 50% 50 ml IV if cause is unknown.
Give diazepam IV or lorazepam IV.

Absence (formerly Petit Mal)

Absence seizures are usually caused by a cortical lesion and generally occur in children between 4 and 12 years old. The child may appear confused and disinterested, have a glassy stare, blink, and make lip-smacking movements. During the seizure the patient may respond to verbal commands.

■ **THERAPEUTIC INTERVENTIONS**
Diazepam IV
Ethosuximide IV

Partial Seizures

Focal (Jacksonian) seizure

Focal or Jacksonian seizures usually occur unilaterally and are caused by a focal brain lesion such as a tumor, abscess, infarction, or eschar. This type of seizure is usually not life-threatening, but it does not respond well to anticonvulsant medications.

■ **THERAPEUTIC INTERVENTIONS**
Diazepam or phenobarbital (although they may not work)
   Be sure to do a brief neurologic examination on all seizure patients once the postictal period has passed.

Status Epilepticus

Status epilepticus is a series of consecutive seizures or a continuous seizure that is not responsive to traditional therapeutic interventions.

■ **THERAPEUTIC INTERVENTIONS**
Try to determine the cause once the seizure is controlled.
Treat the cause if possible.
Clear the airway.
Provide oxygen (consider 100% oxygen and endotracheal intubation if seizure is prolonged).
Consider IV.
Consider naloxone.
Consider dextrose 50%—50 ml.
Consider thiamine 50 to 100 mg if possibility of alcoholism exists.
Consider diazepam 2.5 mg increments IV, ET, or per rectum (to 15 mg) adult dose.
Consider fosphenytoin sodium injection 15 to 20 mg PE/kg at a rate of 100 mg PE/min to 150 mg PE/min for status. May be diluted in D_5W or NS. Orders must always include a PE unit, which stands for *phenytoin equivalent.* Cardiac monitoring and observation for hypotension are essential. May be given IV or IM.
Consider phenytoin 25 to 50 mg/min loading dose (to 1 g) adult dose; be sure to give phenytoin via *normal saline solution,* not D_5W. Patient should also be on a cardiac monitor.
Consider phenobarbital 130 mg every 10 to 15 minutes (to 1 g)—adult dose.
Consider paraldehyde 1 to 4 ml IV or 5 to 10 ml IM—adult dose.
Consider general anesthesia if status has not responded to any of these.

STROKE (CEREBROVASCULAR ACCIDENT)

Stroke is caused by the occlusion or rupture of a cerebral blood vessel by occlusion or hemorrhage.

Occlusion

Embolus—From the heart or large arteries, caused by atrial fibrillation, myocardial infarction, or surgery; sudden onset.
Thrombosis—Often the cause of a transient ischemic episode; gradual onset.
It is often caused by hypertension, age, diabetes, smoking, or elevated lipids.

Hemorrhage

Intracerebral bleeding—sudden onset; usually resulting from hypertension.
Subarachnoid bleeding—sudden onset; there are no known risk factors.
Cerebellar bleeding—sudden onset; usually resulting from hypertension.

■ **SIGNS AND SYMPTOMS**

Headache
Vertigo
Ataxia
Nausea and vomiting
Sudden neurologic deficit
Unequal pupils
Hemiparesis
Aphasia/dysphasia
Dysphagia
Decerebrate posturing
Sleepiness
Coma
Decreased BP on left side (left subclavian artery occlusion)
Frequently occurs in early morning hours
Find out if the patient has a history of any of the following:

Hypertension	Subacute bacterial endocarditis
Hyperlipidemia	Prosthetic heart valve
Diabetes	Collagen disease
Smoking	Use of birth control pills
Heart problems	Recent neck trauma
Atrial fibrillation	

■ **THERAPEUTIC INTERVENTIONS**

Ensure ABCs.
Keep the patient lying flat. This causes loss of autoregulation and a decreased mean arterial pressure. (Remember, cerebral perfusion pressure is equal to mean arterial pressure minus intracranial pressure.)
Decrease blood pressure—usually with nitroprusside.
Correct dysrhythmias.
Consider anticoagulants.
Consider aspirin.
Consider surgery.
Consider osmotic diuretics to decrease cerebral edema.
Consider steroids.
Consider antipyretics.
Consider seizure prophylaxis.

NOTE: If diagnosis of stroke is certain, do not administer dextrose 50%.

It is important to recognize the signs and symptoms of a CVA early, especially within the first 3 hours of onset of symptoms. These patients should be triaged emergent, stat head CT done, and consideration of Alteplase (TPA) to reduce the damage.

Categories of Cerebrovascular Accident

Transient ischemic attack

A transient ischemic attack (TIA) is a neurologic deficit that lasts for less than 12 hours. Most last only about 5 to 30 minutes. There are two causes, thrombosis and embolus. A TIA may be a prodrome to a cerebrovascular accident.

Reversible ischemic neurologic deficit

Symptoms will occur over 24 hours and may last for weeks. The patient may have minimal, partial, or no permanent deficit.

Stroke in evolution

Symptoms last longer than 24 hours with an increasing neurologic deterioration, with residual deficits present.

Completed stroke

There will be permanent neurologic damage.

■ **THERAPEUTIC INTERVENTIONS**
Ensure ABCs.
Consider anticoagulants.
Consider surgery.

UNCONSCIOUSNESS

Unconsciousness is by definition the opposite of consciousness. It is the depression of consciousness or the lack of awareness of self or anything surrounding self. This condition continues despite attempts to provide a stimulus. There are two causes of coma—structural lesions and metabolic or toxic states.

Examine the patient to determine if the coma is focal or diffuse and if it seems to be organic (as it is 95% of the time) or functional. Ascertain whether the patient is improving or getting worse with each passing minute. Pay strict attention to the ABCs. Perform a brief neurologic examination.

■ **THERAPEUTIC INTERVENTIONS**
The main purpose of therapeutic intervention is to protect the patient from further deterioration and to try to isolate the cause of the unconsciousness.

ABCs
Naloxone 0.8 mg IV, to rule out narcotic overdose
Dextrose 50% 50 ml IV, to rule out hypoglycemia and to protect the brain from hypoglycemia
Thiamine 50 to 100 mg IV, if alcohol abuse is suspected, to prevent Wernicke Korsakoff syndrome
Flumazenil to rule out benzodiazepine overdose
Left lateral swimmer's position with head dependent to prevent aspiration
Cervical spine precautions, if trauma is a possibility
Hyperventilate with 100% oxygen if head trauma is suspected as the cause
Other treatment depends on findings.

The causes of unconsciousness can be remembered using a simple mnemonic:

A = Alcoholism
E = Epilepsy/environmental conditions
I = Insulin (too much or too little)
O = Overdose (or underdose)
U = Uremia (or other metabolic causes)
T = Trauma or tumors
I = Infection or ischemia
P = Psychiatric

S = Stroke (that is, CVA or other neurologic or cardiovascular causes)

In the differential diagnosis process, be sure to assess the following:

Temperature	Presence of paralysis
Respirations	Occurrence of trauma
Blood pressure	Abdomen
Pulse	Extremities
Skin vital signs (color, temperature, moistness)	Presence of Babinski's reflex
Pupils	Presence of Battle's sign
Breath odor	Presence of hematotympanum
Presence of needle tracks	Presence of raccoon eyes
Presence of petechiae	Presence of Brudzinski's sign
Lung sounds	Presence of Kernig's sign
Deep tendon reflexes	Presence of incontinence
Presence of posturing	Presence of tongue lacerations

Consider the following laboratory tests to assist with diagnosis:

CBC	Urinalysis
Platelet count	Monitor:
Electrolyte levels	ECG
Glucose levels (serum and urine)	Cerebrospinal fluid pressure
BUN	X-ray examinations:
Creatinine levels	skull
Toxicology screen	face
Cholesterol level	chest
Magnesium level	abdomen
Calcium level	Scan:
Phosphorus level	head
Bilirubin level	lungs

BOTULISM

Botulism is caused by the ingestion of foods that have been improperly canned (high bacteria content before canning), especially those with low acid content, such as green beans. It can also occur in infants who have been fed unprocessed raw honey.

■ SIGNS AND SYMPTOMS

Usually develop 12 to 36 hours after ingestion of contaminated food, but may be delayed up to 4 days.

Dilated fixed pupils/limited eye movement
Dry mouth/sore throat
Diplopia
Urinary retention
Distended abdomen
Postural hypotension
Difficulty swallowing
Constipation
Headache
Decreased deep tendon reflexes
Difficulty chewing
Nasal tone to voice
Respiratory paralysis
Patient remains awake and alert throughout

NOTE: May mimic stroke, Guillain-Barré syndrome, myasthenia gravis, or arsenic intoxication.

■ **LABORATORY TEST**
Blood specimens for determination of presence of toxins
■ **THERAPEUTIC INTERVENTIONS**
ICU admission
ABCs (especially good respiratory support)—may require tracheostomy and ventilator assistance
Gastric lavage or emesis if ingestion is recent—then magnesium sulfate, as toxin is slowly absorbed
Antitoxin
Reporting to CDC in Atlanta

GUILLAIN-BARRÉ SYNDROME

Guillain-Barré syndrome is an acute paralytic disease that causes a decrease of myelin in the nerve roots and the peripheral nerves.
■ **SIGNS AND SYMPTOMS**
Tingling sensation in the extremities (for hours to weeks)
Severely decreased deep tendon reflexes
Symmetrical paralysis, usually beginning in lower extremities and gradually ascending to respiratory muscles
■ **THERAPEUTIC INTERVENTIONS**
ABCs (consider endotracheal intubation and ventilator)
General supportive care

MYASTHENIA GRAVIS

Myasthenia gravis is a defect in neuromuscular transmission. It is most common in persons in their twenties and thirties, and occurs more frequently in females than males. Myasthenia gravis usually affects only the facial and neck muscles; in a myasthenia crisis there is a sudden onset that may cause respiratory paralysis.
■ **SIGNS AND SYMPTOMS**
Increasing fatigue
Delayed recovery of muscle strength
Weak eye muscles
Weak facial muscles
Weak jaw muscles
Weak pharyngeal muscles
Diplopia
Dysphagia
Inability to handle secretions
Possible aspiration
■ **THERAPEUTIC INTERVENTIONS**
ABCs (consider endotracheal intubation)
Neostigmine 1 mg IV in myasthenia crisis
Medications that precipitate myasthenia include:
    Barbiturates
    Opiates
    Quinidine
    Quinine
    Any muscle relaxants
    Adrenocorticotropic hormone (ACTH)
    Steroids
    Aminoglycosides
    Certain antibiotics

PARALYTIC SHELLFISH POISONING

Saxitoxin is a toxin produced by marine protozoans that interferes with neuron membrane permeability to sodium ions. The toxin is consumed by shellfish such as oysters, clams, and sea snails that produce the phenomenon known as *red tide*. When these shellfish are consumed by humans, they cause paralytic shellfish poisoning.

■ **SIGNS AND SYMPTOMS**
Paresthesias (progressive)
Paresthesias of the mouth and head only
Dysphagia
Tremors
Vertigo
Flaccid quadriplegia
Dysarthria
Respiratory paralysis

■ **THERAPEUTIC INTERVENTIONS**
ABCs (consider endotracheal intubation and ventilator)
Good supportive care
The prognosis for paralytic shellfish poisoning is usually good after 24 hours.

SUMMARY

As is obvious from the headings in this chapter, neurologic emergencies covers a wide variety of topics from the not-so-serious to the life-threatening. It is extremely important for emergency nurses to be familiar with all aspects of neurologic emergencies to be better able to intervene in the life-threatening events.

SUGGESTED READINGS

Acute stroke treatment guidelines: background information on the NINDS t-PA trial, National Institute of Neurological Disorders and Stroke, National Institutes of Health, Bethesda, MD. http://www.ninds.nig.gov/healinfo/disorder/stroke/ntpabg.ktm

Aitken Neuroscience Center, New York. tel: (212) 772-0608. http://www.aitken.org/

American College of Rehab Medicine: Recommendations for use of uniform nomenclature pertinent to patients with severe alterations in consciousness, *Arch Phys Med* 76(4): 205, 1995.

Bates D: Neurologic emergencies, Hughes RAC, Ed, 1994, BMJ Publishing Group.

Cherington M et al: Lightning strikes: nature of neurological damage in patients evaluated in hospital emergency departments, *Ann Emerg Med,* 21(5):575, 1992.

Chiocca E: Bacterial meningitis, *Nurs 97* 27(9): 33, 1997.

Johns Hopkins Healthline, Intellhealth MEDLINE. http:intellhealth.silverplatter.com

McNew CD, Hunt S, Warner LS: How to help your patient with epilepsy, *Nurs 97* 27(9): 56-62, 1997.

Nachtman A et al: Cheyne-Stokes respirations in ischemic stroke, *Neurology* 45(4): 820, 1995.

Rowland LP, editor: *Merritt's textbook of neurology,* Baltimore, 1995, Williams & Wilkins.

Wolfe R, Brown D: Coma. In Rosen P et al: *Emergency medicine,* ed 4, St Louis, 1998, Mosby.

Abdominal Pain

Benjamin E. Marett

Abdominal pain is a symptom, not a diagnosis. The fact that the patient is complaining of abdominal pain is indicative of something happening that is causing this symptom to appear. Some conditions change so quickly that approximately one half of presenting diagnoses are changed by the time patients receive appropriate treatment. There are three types of abdominal pain—visceral, parietal, and referred.

Visceral Pain

Visceral pain may be caused by the stretching of a viscus. The patient usually describes abdominal cramping or gas pain. It is pain that intensifies and then decreases and is usually centered around the midline of the abdomen. It is a diffuse pain that is difficult to localize on examination. In response to the pain, the patient may be diaphoretic and experience nausea and vomiting, decreased blood pressure, tachycardia, and spasms of the abdominal wall muscles. Many inflammatory conditions begin with the signs and symptoms of visceral pain. Some of these more common conditions include:

Appendicitis
Cholecystitis
Pancreatitis
Intestinal obstruction

Parietal Pain

Parietal pain develops after visceral pain. It is a steady aching pain that is caused by inflammation. Parietal pain is stimulated by palpation or any tension in the peritoneal area. The pain is more localized. Parietal pain is associated with appendicitis.

Referred Pain

Referred pain is pain felt away from the original source of the pain. One theory is that this occurs as a result of fetal development and nerve growth or relocation.

PROBLEM AREA	PAIN REFERRED TO
Fluid collected under diaphragm	Top of shoulder
Ruptured peptic ulcer	Back
Pancreas	Midline back or directly through to back
Biliary tract	Around right side to scapula
Dissecting or ruptured aneurysm	Low back and thighs
Renal colic	Groin and external genitalia
Appendix	May be epigastric region
Uterine disease	Low back
Rectal disease	Low back

It is important for the caregiver to note that each individual reacts differently to pain. Someone whose condition would normally show a demonstration of severe pain may not demonstrate it. Someone whose condition would lead one to believe that the expression of pain should be minimal may complain of severe pain. Each patient should be treated individually, in accordance with the perceived expression of pain.

ASSESSMENT OF THE PATIENT WITH ABDOMINAL PAIN

The examiner should determine the following in a patient with abdominal pain:
- the possible diagnosis
- the necessity for hospital admission
- the necessity for surgery

When assessing the patient with a complaint of abdominal pain, the caregiver should use a format that is easy to remember and one that will provide a complete assessment. A tool that could be used is the "PQRST" mnemonic:

- **P** = Provokes

  What provokes the pain?

  Is there anything that makes it better?

  Is there anything that makes it worse?

- **Q** = Quality

  Ask the patient to describe the pain. Do not make suggestions unless the patient is unable to describe the pain. If the patient needs some help, suggest words such as "sharp," "dull," or "pressure." If the pain is caused by an event in the hollow viscus, the patient may describe the pain as "like being punched in the gut."

DESCRIPTION	POSSIBLE CAUSE
Severe, sharp	Infarction or rupture
Severe, controlled by medication	Pancreatitis, peritonitis, small bowel obstruction, renal colic, biliary colic
Dull	Inflammation, low-grade infection
Intermittent pain	Gastroenteritis, small bowel obstruction

- **R** = Radiates

  Ask the patient to point to the location of the pain. Ask if the pain radiates to any other place.

- **S** = Severity

  Ask the patient, "On a scale of 1 to 10, with 1 being the least and 10 being the worst, give the pain a number." This is a very subjective finding and will vary in accordance with how the patient tolerates pain.

- **T** = Time

  Ask the patient how long he or she has had the pain. Ask when it started and when it ended. Ask if this pain has ever been felt before. Pain of sudden onset is usually associated with rupture, torsion, strangulation, or vascular problems. Pain that is gradual in onset is usually caused by an inflammatory or obstructive process, such as pain that occurs with appendicitis or intestinal obstruction. Generally, the more acute the underlying process, the more acute the pain.

ASSOCIATED SIGNS AND SYMPTOMS

Nausea, Vomiting, and Anorexia

When nausea and vomiting appear to be the highlights of the clinical findings, the most likely causes are gastroenteritis, acute gastritis, pancreatitis, or an obstruction located high in the intestinal structure. If vomiting is intractable or feces are present in the vomitus, this suggests an intestinal obstruction in progress. If there is blood in the vomitus, this suggests gastritis or gastric ulcer. If abdominal pain precedes vomiting, this suggests appendicitis.

Diarrhea and Constipation

When there is acute abdominal involvement, changes in bowel content may be evident.

DESCRIPTION	POSSIBLE CAUSE
Diarrhea	Inflammatory disease
Constipation (or no flatus)	Dehydration, paralytic ileus, intestinal obstruction
Clay-colored stool	Biliary obstruction
Melena (black tarry stool)	High intestinal bleeding
Bright red blood	Low intestinal bleeding
Bloody diarrhea	Amebic dysentery, Crohn's disease, ulcerative colitis

Fever and Chills

Repeated fever and chills indicate bacterial infection, pyelonephritis, or appendicitis. Intermittent fever and chills may indicate acute cholecystitis.

Urinary Tract Symptoms

SYMPTOM	MAY INDICATE
Burning on urination	Urinary tract infection
Pain on urination	Obstruction somewhere in urinary tract
Hematuria or dysuria	Urinary tract infection or renal colic

Gynecologic Symptoms

Most gynecologic symptoms indicate gynecologic problems, such as pelvic inflammatory disease, ruptured ectopic pregnancy, ruptured ovarian cyst, or ruptured corpus luteum. Vaginal bleeding may indicate miscarriage, ruptured ectopic pregnancy, or one of many other gynecologic disorders.

Gastrointestinal Upset

If a meal was consumed by several people but only one person complains of associated signs and symptoms, the caregiver should rule out the possibility of gastroenteritis. If many persons complain of GI problems, there is a possibility of food poisoning. If there is a history of ingestion of fatty foods followed by abdominal pain, this may indicate acute cholecystitis. If there is a history of alcohol abuse, the caregiver must be sure to rule out pancreatitis. If abdominal pain starts just before eating and eating causes relief of pain, the caregiver should assume that the problem may be caused by a gastric ulcer or associated gastric disorder.

Age-Related Factors

Intussusception is rarely seen in persons over age 2. Intestinal obstruction is rarely seen in persons under age 40. Appendicitis occurs most frequently in persons between the ages of 5 and 45.

With major blood loss and hypovolemia, the signs of abdominal pain may be obscured.

PAIN IN THE FOUR QUADRANTS OF THE ABDOMEN

Physical Examination and Laboratory Analysis

The patient's physical appearance offers clues to the diagnosis.
• The patient's position
• Vital signs

Temperature will often be normal for a while and then elevate in the course of the disease process. Temperature will elevate if there is peritonitis or when an infection is fulminant.

Pulse will usually be evidenced as tachycardia.

Respirations will be shallow, and there will be very little motion of the abdominal wall when there is peritonitis. Rapid respirations may indicate acute abdominal infection such as pancreatitis or peritonitis.

Hypotension may indicate an acute condition that may require surgery.

Inspection

Observe the patient's abdomen.

Check for abdominal wall movement.

If the patient's hips are flexed and the knees drawn up toward the chest, this may be suggestive of appendicitis, a pelvic abscess, or a psoas abscess.

If peristaltic movements or abdominal distension are observed, this may be suggestive of intestinal obstruction.

Ascites may be indicative of liver disease.

An abdominal aneurysm may be evidenced by a visible or palpable abdominal mass.

Auscultation

Bowel sounds are difficult to assess in the emergency care setting because it takes a full 3 to 5 minutes of auscultation before the absence of bowel sounds can be established. Normally, there are 10 to 20 peristaltic sounds per minute (Figure 13-1). Auscultation should occur before manual examination of the abdomen.

Palpation

Palpate the abdomen as gently as possible. Check for spasms, tenderness, and any masses. Be sure to observe the patient's face during this examination, as this may be a clue to the patient's level of pain. Remember to palpate the area that hurts the most last so the examination can be completed without interruption.

Percussion

Percussion is probably the least useful of all examination tools because it is difficult to assess the findings. Areas that are normally dense will produce dull sounds.

Tympany

Tympany is a sign that gas is present. Conditions that sometimes present with this sign are appendicitis and sigmoid colon obstruction. Urinary retention offers the sign of dullness over the suprapubic area.

Ascites

Ascites (shifting dullness) is the presence of fluid where it normally should not be. Ascites could also suggest a tumor, congestive heart failure, or blood in the peritoneal cavity. If you suspect the patient to have ascites remember to measure the abdominal girth with a tape measure and mark the area. After percussion, proceed to palpation. Start the initial abdominal examination with auscultation first, then proceed to percussion.

Laboratory tests and x-ray examination

Perform the following laboratory tests on the patient with abdominal pain:

Serum electrolytes

Serum amylase

Urinalysis

Urine amylase

Complete blood count (including hematocrit and hemoglobin)

Blood urea nitrogen

The Four Quadrants of the Abdomen

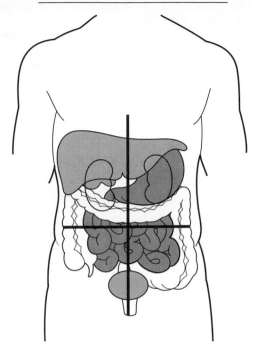

Right Upper Quadrant

Cholecystis
Hepatitis
Hepatomegaly
Biliary Colic
Pancreatitis
Perforated Duodenal Ulcer
Right–sided Nephrolithiosis
Myocardial Ischemia
Right Lung Pneumonia

Left Upper Quadrant

Pancreatitis
Gastric Ulcers
Gastritis
Splenic Rupture
Diverticulitis
Left–sided Nephrolithiosis
Myocardial Ischemia
Left Lung Pneumonia
Pulmonary Embolism
Pericarditis

Right Lower Quadrant

Appendicitis
Intestinal Obstruction
Crohn's Disease
Diverticulosis
Fecal Perforation
Ectopic Pregnancy
Ovarian Cyst
Salpingitis
Strangulated Hernia
Kidney or Ureteral Stone

Left Lower Quadrant

Early Appendicitis
Sigmoid Perforation
Sigmoid Diverticulitis
Colon Perforation
Ulcerative Colitis
Salpingitis
Ovarian Cyst
Ectopic Pregnancy
Strangulated Hernia
Kidney or Ureteral Stone

FIGURE 13-1. The four quadrants of the abdomen.

The following x-ray studies may be obtained:
    Upright chest
    Upright abdominal
    Left lateral decubitus
    Plain abdominal film
    Intravenous pyelogram (IVP)
    Intravenous cholangiogram
    Upper GI series
    Lower GI series
Conditions where surgery should be considered:

Appendicitis   Cholecystitis (may consider lithotripsy)
Bowel obstruction   Pancreatitis
Bowel infarction   Salpingitis
Ruptured ectopic pregnancy   Perforation of viscus
Ureteral stone   Ruptured intraabdominal aneurysm
Peritonitis   Massive GI bleed
Diverticulitis

Chronic conditions where abdominal pain is a major symptom:

Ulcerative colitis	Irritable bowel syndrome
Crohn's disease	Regional enteritis
Reflux esophagitis	

Conditions outside the abdomen that may present with the symptom of abdominal pain:

Hepatitis	Empyema
Rheumatic fever	Pleurisy
Myocardial infarction	Hip joint disease
Pneumothorax	Spinal tumor
Pneumonia	

INFLAMMATORY CONDITIONS THAT CAUSE ABDOMINAL PAIN

Acute Appendicitis

■ **SIGNS AND SYMPTOMS**
Anorexia
Nausea and vomiting
Pain in right lower quadrant, at McBurney's point
Afebrile (unless ruptured)
Guarding posture (fetal position, hips flexed and knees drawn up)
Elevated white blood cell count

■ **THERAPEUTIC INTERVENTIONS**
IV Ringer's lactate
Surgical consultation
Pain management
Antibiotic administration
If ruptured:
    Nasogastric tube
    Rectal acetaminophen for fever control

Acute Pancreatitis

■ **SIGNS AND SYMPTOMS**
Severe epigastric pain following ingestion of alcohol or large amounts of food
Nausea and vomiting
Abdominal distension
Abdominal tenderness
Abdominal rigidity

■ **THERAPEUTIC INTERVENTIONS**
IV Ringer's lactate
Analgesia for pain management
Nasogastric tube
Antibiotics
Chest x-ray film (20% to 50% of patients with pancreatitis have associated pulmonary complications)

Ulcerative Colitis

■ **SIGNS AND SYMPTOMS**
Bloody diarrhea
Frequent stools (usually more than 20 per day)
Abdominal cramps
Weight loss
Weakness
If perforated:
  Fever
  Tachycardia
  Generalized signs of sepsis
■ **THERAPEUTIC INTERVENTIONS**
IV Ringer's lactate or normal saline
Antibiotics
Hospital admission

Toxic Megacolon

Toxic megacolon is a severe dilation of the colon associated with colitis.
■ **SIGNS AND SYMPTOMS**
Fever
Explosive diarrhea
A quiet abdomen
Prostration
Possible shock-like state
■ **THERAPEUTIC INTERVENTIONS**
IV Ringer's lactate
Hospital admission

Esophagitis

Esophagitis is an inflammation of the hiatal esophagus usually caused by the regurgitation of gastric acids. It is often accompanied by a hiatal hernia or gastric ulcer. It may also be caused by the ingestion of a caustic substance such as lye or another strong alkali or acid.
■ **SIGNS AND SYMPTOMS**
Steady, substernal pain that is increased by swallowing
Occasional vomiting
Weight loss
Obstruction
Bleeding
Foul breath
■ **THERAPEUTIC INTERVENTIONS**
Bland diet
Antacids
Surgery to correct anatomic defect, if present
If caused by caustic ingestion:
  ABCs
  Dilation of the esophagus
  Antibiotics

Gastritis

Gastritis is an inflammation of the gastric mucosa. It can occur as a result of ingestion of a gastric irritant, hyperacidity, bile reflux, or shock.

■ **SIGNS AND SYMPTOMS**
Epigastric pain
Nausea and vomiting
Mucosal bleeding
Epigastric tenderness on palpation

■ **THERAPEUTIC INTERVENTIONS**
Antacids
Bland diet
Sedative (if nausea is severe)
Nasogastric tube
Fluid replacement
Anticholinergic medications

Peptic Ulcer

A peptic ulcer can occur in the stomach and the duodenum. It is usually caused by hyperacidity.

■ **SIGNS AND SYMPTOMS**
Burning pain in the epigastric region, usually occurring early in the morning and just before meals
Pain relieved by antacids, bland foods, or vomiting
Symptoms that occur during stressful periods when production of gastric acids is increased

■ **THERAPEUTIC INTERVENTION**
Antacids
Bland diet
Sedation
Nasogastric tube if severe vomiting
Fluid and electrolyte replacement

OBSTRUCTIVE CONDITIONS THAT CAUSE ABDOMINAL PAIN

Intestinal Obstruction

An intestinal obstruction may be caused by a large variety of syndromes. Intestinal obstruction may be caused by a hernia, fecal impaction, adhesions, tumors, paralytic ileus, intussusception, regional enteritis, volvulus, gallstones, abscesses, and hematomas. There may be a primary mechanical obstruction or a secondary obstruction caused by an inflammatory condition or a nervous system problem. The primary danger of an intestinal obstruction is dehydration. Other dangers include infarction and perforation of the bowel.

■ **SIGNS AND SYMPTOMS**
Nausea and vomiting
Abdominal pain
Constipation/obstipation
Abdominal distension

■ **THERAPEUTIC INTERVENTIONS**
IV Ringer's lactate or normal saline
Antibiotics
Nasogastric tube
Possible surgery

Cholecystitis

Cholecystitis is an inflammation of the gallbladder that may be exacerbated by the presence of gallstones.

■ **SIGNS AND SYMPTOMS**

Abdominal pain of sudden onset (especially following ingestion of fried or greasy foods) in the epigastric region, radiating to the right upper quadrant

Low-grade fever (100.4° F [38° C])

Nausea and vomiting

Local and rebound tenderness

Referred pain into the right subclavicular area

Slight jaundice

Usually overweight, over 40 years old, and female

■ **THERAPEUTIC INTERVENTION**

Nasogastric tube

IV Ringer's lactate or normal saline

Possible surgery

Esophageal Obstruction

Most of the time an esophageal obstruction is the result of a foreign body ingestion.

■ **SIGNS AND SYMPTOMS**

History of foreign body ingestion

Cervical subcutaneous emphysema (if there is a perforation)

Patient complains of "something stuck" in his throat

■ **THERAPEUTIC INTERVENTIONS**

If the object does not have sharp edges and can pass into the stomach, it can usually pass through the intestines without difficulty.

Retrieval of the object through esophagoscopy.

Incarcerated Hernia

An incarcerated hernia is a protrusion of bowel or other abdominal contents through the abdominal musculature but not through the skin. There is usually a good blood supply to the hernia unless it is incarcerated. Hernias are most commonly found in the inguinal, femoral, and umbilical areas.

■ **SIGNS AND SYMPTOMS**

The patient notices the herniation.

Pain in the abdominal wall following exertion.

■ **THERAPEUTIC INTERVENTIONS**

If the hernia is not incarcerated, manual attempt, by a surgeon, at replacement

If incarcerated, surgery

HEMORRHAGIC CONDITIONS THAT CAUSE ABDOMINAL PAIN

Upper GI Bleeding

There are several causes of upper GI bleeding, or bleeding proximal to the ligament of Treitz.

■ **SIGNS AND SYMPTOMS**

Hematemesis

Melena (blood and stomach acids mix with stool)

Possible shock

Possible history of chronic alcohol ingestion

Epigastric tenderness
Possible jaundice, an enlarged spleen, and an enlarged liver

Specific Causes

Bleeding peptic ulcer

Two thirds of all cases of upper GI bleeding are caused by peptic ulcers. The bleeding is caused by the granulation of the ulcer that erodes into a vessel during the healing process.

■ **THERAPEUTIC INTERVENTIONS**
ABCs
IV Ringer's lactate or normal saline
Bedrest
Oxygen
Cooled-saline gastric lavage through a large gastric tube
Surgery if bleeding is uncontrolled and the patient shows signs and symptoms of shock
Blood replacement

Bleeding Esophageal Varices

Patients with liver disease have a high risk of developing esophageal varices. Portal hypertension causes collateral vessels to develop between the stomach and the systemic veins of the lower esophagus. Rupture of these vessels can rapidly cause death. It is the cause of death in over one third of patients with cirrhosis of the liver.

■ **SIGNS AND SYMPTOMS**
Massive bleeding from the upper GI tract
History of chronic alcohol ingestion or portal hypertension
■ **THERAPEUTIC INTERVENTIONS**
ABCs
Balloon tamponade with a Sengstaken-Blakemore tube (Figure 13-2)
Intraarterial vasopressin
Surgery
IV fluid and/or blood replacement as indicated

Mallory-Weiss syndrome

This syndrome is usually caused by retching and vomiting that is not synchronized with gastric regurgitation. This causes bleeding at the cardioesophageal junction.

■ **SIGNS AND SYMPTOMS**
History of retching and vomiting with normal gastric content emptying, followed by hematemesis on subsequent vomiting episodes
■ **THERAPEUTIC INTERVENTIONS**
Whole blood transfusions
Balloon tamponade with a Sengstaken-Blakemore tube (see Figure 13-2)
Intraarterial vasopressin
Surgery
IV fluid and/or blood replacement as indicated

Borhave's syndrome

Borhave's syndrome is the term for small tears of the esophagus that are caused by vomiting following a large meal. It is thought to be caused by distension of the esophagus.

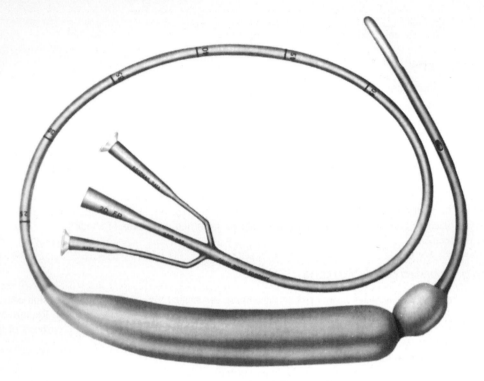

FIGURE 13-2. Sengstaken-Blakemore tube.

■ **SIGNS AND SYMPTOMS**
Bloody expectoration when the patient clears vomitus
Possible massive bleeding if tears are severe
Pain in the esophagus
■ **THERAPEUTIC INTERVENTIONS**
ABCs
Close observation
Surgery if bleeding is heavy and uncontrolled

Lower GI Bleeding

Bleeding from the large bowel and rectum is usually caused by ruptured diverticula, ulcerative colitis, tumors, cecal ulcers, ruptured hemorrhoids, or polyps.
■ **SIGNS AND SYMPTOMS**
Bright red blood from the rectum
■ **THERAPEUTIC INTERVENTION**
Control of bleeding (depends on the source)
Possible surgery
Possible IV fluid and/or blood replacement as indicated

HOW TO INSERT A NASOGASTRIC TUBE

1. Measure the length of the tube required by measuring from the tip of the patient's earlobe to the tip of the nose and from the tip of the nose to the umbilicus; mark the tube at this point.
2. Explain the procedure to the patient.
3. Lubricate the tube at the tip and a few inches up from the distal end with a water-soluble lubricant.
4. Place the patient in high Fowler's position.
5. Have the patient place his or her head in a sniffing position.
6. Check the patient for a deviated septum.
7. Insert the tube via the nares, instructing the patient to swallow as the tube is being passed; using a small amount of water and having the patient sip and swallow during this process usually helps (unless water is contraindicated).
8. Continue to pass the tube until it is at the level previously marked; if the patient begins to choke or cough during the procedure, stop and allow the patient to rest; if coughing and choking continue, remove the tube and begin again, as the tube may have inadvertently passed into the trachea.
9. Check to be sure the tube is in the stomach (while air is being injected into the tube, auscultate the epigastric region for the sound of air movement or aspirate the tube for the presence of stomach contents).
10. Secure the tube by taping it to the nose and the forehead.
11. Connect the distal end of the tube to intermittent suction if the tube is single lumen and to continuous suction if the tube is double lumen. (Single-lumen tubes are uncommon in current practice.)

HOW TO INSERT A SENGSTAKEN-BLAKEMORE TUBE

1. Explain the procedure to the patient.
2. Check the tube balloons for patency.
3. The pharynx may be anesthetized.
4. Lubricate the tube with a water-soluble lubricant at the tip and several inches up from the distal end.
5. Insert the tube via the nares for approximately 50 cm.
6. Check to be sure the tube is in the stomach; while air is being injected into the tube, auscultate the epigastric region for the sound of air movement or aspirate the tube for the presence of stomach contents.
7. Fill the gastric balloon with 200 to 250 ml of radiopaque (Hypaque) dye and double-clamp it.
8. Apply gentle traction to check for placement and to wedge the balloon into the cardioesophageal junction.
9. Aspirate the stomach contents to check for continued bleeding; if bleeding is present, inflate the esophageal balloon to a pressure between 25 and 45 mm Hg by attaching the distal end of the balloon to a sphygmomanometer.
10. Double-clamp the tube.
11. Obtain an abdominal x-ray film to verify the tube's position.
12. A small nasogastric tube may be passed to the upper end of the gastric balloon to allow upper esophageal aspiration if required.
13. The esophageal balloon should be deflated every 8 hours to avoid necrosis.
14. Be sure to monitor the patient closely for airway obstruction and keep equipment close by in case the balloons must be deflated rapidly.

SUGGESTED READINGS

Grendell JH: Miscellaneous disorders of the stomach and small intestine. In Grendell JH et al, editors: *Current diagnosis and treatment in gastroenterology,* Stamford, Conn, 1996, Appleton & Lange.

Newbury L, Emergency Nurses Association: *Sheehy's emergency nursing,* ed 4, St Louis, 1998, Mosby.

Pace S, Burlae TF: Intravenous morphine for early pain relief in patients with acute abdominal pain, *Acad Emerg Med* 3: 1086, 1996.

Rusnak RA, Borer JM, Fastow JS: Misdiagnosis of acute appendicitis: common features discovered in cases after litigation, *Am J Emerg Med* 12: 397, 1994.

Wright JA: Seven abdominal assessment signs every emergency nurse should know, *J Emerg Nurs* 23(5): 446-450, 1997.

Blood Disorders

Benjamin E. Marett

There are several disorders of the blood, but only the three most common will be discussed here: sickle cell disease and crisis, hemophilia, and anemia.

SICKLE CELL DISEASE

Sickle cell disease is an inherited disorder that occurs in 7% of West Africans and African Americans. It is an autosomal recessive disease with an altered hemoglobin molecule. A person with sickle cell disease has two sickle cell genes and rarely lives past early adulthood. A person who has sickle cell *trait* has one sickle cell gene, and the disease remains clinically inactive.

SICKLE CELL CRISIS (VASO-OCCLUSIVE CRISIS)

Sickled cells carry a normal amount of hemoglobin, but the cells have a tendency to clump together because of their sickled shape. As these cells clump, obstruction occurs and oxygen and other nutrients do not reach capillaries distal to the blockage, resulting in ischemia.

This causes severe pain and leads to chronic and acute organ dysfunction and frequent infections.

Sickle cell crisis may be precipitated by cold, stress, infection, metabolic or respiratory acidosis, high altitude, or unknown factors. It usually occurs more frequently at night. If the ischemic state is not corrected, local tissue necrosis occurs.

Common sites of sickle cell crisis/pain in children are the hands, feet, and abdomen (mimicking appendicitis). In adults, pain commonly occurs in the long bones, large joints, and the spine.

■ SIGNS AND SYMPTOMS
Pain (episodic and in target areas)
History of sickle cell disease
Weakness
Pallor

■ THERAPEUTIC INTERVENTIONS
Analgesia
    Acetaminophen or codeine for mild-to-moderate pain
    Ketorolac or morphine sulfate for moderate-to-severe pain
Oxygen
IV D5% in ½ normal saline or D_5W for hydration
Antibiotics for the infection
Local heat
Warm environment
Emotional support

■ COMPLICATIONS

Recurrent crisis
Chronic hemolytic anemia
Frequent infections
Transient aplastic crisis
Cholelithiasis and cholecystitis
Delayed sexual maturation
Priapism
Renal disease/failure
Bone disease (infarction leading to avascular necrosis of femoral heads)
High-output cardiac failure
Autosplenectomy
Pneumonia
Meningitis
Osteomyelitis
Pulmonary embolus
Cor pulmonale
Chronic skin ulcers
High incidence of spontaneous abortion, perinatal mortality, maternal mortality
Hepatomegaly
Hepatic infarction
Jaundice
Coma
Death

HEMOPHILIA

In its simplest expression, hemophilia can be viewed as a bleeding disorder caused by the absence of a clotting factor. However, hemophilia is actually a catch-all term for a number of bleeding disorders.

Hemophilia (factor VIII deficiency or factor IX deficiency) is an X chromosome, sex-linked disorder that occurs recessively in males and is transmitted by females. The level of bleeding disorder can be quite variable. Factor VIII (antihemophilia factor) deficiency occurs in 1 of 10,000 people. Factor IX deficiency occurs in 1 of 40,000 people. Both are usually manifested by hemarthrosis of the knees, elbows, and ankles, but bleeding can also occur in the central nervous system, the oral or nasal mucosa, the urinary tract, or the GI tract. It may first be seen in infancy when excessive bleeding occurs on circumcision, with bleeding gums, and/or epistaxis.

Figure 14-1 schematically depicts the primary clotting mechanism. Each factor is a protein or glycoprotein that circulates in the plasma. Clotting factors circulate in an inactive form. Initiation of clotting factors first requires factor activation. This occurs whenever a cut or bruise is sustained. The subsequent factors are activated in a domino-like fashion until fibrinogen becomes fibrin and a clot is formed. If any one of these factors is removed from the sequence or inactivated, clotting will not take place.

Hemophilia Type A (Factor VIII Disorder)

Hemophilia type A is a factor VIII disorder. In the majority of patients, factor VIII may be present but not functional, or is functioning at less than normal capacity. The actual severity of the disease depends on the functional activity of the factor in each patient.

In type A hemophilia, the functional level of factor VIII can be augmented by transfusion with fresh frozen plasma, fresh plasma, cryoprecipitate (from pooled plasma), or factor VIII concentrate. The amount of factor VIII in the plasma is small. Consequently, the patient may be at risk of fluid overload and infectious diseases. Cryoprecipitate and factor VIII concentrate are smaller in volume but carry a high risk of hepatitis and the human immunodeficiency virus (HIV). Current preparations and modifications have noticeably reduced this

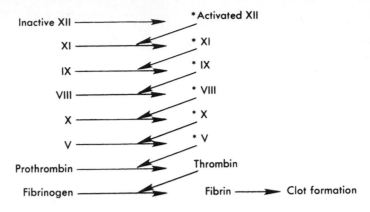

FIGURE 14-1. Clotting factors (intrinsic mechanisms).

risk. D-Desaminoarginine vasopressin (DDAVP) stimulates the release, but not the formation, of factor VIII and may be used for mild hemophilia bleeds.

Hemophilia Type B (Christmas Disease)

The less common form of hemophilia, known as type B hemophilia or Christmas disease, is the absence or functional defect of factor IX. Bleeding caused by factor IX deficiencies can be treated with fresh frozen or fresh plasma or factor IX concentrate. Cryoprecipitate cannot be used because it does not contain factor IX.

Episodes of hemarthrosis that result from type A or B hemophilia are usually self-limiting; the joint capsule can only distend to a certain point before the bleeding eventually is tamponaded. Treatment includes immobilization, elevation, and ice application over a light pressure dressing. After administering therapeutic products that correct coagulation problems, joint aspiration may be considered. Discharge instructions include limited weight-bearing and range-of-motion exercises. A hematologic and orthopedic follow-up should be arranged.

A third type of bleeding disorder that is not really hemophilia is von Willebrand's disease. It is a decrease in von Willebrand factor, a plasma protein necessary for platelet function. It is usually evidenced by mucocutaneous bleeding, such as epistaxis or excessive vaginal bleeding during menstruation. Bleeding problems are treated with fresh frozen or fresh plasma, cryoprecipitate, or DDAVP.

Treatment for all hemophilia and von Willebrand's disorders is rapid factor replacement or other therapeutic intervention mentioned above and close observation for further bleeding.

ANEMIA

Anemia is defined as a hemoglobin less than 50% of normal value. Normal hematocrit at sea level in a male should range between 42% and 53%. Normal hematocrit at sea level in a female should range between 37% and 47%.

Identify the cause of the anemia and treat the cause. Remember, when an acute bleed occurs, hematocrit and hemoglobin will remain the same as normal until some rehydration occurs. Acute bleeding may not demonstrate immediate changes in hematocrit and hemoglobin.

■ TYPES OF ANEMIA

Macrocytic hypochromic
Macrocytic
Normocytic normochromic

■ **SIGNS AND SYMPTOMS**
Weakness and fatigue
Syncope
Dyspnea on exertion
Palpitations
Possible CHF
Possible myocardial infarction
Possible shock
The diagnosis of anemia can be made on the basis of history as well as:
    Orthostatic vital signs
    Abnormalities in
        CBC
        Reticulocyte count
        Wright's stain

■ **THERAPEUTIC INTERVENTIONS**
Folate (oral)
Treat underlying condition
Three of the most common blood disorders have been briefly discussed. For a more in-depth evaluation, the reader is referred to the suggested reading list.

SUGGESTED READINGS

Alaui JB: Sickle cell anemia, *Emerg Med Clin North Am* 68: 545, 1984.

Charache S, Koshy M, Milner PF: Care of patients with sickle cell anemia in the adult emergency department. In Bell WR, editor: *Hematologic and oncologic emergencies,* New York, 1993, Churchill Livingstone.

Fitzpatrick L, Fitzpatrick T: Blood transfusions: keeping your patient safe, *Nurs 97* 27(8): 34-42, 1997.

Newbury L, Emergency Nurses Association: *Sheehy's emergency nursing principles and practice,* edition 4, St Louis, 1998, Mosby.

Pfaff JA, Geninatti M: Hemophilia, *Emerg Med Clin North Am* 11(2): 337, 1993.

USDHHS: *Sickle cell disease: screening diagnosis, management and counseling in newborns and infants, AHCPR Publication 93-0562,* Rockville, Md, 1993, USDHHS.

Metabolic Emergencies

Jaye M. Sengewald

ENDOCRINE EMERGENCIES

Overproduction or underproduction of certain hormones may result in endocrine emergencies. Often a stressful event triggers a crisis of the endocrine system.

DIABETES EMERGENCIES

Diabetes mellitus is a chronic condition in which the body is unable to metabolize glucose, the body's major source of energy, because of a lack of effective insulin. There are two major types of diabetes: type I (also called insulin-dependent diabetes mellitus or juvenile onset diabetes), characterized by insulin deficiency, and type II (also called noninsulin-dependent diabetes mellitus or adult onset diabetes), characterized by insulin resistance. The goal in treatment of diabetes is to balance food intake/energy output (exercise) and the use of insulin (which may be endogenous or exogenous) to maintain the blood glucose levels at or near the normal range. When that balance is not achieved, diabetes emergencies may occur.

Hypoglycemia

Hypoglycemia is the most common acute complication of diabetes and the most common side effect of insulin and oral hypoglycemic agents. As more and more individuals with diabetes follow intensive therapy regimens (three or more insulin injections per day or use of an insulin pump, as recommended by the American Diabetes Association based on the results of the Diabetes Control and Complications Trial),[1] it is likely that there will be an increase in the frequency of severe hypoglycemia seen in the Emergency Department. Severe hypoglycemia is defined as a condition in which assistance is needed to obtain treatment. Mild and moderate hypoglycemia are common self-treated conditions.

The normal blood glucose range is 80 to 120 mg/dl (4.4 to 6.6 mmol/L). Hypoglycemia, or low blood glucose, is defined as a blood glucose level below 50 mg/dl (2.8 mmol/L). In an individual whose blood glucose normally runs very high, or with a very sudden drop in blood glucose, symptoms of hypoglycemia may be present at higher blood glucose levels (>50 mg/dl).

All those who take sulfonylureas for their diabetes are at risk for hypoglycemia. Biguianides and alpha-glucosidase inhibitors, when used alone, do not cause hypoglycemia. An increased risk exists for those with type I diabetes practicing intensive therapy (three or more insulin injections a day or use of an insulin pump) and those with type II diabetes taking a long-acting oral hypoglycemic agent, such as chlorpropamide (Diabinese).

Other conditions associated with hypoglycemia:

Onset of menses

Immediate postpartum period

Autonomic neuropathy

■ **CAUSES**

Too much insulin*

Too much exercise/activity

Too little food

Alcohol

■ **SIGNS AND SYMPTOMS**

Mild hypoglycemia. Characterized by adrenergic symptoms:†

Shaking

Sweating

Tachycardia

Hunger

Pallor

Tingling of lips

Anxiety

Palpitations

Restlessness

Moderate hypoglycemia. Characterized by neuroglycopenic symptoms:

Irritability

Inability to concentrate

Behavior change

Drowsiness

Confusion

Slurred speech

Staggered gait

Weakness

Blurred vision

Headache

Severe hypoglycemia. May result in:

Unconsciousness

Seizures

Rarely, death

Hypoglycemia unawareness, a result of autonomic neuropathy, eliminates the individual's ability to recognize early signs and symptoms.

■ **THERAPEUTIC INTERVENTIONS**

Box 15-1 lists treatments for hypoglycemia.

Treatment of hypoglycemia in the conscious patient

- Recognize symptoms.
- Confirm blood glucose level (a fingerstick, blood glucose test performed with a light-reflectance meter is adequate to begin treatment if the equipment is functioning properly and the operator has been well-trained in the procedure).
- Obtain laboratory analysis of blood glucose for confirmation of the meter result.
- Administer 15 g of rapid-acting carbohydrate (see examples in the box below).
- If no improvement in 10 minutes, as evidenced by blood glucose level, repeat administration of 15 g of carbohydrate. Neurogenic symptoms may continue for an hour or more with blood glucose levels above 100 mg/dl.

*Too much insulin may include accidental or intentional overdoses of insulin or oral hypoglycemic agents.

†These symptoms may be masked with long-standing diabetes, autonomic neuropathy (specifically, hypoglycemic unawareness), beta blockers or alcoholism.

BOX 15-1   Treatment of Hypoglycemia

Each of the following contain 15 g of carbohydrate
½ cup orange juice
1 cup milk
⅓ cup apple juice
½ cup regular soda (not diet soda)
½ oz box raisins
10 jelly beans
3 tsp honey or syrup
3 glucose tablets
8 Lifesavers
8 small sugar cubes
4 tsp sugar
1 small tube cake frosting
1 small tube glucose gel

Treatment of hypoglycemia in the semiconscious or unconscious patient
• Confirm blood glucose level, as above.
• Administer 50% dextrose 25 to 50 ml IV.
• A continuous infusion of D_5W or $D_{10}W$ to maintain blood glucose in the normal range may be necessary.
              or
• Administer glucagon 1 mg IM (0.5 mg in children ages 3 to 5, 0.25 mg in children less than 3 years).
• If no improvement in 20 minutes, repeat the glucagon.
• Once the patient can swallow, give 20 g of carbohydrate by mouth to prevent a recurrence and to restock depleted glycogen stores.
• Vomiting is common following the administration of glucagon, so position the patient to avoid aspiration.
• Glucagon may not be effective if the liver glycogen stores have been depleted.
• Monitor blood glucose levels, vital signs and neurological status.

Following successful treatment of hypoglycemia, it is helpful for the patient to reflect on possible causes as an aid to prevention of hypoglycemia in the future. Recalling past insulin doses (Table 15-1), time of injection, food intake, activity, and special circumstances may help to identify the cause of hypoglycemia. Frequent or prolonged hypoglycemia may result in permanent neurologic damage. Early recognition of symptoms and prompt treatment is the key. Recommend to the patient that identification, such as a Medic-Alert necklace or bracelet, be worn.

Reactive Hypoglycemia

Reactive, or postprandial, hypoglycemia is described as hypoglycemia that occurs in response to a meal, generally 1 to 2 hours after eating. This occurs in people who do not have diabetes.

■ CAUSES
Altered GI motility after gastric surgery
Fructose intolerance
Impaired glucose tolerance
Insulinoma
Idiopathic

■ THERAPEUTIC INTERVENTIONS
Administer oral glucose.
Refer for further work-up of etiology and treatment plan.

TABLE 15-1   Types of Insulin—Onset, Peak, and Duration of Action

TYPE	ONSET*	PEAK*	DURATION*
Insulin analog (insulin lispro)	¼-½	1-2	3-4
Short-acting			
Regular	½-1	2-4	6-8
Semilente	1-2	3-8	10-16
Intermediate-acting			
NPH	1-2	6-12	18-24
Lente	1-3	6-12	18-24
Long-acting			
Ultralente	4-6	8-20	24-28

*In hours following subcutaneous administration. These times are approximate and are based on biosynthetic human insulin. Animal insulins tend to have slightly longer action times. Individual variations in insulin absorption and action may be caused by many factors, including dose, injection technique, injection site, temperature of insulin, exercise following injection, and insulin antibodies.

Hyperglycemic Emergencies
Diabetic ketoacidosis

Diabetic ketoacidosis (DKA) is the most common endocrine emergency and accounts for about 80% to 90% of hyperglycemic emergencies. This is an acute complication of diabetes and in some cases may be the initial presentation of new-onset diabetes. DKA is characterized by dehydration, electrolyte losses, ketonuria, and acidosis, resulting from an inadequate amount of available insulin. When insulin is unavailable for the transport of glucose into cells, fatty acids are metabolized into ketone bodies in the liver. An accumulation of ketones results in metabolic acidosis.

DKA usually occurs only in type I diabetes, but under conditions of extreme stress may be seen in type II diabetes. There is a 6% to 10% mortality rate associated with the precipitating cause, the DKA itself or complications of the treatment.

■ **CAUSES**
Omission of insulin injection(s)
Inadequate insulin dose
New-onset diabetes
Illness
Infection
Myocardial infarction
Cerebrovascular accident
Trauma
Surgery
Steroids
Pancreatitis
Pregnancy
Emotional stress
Unknown etiology
■ **SIGNS AND SYMPTOMS**
Nausea
Vomiting
Anorexia

Blurred vision

Hypothermia

Diminished bowel sounds

Hyporeflexia

Kussmaul respirations (rapid, deep breathing)

Acetone on the breath (fruity-smelling breath)

Abdominal pain

Drowsiness

Weakness

Thirst

Polyuria

Tachycardia

Orthostatic hypotension

Poor skin turgor

Dry mucous membranes

Hyperglycemia (>250 mg/dl)

pH <7.3

Serum bicarbonate <15 mEq/L

Ketonuria

Glucosuria

Mental status ranging from normal to coma

■ DIFFERENTIAL DIAGNOSIS

Alcoholic ketoacidosis

Hyperglycemic hyperosmolar nonketotic coma

Starvation ketosis

Uremia

Lactic acidosis

Toxin ingestion

■ THERAPEUTIC INTERVENTIONS

The goals of treatment are fluid and electrolyte replacement, reversal of ketonemia and hyperglycemia, and determination and treatment of the precipitating cause. Correction that occurs too rapidly may result in cerebral edema, hypoglycemia, or hypokalemia.

Laboratory evaluation

Obtain a blood glucose level. If unable to do so rapidly, give an unconscious patient 25 g of dextrose to rule out hypoglycemia, the most common cause of altered mental status in a person with diabetes. (This small amount of glucose would not be harmful to a person in DKA.)

Obtain urine ketones, serum glucose, electrolytes, ketones, BUN, creatinine, phosphate and amylase levels.

Obtain arterial blood gases.

Additional studies may be needed to determine precipitating cause.

Fluid replacement

Administer normal saline at 1 L/hr for 1 to 2 hours, then 100 to 500 ml/hr.

Change to ½ normal saline when the patient is no longer hypovolemic.

The total fluid deficit generally averages 6 L.

Insulin

Administer insulin following the first liter of saline (see Table 15-1).

IV insulin is recommended, as IM or SC insulin is erratically absorbed in the presence of hypovolemia.

A bolus of 5 to 10 units of regular insulin may be given, or a continuous infusion may be started (remember to prime the tubing and discard the first 30 to 50 ml of the insulin/NS solution).

The rate of infusion should be titrated for a reduction in the patient's blood glucose of 100 mg/dl/hr.

For children, first hour replacement should be 20 ml/kg of body weight.

Insulin therapy must be aggressive until ketogenesis stops.

When the blood glucose level falls to 250 mg/dl or below, the IV fluid should be changed to fluid containing 5% dextrose.

Subcutaneous insulin must be given 1 to 4 hours before discontinuing the insulin infusion.

Electrolyte replacement

Initially, the potassium level may be high.

Fluid resuscitation, insulin, and correction of acidosis all reduce extracellular potassium.

Replace potassium, after documented urine output, at 20 to 40 mEq/L.

Phosphate replacement may be necessary.

Sodium bicarbonate may be necessary if the arterial blood pH is ≤7.1.

Monitor electrolytes every 2 to 4 hours.

Follow-up

Determine the precipitating cause and plan treatment.

Patient and family education is needed if the cause was the omission of an insulin dose during illness.

Hospital admission is usually indicated. In mild cases of DKA the patient may be discharged home from the Emergency Department following treatment if the following conditions have been met:

Vital signs are normal.

Patient tolerates po fluids.

Blood glucose is <300 mg/dl.

There is a normal pH.

Bicarbonate is >15 mEq/L.

The precipitating cause has been determined and corrected.

Follow-up with the patient's private medical doctor has been arranged.

Hyperosmolar hyperglycemic nonketotic coma

Hyperosmolar hyperglycemic nonketotic coma (HHNC) accounts for about 10% to 20% of hyperglycemic emergencies. This is an acute complication of type II diabetes and is characterized by dehydration, extreme hyperglycemia, electrolyte imbalances, and altered mental status. Acidosis is not present in HHNC, in contrast to DKA (Table 15-2). This may represent the initial presentation of type II diabetes. The high mortality rate

TABLE 15-2   Diabetic Ketoacidosis (DKA) and Hyperosmolar Hyperglycemic Nonketotic Coma (HHNC): Comparison of Some Salient Features

FEATURE	CONDITIONS	
	DKA	HHNC
Age of patients	Usually <40 years	Usually >60 years
Duration of symptoms	Usually <2 days	Usually >5 days
Glucose level	Usually <600 mg/dL (<33.3 mmol/L)	Usually >800 mg/dL (>44.4 mmol/L)
Sodium concentration	More likely to be normal or low	More likely to be normal or high
Potassium concentration	High, normal, or low	High, normal, or low
Bicarbonate concentration	Low	Normal
Ketone bodies	At least 4+ in 1:1 dilution	<2+ in 1:1 dilution
pH	Low	Normal
Serum osmolality	Usually <350 mOsm/kg (<350 mmol/kg)	Usually >350 mOsm/kg (>350 mmol/kg)
Cerebral edema	Often subclinical; occasionally clinical	Subclinical has not been evaluated; rarely clinical
Prognosis	3% to 10% mortality	10% to 20% mortality
Subsequent course	Insulin therapy required in virtually all cases	Insulin therapy not required in many cases

may be caused by the existence of severe underlying conditions, the lack of aggressive treatment, or a delay in establishing the diagnosis. With an increase in the elderly population, it is likely that HHNC will be seen more frequently in the future. Potential complications of treatment include cerebral edema, systemic hypoperfusion, cerebral infarction, and hypokalemia.

■ **CAUSES**

Illnesses
Chronic renal insufficiency
Severe diarrhea
Gram-negative pneumonia
Gram-negative urinary tract infection
GI bleed
Gram-negative sepsis
Myocardial infarction
Uremia
Vomiting
Acute viral illness
Pulmonary embolism
Subdural hematoma
Cerebrovascular accident
Pancreatitis
Burns
Heat stroke

Medications
Thiazide diuretics
Steroids
Phenytoin
Propranolol
Cimetidine
Immunosuppressive agents

Other causes
Hyperalimentation
Tube feeding without sufficient free water
Dialysis
Recent cardiac surgery

■ **SIGNS AND SYMPTOMS**
Dehydration
Hyperglycemia (>600 mg/dl)
Hyperosmolality (>300 mOsm/L)
Absent or minimal ketones
pH >7.3
Serum bicarbonate >20 mEq/L
Mental status ranges from drowsy to unresponsive
Seizures

■ **DIFFERENTIAL DIAGNOSIS**
DKA
Alcoholic ketoacidosis
Lactic acidosis
Other causes of altered mental status

■ **THERAPEUTIC INTERVENTIONS**
The goals of treatment are rehydration, correction of electrolyte imbalances, reduction of glucose, and determination and treatment of precipitating cause.

Laboratory evaluation

Blood sugar level

Serum glucose, electrolytes, BUN, creatinine

CBC

Urinalysis

Arterial blood gases

Other studies may be necessary to determine underlying cause

Serum osmolality may be calculated as follows:

$$\text{Osmolality (mmol/L)} = \text{serum sodium} \times 2 \\ + \text{blood glucose}/18 + \text{BUN}/2.8$$

Fluid replacement

Begin fluid resuscitation with normal saline. Give 1 L over the first hour.

Change to ½ NS and reduce the rate when the patient's blood pressure responds and urine output is adequate. Exhibit caution when rehydrating elderly patients with saline.

When the blood glucose drops to 250 mg/dl or below the fluid should contain 5% dextrose.

The average fluid deficit is 9 to 12 L.

Insulin

The goal is to reduce the blood glucose level by 100 mg/dl/hr.

With acidosis, hyperkalemia, or renal failure, insulin is needed and should be given IV or IM until the blood glucose has dropped to 250 mg/dl or the osmolality has been reduced to 315 mmol/L.

In some cases insulin is not necessary because the fluid replacement is adequate to reduce the blood glucose levels.

Electrolyte replacement

After urine output is documented and before insulin is given, begin potassium replacement, initially at 10 mEq/hr, then by adding 20 to 30 mEq/L IV fluid.

Check the potassium level every 2 hours until it is stable.

Follow-up

Admission to an intensive care unit is indicated.

Determination and treatment of the precipitating cause is essential.

Diabetes insipidus

In diabetes insipidus the kidneys are unable to resorb water because the action of antidiuretic hormone (ADH) is not effective in increasing the permeability of the renal tubules. Thus the kidneys are unable to concentrate urine appropriately, and excessive amounts of dilute urine are excreted. The condition may be temporary or permanent, depending upon the amount of hypothalamic secretory tissue remaining.

Nephrogenic diabetes insipidus may occur, resulting in a lack of response of the renal tubules to appropriate levels of ADH. This situation may be caused by familial conditions, renal disease, electrolyte imbalances, or lithium carbonate. This condition does not respond to ADH replacement therapy, so it must be treated with dietary sodium and protein restrictions, thiazide diuretics, and nonsteroidal antiinflammatory drugs. The condition has no association with diabetes mellitus, other than some similarity of symptoms.

■ **CAUSES**

Tumors in the hypothalamus/pituitary region

Head trauma

Surgical trauma

Ischemia of the hypothalamus/pituitary gland

CNS infections

Phenytoin

■ **SIGNS AND SYMPTOMS**

Polyuria (3 to 15 L/day)

Polydipsia

Specific gravity <1.005
Urine osmolality <300 mOsm/L
Serum osmolality >295 mOsm/L
Serum sodium >145 mEq/L
Weight loss
Fatigue
■ **THERAPEUTIC INTERVENTIONS**
Fluid replacement
Replacement of ADH
    Vasopressin tannate in oil
    Lysine vasopressin spray
    Desmopressin acetate (DDAVP)

SYNDROME OF INAPPROPRIATE ANTIDIURETIC HORMONE

Secretion of ADH is sustained and abnormal in the syndrome of inappropriate antidiuretic hormone (SIADH), resulting in water intoxication. This condition is characterized by hyponatremia and hypotonicity.

■ **CAUSES**
Malignancies
Pulmonary disease
Adrenal insufficiency
CNS disorders
Pain
Stress
General anesthesia
Oral hypoglycemic agents
Psychotropic drugs
Antineoplastic agents
Narcotics
More common in elderly
■ **SIGNS AND SYMPTOMS**
Fatigue
Headache
Confusion
Decreased level of consciousness
Nausea and vomiting
Diminished tendon reflexes
Seizures
Weight gain without edema
Dilutional hyponatremia
Decreased plasma osmolality
Increased urine osmolality
Increased urine sodium
Increased specific gravity
■ **THERAPEUTIC INTERVENTIONS**
Hypertonic saline and furosemide (check serum sodium every hour)
Fluid restriction
IV normal saline or oral salt supplements
Potassium replacement

THYROID EMERGENCIES

The thyroid hormone has an effect on nearly every organ system. Severe thyroid dysfunction, both hypothyroid and hyperthyroid, presents a significant medical emergency.

Thyroid Storm (Hyperthyroid Crisis)

Thyroid storm, a hyperthyroid crisis, may occur in a previously undiagnosed hyperthyroid patient who is under significant stress. If not promptly diagnosed and treated, this condition may progress to exhaustion, cardiac failure, and death. Death may occur within 2 hours if this condition goes untreated. The mortality rate is 20% to 60%. Thyroid storm is four times more likely to occur in women than in men.

■ **CAUSES**
Stress
Severe drug reaction
MI
Infection
DKA
Embolism
Surgery
Trauma
Manipulation of the thyroid gland

■ **SIGNS AND SYMPTOMS**
Fever
Anxiety
Agitation
Tremors
Nausea, vomiting
Tachydysrhythmias
Tachypnea
Hypertension
Diaphoresis
Flushing
Abdominal pain
Muscle weakness
Exophthalmos
Decreased level of consciousness
Psychosis
Pulmonary edema
Cardiac failure
Hypercalcemia
Hyperglycemia
Metabolic acidosis

■ **THERAPEUTIC INTERVENTIONS**
The goals of treatment are to reduce the fever and prevent life-threatening arrhythmias.
Cooling blanket
Acetaminophen (not aspirin)
Cardiac monitor
Oxygen
Elevate head of bed
Corticosteroids
IV fluids containing dextrose

B vitamins
Propranolol
Propylthiouracil
Iodine—sodium iodide, potassium iodide, or Lugol's solution
Treatment of underlying illness

Myxedema Coma (Hypothyroid Coma)

Myxedema coma is the very rare, very serious crisis of hypothyroidism. It occurs most often in older patients with underlying pulmonary and vascular disease. Respiratory failure is the usual cause of death from myxedema coma. The mortality rate is 30% to 80%.

■ **CAUSES**
Infection
Congestive heart failure
General anesthesia
Surgery
Trauma
Sedatives
Narcotics
Antidepressants
Exposure to cold temperatures
Stress

■ **SIGNS AND SYMPTOMS**
Hypothermia without shivering
Bradycardia
Hypoventilation
Hypotension
Hyponatremia
Hypoglycemia
Water intoxication
Dry skin
Respiratory or metabolic acidosis
Fatigue
Seizures
Lethargy
Stupor
Coma

■ **THERAPEUTIC INTERVENTIONS**
Oxygen
Thyroid hormone replacement
Glucocorticoids
Gentle hydration
Sodium replacement
Passive warming
Vigorous treatment of infection
Possible intubation and ventilation

Thyroiditis

Thyroiditis is usually characterized by anterior neck pain that comes on gradually or suddenly after an upper respiratory infection. It is most often caused by a viral infection.

■ **SIGNS AND SYMPTOMS**
Increased neck pain when the head is turned
Fever
Malaise
Hoarse voice
Elevated pulse
Increased neck pain on swallowing
Firm or nodular thyroid
■ **THERAPEUTIC INTERVENTIONS**
Aspirin or acetaminophen
Bedrest
Antibiotics
Propranolol
Glucocorticoids
Possible surgery

ADRENAL EMERGENCIES

The adrenal cortex produces corticosteroids, which control metabolism and fluid and electrolyte balance. The adrenal medulla produces epinephrine and norepinephrine, which affect the autonomic nervous system.

Acute Adrenal Insufficiency

Acute adrenal insufficiency, or Addison's disease, is a decreased secretion of cortisol and aldosterone. The onset of this condition is often triggered by an underlying illness or stress. Long-term steroid use causes adrenal atrophy; thus rapid discontinuation of steroids may result in acute adrenal insufficiency.

■ **CAUSES**
Immune disorders
Infection
Metastatic malignancy
Adrenal hemorrhage
■ **SIGNS AND SYMPTOMS**
Nausea and vomiting
Abdominal cramping
Amenorrhea
Hypovolemic shock
Diarrhea
Headache
Fever
Hypotension
Weakness
Irritability
Fatigue
Lethargy
Dehydration
Tachycardia
Weight loss
Anorexia
Truncal obesity
Hyperpigmentation, particularly over knuckles, in creases of hands, in axilla, in the gums, and in recent scars
Moon face

Hyponatremia
Hyperkalemia
Hypercalcemia
Hypoglycemia
Hypochloremia
Azotemia

■ **THERAPEUTIC INTERVENTIONS**
Laboratory evaluation
 Cortisol
 ACTH
 Electrolytes
 Glucose
Fluid and electrolyte replacement
Administration of hydrocortisone
Cardiac monitoring
Determination and treatment of precipitating cause

Pheochromocytoma

Pheochromocytoma is a tumor of the adrenal gland that is usually benign. The tumor stimulates excessive secretion of catecholamines and produces active peptides. The hallmark symptom of this condition is extreme hypertension, which may be persistent or paroxysmal.

■ **SIGNS AND SYMPTOMS**
Hypertension
Headache
Anxiety
Fatigue
Visual disturbances
Diaphoresis
Pallor
Tremor
Chest pain
Abdominal pain
Palpitations
Mental status changes

■ **THERAPEUTIC INTERVENTIONS**
Control the hypertensive crisis.
Maintain volume status.
Observe for cardiac arrhythmias.
Stabilize for surgery.
Disruptions in the production of endocrine hormones result in medical emergencies that require prompt assessment, diagnosis, and correction, along with determination and treatment of a precipitating cause.

ELECTROLYTE DISORDERS

Electrolytes, ions that conduct electrical current, are essential for properly functioning cells and maintenance of fluid balance and acid-base balance. An excess or deficit of any of the vital electrolytes may result in a life-threatening crisis.

CALCIUM PROBLEMS

Hypocalcemia

Hypocalcemia is an unusual diagnosis in the emergency setting. It is uncommon and usually a chronic condition. It occurs in approximately 20% of patients with gram-negative bacterial sepsis. If there is a deficiency of parathyroid hormone (PTH) or if there is PTH impairment, serum calcium levels are reduced.

■ **SIGNS AND SYMPTOMS**

Laryngeal spasm with stridor
Numbness and tingling (circumorally and in distal extremities)
Tetany
Dysrhythmias
Seizures
Muscle cramps
Abdominal pain
Hyperactive reflexes
Chvostek's sign (contraction of facial muscle when facial nerve is tapped against the bone anterior to the ear)
Trousseau's sign (occlusion of brachial artery for 3 minutes with B/P cuff results in carpal spasm)

■ **THERAPEUTIC INTERVENTIONS**

Acute

Administer a calcium gluconate IV 10% solution over 10 to 15 minutes (rapid administration could cause hypotension). Calcium chloride may be substituted, but **be aware that local tissue necrosis may occur.**
Seizure precautions
Calcifediol

Chronic

Ergocalciferol
Vitamin D treatment
Increased dietary intake of calcium
Oral calcium

Hypercalcemia

Hypercalcemia is usually a complication of a malignancy, but may also be caused by hyperparathyroidism, thiazide diuretics, hypervitaminosis D, hyperthyroidism, or Addison's disease. Over-ingestion of calcium for osteoporosis prevention should be considered. It is usually not acute or life-threatening. The goals of treatment are to decrease the serum calcium level, which can usually be accomplished by rehydration, and to detect and treat the underlying cause.

■ **SIGNS AND SYMPTOMS**

Nausea and vomiting
Constipation
Thirst
Dry nose
Dysrhythmias and shortened QT interval
Weakness
Itching
Dehydration from polyuria
Postural hypotension
Elevated BUN
Lethargy to coma
Confusion

■ **THERAPEUTIC INTERVENTIONS**

Administer an IV of normal saline at 200 ml/hr (or in accordance with CVP).

Furosemide may be given to prevent fluid overload.

Furosemide and thiazides can worsen hypercalcemia unless adequate amounts of saline are administered.

MAGNESIUM PROBLEMS

Hypomagnesemia

Magnesium is contained primarily in green vegetables. It is absorbed at the small bowel level and is excreted by the kidneys. Many enzyme systems that control the permeability of cell membranes, muscle contractions, oxidative phosphorylation, fat and nucleic acid synthesis, and the stabilization of nuclear proteins are activated by magnesium.

Decreased magnesium is caused by poor dietary intake or when magnesium needs are increased, such as in pregnant women, nursing mothers, and growing children. It can also be caused by chronic alcohol use, malabsorption syndromes, nasogastric suctioning, vomiting, diarrhea, or by renal loss. Decreased magnesium can also occur as a result of hypoparathyroid or hyperparathyroid disease, hyperthyroidism, or during treatment of diabetic ketoacidosis. Hypomagnesemia should also be considered in patients who have received massive transfusions with citrated blood, those with acute pancreatitis, and those who have recently had a cardiopulmonary bypass. Other causes include administration of cisplatin and nephrotoxic agents such as aminoglycosides and amphotericin B.

■ **SIGNS AND SYMPTOMS**

Nausea, vomiting, and diarrhea

Anorexia

Decreased level of consciousness

Muscle fibrillation, tremors, hyperreflexia

Ataxia

Hypertension

Vertical nystagmus

Tetany

Positive Babinski

Psychosis

Hallucinations

Dysrhythmias

Paroxysmal supraventricular tachycardia

Ventricular tachycardia

Ventricular fibrillation

Apathy

Leg cramps

Insomnia

Confusion

■ **THERAPEUTIC INTERVENTIONS**

Administer oral, IM, or IV magnesium

Hypermagnesemia

Hypermagnesemia is a life-threatening condition. Fortunately, it is uncommon. Usually hypermagnesemia results from iatrogenic excessive administration of magnesium-containing products such as antacids, enemas, dialysate solution, or in patients with renal failure or overdoses of lithium. It may also be seen in patients with diabetic ketoacidosis, Addison's disease, viral hepatitis, or hypothermia.

■ **SIGNS AND SYMPTOMS**
Mild (3 to 5 mEq/L)
Bradycardia
Nausea and vomiting
Decreased deep tendon reflexes
Hypotension
Red, warm skin
Diaphoresis
Muscular weakness
Moderate (5 to 10 mEq/L)
Decreased level of consciousness
Prolonged P-R interval, QRS complex, and QT interval
Paralysis
Severe (>10 mEq/L)
Third-degree heart block
Paralysis of respiratory muscles
Asystole

■ **THERAPEUTIC INTERVENTIONS**
ABCs
Decreased magnesium intake
Administer an IV of 0.45% normal saline and diuretics to enhance excretion (if normal renal function)
If greater than 5 mEq/L, give calcium chloride, 5 ml of a 10% solution over 30 seconds (may be repeated)
Consider renal dialysis with magnesium-free dialysate

PHOSPHORUS PROBLEMS

Hypophosphatemia

In humans 80% to 85% of phosphate is in bones and teeth and 15% to 20% is intracellular. The main source of phosphate is food products. It is important to cellular structure and function, serum calcium levels, and glycolysis and oxygen delivery. It is excreted by the kidneys. Hypophosphatemia is more common in diabetes, chronic alcohol use, chronic bowel disease, and after severe burns.

Signs and symptoms begin when serum phosphorus is less than 2 mg/100 ml and becomes life-threatening when levels are less than 1 mg/100 ml. Hypophosphatemia results from loss of the mineral through the intestines or kidneys or intracellular phosphate shifts caused by sepsis, respiratory alkalosis, epinephrine administration, or hepatic failure. COPD and asthma patients may experience hypophosphatemia as a reversible cause of respiratory muscle hypocontractility and impaired tissue oxygenation.

■ **SIGNS AND SYMPTOMS**
Moderate decrease
Weakness
Anorexia
Fractures
Confusion
Tremors
Pain in bones
Joint stiffness
Chest pain
Muscle pain
Tingling of fingers and circumoral area

Severe decrease

Hemolytic anemia

Seizures

Anisocoria (unequal pupils)

Impaired oxygen delivery

Paralysis

Coma to death

■ **THERAPEUTIC INTERVENTIONS**

Decrease intake of substances that cause decreased phosphorus, such as phosphorus-binding antacids.

Replace with oral or (if severe) IV phosphorus. IV replacement of phosphate can lead to a rapid decrease in calcium levels.

Hyperphosphatemia

Hyperphosphatemia is considered present when serum phosphorus levels are above 4.5 mg/100 ml. It is most commonly caused by lack of phosphorus excretion at the renal level and can occasionally be caused by phosphorus moving from the intracellular to the extracellular spaces as a result of cellular tissue destruction. Other causes include endocrine diseases such as acromegaly and hypoparathyroidism and excessive intake of phosphate-containing laxatives or enemas.

■ **SIGNS AND SYMPTOMS**

Pruritis

Tetany

Calcium phosphate deposits in joints and blood vessels

Nausea, vomiting, anorexia

Muscle weakness

Tachycardia

■ **THERAPEUTIC INTERVENTIONS**

Administer phosphate binding agents, such as magnesium, or calcium antacids.

Decrease dietary intake of phosphorus.

If severe, dialysis may be necessary.

POTASSIUM PROBLEMS

Hypokalemia

Hypokalemia is defined as a serum potassium level below 3.5 mEq/L. It results from excess potassium excretion in urine that could be caused by use of diuretics, excess potassium excretion in feces resulting from diarrhea or malabsorption, metabolic alkalosis, intracellular shift of potassium, or a magnesium deficiency. Trauma patients may experience short-term hypokalemia because of elevated serum epinephrine. Normal serum potassium levels are 3.5 to 5 mEq/L.

■ **SIGNS AND SYMPTOMS**

Muscle weakness

Rhabdomyolysis

Fatigue

Leg cramps

Nausea, vomiting

CNS irritability

Paresthesias

Paralysis

Decreased reflexes

Paralytic ileus

Polydipsia

Dysrhythmias (PVCs, atrial tachycardia, nodal tachycardia, ventricular tachycardia, ventricular fibrillation)

Respiratory or cardiac arrest

■ **THERAPEUTIC INTERVENTIONS**

Replace potassium orally with potassium chloride.

IV infusion rate

    <10 to 20 mEq/hr; in severe deficiency may infuse up to 40 mEq/hr.

    Concentration <30 to 40 mEq/L

    May irritate vein

    Do not give as IV bolus.

Closely monitor for dysrhythmias.

Monitor serum potassium and other electrolytes.

Monitor hourly urine output.

Consider potassium-sparing diuretics.

Magnesium deficiency makes it more difficult to correct hypokalemia.

Hyperkalemia

Hyperkalemia (serum potassium levels above 5 mEq/L) may be caused by insulin deficiency, major crush injuries, severe electrical burns, major thermal burns, severe acidosis (potassium increases by 0.6 mEq/L with each decrease of 0.1 U of pH), renal failure, potassium overdose, increased potassium intake, decreased urinary excretion, extracellular shift, overuse of salt substitutes, lupus, sickle cell disease, amyloidosis, or gastrointestinal disorders. Clenching and unclenching a fist during venipuncture causes local release of potassium from forearm muscles, and can raise the level by 1 to 2 mEq/L.

■ **SIGNS AND SYMPTOMS**

Dysrhythmias

    Sinus bradycardia, sinus arrest, first degree heart block, junctional rhythms, idioventricular rhythms, ventricular tachycardia, ventricular fibrillation, asystole

Decreased reflexes

Paresthesias

Paralysis

Irritability

Anxiety

Abdominal cramping

Diarrhea

Weakness

Respiratory and/or cardiac arrest

■ **THERAPEUTIC INTERVENTIONS**

Therapeutic intervention is aimed at increasing cellular uptake of potassium.

Administer calcium gluconate 10 to 20 ml of 10% solution IV slowly.

    Rapid acting; lasts 30 to 60 minutes.

    Antagonizes potassium at the cell membrane.

    Especially useful in dialysis patients, particularly in cardiac arrest situations resulting from hyperkalemia.

    Not recommended for use in patients who are on digitalis.

                or:

Administer sodium bicarbonate 44 mEq (1 amp) IV slowly.

Causes cells to absorb potassium immediately; lasts 1 to 2 hours.

                 or:

Administer insulin and glucose.

    D_{10} (500 ml) with 10 to 20 U regular insulin over ½ to 1 hour.

Takes about 30 minutes to start working, but lasts 4 to 6 hours.
Check serum glucose. Observe closely for hypoglycemia.
or:
Administer kayexalate (a cation exchange resin).
25 g retention enema (followed by 15 ml of 70% solution of sorbitol to promote diarrhea)
Takes about 2 hours to start working
or:
Administer furosemide and saline
40 mg Lasix in normal saline at 100 ml/hr
Problem: Has a slow onset and causes an excessive electrolyte excretion.
or:
For patients on hemodialysis
Nebulized albuterol can reduce serum k^+ 0.5-1 mEq/L within 30 minutes for duration of over 2 hours.
or:
Renal dialysis
Efficient/effective

SODIUM PROBLEMS

Hyponatremia

Intracellular and extracellular fluids normally have the same osmolality. The electrolyte that controls the extracellular osmolality is sodium. A serum sodium level of less than 135 mEq/L is considered hyponatremia. This can occur when there is an actual decrease in the volume of extracellular sodium or an increase in the volume of extracellular fluid, resulting in dilutional hyponatremia. Excessive extracellular fluid may be caused by congestive heart failure, hepatic failure, or subnormal availability of antidiuretic hormone (ADH). Sodium loss can be caused by use of diuretics, vomiting, severe burns (third spacing), and lack of dietary sodium. Up to 50% of hospitalized AIDS patients and 20% of ambulatory AIDS patients exhibit hyponatremia.

■ SIGNS AND SYMPTOMS
Severity of signs and symptoms depends on the level of serum sodium, affecting the amount of brain cell edema.
Lethargy
Postural hypotension
Tremors
Cool, clammy skin
Headache
Edema
Confusion
Seizures
Coma

■ THERAPEUTIC INTERVENTIONS
Treat cautiously, overtreatment is dangerous.
Consider IV fluid and sodium replacement.
Replace other electrolyte losses.

Hypernatremia

Hypernatremia is defined as a serum sodium level above 145 mEq/L. It can result either from an increase in sodium or a decrease in fluid. Fluid decrease is the most common cause. Fluid loss may occur as a result of renal causes, fever, hyperventilation, or excessive perspiration.

An increase in extracellular sodium causes fluid to move from the intracellular spaces to the extracellular spaces in an attempt to achieve osmotic equilibrium. The resulting cellular "dehydration" causes CNS depression and possibly intracerebral hemorrhage.

■ **SIGNS AND SYMPTOMS**

Thirst
Fatigue
Orthostatic hypotension
Oliguria
Hyperthermia
Lethargy
Confusion
Coma

■ **THERAPEUTIC INTERVENTIONS**

Treat the underlying cause and bring serum sodium levels to within normal limits.

Ensure hypotonic replacement (gradually), usually with D_5W and/or 0.45% normal saline solution, in accordance with calculations, correct slowly to avoid cerebral edema.

Consider hemodialysis.

ALCOHOL EMERGENCIES

Acute alcohol intoxication or other alcohol-induced problems may create a medical emergency. Acute intoxication or acute withdrawal from alcohol can be life-threatening. It is essential to determine that there is no underlying cause of illness or injury other than alcohol intoxication, such as head trauma, diabetic ketoacidosis, or overdose.

Obtain a good history whenever possible:

• When was the patient's last drink?
• How much did the patient drink? (Remember that it is the *amount* of alcohol and not the type that affects the blood alcohol level.)
• How much does the patient usually drink each day? How much each week?
• When was the last time the patient ate?
• Is the patient taking any medications?
• Has the patient taken any medications or drugs? (Specifically ask about disulfiram [Antabuse] and metronidazole [Flagyl].)
• Does the patient have any other medical illness?

Acute Intoxication

Acute intoxication is caused by consumption of a large amount of alcohol over a short period of time. Acute intoxication can occur at various levels, depending on the patient's drinking frequency, the amount of food consumed with the alcohol, and the physiologic tolerance of the drinker (Table 15-3).

■ **SIGNS AND SYMPTOMS**

Hypothermia or hyperthermia
Tachycardia
Hypotension
Hypovolemia
Arrhythmias
Respiratory depression
Aspiration (common)
Nausea/vomiting
Abdominal pain
Hypoglycemia

TABLE 15-3   Blood Alcohol Levels and Associated Signs and Symptoms

BLOOD ALCOHOL PERCENTAGE IN 70 KG PERSON	SIGNS AND SYMPTOMS
0.05%	Very few
0.10% (legally intoxicated in most states)	Giddy; decreased muscle coordination; decreased inhibitions
0.15%	Decreased sensory level; slurred speech; vertigo; ataxia; elevated pulse; diaphoresis
0.20%	Very decreased sensory level; marked decrease in reaction to stimuli; inability to walk; nausea, vomiting
.30% (confusion, stupor)	
0.40%	No response to stimuli; decreased deep tendon reflexes; decreased blood pressure; elevated pulse; cool, clammy, moist skin; seizures
0.50%	Death from primary respiratory arrest caused by blocking respiratory functions of medulla

Lactic acidosis
Decreased muscle coordination
Dehydration
■ **THERAPEUTIC INTERVENTIONS**
Airway management **(aspiration is a major cause of death in the acutely intoxicated)**
Oxygen
Cardiac monitor
ABCs, alcohol level, lytes, CBC, glucose
Drawing blood for medical/forensic purposes
Warming blanket
Chest x-ray film
Ipecac, if necessary, if alcohol was consumed within 1 to 2 hours, especially in children
Gastric lavage with charcoal if necessary
Control of seizures with diazepam (Valium)
IV D_5W or RL or D_5NS if hypovolemia or alcoholic ketoacidosis is suspected
Dextrose 50% and thiamin 100 mg (to prevent Wernicke-Korsakoff syndrome), naloxone, dextrose, and thiamine
Possible renal dialysis
Electrolyte replacement
Ruling out other causes of current status
Other appropriate therapeutic intervention, depending on findings (Figure 15-1)

Rum Fits/Alcohol Seizures

Rum fits are seizures that are concurrent with drinking alcohol, generally following 8 to 36 hours of abstinence. Typically 1 to 3 grand mal seizures occur over a 6-hour period. They may be caused by a severely decreased blood alcohol level, a decreased glucose level, or an electrolyte imbalance. The patient may progress to delirium tremens without intervention.
■ **THERAPEUTIC INTERVENTIONS**
ABCs
Oxygen
Arterial blood gases
Diazepam
IV D_5W

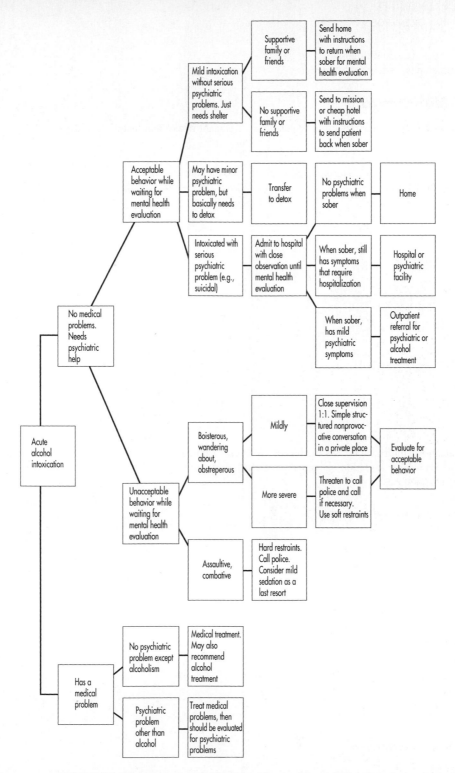

FIGURE 15-1. Plan for triage of a patient with acute alcohol intoxication.

Naloxone, dextrose, and thiamine
Use of anticonvulsants is controversial

Alcohol Withdrawal

Begins 6 to 48 hours after reduction or cessation of ethanol intake and lasts 2 to 7 days.

Minor

Less than 24 hours after cessation or reduction of alcohol consumption.

■ **SIGNS AND SYMPTOMS**
Hangover
Hyperalert
Headache
Shaking
Nausea and vomiting
Insomnia
Irritability
Anxiety
Tachycardia
Mild ataxia
Hypertension

■ **THERAPEUTIC INTERVENTIONS**
Rest
Aspirin
Rehydration

Major

Severe alcohol withdrawal occurs in chronic alcoholics who have been without alcohol. It occurs from 24 hours to 5 days after cessation or reduction of alcohol consumption.

■ **SIGNS AND SYMPTOMS**
Seizures
Decreased level of consciousness
Nausea, vomiting, anorexia
Photophobia
Hallucinations (auditory and visual)
Slight lateral nystagmus
Diaphoresis
Ataxia
Fever
Disorientation
Anxiety
Irritability
Tremor
Tachycardia
Hyperreflexia
Hypertension
Delirium

■ **THERAPEUTIC INTERVENTIONS**
ABCs
Fluid and electrolyte replacement
Thiamine and dextrose IV

Multivitamins
Benzodiazepines
Dextrose 50%
Diazepam
Reassurance
Reorientation

Delirium Tremens

Delirium tremens (DTs) occurs after a severe drop in the amount of alcohol consumed by an alcoholic usually after third day without alcohol. Delirium tremens is an acute medical emergency resulting in a 10% to 15% mortality rate. Death typically results from hyperthermia or peripheral vascular collapse.

■ **SIGNS AND SYMPTOMS**

Gross tremors
Increasing agitation
Diaphoresis
Tachypnea
Hallucinations (auditory and visual)
Confusion
Fever
Incontinence
Mydriasis
Seizures
Decreased blood pressure
Elevated pulse
Dysrhythmias

■ **THERAPEUTIC INTERVENTIONS**

Haloperidol
Chlordiazepoxide
Careful airway management
Protection of head and limbs (padded bedsides)
IV with electrolyte additions

Disulfiram Reactions

Disulfiram is a drug given in some alcohol detoxification programs. Disulfiram may react with foods or medications containing alcohol, including cough syrups, fermented vinegar, and perhaps even the odor of rubbing alcohol or aftershave.

■ **SIGNS AND SYMPTOMS**

Severe nausea and vomiting (5 to 15 minutes following contact with alcohol) that may continue for 6 to 12 days

Flush of face, chest, and neck
Perspiration
Reddened conjunctiva
Headache
Increased pulse
Increased respirations
Decreased blood pressure
Decreased level of consciousness
Chest and abdominal pain
Vertigo

■ **THERAPEUTIC INTERVENTIONS**
ABCs
Oxygen
IV normal saline
Consider ascorbic acid
Chlorpheniramine
Diphenhydramine
Antiemetics
Metabolic emergencies require careful assessment, prompt diagnosis, and aggressive treatment of the acute problem. Follow-up management must include determination and treatment of the precipitating cause. Prevention of a future episode necessitates continued health care management and patient and family education. Emergency medical identification should be worn by individuals with chronic conditions that predispose them to acute metabolic crises.

REFERENCES
American Diabetes Association: Implications of the diabetes control and complications trial, *Clin Diabetes* 11(4):91, 1993.

SUGGESTED READINGS
Brown KA: Nursing rounds: malignant hyperthermia, *AJN* 97(10):33-34, 1997.
Wogan JM: Endocrine disorders. In Rosen P et al, editors: Emergency medicine, St Louis, 1998, Mosby.

Toxicologic Emergencies

Susan F. Strauss

Toxicology is the science of poisons and their effects on living organisms. According to the American Association of Poison Control Centers (AAPCC) in 1996 over 2 million people were exposed to toxic substances, an increase of 6.6% over the previous year.[1] Exposure to these substances can occur at work, school or in health care facilities, though over 90% of poisoning occur at a residence. Children younger than 3 years of age were involved in 39.3% of cases, and 52.8% occur in children younger than 6 years. The vast majority of poison exposures are unintentional and relatively mild in nature and do not require emergency services. Treatment in a health care facility is required in 25% of patients contacting poison control centers and over 12% of these patients require hospitalization and critical care management.[1]

Principles for therapeutic interventions are:

- Prevent further absorption
- Promote excretion
- Provide appropriate antidote
- Provide physiologic and psychologic support
- Educate patient, family and significant others

Support care guidelines in all toxic overdoses/poisonings include:

- ABCs—airway protection is critical
- Oxygen
- IV of Ringer's Lactate or normal saline
- Naloxone 0.4 mg up to 2 mg IV, ET, IO
- Dextrose 50% 50 ml
- Thiamine 50 to 100 mg
- ECG and cardiac monitoring
- Frequent VS
- Monitoring of urinary output
- Monitoring ABGs as indicated

To determine the best interventions in the prevention of absorption and promotion of excretion it is important to understand the nature of the toxin. Knowing how it is absorbed, catabolized, excreted and detected will assist in establishing the appropriate treatment modality. History and investigation concerning the toxin is vital to appropriate treatment. The history should include:

- Time of ingestion
- Amount of substance ingested
- Treatment prior to arrival
- PMH—especially cardiac, hepatic, and renal disorders
- Current signs and symptoms
- Psychological, social, and environmental risk factors

TABLE 16-1   Growth of the AAPCC Toxic Exposure Surveillance System

YEAR	NO. OF PARTICIPATING CENTERS	POPULATION SERVED (MILLIONS)	HUMAN EXPOSURES REPORTED	EXPOSURES/THOUSAND POPULATION
1983	16	43.1	251,012	5.8
1984	47	99.8	730,224	7.3
1985	56	113.6	900,513	7.9
1986	57	132.1	1,098,894	8.3
1987	63	137.5	1,166,940	8.5
1988	64	155.7	1,368,748	8.8
1989	70	182.4	1,581,540	8.7
1990	72	191.7	1,713,462	8.9
1991	73	200.7	1,837,939	9.2
1992	68	196.7	1,864,188	9.5
1993	64	181.3	1,751,476	9.7
1994	65	215.9	1,926,438	8.9
1995	67	218.5	2,023,089	9.3
1996	67	232.3	2,155,952	9.3
Total			20,370,415	

Litovitz et al: AAPCC report, *American Journal of Emergency Medicine* 15(5):448, 1997.

POISON INFORMATION

Toxicology is a rapidly evolving science, and the standard of care changes as new interventions are found. Poison centers have assumed an increased role in the identification and management of poisonings and overdoses. Poison centers are located throughout every state and have access to information that is updated every three months on Poisindex and to other current toxicologic references. Poison centers should be contacted for each poisoned patient. The poison center will help the clinician assess the patient and implement the most current standard of care.

The Toxic Exposure Surveillance System (TESS) data are compiled by the AAPCC in cooperation with the majority of US poison centers (Table 16-1). The data is used to identify hazards early, focus on prevention education, guide clinical research, and direct training. TESS data have prompted product reformulation, repackaging, recalls, and bans, and are used to support regulatory action and form the basis of post-marketing surveillance of newly released drugs and products.

THERAPEUTIC INTERVENTIONS FOR POISONINGS AND OVERDOSES

Induced Emesis

In 1985, 15% of all poisoning victims were treated with syrup of ipecac. In 1992 the use of syrup of ipecac was down from 71% to 4.3% and in 1996 to 1.8% of all poisoning cases.[2] Although its role has significantly decreased, emesis remains a useful methods of gastric emptying in ingestion of less than 1 hour in duration.

Emesis is induced with syrup of ipecac, an emetic agent that causes irritation of the stomach lining and stimulates the emetic center in the medulla. It should only be given to patients with a gag reflex. Syrup of ipecac administration is contraindicated: (1) if there is altered mental status; (2) if there is predictable severe central nervous system depression within 30 minutes resulting in airway compromise; (3) if the substance can cause seizures to ensue at the same time ipecac begins to work; (4) in cases of acid ingestion; (5) in cases of alkali ingestion; (6) in cases of petroleum distillate ingestion; (7) in cases of aliphatic hydrocarbon ingestion; (8) when there are preexisting health problems—seizure disorder, cardiac history, or pregnancy; (9) when vagal reflexes from vomiting may worsen bradydysrhythmias in certain drugs, i.e., beta blockers, digoxin, calcium antagonist; (10) in children under the age of 6 months because of immature gag reflex; (11) in patients over the age of 70; (12) in which potentially fatal quantities of a substance for which there is an oral antidote have been ingested; and (13) in the ingestion of a foreign body.

Conflict continues over oral fluid administration with the use of syrup of ipecac. Studies show that the there is no significant change in onset or effectiveness of syrup of ipecac regardless of temperature or amount of fluid.[3,4] Compliance may actually be enhanced in children by administration of ipecac with a clear carbonated beverage.

Therapeutic use of syrup of ipecac is rarely associated with adverse effects. The most significant drawback to administration is the lasting effects of vomiting. It may take 2.2 to 4.2 hours after cessation of vomiting to tolerate oral fluids.[3] Reported but rare complications include Mallory-Weiss tears or rupture of the esophagus, gastric rupture, pneumothorax, and bradycardia.

Syrup of ipecac dosage

	Ipecac	Fluids
1 year old	10 ml	15 ml/kg
1 to 12 years old	15 ml	4 to 6 oz
>12 years old	30 ml	6 to 8 oz

Gastric Lavage

Gastric lavage is more effective than ipecac-induced emesis if a large-bore tube is used in conjunction with large fluid volumes and frequent repositioning.[3] Lavage allows the use of activated charcoal without delay.

Follow this procedure:

1. Protect the patient's airway.
   a. Consider endotracheal intubation if the patient has altered consciousness (CNS depression) or has no gag reflex.[4]
   b. Have suction readily available.
2. Select the proper size gastric tube.
   a. Preferably a 36-40 French gastric tube inserted via the oral route.
   b. Use a 24-32 French gastric tube for a child.
3. Lubricate the tube with a water-soluble lubricant.
4. If possible, have the patient cooperate by sitting up and taking sips of water while swallowing the tube.
5. Advance the tube.
6. Auscultate over the epigastric area while forcing some air into the tube to ensure proper placement.
7. Secure the tube with tape.
8. Place the patient in a left lateral position with the head dependent.
9. Lavage with warmed normal saline solution (150 to 200 ml per rinse in an adult and 10 ml/kg in a child).
10. Allow for fluid return by gravity.
11. Repeat lavage until the fluid returned is clear.
12. Provide oral hygiene.

Activated Charcoal

Activated charcoal is usually given by mouth or nasogastric tube following emesis or lavage. It adsorbs many substances and may even bind some agents in the proximal small bowel.

During the last decade extensive research conducted on the efficiency of activated charcoal reveals that the use of activated charcoal alone may be equivalent to or even superior to the conventional treatment modalities.[5,6] However, the sole use of activated charcoal does not have universal application and research is being identified to the specific indications for its use. Specific contraindications to the use of charcoal are 1) corrosive ingestion, 2) decreased or absent bowel sounds, 3) toxins not bound by charcoal (metals).

The number of cases of adverse reactions associated with activated charcoal are isolated, but have become more apparent as the use of activated charcoal grows.

Recommendations for the administration of activated charcoal:

Aggressive attention in protection of the airway; consider intubation in high risk patients; visualization of the epiglottis after vomiting of activated charcoal is grossly diminished.

Anchor N-G tube to prevent retraction from the stomach to the esophagus.

Placement of the N-G tube *must* be determined immediately prior to administration

Shake the slurries thoroughly to eliminate clumping

Use more dilute slurries

Small intermittent doses may reduce vomiting

Delay the administration of cathartics

Should not be administered for 60 to 90 minutes after ipecac-induced emesis subsides

Aggressive suctioning of the activated charcoal appears to improve the outcomes of patients who have aspirated charcoal.

Multiple Dose Activated Charcoal

Multiple doses of activated charcoal have been shown effective in enhancing total body clearance and elimination in these drugs:

• Tricyclic antidepressants
• Phenobarbital
• Theophyllin
• Digoxin
• Phenytoin
• Carbamezapine
• Sustained release preparations

Repeat every 2 to 6 hours. Give 20 to 50 g in an adult and half that dose in a child.

Cathartics

Cathartics such as magnesium sulfate, magnesium citrate, sodium citrate, or sorbitol are used to enhance excretion of poisons. One study in poisoned patients demonstrated a direct correlation between the amount of sorbitol in the product and the incidence of vomiting (31% to 57% of patients).[7] To reduce the potential of vomiting it may be judicious to delay the use of sorbitol until drug-induced vomiting has subsided. Overuse of cathartics may cause diarrhea and dehydration. Cathartics should not be given to children less than 1 year old or if bowel sounds are absent.

Whole Bowel Irrigation

Whole bowel irrigation involves the use of an electrolyte solution administered orally at approximately 2 liters an hour until the bowel is purged. This therapy is useful in the treatment of time-release agents and in poisonings that have delayed absorption. Commercially available solutions are Colyte or Golytely. Whole bowel irrigation produces a rapid catharsis, cleaning most matter from the GI tract in hours. Though it is not a substitute for activated charcoal, it seems to be most useful in agents not well adsorbed via charcoal (iron, lead, lithium, zinc).

Charcoal Hemoperfusion and Dialysis

Charcoal hemoperfusion is an extracorporeal technique that involves percolating blood through a cartridge containing activated charcoal. Hemodialysis is indicated in the patient who has severe metabolic acidosis, electrolyte abnormalities or renal failure in addition to toxic levels of a poison. Dialysis is not indicated 1) in a patient who has ingested a substance that is markedly protein bound, 2) in a drug ingestion where the agent is rarely lethal, or 3) where the action of the agent is reversible. Peritoneal dialysis can be useful for short term treatment.

Prevention and Education

The Poison Prevention Act of 1970 has been successful in reducing the number of pediatric poisonings as well as mortality. "Child-proof" containers are a fallacy. They are child resistant. However, child resistant containers should not replace prevention education and aggressive poison-proofing of homes frequented by young children.

Recently, Denatonium Benzoate (Bitrex), a taste aversive agent, has been added to products to dissuade children from drinking toxic quantities of household products. Expanding the use of this product in more toxic agents may further decrease the incidence of pediatric poisonings.

The prolific use of "recreational" alcohol and drugs has skyrocketed. Prevention campaigns by groups such as Emergency Nurses Cancel Alcohol Related Emergencies (EN CARE) are educating the public as to the tragedies associated with alcohol and drugs.

The emergency nurses are in an excellent position to educate their patients and communities in the proper use of medications, safe storage of potentially toxic substances, and risks of drug and alcohol abuse.

Analgesics

The nonprescription analgesics acetaminophen, aspirin, and ibuprofen account for more exposure calls to poison control centers than any other category of medications. These medications come in a variety of dosage strengths, colors, sizes and forms, often leading to misdosing and mismanagement of overdoses. Complacency and availability add to the high incidence of exposures (Table 16-2).

Acetaminophen

Acetaminophen, a metabolite of phenacetin, is found in varying quantities in more than 200 miscellaneous remedies for pain, sleep, cough, and colds.

The toxic metabolites of acetaminophen destroy hepatocytes, resulting in hepatic necrosis and massive liver damage. Hepatotoxicity is seen in ingestion of >140 mg/kg. Patients with a history of alcohol abuse are at increased risk for acetaminophen toxicity.

■ SIGNS AND SYMPTOMS
Initial stage (0 to 24 hours after ingestion)
Symptoms may be absent early even if severely toxic
GI irritation (nausea, vomiting, anorexia)
Lethargy
Diaphoresis
Coma and metabolic acidosis have developed in rare cases of poisoning when the 4° blood level is
>800 mg/L
Middle stage (24 to 48 hours after ingestion)
This may be a symptom-free stage of toxicity.
Hepatic abnormalities of AST (SGOT), ALT (SGPT) bilirubin, and prothrombin time will develop.
Right upper quadrant pain.

TABLE 16-2 Categories with Largest Numbers of Deaths

CATEGORY	NO.	% OF ALL EXPOSURES IN CATEGORY
Analgesics	228	0.109
Antidepressants	146	0.241
Stimulants and street drugs	120	0.323
Cardiovascular drugs	102	0.278
Alcohols	89	0.161
Sedative/hypnotics/antipsychotics	83	0.124
Gases and fumes	49	0.105
Chemicals	36	0.066
Anticonvulsants	25	0.136
Insecticides/pesticides (includes rodenticides)	20	0.023
Cleaning substances	17	0.008
Antihistamines	16	0.035
Asthma therapies	15	0.082
Automotive products	14	0.097
Hydrocarbons	10	0.015
Cold & cough preparations	10	0.009

Litovitz et al: AAPCC report, *Am J Emerg Med* 15(5):448, 1997.

Hepatic stage (48 to 96 hours after ingestion)

Progressive hepatic encephalopathy develops characterized by:

Vomiting	Confusion
Jaundice	Lethargy
Right upper quadrant pain	Coma
Bleeding	

Hypoglycemia
Transient high levels of liver enzymes
Renal damage

Obtain baseline liver enzymes, prothrombin time, BUN, and blood sugar.

■ **SPECIFIC INTERVENTION**

1. Supportive care.
2. Gastric decontamination using ipecac or lavage should be done if ingested dose is >7.5 g in an adult or >140 mg/kg in a child. If there is a delay in GI decontamination (>30 minutes), lavage is preferred.
3. Activated charcoal.
4. Draw quantitative level at 4 hours postingestion and plot it on the Rumack/Matthews nomogram. Levels drawn before 4 hours have no clinical value.
5. Baseline hepatic and renal functions.
6. Antidote N-acetylcysteine (NAC).
   a. If plasma level is toxic—N-acetylcysteine is preferably initiated within 10 hours of ingestion, but has statistical efficacy when given up to 24 hours postingestion.
   b. NAC dosage
      Loading dose: 140 mg/kg orally as a 5% solution in cola, Fresca, orange juice, or grapefruit juice.
      Maintenance dose: 70 mg/kg orally as 5% solution every 4 hours for a total of 17 doses.
   c. NAC should be completely administered until the entire 17 doses are completed.
   d. If there are problems with retention of NAC:
      I. Metoclopramide may be given.

II. Insert a gastric tube and drip in slowly.

III. If any dose is vomited within 1 hour, the dose should be repeated.

Salicylates

Salicylate poisoning has decreased over the last decade with the emergence of other analgesics and the development of Reye's syndrome in children. Aspirin interferes with a variety of organ systems. It stimulates the respiratory center producing a respiratory alkalosis and compensatory renal loss of bicarbonate. It interferes with lipid/carbohydrate metabolism and produces a concurrent metabolic acidosis. Aspirin has a long half-life. The generally accepted toxic dose is 150 mg/kg.

■ **SIGNS AND SYMPTOMS**

Mild to moderate toxicity (150 to 300 mg/kg)

Tachypnea	Fever
Tinnitus	Dehydration
Nausea, vomiting	Abdominal pain
Tachycardia	Hypoglycemia
Electrolyte imbalance	

Severe toxicity (greater than 300 mg/kg)

Altered mental status
Seizures
Noncardiac pulmonary edema
Hemorrhagic gastritis
Coagulation abnormalities

■ **THERAPEUTIC INTERVENTIONS**

Supportive care

Gastric emptying may be effective for several hours because of bezoar formation

Activated charcoal has a high affinity for aspirin. Multiple dosing is recommended

Quantitative serum salicylate level initially and at 6 hours postingestion. Dome nomogram at 6 hours is of prognostic value. Levels should be obtained every 6 to 12 hours because of the long half-life of aspirin and bezoar formation.

Alkalization of serum and urine

Correct fluid and electrolyte imbalances

Conventional treatment for hypoglycemia, seizures, and pulmonary edema

Fever usually subsides with rehydration and external cooling

Hemodialysis in severe poisonings. This aids in the treatment of fluid and electrolyte disturbances as well as removal of salicylate

■ **PREVENTION AND EDUCATION**

See *Acetaminophen.*

Ibuprofen

Introduced in 1984 as a nonprescription analgesic, Ibuprofen has increased in popularity and use. Ibuprofen has a short half-life and is rapidly absorbed and eliminated. Acute ingestion of less than 100 mg/kg is considered nontoxic. Ingestion of >300 mg/kg is considered severe. Ibuprofen appears to have a relatively high safety profile when compared to the fatality incidence associated with acetaminophen and aspirin.

■ **SIGNS AND SYMPTOMS**

Drowsiness and lethargy
Gastrointestinal irritation
Hypotension

Bradycardia
Renal failure
Hepatotoxicity
Apnea
Seizures—in children who ingest 400 mg/kg
Metabolic acidosis
■ **THERAPEUTIC INTERVENTIONS**
Supportive care
Quantitative ibuprofen level—There is a nomogram similar to the Rumak-Matthew nomogram for prognostic assessment only.
Syrup of ipecac in adults—This may depend on time of ingestion and patient's LOC
Lavage
Multiple dose activated charcoal
Alkaline diuresis
Seizure precautions in children
Cardiac monitoring in significant overdoses
■ **PREVENTION AND EDUCATION**
See *Acetaminophen.*
Keep medication out of the reach of young children
Take only the amount recommended on the bottle label. If symptoms persist, seek the advice of your healthcare practitioner.
Read bottle labels to see if medication contains aspirin. Aspirin products should never be administered to children.
Do not take multiple OTC medications without the advice of a healthcare professional.

PRESCRIPTION MEDICATIONS

Calcium Channel Antagonists

Sustained-release calcium channel antagonists, primarily verapamil, continue to represent a unique and problematic profile including late onset of toxicity, waxing and waning deterioration, and often with death more than 24 hours after the overdose.[1] Symptoms are frequently rapid in their progression and resistant to conventional therapies.

As implied in the name, calcium channel antagonists prevent the influx of calcium through the slow calcium channels in the cardiac and vascular smooth muscle. They prolong the refractory period and depress impulses in conduction, thereby reducing heart rate. Drugs in this category can produce a variety of negative chronotropic, dromotropic and inotropic properties. These drugs are metabolized by the liver and extensively protein-bound, therefore not dialyzable. Quantitative levels are of little value in the management of acute toxicity.

■ **SIGNS AND SYMPTOMS**
Hypotension
Cardiac disturbances, especially conduction abnormalities and bradycardia
Confusion, altered mental status
Nausea and vomiting
CHF
Syncope
Hyperglycemia
■ **THERAPEUTIC INTERVENTIONS**
Supportive care
Lavage
Activated charcoal and cathartic
Multiple dose activated charcoal and whole bowel irrigation for sustained-release products

Cardiac monitor and ECG

Cardiac pacing

Antagonist

Calcium—increases concentration gradient in serum, thereby lowering intracellular calcium flow. Effective in small or therapeutic overdoses. Relatively ineffective in massive overdoses. Should be administered to all patients although effects may not be dramatic.

Atropine—treatment of bradycardia at the SA node. Will not affect the A-V blockade effects.

Glucagon—may reverse myocardial depression, Glucagon is an antidote for drugs that reduce intracellular calcium.[4]

Catecholamine—Beta-1 agonists such as isoproterenol may be effective by increasing heart rate and contractility. Norepinephrine can be used for hypotension.

Aminopyridine—directly enhances transmembrane calcium influx and has a positive inotropic effect.

Charcoal hemoperfusion in children has had some results.[8]

Extracorporeal treatment (ECMO)/cardiac bypass (these treatments are not readily available in all institutions).

Cyclic Antidepressants

Tricyclic antidepressants (TCA) are the second most frequent cause of death in overdoses. Onset of action is rapid and symptoms may peak as soon as 60 minutes after ingestion. TCAs are highly protein bound and lipid soluble. This results in falsely low serum levels, poor hemodialyzability and long elimination half-life. The three pharmacologic features responsible for the toxic manifestations most commonly observed in TCA are:

1) anticholinergic activity (little impact on morbidity and mortality) (Table 16-3).

2) membrane stabilization effects on myocardial tissue decreasing cardiac conduction (most significant effect).

3) adrenergic compromise with alpha adrenergic blocking properties and depletion of catecholamine.

■ **SIGNS AND SYMPTOMS**

Anticholinergic effects (Table 16-3)

Nausea and vomiting

Tachyarrhythmias, prolonged PR interval, widening of QRS, heart blocks, asystole

Hypotension

Seizures/coma

■ **THERAPEUTIC INTERVENTIONS**

Supportive care

Quantitative serum level (may be falsely lower)

Gastric lavage—Ipecac is contraindicated because of the rapid onset of toxic symptoms

Multiple dose activated charcoal (check for presence of ileus)

TABLE 16-3   The Anticholinergic Toxidrome: Common Signs and Symptoms

PERIPHERAL ANTICHOLINERGIC EFFECTS	CENTRAL NERVOUS SYSTEM EFFECTS
Reduced secretions	Delirium
Dry mouth	Anxiety
Dry skin	Disorientation
Flushed skin	Hallucinations
Fever	Confusion
Dilated pupils	Paranoia
Blurred vision	Incoherent speech
Increased heart rate	Impaired recent memory
Urinary retention	Purposeless movements
Decreased bowel motility	

Cathartics

Cardiac arrhythmias—Lidocaine and phenytoin may be used

> Sodium bicarbonate (Mild alkalosis appears to resolve arrhythmias and may have prophylactic value. Keep serum PH 7.5)

Hypotension may resolve with fluid or may require the use of norepinephrine

Seizures—Diazepam for static, isolated seizure activity may not require treatment.

Physostigmine—Once the standard of care, now relatively contraindicated.[9] Usefulness is limited and toxicity is high.

Research is ongoing in the development of a specific antibodies similar to Digoxin immune fab.

Digoxin

Digitalis has been used to treat congestive heart failure, as well as reducing ventricular responses in certain supraventricular tachycardia. This is accomplished through slowing A-V nodal conduction and increasing contractibility (positive inotropic). Concurrent cardiac drugs, diuretics and hypokalemia, may increase the incidence of mild toxicity in patients receiving therapeutic doses. The peak manifestation of cardiac toxicity following acute ingestion may be as little as 30 minutes or as great as 12 hours.

■ **SIGNS AND SYMPTOMS**

Mild	*Severe*
Anorexia	Blurred vision
Premature ventricular contractions	Disorientation
Bradycardia	Diarrhea
Nausea and vomiting	SA or AV block
Headache	Ventricular tachycardia
Malaise	Ventricular fibrillation
Visual disturbances (i.e., see halos and yellow)	

■ **THERAPEUTIC INTERVENTIONS**

Supportive care

Discontinue digoxin and diuretics

Lavage

Multiple dose activated charcoal

Careful correction of electrolyte imbalances

Quantitative serum digoxin level immediately and at 6 hours post acute ingestion

Antidote—Digoxin immune fab (Digibind)

Indications

Severe arrhythmia that is not responsive to treatment

Large ingestions in previously healthy individuals (adults 10 mg, children 4 mg)

Digoxin levels in excess of 10 ng/ml and hyperkalemia > 5mEq/L

Precautions

Excellent safety profile, though allergic reaction are possible

Monitor for precipitous drop in potassium levels

Monitor ECG for symptoms of CHF and arrhythmias in patients using digoxin therapeutically

Further digoxin levels are of no value

Theophylline

Theophylline is a bronchodilator most commonly used in the treatment of asthma and chronic pulmonary disease. It has a narrow therapeutic index, which results in the development of toxicity from seemingly modest overdoses and iatrogenic causes. Chronic overdose is the most common form of theophylline poisoning.[1,7] The patient already has a body burden of theophylline that is not truly reflected by serum level. Serum concentrations that create only minor adverse effects in the acute overdose patient may produce life-threatening effects in the chronic overdose patient.

■ **SIGNS AND SYMPTOMS**

Gastrointestinal
Protracted nausea and vomiting
Abdominal pain

CNS
Agitation
Tremors
Seizures, and rarely coma

Cardiovascular
Sinus tachycardia (most common), and premature ventricular contractions
Ventricular tachycardia
Hypotension
Hypokalemia

■ **THERAPEUTIC INTERVENTIONS**

Supportive care
Lavage (pill size may be too large to fit through orogastric tube)
Multiple dose activated charcoal is the treatment of choice and may be repeated every 2 to 6 hours
Use of antiemetic (imperative to prevent vomiting of activated charcoal)
Consider cathartics
Quantitative theophylline level
    Risk of seizures in the chronic overdose: 20 to 60 mcg/ml
    Risk of seizures in the acute overdose: 60 to 100 mcg/ml
Charcoal hemoperfusion
Hemodialysis

■ **PREVENTION AND EDUCATION**

(For all prescription drugs)
Keep all prescription medications out of reach of children
Patients and caregivers should be informed of early warning signs of toxicity.
Serum blood levels should be routinely monitored
Know what medication you are currently taking and inform your healthcare provider of any changes in health status or medications.
Dosages of medication should not be changed without your healthcare provider's knowledge.

ENVIRONMENTAL POISONING

In the course of a day we are exposed to a variety of elements that can produce toxic effects. At home the potential toxins are infinite. Cosmetic and personal care products are the number one cause for calling a poison control centers for children under the age of 6 years (see Table 16-4).

Household plants have been maligned over the years as a source of potential toxins. Of all reported plant exposures, 98% resulted in the development of no toxicity or only minor toxicity.[1]

The workplace contains chemicals and toxins that may not be commonplace, especially toxic gases and vapors. The Occupational Safety and Health Administration (OSHA) places strict safeguards on the handling, disposal and use of toxins in the workplace unlike the home. Even with these guidelines misfortunes occur in the workplace. The following are just a few of the most common toxic environmental poisonings.

Carbon Monoxide

Carbon monoxide is emitted in the act of combustion. All fossil fuels, such as coal, gasoline, and natural gas, release carbon monoxide during combustion. Carbon monoxide released from wood and other material in house fires is a principal cause of death from smoke inhalation. Smoke inhalation also presents an inherent risk of

TABLE 16-4   Substances Most Frequently Involved in Pediatric Exposures (Children Under 6 Years)

SUBSTANCE	NO.	%*
Cosmetics and personal care products	137,225	12.1
Cleaning substances	126,511	11.1
Analgesics	86,936	7.6
Plants	79,362	7.0
Cough and cold preparations	70,632	6.2
Foreign bodies	60,579	5.3
Topicals	57,673	5.1
Pesticides (includes rodenticides)	45,897	4.0
Antimicrobials	40,220	3.5
Vitamins	37,932	3.3
Gastrointestinal preparations	37,027	3.3
Arts/crafts/office supplies	29,010	2.6
Hydrocarbons	27,632	2.4
Hormones and hormone antagonists	21,161	1.9
Food products/food poisoning	20,143	1.8

NOTE: Despite a high frequency of involvement, these substances are not necessarily the most toxic, but rather may only be the most readily accessible.
*Percentages are based on the total number of exposures in children under six years, rather than the total number of substances.
Litovitz et al: AAPCC report, *American Journal of Emergency Medicine* 15(5):454, 1997.

concurrent cyanide poisoning. Improperly vented hot water heaters, stoves, and furnaces are also a source of CO poisoning.

Clinical manifestations of carbon monoxide poisoning are produced by tissue hypoxia and direct cellular toxicity. Carbon monoxide inhalation results in formation of carboxyhemoglobin, displacing oxygen from hemoglobin. This binding does not allow the release of oxygen to the tissues. Furthermore, carbon monoxide causes the oxygen dissociation curve to shift to the left, which subsequently results in even less oxygen reaching the tissues. The half life of COHgb is approximately 5 hours. Organs that are most sensitive to hypoxia, the central nervous and cardiovascular systems, are greatly affected. Children and those with underlying cardiac and pulmonary disease are at greatest risk. In pregnancy, fetal COHgb levels rise more slowly than maternal levels and persist for prolong periods of time.[10]

■ **SIGNS AND SYMPTOMS**
Mild (COHgb level 10% to 20%)
Nausea
Vomiting
Mild throbbing headache
Malaise
Mimics flulike illness
Should be suspect in outbreaks of "food poisoning"
Moderate (COHgb level 20% to 30%)
Dyspnea with less exertion
Exacerbation of underlying coronary artery disease
Dizziness
Increase severity of mild symptoms
Confusion/agitation
Severe (COHgb levels 30% to 50%)
Seizures
Coma

Respiratory failure

Hypotension/dysrhythmia

■ **THERAPEUTIC INTERVENTIONS**

Removal from contaminated area

Give 100% oxygen by tight-fitting mask

ECG and cardiac monitoring

COHgb levels are only a guide and may not correlate with the severity of poisoning

Dexamethasone for toxic symptoms

Consider mannitol, urea, and glycerol for treatment of cerebral edema

Hyperbaric oxygen therapy (HBO)

    HBO can reduce the half life 4 to 5 times more rapidly than normobaric oxygen

    Indications for HBO include COHgb levels >25%, patients with altered mental status, pregnant patients, exacerbation of symptoms in cardiac and pulmonary patients.

■ **PREVENTION AND EDUCATION**

In 1996, 97% of all carbon monoxide cases reported to TESS were unintentional inhalations. The routine installation of smoke and carbon monoxide detectors in home and industry could reduce this number. Education as to sources of carbon monoxide exposure, especially in the winter months, is also important.

Food Poisoning

Bacterial contamination of food is the most common cause of food poisoning.[11] Most cases of food poisoning occur from improper handling of foods and failure to maintain foods at a proper temperature. Over 70,000 cases of poisonings from food were reported to poison control centers in 1996.[1] Because of the self-limiting nature of this illness, the number is probably much greater. The most common causative organisms are *Staphylococcus aureus, Salmonella, Escherichia coli, Clostridium perfringens, Campylobacter jejuni* and *Bacillus cereus. E. coli* has received increased notoriety because of illness and deaths related to contaminated and undercooked beef products.

    A high index of suspicion and a careful history regarding eating habits and recent travel may help to diagnose food poisonings of a nonbacterial nature (Table 16-5).

■ **SIGNS AND SYMPTOMS**

Nausea and vomiting

Diarrhea (may be watery or contain mucus or blood)

Abdominal cramping

Fever or subnormal temperature

Headache

Dehydration

Hemolytic uremic syndrome (seen in *E. coli* contaminations)

■ **THERAPEUTIC INTERVENTIONS**

Oral fluids if tolerated

IV hydration for symptoms of dehydration

Appropriate cultures

Antibiotic for Shigella and Streptococcus or in immunocompromised patients

Antiemetic

Electrolyte replacement

■ **PREVENTION AND EDUCATION**

Wash hands well before handling food or eating

Wash all utensils and cutting surfaces between food preparations

Wash all fresh fruits and vegetables

Thoroughly cook all meat and poultry

Maintain foods at 140 degrees during periods of prolonged serving

Check expiration dates on all products

TABLE 16-5 Differential Diagnosis of Bacterial Etiologies for Diarrhea and Food Poisoning

BACTERIAL DIARRHEA	PATHOGENESIS	SYMPTOMS					INCUBATION PERIOD	EFFECT OF HEAT	AGE GROUP	TRANSMISSION PATTERN	EXTRAINTESTINAL SYMPTOMS	CULTURE
		FEVER	DIARRHEA	DYSENTERY*	ABDOMINAL PAIN	VOMITING						
Clostridium perfringens	Enterotoxin	−	+†	+	++	±‡	8-24 hr	Thermostable organism Thermolabile toxin	Adults	Poultry, heat-processed meats (stews)	Volume depletion	Food, stool, vomitus
Escherichia coli	Enterotoxin	−	±	±	±	0§	24-72 hr	Thermostable toxin; capsular-thermolabile toxin	All	Contact	Volume depletion	Stool
Salmonellae	Bacteria (endotoxin)	+	+	±	±	±	8-48 hr	Thermolabile organism	All	Prepared foods, poultry, egg products, pet turtles and chicks	Headache, bacteremia	Food, stool, blood
Shigellae	Bacteria (endotoxin)	±	+	+	+	±	24-72 hr	Thermolabile organism; thermolabile toxin	All	Institutions	Seizures, meningismus	Food, stool

Staphylococci	Enterotoxin	−	+	0	+	+	2–6 hr	Thermostable toxin	All	Prepared food (salami, varied salads), fowl, pastry	Volume depletion	Food, stool
Streptococci	Bacteria	+	±	−	−	−	24–72 hr	Thermolabile organism	All	Proteinaceous foods	Influenza-like pharyngitis	Food, stool, blood
Vibrio cholerae	Enterotoxin	±	+	0	±	±	24–72 hr	Thermolabile toxin	All	Water, food	Hypokalemic nephropathy	Stool
Clostridium botulinum	Neurotoxin	−	−	−	±	±	12–36 hr	Thermostable spore; thermolabile toxin	All	Diverse canned foods	Dysphagia, descending paralysis	Serum, stool, vomitus for toxin
Bacillus cereus												
Type I	Enterotoxin	−	+	−	+	++	1–6 hr	Thermolabile toxin	All	Fried rice	Limited	Food, stool
Type II	Enterotoxin	−	++	−	+	±	10–12 hr	Thermolabile toxin	All	Meats, vegetables	Volume depletion	Food, stool
Campylobacter jejuni	Enterotoxin	+	+	−	+	+	1–7 days	Thermolabile toxin	All	Poultry, meats, dairy produce	Limited	Food, stool, blood

*Dysentery = diarrhea with blood and mucus.
† + = Occurs regularly. §0 = Does not occur.
‡ ± = May or may not occur.
(Modified from Grady GF, Keusch GT: Pathogenesis of bacterial diarrheas, *N Engl J Med* 285:831–841, 891–900, 1971.)

Dispose of canned goods whose integrity is in question or that are bulging
Refrigerate all dairy products or susceptible foods at 40 degrees or less

Botulism

Botulism is a paralytic illness produced by neurotoxins from *Clostridium botulinum*. Botulism is relatively rare, but occurs typically as a sporadic outbreak within a family or other group. This toxic syndrome can result from the ingestion of the toxin or from contamination of a wound or gastrointestinal tract. Endotoxins are classified as A through G. The most common in humans are A, B, and E.

The typical cause of botulism is poorly processed or spoiled home-canned vegetables, especially the nonacid types, such as green beans. Bulging can lids (resulting from expanding gases as the organisms grow) are often mentioned in the history-taking phase.

Signs and symptoms usually develop 8 to 36 hours following ingestion of contaminated food, but may be delayed for as long as 4 days.

■ SIGNS AND SYMPTOMS

Presenting signs and symptoms are often vague.

Lethargy/weakness
Constipation
Visual disturbances (double vision)
Impaired speech
Headache
Afebrile or subnormal temperature
Dry, sore throat with hoarseness; inability to swallow
Limited eye movement
Dilated pupils
Decreased tendon reflexes
Descending paralysis

■ THERAPEUTIC INTERVENTIONS

1. Ensure ABCs (the patient may require a tracheostomy and ventilatory assistance).
2. Induction of emesis may be of benefit in patients immediately following food *known* to contain botulism toxin.
3. Symptomatic patients should not be lavaged or made to vomit.
4. If several hours have elapsed, administer sodium sulfate (250 mg/kg) orally or magnesium sulfate (250 mg/kg) orally as a cathartic because this toxin is slowly absorbed.
5. If the patient is asymptomatic or exposure is questionable, may follow closely as an outpatient.
6. Asymptomatic and probably exposed patients should be hospitalized under close observation and treated with antitoxin on appearance of symptoms. Symptomatic patients should be admitted to ICU, the toxin type determined, and treated with the antitoxin.
7. Specific trivalent (A, B, E) horse serum antitoxins are available from the Center for Disease Control and Prevention. They will stop the progression of the neuropathology but will not antagonize existing problems.

■ PREVENTION AND EDUCATION

See *Food Poisoning*.

Iron

The most common ingestion of iron is through vitamins. Over 25,000 calls were made concerning ingestion of vitamins containing iron in 1996. There is no physiological mechanism for iron excretion. Normal serum iron levels range from 50 to 175 mcg/100ml. Ingestion of >20 ml/kg is thought to be potentially toxic. Ingestion of 300 mg/kg is lethal.

■ **SIGNS AND SYMPTOMS**

Initial (within 2 hours of ingestion)
Nausea and vomiting
Hematemesis
Bloody stools
Abdominal pain
Hyperglycemia

Second stage
Resolution of GI symptoms
Dehydration may be the only symptom

Third stage (48 to 96 hours)
Metabolic acidosis
Disturbances in clotting mechanisms
Hemorrhage and shock
Hepatic and renal failure
Hypoglycemia

■ **THERAPEUTIC INTERVENTIONS**

Supportive care
Induced emesis (preferred in children)
Gastric lavage (most adult strength pills will not fit through lavage tubes)
Cathartic
Abdominal x-ray—Iron tablets occasionally form bezoars or concretions in the gut; chewable vitamins containing iron will not be radiopaque
Whole bowel irrigation—should be initiated if there is radiographic evidence of iron tablets past the pylorus or if there is evidence of iron in the stomach after other attempts at decontamination
Serum Iron levels at 4 to 6 hours postingestion
Chelation therapy should be initiated in:
    Symptomatic patients
    Ingestion of >20 mg/kg of elemental iron
    Serum iron levels >350 mcg/100 ml
    Deferoxamine—15 mg/kg/hr IV until the vin rose color of the urine disappears.
Emergency gastrotomy for removal of bezoar formation in the GI tract. Bezoars can cause necrosis and perforation in the GI tract
Exchange transfusions (rarely indicated)

Lead

It is estimated that there are five million tons of lead in the paint in United States homes and that up to 70% of homes built before 1960 have some surfaces covered with lead-based paint.[12] Although leaded paint is the most visible source of lead, it should not be regarded as the only source. Lead poisoning does not produce a classic toxidrome that facilitates an easy diagnosis. The symptoms in children may range from subtle behavioral changes to acute encephalopathy and death. Peak incidence of lead poisoning occurs in the summer months. Lead is compartmentalized into three main areas: bone, soft tissue (including the brain) and blood. Excretion occurs slowly through urine, feces, and sweat. Organic lead is rapidly assimilated by the central nervous system and can produce a host of neuropsychiatric manifestations.

■ **SIGNS AND SYMPTOMS**

Gastrointestinal
Viral symptoms
Nausea and vomiting

Abdominal pain or colic
Changes in bowel habits
Anorexia
Neuropsychiatric
Motor/coordination difficulties
   Delayed reaction times
Impaired cognitive skills
Changes in behavior and attention disorders
   Headache, encephalopathy
   Mental retardation
Miscellaneous
Microcytic anemia
Renal dysfunction (proximal tubular acidosis)
Urination of porphyrins
Long bone changes (radio dense) in children

■ **ROUTE OF ENTRY**

Oral: "pica" or the craving for and eating of paint chips; glazed pottery leaching or ingestion of glazing material; cultural herbal medicines, especially Mexican-American, Indian, and Chinese folk medicines; dust particles from lead-filled homes or renovations; water contaminated by lead piping

Inhalation—sniffing of leaded gasoline produces the sequelae of gasoline abuse and lead intoxication; fumes or dust particle during renovations; occupational exposure

Drugs of abuse—samples of heroin, cocaine, and methamphetamine have been reported to contain as much as 60% lead by weight;[12] homemade alcoholic beverages, especially moonshine, and wine, from still piping and lead salts.

■ **THERAPEUTIC INTERVENTIONS**
Acute ingestion
Whole bowel irrigation, and cathartics for ingestion of lead glazes or lead products
Radiograph of abdomen
Chronic exposure
Blood lead level (acceptable levels are now 10 ug/dl [was 25 ug/dl])
Radiographs of abdomen, wrist, knees
Erythrocyte protoporphyrin level
Chelation therapy recommended for levels >45 ug/dl or in symptomatic children
BAL or Ca EDTA—Parenteral, require hospitalization
Succimer (2,3 dimercaptosuccinic acid) is approved for oral chelation therapy
   Dose: 30 mg/kg for 7 days

■ **PREVENTION AND EDUCATION**

Ascertain if children have had lead levels checked. Household risks—Houses built before 1960; renovations; pica eating; imported ceramic plates
Never store food in lead containers
Water should be tested for contamination
Adherence to OSHA standards in the workplace

Mushrooms

Mushroom species range from delectable to lethal. The typical ingestion of mushrooms by inquisitive children is nontoxic. Only 8 mushroom fatalities out of more than 100,000 mushroom exposures have been reported by the AAPCC in the last 10 years. Most fatalities involve adults who fail to properly identify mushrooms before consuming them. Other tragic cases are individuals who seek hallucinogenic mushrooms, but mistakenly pick one with profound hepatotoxicity. Only highly suspicious mushrooms or symptomology in a patient require identification of the mushroom by a mycologist.

- **SIGNS AND SYMPTOMS**

  May mimic food poisoning in toxic and nontoxic ingestion

  Development of symptoms within two hours of ingestion are unlikely to be fatal

  Development of symptoms at 6 hours or more is suggestive of containing highly toxic amatoxins

  Hepatotoxicity

  CNS (vertigo, seizures, incoordination)

  Hepatorenal syndrome

- **THERAPEUTIC INTERVENTIONS**

  Supportive care

  If the mushroom is not available, obtain a detailed description of its appearance

  If a sample of the mushroom is available, save it in a *paper* bag in refrigerator

  Interventions will be determined by identification of the mushroom

  Emesis if recent ingestion

  Activated charcoal and cathartic

  Save all emesis and stools in refrigerator (do not freeze) for possible microscopic study and analysis

  Observation for seizures, hypotension

  Possible analgesics, sedatives, antispasmodics, and antiemetics

- **PREVENTION AND EDUCATION**

  Unless assured of the identity of a plant, flower, or mushroom, do not eat it.

Pesticides

Organophosphates and carbamates are two very common pesticides available that can cause serious toxicity. They have similar symptoms, but duration of symptoms is usually less with carbamates. Organophosphates bind acetylcholinesterase, allowing accumulation of acetylcholine at the neuroreceptor sites and produce a cholinergic crisis.

These can be absorbed by all routes of administration—inhalation, dermal, and oral.

- **SIGNS AND SYMPTOMS**

  See Box 16-1.

BOX 16-1   Clinical Effects of Organophosphate Poisoning (Acetylcholine Excess)

Muscarinic effects

Sweat glands	Sweating
Pupils	Constricted
Lacriminal glands	Lacrimation
Salivary glands	Excessive salivation
Bronchial tree	Wheezing
Gastrointestinal	Cramps, vomiting, diarrhea, tenesmus
Cardiovascular	Bradycardia, fall in blood pressure
Ciliary body	Blurred vision
Bladder	Urinary incontinence

Nicotinic effects

Striated muscle	Fasciculations, cramps, weakness, twitching paralysis, respiratory embarrassment, cyanosis, arrest
Sympathetic ganglia	Tachycardia, elevated blood pressure
CNS	Anxiety, restlessness, ataxia, convulsions, insomnia, coma, absent reflexes, Cheyne-Stokes respirations, respiratory and circulation depression

■ **THERAPEUTIC INTERVENTIONS**
Decontamination of patient and prevention of personnel exposure
Supportive care
Antidotes
   Atropine—may need to be given for up to 24 hours, until secretions are minimal and cessation of bradycardia
   Pralidoxime (2-PAM)—in severe organophosphate poisonings, effects are often dramatic. 2-PAM is usually given only with organophosphate, but many exposures are mixed exposures. 2-PAM is synergistic with atropine, so use only with severe organophosphate poisoning and when exposure is unknown.

■ **PREVENTION AND EDUCATION**
Use only nonleather gloves
Protective coverings and eyewear should be used when handling pesticides
Use pesticides only in well-ventilated areas and spray or spread down wind
Read label on product before use.

Petroleum Distillates

Kerosene, charcoal lighter fluid, mineral oil, furniture polish, turpentine, gasoline, and many insecticides have petroleum-distillate bases. Complications usually occur as a result of aspiration or other pulmonary problems. Aspiration of hydrocarbons may also result in transient CNS depression or excitation.

■ **SIGNS AND SYMPTOMS**
Respiratory difficulty
Infiltrates on chest x-ray
Abnormal arterial blood gases
Dysrhythmias

■ **THERAPEUTIC INTERVENTIONS**
ABCs; intubate if necessary.
Give oxygen.
Wash surface areas that have been contaminated.
Gastric emptying is not indicated unless there is a history of large ingestion of hydrocarbons that may produce renal, liver or CNS toxicity (i.e., halogenated hydrocarbons or petroleum or petroleum distillates with additives).
Monitor ABGs in symptomatic patients (for example, coughing, choking).
Obtain a chest x-ray film (should be diagnostic within 6 hours after ingestion).

SUBSTANCE ABUSE

Prevention and education is the means for decreasing morbidity and mortality in drugs of abuse. Community referral to agencies specializing in the treatment and counciling of drug abuses should be made for patients presenting to the emergency department. Drugs of abuse vary in different parts of the country. With the number of available illicit drugs increasing at a rapid rate, the poison center may be the only source of information for an overdose or poisoning with a brand new "designer" drug. The use of a nonjudgmental approach and maintenance of the patient's dignity may enhance identification of the substance of abuse.

Aggressive, and at times, unpredictable behavior is frequently seen in drug and alcohol abuse and withdrawal. Safety of the patient and emergency department staff should be assured at all times.

Alcohols

Alcohol is the most common drug taken by patients today. Different forms of alcohol—ethanol, isopropanol, methanol, and ethylene glycol—have varying degrees of toxicity. Table 16-6 shows varying degrees of toxicity.

TABLE 16-6 Alcohols

FORMULATIONS AND USES:

Use	Approx. conc.
1. Methanol: Gas line antifreeze	95
Windshield washer fluid	35-95
Antifreeze	Varied
Industrial solvents (e.g., paint & varnish remover, shellac)	
Sterno	
Dry gas	
2. Ethanol/Isopropanol	(proof/2 = % ETOH)
Ethanol: Beverages	
A) Beer	4-6
B) Wine	10-20
C) Spirits	20-50
Rubbing alcohol	70
Aftershaves/colognes	40-60
Mouthwashes	Up to 75
Medicinal preparations	Varied
Isopropanol: Rubbing alcohol	70
Pine disinfectants	5-30
Solvents	Varied
3. Ethylene glycol: car radiator antifreeze	95

Note: Longer-chain glycols (i.e., propylene glycol, polyethylene glycol) are relatively nontoxic orally.

	METHANOL	ETHANOL/ISOPROPANOL	ETHYLENE GLYCOL
Comparison of toxicity	"Highly toxic" By history death has been reported after 15 ml 40% methylhydroxide; blindness reported after 4 ml. Ex. 1.5 ml of 100% methanol in a 10 kg child produces a potential level of 20 mg%; one gulp (2-8 ml) can produce levels of 26-105 mg% **Blood levels** All are potentially toxic depending on the time of ingestion and presence of signs and symptoms.	Isopropanol is approximately twice as intoxicating as ethanol at equivalent blood levels. (Severe toxicity with blood levels >150 mg%) Ethanol (blood levels) 50-100 mg% = mild toxicity 100-300 mg% = moderate toxicity >300 mg% = severe toxicity, but 1 ml/kg of pure ethanol will result in a blood level of approximately 100 mg% at 2 hours postingestion.	"Highly toxic" Ex 3.0 ml of 100% ethylene glycol in a 10 kg child produces a potential level of 50 mg%; one gulp (2-8 ml) can produce levels of 34-135 mg% **Blood levels** All are potentially toxic depending on the time of ingestion and presence of signs and symptoms.

*New York City Poison Center: *Syllabus,* 1993.

Continued

TABLE 16-6 Alcohols—cont'd

	METHANOL	ETHANOL/ISOPROPANOL	ETHYLENE GLYCOL
Presentation and onset of symptoms	Toxicity *delayed:* Usual latent period is 12-24 hrs (may be delayed during concurrent ethanol ingestion). Gastritis and "hang-over"-like effect followed by visual disturbances and an anion gap metabolic acidosis. Anion gap = *Na minus (HCO3 + CL). Normal = 12 ± 4 Mnemonic for an anion gap metabolic acidosis. M-U-D-P-I-L-E-S Methanol Uremia **Diabetic ketoacidosis** Paraldehyde; phenformin Iron, isoniazid Lactic acidosis Ethylene glycol, ethanol ketoacidosis Salicylates, sympathomimetics	Rapid onset of intoxication (30-60 min) Gastritis possible from high concentrations.	**Phase I (½-12 hr)** CNS ethanol-like inebriation (no odor) Anion gap metabolic acidosis Calcium oxaluria **Phase II (2-36 hr)** Tachypnea, tachycardia **Phase III (2-3 days)** Renal failure
Toxicology	Metabolized by the liver via alcohol dehydrogenase, to formaldehyde, and then very quickly to formic acid. It is these two metabolites, rather than the methanol, that causes the visual and metabolic changes.	*Ethanol:* Direct-acting CNS (reticular activating system) depressant. *Isopropanol:* Direct-acting CNS depressant. Causes local gastritis. The metabolite acetone acts to prolong CNS effects. Produces a ketosis without an acidosis	Neurologic symptoms Due to parent compound. Renal toxicity due to formation of oxalic acid metabolite.
Home management	Consider emesis while en route to hospital. All but minute amounts of dilute concentrations must be referred to hospital.	If ingestion accidental, home assessment for CNS changes.	Consider emesis while en route to hospital. All but minute amounts of dilute concentration: refer to hospital.
Referral to medical facility	All suicide gestures. All symptomatic patients. All but minute amounts of dilute concentrations.	All suicide gestures. Symptomatic patients with calculated ethanol level >100 mg%.	All suicide gestures. All symptomatic patients. All but minute amounts of dilute concentration.

Hospital management	(1) ABCs (2) Gut decontamination (time dependent) (3) Labs, diagnostic Blood methanol Lytes ABCs Calculate anion gap Blood ethanol Fundoscopic exam of the eye (4) Ethanol therapy: (A) Loading dose followed by maintenance dose. (Ethanol has 20× the affinity for alcohol dehydrogenase compared to methanol.) *Indications* (B) (+) Blood methanol level OR (C) Symptomatic patient and strong suspicion. *Load* 7.6-10 ml/kg IV of 10% ethanol in D5W over 30 minutes to achieve blood ethanol level of 100 to 130 mg%. Oral route acceptable. **Maintenance** 1.4 ml/kg/hr of 10% ethanol IV. Requirements increase in chronic alcoholics and during hemodialysis. Treat until level of methanol is zero. (5) Hemodialysis (6) Folinic or folic acid.	(1) ABCs (2) Gut decontamination (time dependent) (3) Labs, diagnostic Ethanol/isopropanol/acetone levels Blood and urine ketones Electrolytes Glucose Calculate anion gap (4) Supportive care	(1) ABCs (2) Gut decontamination (time dependent) (3) Labs Ethylene glycol (if possible) Electrolytes—including calcium ABG Calculate anion gap ECG Urine analysis for oxalate or hippurate crystals Some brands of antifreeze may be fluorescent under Woods' lamp. Ethanol therapy—loading dose followed by maintenance. (Same indications and dosing as in methanol management.) (5) Hemodialysis. (6) Possibly thiamine and pyridoxine.
Physician consultant	All patients in hospital.	All patients with unstable vital signs (or acidosis-unrelated). Suspect MEOH or ethylene glycol.	All patients in hospital.

*New York City Poison Center: *Syllabus,* 1993.

■ **PREVENTION AND EDUCATION**

All patients presenting with ethanol alcohol intoxication should be given a referral to an alcohol/substance abuse program. Become involved in EN CARE or other prevention program. Keep all toxic products out of the reach of children.

Cocaine

The National Institute on Drug Abuse indicates that over 30 million people have used cocaine and that 5 million people use cocaine regularly. The use of this drug spans all racial, economic and social boundaries. Cocaine is frequently cut with other metabolites to increase potency, mixed with unknown additives, or used in combination with other "designer" drugs. Cocaine can be injected, smoked, inhaled (snorted), or rubbed on mucous membranes. Drug smugglers or "packers" are known to swallow large qualities of cocaine wrapped in latex that can leak or rupture.

Acute MI has been reported up to 14 days after cocaine use in patients with and without preexisting cardiac disease, some as young as 19 years.[13] Cocaine crosses the placental barrier and is excreted in breast milk for up to 36 hours after use. It is estimated that up to 10% of pregnant women use cocaine at least once during their pregnancy, placing these children at risk.

■ **SIGNS AND SYMPTOMS**

See Box 16-2.

BOX 16-2   Medical Complications of Cocaine Use

Cardiovascular
Arrhythmias
Hypertension
Myocardial ischemia/infarction
Contraction band necrosis
Deep venous thrombosis
Central nervous system
Agitation
Headaches
Seizures
Cerebral infarction
Pulmonary
Pulmonary edema
Hemoptysis
Pneumomediastinum (crack lung)
Cough
Obstetric/perinatal
Abortion
Abruptio placentae
Neonatal cerebral infarction
Breast-feeding complications
Others
Psychiatric
Infectious disease
Rhabdomyolysis
Renal failure

■ THERAPEUTIC INTERVENTIONS

Ingestion

Abdominal x-rays may reveal latex packages

Activated charcoal and cathartic

Whole bowel irrigation

Rarely endoscopy or surgical removal of packets

Inhalation

CXR may show pneumomediastinum from rupture of alveoli

Mediastinal/chest tube placement

Supportive care

Administer benzodiazepine for sedation and seizures

Acetaminophen and external cooling of hyperthermia

ECG and cardiac monitoring

Baseline cardiac enzymes

Treatment of arrhythmias—*Lidocaine is relatively contraindicated* because of potential increase effects.[14]

Narcotic/Opiates

Heroin abuse continues to be a significant problem in the United States as well as throughout the world. Nearly all reported heroin related fatalities involve parenteral use, which is the primary route of administration in the United States. Like other illicit drugs, the introduction of other chemicals may complicate management. Iatrogenic overdoses of narcotics are reported annually, and the emergency nurse should be diligent in monitoring all patient receiving narcotic. Patients with significant opioid overdose merit close observation and supportive care for 24 to 48 hours.

■ SIGNS AND SYMPTOMS

Depression of all vital signs

Miosis

Hypotension

Mental status depression

Respiratory depression is most critical problem

Nausea/vomiting

■ THERAPEUTIC INTERVENTIONS

Supportive care

Gastric lavage

Activated charcoal and cathartic

Multiple-dose activated charcoal

Naloxone (Narcan)—up to 2 mg may be required

Inhalant Abuse

The National Institute on Drug Abuse reported in 1996 that one in five American teenagers has used inhalants to get "high." A variety of agents are used: nail polish remover, marking pens, paint thinner, gasoline, butane lighters, and aerosol sprays are just a few. Many of the inhalants contain chlorofluorocarbons (CFCs). Inhalant abuse can cause severe hypoxia and chronic inhalation abuse can cause permanent end-organ damage.

■ SIGNS AND SYMPTOMS

Unusual breath odor

Slurred speech, disorientation

Red or runny nose and eyes

Nausea

Anxiety, irritability

Behavioral changes

TABLE 16-7 Antidote Chart

POISON	ANTIDOTE	COMMENTS
Black widow spider	Antivenin	Latrodectus-mactans venom neutralizer; 1-2 vials IV over 1 hour
Rattlesnake		Crotalidae Polyvalent venom neutralizer; see P'dex for dosage.
Carbamates Organophosphate Physostigmine excess Synthetic choline esters and inocybe Mushrooms (clitocybe and inocybe)	Atropine	Antagonizes cholinergic stimuli at muscarinic receptors.
Neuroleptic drugs (Haloperidol, Phenothiazines, Thioxanthenes) and Metoclopramide	Benztropine	Reverses drug-induced dystonias through competitive inhibition of muscarinic receptors & blockade of dopamine reuptake.
Botulism	Botulism antitoxin	Contact CDC—404-329-3753; after hours—404-329-3644. Draw 10 ml of serum for determination of toxin before treatment is started.
Calcium channel blockers	Calcium chloride (drug of choice unless patient is acidotic) Calcium gluconate (use if patient is acidotic)	Large amounts may be required. Keep serum $Ca^{++} < 11$.
Hydrofluoric acid burns Hyperkalemia Hypermagnesemia	Calcium gluconate	2.5% gel for dermal exposure (calcium gluconate). 10% calcium gluconate local infiltration or arterial infusion for HF burns. IV calcium gluconate for hyperkalemia & hypermagnesemia
Lead Cadmium Zinc Copper	CaEDTA Calcium disodium edetate	Precautions: adequate fluids, monitor urine output; avoid rapid IV. Not effective on mercury, gold or arsenic.
Cyanide Hydrogen sulfide (H_2SO)	Cyanide kit	Instructions are explicit in kit. Oxygen and methemoglobin levels need to be monitored closely.* Do not use methylene blue if excessive methemoglobinemia occurs. H_2SO. DO NOT use NaThiosulfate. Use nitrites only.
Iron	Deferoxamine	Deferoxamine mesylate forms excretable ferrioxamine complex. This red complex is water soluble and readily excreted by the kidneys. Passing of vin rosé urine indicates Fe present.

Toxin	Antidote	Comments
Cocaine LSD	Diazepam	
Digitalis Oleander Foxglove	Digoxin Immune Fab (Digibind®)	Antigen-binding fragments bind with digoxin for digitalis overdose.
Arsenic Lead encephalopathy Gold Mercury	Dimercaprol (Bal)	Heavy metals inhibit sulfhydryl containing enzymes; the resulting chelated mercaptide product is less toxic and more easily excreted from the body than the heavy metals.
Phenothiazine Allergic reactions	Diphenhydramine	Will reverse drug-induced extrapyramidal effects.
Lead	DMSA (Dimercaptosuccinic acid)	Oral active chelating agent indicated for treatment of lead poisoning in children with lead levels >45 µg/dl.
Arsenic Lead Mercury Bismuth	D-Penicillamine	Contraindicated for penicillin allergic patients.
Methanol Ethylene glycol	Ethanol for IV administration	Reduces formation of toxic metabolites. Competitive inhibitors of alcohol dehydrogenase. Monitor blood glucose. Adjust dose if dialysis is performed.
Benzodiazepines	Flumazenil	Use caution if unknown drug ingestion. Seizures can occur with reversal of BZP effects, especially with TCA coingestion.
Methanol	Folic acid & Leucovorin	May be effective in adjunctive therapy stimulating the pathway for methanol metabolites. Allergic reaction may occur.
Beta-blocker	Glucagon	Bypasses beta adrenergic blockades by activating nonbeta receptors; increasing contractility.
Aniline Nitrites Local anesthetics	Methylene blue	Reducing agent to convert methemoglobin to methemoglobin hemoglobin.
Acetaminophen	N-Acetylcysteine	Gluthathione substitute that prevents the formation of toxic intermediary metabolites. Best when given within 8 hours of ingestion; can be given within 24 hours of ingestion.

continued

Modified from New Hampshire Poison Center's Protocols.

TABLE 16-7 Antidote Chart—cont'd

POISON	ANTIDOTE	COMMENTS
Opioids Ethanol-induced coma Clonidine Propoxyphene Diphenoxylate Pentazocine	Naloxone	Opioid antagonist that reverses the CNS and respiratory depressant effects.
Vacor Streptozocin	Nicotinamide	For best results should be given within 30 minutes of vacor ingestion.
Carbon monoxide	Oxygen	Administer 100% oxygen by tight-fitting mask to reduce half life of CO.
Anticholinergic (rarely) TCA (last resort)	Physostigmine	Inhibits the destructive action of acetylcholinesterase. Should not be used routinely for OD because of its potential adverse effects.
Warfarin Long-acting anticoagulants	Phytonadione (Vit K$_1$)	Reverses the inhibitory action of warfarin on blood clotting factors II, VII, IX & X in the liver.
Organophosphate	Pralidoxime	Cholinesterase reactivator for organophosphate OD. Should be given after adequate atropine therapy.
Heparin	Protamine	Protamine reacts with heparin to form a stable salt resulting in neutralization of heparin anticoagulant activity.
Isoniazid Monomethylhydrazine mushrooms	Pyridoxine	Pyridoxine is used to prevent and control isoniazid-induced seizures. Pyridoxine may reverse neurologic symptoms with this mushroom ingestion.
TCA	Sodium bicarbonate	Aside from gastric decontamination NaHCO$_3$ is the most useful single intervention for management of TCA.

Modified from New Hampshire Poison Center's Protocols.

Cardiotoxic and neurotoxic effects
V-fibrillation ("sudden sniffer's death")
■ **THERAPEUTIC INTERVENTIONS**
Oxygen
Supportive care
Determination of substance may give some additional interventions
Symptomatic treatment

BOX 16-3   Diagnostic Clues in Unknown Ingestions

Metabolic acidosis (mudpiles)
Methanol
Uremia
Diabetes ketoacidosis
Paraldehyde
Isoniazid, iron
Lactic acidosis
Ethanol, Ethylene glycol
Salicylate, sympathomimetics
Glucose

Increased	*Decreased*
Salicylate	Salicylate
Isopropyl alcohol	Acetaminophen
Isoniazid	Isoniazid
Iron	Methanol
	Insulin
	Ethanol

Urine color
Red: hematuria, hemoglobinuria, myoglobinuria, pyrvinium (Povan), phenytoin (Dilantin), phenothiazine, mercury, lead, anthrocycan (food pigment in beets and blackberries)
Brown-black: hemoglobin pigments, melanin, methyldopa (Aldomet), cascara, rhubarb, methocarbamol (Robaxin)
Blue, blue-green: amitriptyline, methylene blue, triamterene (Dyazide), Clorets, *Pseudomonas*
Brown, red-brown: Porphyria, urobilinogen, nitrofurantoin, furazolidone, metronidazole, aloe, seaweed
Orange: rifampin, phenazopyridine (Pyridium), sulfasalazine (Azulfidine)
Radiographic medication—(CHIPE)
Chloral Hydrate
Heavy metals
Iron
Phenothiazine
Enteric coated tablets
Breath odor
Alcohol: ethanol, chloral hydrate, phenols
Acetone: acetone, salicylate, isopropyl alcohol
Bitter almond: cyanide
Coal gas: carbon monoxide
Garlic: arsenic, phosphorus, organophosphate
Nonspecific—consider inhalation abuse
Oil of wintergreen: methylsalicylates

Jimsonweed

Jimsonweed has been abused for its hallucinogenic effect for centuries. All parts of the jimsonweed plant are toxic.[15] It is usually ingested in a tea form or by eating the seeds. The clinical manifestations are of classic atropine poisoning. The half-life is long and symptoms may persist for hours to days. Other plants, such as nightshade, angel trumpet, thornapple, and moonflower, contain belladonna, alkaloids, atropine, scopololamine, and hyoscyamine.

■ **SIGNS AND SYMPTOMS**

Consistent with anticholinergic drugs (see Table 16-3).

■ **THERAPEUTIC INTERVENTIONS**

Supportive care
Gastric lavage when indicated
Multiple dose activated charcoal (cautiously in the presence of decreased bowel sounds)
Whole bowel irrigation
Small incremental doses of physostigmine in severe anticholinergic toxicity

---

CURRENTLY AVAILABLE ANTIDOTES

An antidote is a physiological antagonist that may reverse the signs and symptoms of poisoning (Table 16-7 and Box 16-3).

This is a very brief guide to some of the more common problems in toxicology. This field is emerging and changing rapidly. For the most current information and help in caring for your patient, contact your local Poison Information Center. They can give you more in-depth guidance for treatment of the poisoned patient.

REFERENCES

1. Litovitz TL et al, 1996 annual report of the American Association of Poison Control Centers national data collection systems, *Am J Emerg Med* 15:447-500, 1997.
2. Wrenn K, Rodewald L, Dockstader L: Potential misuse of ipecac, *Ann Emerg Med* 22:1408-1412, 1993.
3. Kornberg AE, Dolgin J: Pediatric ingestions: charcoal alone versus ipecac and charcoal, *Ann Emerg Med* 20:648-651, 1991.
4. Goldfrank L: *Goldfrank's toxicologic emergencies,* ed 5, Norwalk, Conn, 1994, Appleton & Lange.
5. Auerbach P, Osterloh J et al: Efficacy of gastric emptying: gastric lavage versus emesis induced by ipecac, *Ann Emerg Med* 15:692-698, 1986.
6. Neuvonen PJ, Vartianainen M, Tokola O: Comparison of activated charcoal and ipecac syrup in prevention of drug absorption, *Eur J Clin Pharmacol* 24:557-562, 1983.
7. *Vet Hum Toxicology* 3:350, 1989.
8. Litovitz TL: *Ann Emerg Med* 15:1221-1224, 1986.
9. Rumak BH, Spoerke DG: *Poisondex toxicologic information systems,* Denver, Micromedex Computerized Information Systems.
10. *J For Sci* 6:1448-1452, 1990.
11. Krenzelok EP: Food poisonings, *Clin Toxic Forum* 5:1-4, 1993.
12. *Environmental Health Perspectives* 89:109-120, 1990.
13. Weiss RJ: Recurrent myocardial infarction caused by cocaine abuse, *Am Heart J* 111:793, 1986.
14. Derlet RW, Albertson TC, Tharratt RS: Lidocaine potentiation of cocaine toxicity, *Ann Emerg Med* 20:135-138, 1991.
15. Centers for Disease Control and Prevention: Jimsonweed poisoning—Texas, New York, and California, *MMWR* 44:41-44, 1994.
16. *JAMA* 263:797-798, 1990.

CHAPTER 17

Environmental Emergencies

Susan Budassi Sheehy

SNAKEBITES

There are over 3000 species of snakes; of these, 375 from five different families are venomous. These families are:

- Crotalidae—copperheads, rattlesnakes, cottonmouths
- Elapidae—coral snakes, cobras, mambas
- Viperidae (true vipers)—puff adders
- Hydrophidae—sea snakes
- Colubridae—boomslangs

Although 45,000 snakebites occur each year in the United States (8000 by poisonous snakes), fewer than 15 deaths result.

Several poisonous snakes have venoms that contain toxins that are cardiotoxic, neurotoxic, or hemotoxic. Venom is injected by the fangs of the snake. The ducts of the fangs are filled with the venom, which is manufactured in the salivary glands.

The most common site for a snakebite is an extremity (that is, an arm or a leg) that is close to the snake.

■ SIGNS AND SYMPTOMS

Signs and symptoms of snakebite depend on several factors:

Species and size of the snake
Location of the bite
Depth of the bite
Number of bites
Amount of venom injected
Age of the patient
Size of the patient
Patient's sensitivity to venom
Number of microorganisms in the snake's mouth

Signs and symptoms can be divided into local and systemic reactions

Local reactions

Fang marks
Teeth marks
Edema (occurs within 5 minutes and may extend to 36 hours)
Pain at the site (usually correlated with the amount of edema)
Petechiae
Ecchymosis
Loss of function of the limb
Necrosis (16 to 36 hours after the bite)

Systemic reactions

Nausea and vomiting	Salivation
Diaphoresis	Difficulty speaking
Syncope	Epistaxis
Metallic or rubber taste in mouth	Hematemesis
Constricted pupil (unilateral or bilateral)	Hemoptysis
Ptosis	Hematuria
Visual disturbances (mostly diplopia)	Melena
Muscle twitching	
Paresthesias	

Severe systemic reactions
Pulmonary edema
Seizures
Severe hemorrhage
Renal failure
Paralysis
Hypovolemic shock

■ THERAPEUTIC INTERVENTIONS
Ensure ABCs
Keep the patient calm
Remove potentially constricting jewelry
Do *not* use ice. (Although cryotherapy has some strong proponents, most experts advise against the application of cold packs. In some cases, *cryotherapy* rather than the bite itself has resulted in amputation.)
Do *not* give alcohol or substances containing caffeine to drink
Do *not* allow patient to smoke
Immobilize the limb
Keep the limb at or below the level of the heart
Place a *loose* constriction band 4 inches proximal to the bite if within 30 minutes of the bite. (Once applied, do not remove in the field.)
Cleanse the wound
Early incision and wound suction. (If done *immediately,* this can remove 25% to 50% of the venom. This is generally not effective after 10 to 15 minutes.) Suction wound with rubber suction cup or syringe. Avoid mouth suction to prevent absorption of venom via open areas in the mouth.
Give analgesics for pain management
Initiate IVs (two) with Ringer's lactate or normal saline solution
Place a central venous pressure line or an arterial pressure line
Ensure current tetanus prophylaxis status
Consider surgical intervention
Consider antivenin therapy
Be sure to record the time of the bite and the times of any subsequent therapies
Identify (or secure the snake) if possible. (DO *NOT* HANDLE THE SNAKE!)

Antivenin. Antivenin administration should be reserved for life-threatening snakebites only, because it carries a high incidence of sensitivity reactions and possible anaphylaxis. It should be administered in the hospital setting, where the patient can be closely monitored. (Antivenin administration is not a prehospital care procedure!) Follow these guidelines:
- Be sure equipment is readily available; be prepared for CPR situations.
- Obtain a careful allergy history.
- Do a conjunctival or skin test to test for sensitivity reaction: A positive reaction occurs within 5 to 30 minutes.

- If a reaction does occur (urticaria, wheezing, cyanosis, edema, anaphylaxis), administer 1:1000 epinephrine (0.2 to 0.5 ml) subcutaneously

Be sure to read the antivenin package insert thoroughly and follow the directions *precisely*.

SPIDER (ARACHNID) BITES

Most spider bites induce local reactions, such as itching, swelling, and stinging pain. Spiders that induce systemic, as well as local complications are the black widow and the brown recluse spiders.

Black Widow Spiders *(Latorodectus Mactans)*

Black widow spiders are usually found in damp, cool places, such as wood piles. They are identified by their black bodies and the red hourglass-shaped figure on their abdomens. The venom of the black widow is *neurotoxic*.

■ SIGNS AND SYMPTOMS
Painful sting at the time of the bite followed by a dull, numb pain
Tiny red marks at the point of entry of the venom
Nausea and vomiting
Hypertension
Elevated temperature
Respiratory distress
Headache
Syncope
Weakness
Chest pain
Abdominal pain
Seizures
Shock

■ THERAPEUTIC INTERVENTIONS
If aggressive supportive therapy is given, signs and symptoms will usually be gone within 48 hours.
  Treat the patient symptomatically
  Cool the area of the bite with ice packs to slow the action of the neurotoxin
  Give muscle relaxants—methocarbamol (Robaxin) or diazepam (Valium)
  Administer calcium gluconate for muscle spasms (use 10 ml of 10% solution mixed in 100 ml of normal saline solution and run it in over 20 minutes)
  Consider narcotic analgesics
  Consider antivenin; read antivenin literature carefully and thoroughly before administering

Brown Recluse Spiders *(Loxosceles Reclusa)*

Brown recluse spiders are usually found in the southeastern, south-central, and south-western states, although there have been recent reports of habitats farther north. They inhabit dark areas such as basements, garages, boxes, and closets. These spiders may be identified by their light brown color and the dark brown fiddle-shaped mark on their thoraxes.

■ SIGNS AND SYMPTOMS
Local reactions
Mild stinging at the time of the bite
Local edema
Bluish ring around the bite appears within 2 to 8 hours after the bite
Bleb formation
Erythema

Local ischemia
Tissue necrosis—appears on third or fourth day
Eschar/open sore—appears in 14 days
Wound healing—appears in 21 days

Systemic reactions

Fever	General malaise
Chills	Arthralgias/joint pain
Nausea and vomiting	Petechiae
Weakness	

Severe systemic reactions (seen in small adults and children)—very rare

Seizures
Disseminated intravascular coagulation (DIC)
Renal failure
Hemolysis
Cardiopulmonary arrest (very rare)

■ **THERAPEUTIC INTERVENTIONS**

Consider antihistamines
Consider antibiotics
Consider systemic or local steroids
Consider local debridement
Consider skin grafting
Rehydration (orally or intravenously)
Consider blood transfusions
Arrange for renal dialysis

Scorpion Stings

Scorpions are found in the desert areas of the southwestern states of California, Arizona, and Texas. The incidence of scorpion stings increases in the cool evening and night hours. Although there are several species of scorpions, *Centuroides sculpturatus* is the only species that injects a lethal venom. The tail of the scorpion contains the telson, in which venom is produced and stored, and the stinger, which injects the venom.

■ **SIGNS AND SYMPTOMS**

Local pain at the sting site	Wheezing/respiratory stridor
Edema	Profuse salivation
Discoloration	Visual disturbances
Hyperesthesia	Ataxic gait
Agitation or drowsiness	Incontinence
Itching	Trismus
Speech disturbances	Nausea and vomiting
Tachycardia	Dysphagia
Hypertension	Seizures
Tachypnea	Anaphylaxis

■ **THERAPEUTIC INTERVENTIONS**

Support ABCs
Treat the patient symptomatically
Ensure tetanus prophylaxis
Consider antivenin therapy
(Avoid narcotic analgesics and barbiturates as these have been shown to increase the toxic effects of the venom)

BEE, WASP, HORNET, AND FIRE ANT (HYMENOPTERA) STINGS

Hymenoptera stings can be as mild as a local reaction or as life-threatening as anaphylactic shock. Reactions can occur immediately or as late as 48 hours after the sting. The greater the incidence of stings, the greater the possibility of a severe reaction.

- **SIGNS AND SYMPTOMS**
  ### Mild local reactions
  Stinging and burning sensation at time of sting
  Local swelling
  Local itching
  ### Severe local reaction
  Total extremity edema
  ### Systemic reactions
  Urticaria
  Pruritus
  Edema (extremities and periorbital region)
  Bronchospasm
  Anaphylactic shock
  Laryngeal edema
  Hypotension

- **THERAPEUTIC INTERVENTIONS**
  ### For mild reactions
  Scrape the stinger in the opposite direction of the penetration angle with a dull object; do not grasp and pull it, because this squeezes the venom sac and causes more toxin to be released
  Cleanse the sting site
  Apply antiseptic cream
  Consider oral antihistamines
  Consider steroids
  Apply ice
  Elevate the limb
  ### For severe reactions
  Support ABCs
  Give epinephrine (1:10,000 IV for anaphylactic shock)
  Initiate IVs
  Apply the PASG
  Consider vasopressors
  Antihistamine doses will vary
  Consider steroids
  Consider theophylline

Fire ants have a painful sting that forms a wheal, which expands into a large vesicle. The area reddens and a pustule forms. As the pustule is reabsorbed, crusting and scar formation follow. This hymenopteran's sting may also cause anaphylaxis. Therapeutic intervention is the same as that for other hymenoptera stings.

- **PREVENTIVE MEASURES AGAINST HYMENOPTERA STINGS**

Avoid areas where hymenoptera are usually present.
Avoid wearing bright colors.
Avoid wearing perfumes outdoors.
Wear shoes when walking outdoors.
People who have a sensitivity to hymenoptera venom should carry an anaphylaxis prevention kit that contains 1:1000 epinephrine and antihistamines. They should also be instructed to wear a Medic-Alert bracelet or some other type of medical identification tag stating their sensitivity. Desensitization is a possibility in some patients; it has been reported as 95% effective.

TICK BITES

Rocky Mountain Spotted Fever

Rocky Mountain spotted fever is a tick-borne disease for which the causative agent is *Rickettsia ricketsii*. Complications include renal failure and shock.

■ **SIGNS AND SYMPTOMS**

Chills

Fever

Severe headache

Myalgias

Hemorrhagic lesions, petechiae

Constipation

Abdominal distention

Decreased level of consciousness

Maculopapular rash (initially on wrists and ankle, then on extremities, trunk, face, palms, and soles of feet)

■ **THERAPEUTIC INTERVENTIONS**

Remove tick

Administer antibiotics

Lyme Disease

Ticks are the vector for the spirochete that causes Lyme disease, so named for the geographic location of its original presentation. Because of the vague viral symptomatology, Lyme disease is often misdiagnosed.

■ **SIGNS AND SYMPTOMS (generally occur 1 week after exposure)**

Fatigue

Lethargy

Myalgias

Headache

Pain in extremity

Target rash (annular lesion with bright red borders and fading center, present in only 25% of cases)

Second stage presentation (4 weeks after the bite)

Bell's palsy (common)

Meningitis

Paresthesias

Syncope/AV block

Third stage presentation (6 months after the bite)

Joint pain

Arthritis, predominantly in large joints

■ **THERAPEUTIC INTERVENTIONS**

Symptomatic treatment (nonsteroidal antiinflammatory medicines)

Doxycycline/tetracycline/Pen-VK/erythromycin for 30 days

INJURIES CAUSED BY COLD

Chilblains

Chilblains are localized areas of itching, painful redness, and recurrent edema, usually on the earlobes, fingers, and toes. Chilblains usually occur in climates that are cool and damp. They are a mild form of frostbite. There is no specific treatment, as the symptoms are usually self-limiting.

Immersion Foot

Immersion foot occurs when there is constant contact of the foot with cold temperatures through moisture inside a boot or shoe. It is a common condition in foot soldiers and hunters who spend some time in the water and then later come to dry ground without changing their wet socks or boots. The foot begins to appear wrinkled and, if the condition is allowed to continue for a prolonged period, may develop tissue sloughing.

■ **THERAPEUTIC INTERVENTIONS**
Warm the affected foot in tepid water
Change into dry socks and shoes

Frostbite

Frostbite is a traumatic condition induced when ice crystals form and expand in the extracellular spaces. The enlarging ice crystals compress the cells, resulting in cell membrane rupture and the interruption of enzymatic activity and metabolic processes. As histamine is released, capillary permeability is increased with red-cell aggregation and microvascular occlusion similar to that seen in burn patients. This is a condition that is not reversible once it has occurred. It is important, however, to protect the areas surrounding the frostbite to prevent further injury.

Frostbite is often accompanied by hypothermia. Depending on the degree of the hypothermia, it may take priority over frostbite for therapeutic intervention.

Superficial frostbite

Superficial frostbite usually involves the fingertips, ears, nose or cheeks, and toes.

■ **SIGNS AND SYMPTOMS**

Burning	Numbness
Tingling	Whitish color

■ **THERAPEUTIC INTERVENTIONS**
Apply warm (104° to 110° F [40° to 43.3° C]) soaks
Do *not* apply friction (rubbing)

Deep frostbite

In deep frostbite the actual cellular temperature of the injured part is lowered. This produces local vascular and tissue changes that can lead to the injury and death of the surrounding cells. Several factors can affect the possibility of sustaining frostbite:

Ambient temperature
Wind-chill factor (Figure 17-1)
Amount of time exposed
Whether or not the patient was wet or exposed to direct contact with metal objects
Type and number of layers of clothing worn

Other factors may contribute to the individual's predisposition to frostbite:

Darker-skinned people are more prone
Lack of acclimatization (moving abruptly from a warm area to a cold area)
Previous frostbite injury
Poor peripheral vascular status
Anxiety
Exhaustion
Frail body type

■ **SIGNS AND SYMPTOMS**
Whitish discoloration of the skin, followed by a waxy appearance
Slight burning pain, followed by a feeling of warmth, then numbness

Estimated wind speed (in mph)	Actual Thermometer Reading (°F)											
	50	40	30	20	10	0	-10	-20	-30	-40	-50	-60
	EQUIVALENT CHILL TEMPERATURE (°F)											
Calm	50	40	30	20	10	0	-10	-20	-30	-40	-50	-60
5	48	37	27	16	6	-5	-15	-26	-36	-47	-57	-68
10	40	28	16	4	-9	-24	-33	-46	-58	-70	-83	-95
15	36	22	9	-5	-18	-32	-45	-58	-72	-85	-99	-112
20	32	18	4	-10	-25	-39	-53	-67	-82	-96	-110	-124
25	30	16	0	-15	-29	-44	-59	-74	-88	-104	-118	-133
30	28	13	-2	-18	-33	-48	-63	-79	-94	-109	-125	-140
35	27	11	-4	-21	-35	-51	-67	-82	-98	-113	-129	-145
40	26	10	-6	-21	-37	-53	-69	-85	-100	-116	-132	-148
(Wind speeds greater than 40 mph have little additional effect)	LITTLE DANGER in <5 hr with dry skin Maximum danger of false sense of security			INCREASING DANGER Danger from freezing of exposed flesh within one minute				GREAT DANGER Flesh may freeze within 30 seconds				
	Trenchfoot and immersion foot may occur at any point on this chart.											

FIGURE 17-1. Cooling power of wind on exposed flesh expressed as an equivalent temperature.

Swelling and burning following numbness

Blisters (usually appear in 1 to 7 days)

Edema of entire extremity

Severe discoloration and gangrene appear later

■ **THERAPEUTIC INTERVENTIONS**

Prehospital (or in the wilderness)

Leave the affected part cold unless the temperature of thawing water can be ensured and maintained, and analgesics are available (thawing is extremely painful).

If the extremity is thawed, do not permit the patient to use it.

Do not use ice or snow and friction to massage the extremity (this causes tissue damage).

Prevent further heat loss:

Remove the patient's wet clothing.

Cover the patient with dry blankets or sheets.

Give warm noncaffeine liquids if the patient is conscious and has a gag reflex.

Protect the injured part from further damage.

Splinting and soft padding are advisable (avoid pressure).

Attempt to get to a place where there is a heat source and a constant supply of warm water.

If in the wilderness and a long hike to obtain help is necessary, the patient may walk on the frostbitten extremity if necessary unless it is thawed or begins to thaw; the patient must *not* walk on a thawed extremity.

In the emergency department

Immerse the frostbitten part in warm (104° to 110° F [40° to 43.3° C]) water that maintains a constant temperature.

Administer warm liquids by mouth if the patient is alert and has a gag reflex.

Cover the patient with warm blankets; be careful not to place any pressure on the frostbitten part.

Administer narcotic analgesics (rewarming is very painful).

After it has thawed, protect the part with bulky sterile dressings.

Ensure tetanus prophylaxis.

Consider antibiotics.

Consider escharotomy if vascular constriction is severe.

Amputation is not an emergency procedure; it may have to be performed several weeks after the injury.

■ **PREVENTIVE MEASURES AGAINST FROSTBITE**

Dress properly for the climate (layers of loose-fitting clothing).

Eat a diet high in carbohydrates and fats (a heat source).

Avoid smoking and drinking alcohol or beverages that contain caffeine.

Avoid bare skin contact with metal objects.

Keep dry.

Avoid exhaustion.

Protect previously frostbitten parts from exposure.

Hypothermia

Hypothermia is defined as a condition in which the core temperature of the body is less than 95° F (35° C) (Table 17-1). Severe hypothermia is defined as a core temperature of 90° F (32.2° C). It is at this temperature that severe physiologic detriments occur. Death usually occurs when core temperature falls below 78° F (25.6° C). Early signs and symptoms of hypothermia are:

Fatigue

Slow gait

Muscle incoordination

Apathy

TABLE 17-1   Signs and Symptoms of Hypothermia

TEMPERATURES	SIGNS AND SYMPTOMS
96°-99° F (35.6°-37.2° C)	Shivering, loss of manual coordination
91°-95° F (32.8°-35° C)	Violent shivering, slurred speech, amnesia
86°-90° F (30°-32.2° C)	Shivering decreases but is replaced by strong muscular rigidity and cyanosis
Below 86° F (30° C)	Possibility of developing rewarming shock, atrial fibrillation
81°-85° F (27.2°-29.4° C)	Irrational, stuporous; pulse and respirations decrease
78°-80° F (25.6°-26.7° C)	Coma, erratic heartbeat
Below 81° F (27.2° C)	Possibility of ventricular fibrillation
Below 78° F (25.6° C)	Cardiopulmonary arrest

Pathophysiology of hypothermia

Many metabolic responses are temperature dependent. When hypothermia occurs, cellular activity drops. As the temperature drops by 18° F (10° C), the metabolic rate decreases by two to three times. Renal blood flow decreases, causing a decrease in glomerular filtration rate. As a result of this, water is not reabsorbed and dehydration occurs. In addition, respirations decrease, carbon dioxide is retained, and hypoxia and acidosis occur. Because of diminished glucose supply, the patient becomes hypoglycemic.

In addition to the cellular changes, the cells of the heart become more sensitive and prone to dysrhythmias as core temperature begins to fall. Osborne waves develop on the ECG. Be very careful not to cause any sudden movement of the hypothermia patient because sudden movement may trigger fibrillation.

Mild hypothermia, in which the patient is shivering and still alert and oriented, should be treated by placing the patient in a warm (104° to 110° F [40° to 43.3° C]) bath and administering warm fluids that contain glucose or other sugar substances by mouth to provide heat through calories.

■ **THERAPEUTIC INTERVENTIONS FOR SEVERE HYPOTHERMIA**

Core rewarming is essential to prevent rewarming shock. Rewarming shock occurs when the peripheral areas are rewarmed faster than the core. This causes a large amount of lactic acid, which was located in the extremities, to be rapidly shunted back to the heart, where fibrillation may occur. It is also possible that peripheral vasodilation and hypotension will occur as a result of relative hypovolemia.

Protection of ABCs

    Avoid endotracheal intubation if possible and manage the airway and breathing with a bag-valve-mask device to avoid excess patient stimulation and the possibility of ventricular fibrillation.

    Warm humidified oxygen

    Core rewarming

by peritoneal lavage   Two cannulas running warmed normal saline or Ringer's lactate solution into the peritoneal cavity and removing it by suction can raise the core temperature 10.8° F (6° C)/hour.

by gastric lavage   Not as effective as peritoneal lavage because of smaller surface area of stomach; there is a risk of ventricular fibrillation when the lavage tube is placed.

by warmed IV solutions   This will not raise core temperature significantly, but will prevent further heat loss.

by warm humidified oxygen with IPPB   This will not raise the core temperature very much, but will prevent further heat loss.

by mediastinal lavage   through two chest tubes or through direct contact of warmed fluids into the mediastinum through a thoracotomy incision; this is used only in the event of intractable ventricular fibrillation in which core temperature elevation is the only hope of survival.

by renal dialysis or heart-lung bypass machine   Although impractical in most emergency settings, this may be done if the equipment is ready and skilled personnel are available to run the equipment.

Correct fluid and electrolyte status.
Administer IV fluids to compensate for hypovolemic state.
Consider administration of steroids.

INJURIES CAUSED BY HEAT

Heat Cramps

Heat cramps occur when a person is doing physical work in hot weather, causing electrolyte loss from excessive perspiration.

■ **SIGNS AND SYMPTOMS**

Cramps (particularly in the shoulders, thighs, and abdominal wall muscles)
Weakness
Nausea
Tachycardia
Pallor
Profuse diaphoresis
Cool, moist skin

■ **THERAPEUTIC INTERVENTIONS**

Sodium chloride by mouth or intravenously (depending on degree of discomfort and clinical status of patient); balanced electrolyte drinks
Cool environment
Rest

Heat Exhaustion

Heat exhaustion occurs when there is a prolonged period of fluid loss (for example, from perspiration, diarrhea, or the use of diuretics) and exposure to warm ambient temperatures without adequate fluid *and* electrolyte replacement. It is particularly common in the very young and the very old.

■ **SIGNS AND SYMPTOMS**

Thirst	Anorexia
General malaise	Anxiety
Cramps in muscles	Syncope
Headache	Dehydration
Tachycardia	Muscle incoordination
Orthostatic hypotension	Possible elevated temperature
Nausea and vomiting	

■ **THERAPEUTIC INTERVENTIONS**

Rest
Cool environment
IV fluids to replenish fluids and electrolytes

Heat Stroke

Heat stroke can be exercise-induced, occurring when a person exercises strenuously in a very hot environment and is unable to dissipate the heat the body produces. It can also be nonexercise-induced, occurring in individuals who are vulnerable to high temperatures. Heat stroke can be precipitated by certain medications that affect heat production (thyroid extracts and amphetamines), decrease thirst (haloperidol), and decrease diaphoresis (antihistamines, anticholinergics, phenothiazines, and propranolol). As the body temperature rises to

---

BOX 17-1   Body Temperature and Metabolism

If body temperature rises to 100.4° F (38° C), metabolism will increase by 13%.
If body temperature rises to 102.2° F (39° C), metabolism will increase by 26%.
If body temperature rises to 104° F (40° C), metabolism will increase by 39%.
If body temperature rises to 105.8° F (41° C), metabolism will increase by 52%.
If body temperature rises to 107.6° F (42° C), there will not be enough oxygen available to meet the increased needs of the cells.

105.8° F (41° C) there is depressed central nervous system, heart, and cellular function. Death will occur if the body temperature is not lowered.

For every 1.8° F (1° C) rise in temperature, the body's metabolism will increase by 13% (Box 17-1).

■ SIGNS AND SYMPTOMS

Tachycardia
Tachypnea
Hyperpyrexia of 105.8° F (41° C) or more
Hypotension
Nausea and vomiting
Diarrhea

Decreasing level of consciousness
Decreased urinary output
Hot, dry skin
Seizures
Decerebrate posturing
Dilated, nonresponsive pupils

■ THERAPEUTIC INTERVENTIONS

ABCs
Rapid cooling
IVs
Other supportive measures
   Control shivering (will cause temperature to rise)
   Chlorpromazine
Hospital admission

DIVING EMERGENCIES

In diving, a person is exposed to pressure greater than he or she is normally exposed to on land. These greater atmospheric pressures bring with them a whole array of medical problems unique to underwater diving and conditions that cause increased atmospheric pressures.

When a person is at sea level, the pressure exerted on the body is 1 atmosphere. At a water depth of 33 feet, the pressure exerted on the body is 2 atmospheres. At a water depth of 66 feet, the pressure is 3 atmospheres.

Water depth (feet)	Pressure (atmosphere)
Sea level	1
33	2
66	3
100	4
133	5
166	6
200	7
300	10
400	13
500	16

Depth of Diver and Effect on Gas Volume

Boyle's law states: The volume of a gas varies inversely with the absolute pressure. In other words, as pressure increases, gas volume decreases. For example, if a normal pair of lungs contains 2000 cc of air at sea level, the volume of air decreases as the diver descends:

Depth	Air in both lungs (cc)
Sea level	2000
33	1000
100	500
233	250

At a depth of 33 feet the total volume of air would be 1000 cc (half of normal), at 100 feet it would be 500 cc (one fourth of normal), and at 233 feet it would be 250 cc (one eighth of normal).

A scuba tank is added to the diver at sea level. If the diver forcefully inhales supplemental air from the tank, the lungs will still contain 2000 cc regardless of the depth.

Depth (feet)	Air in both lungs (cc)
Sea level	2000
33	2000
100	2000
233	2000

If the diver ascends but forgets to exhale on the way up, the atmospheric pressure will decrease as he ascends and the gas in his lungs will expand.

Depth (feet)	Air in both lungs (cc)
233	2000
100	4000
33	8000
Sea level	16000

It is easy to see what will happen—as the gas expands, the lungs expand, to a limit. Then the lungs rupture, a spontaneous pneumothorax results, and air escapes into the circulation, producing an air embolism. The mechanism of injury is breath holding on ascent because gas expansion occurs.

Air Embolism

■ **SIGNS AND SYMPTOMS**
Chest tightness
Shortness of breath
Pink frothy sputum
Vertigo (loss of visual point of reference)
Limb paresthesias or vertical (one-sided) paralysis
Seizures
Loss of consciousness
Signs and symptoms of pneumothorax
This is an extremely serious condition. The diver must receive extremely prompt therapy.

■ **THERAPEUTIC INTERVENTIONS**
Oxygen under positive pressure
If tension pneumothorax is present, needles inserted into anterior chest wall
Trendelenburg's position in left lateral decubitus position to avoid cerebral embolization
Urgent recompression in hyperbaric chamber

Nitrogen Narcosis

Nitrogen narcosis is a condition in which, in accordance with Henry's law,* nitrogen (which is 79% of air) is dissolved in solution because the person is breathing nitrogen under greater pressure than normal. Dissolved nitrogen produces effects similar to those of alcohol. The deeper one dives, the greater the narcosis. After 1 hour, the effects of nitrogen at various depths are as follows:

Depth	Effects
125 to 150 ft	Narcosis begins
150 to 200 ft	Drowsiness, decreased mental functions
200 to 250 ft	Decreased strength, decreased coordination
300 ft	Diver's mental function and movement deteriorate
350 to 400 ft	Unconsciousness, death

Therapeutic intervention consists of a gradual ascent to shallow water, with decompression stops along the way, so that nitrogen can slowly reabsorb.

Decompression Sickness

If a diver is at a depth long enough for nitrogen to be dissolved and then ascends rapidly, there is not enough time for the nitrogen to reabsorb, and nitrogen bubbles form, producing decompression sickness (the bends, dysbarism, caisson disease, diver's paralysis). Exercise (such as swimming toward the surface) causes a rapid release of nitrogen bubbles, similar to the effect of shaking a bottle of a carbonated beverage, causing gas to be released from solution.

■ SIGNS AND SYMPTOMS

Itch	Crepitus
Rash	Visual loss
Fatigue	Joint soreness
Dizziness	Shortness of breath
Paresthesias or paralysis	Unconsciousness
Seizures	

■ FACTORS INCREASING SEVERITY OF SIGNS AND SYMPTOMS

Extremes of water temperature	Poor physical condition
Increased age	Alcohol consumption
Obesity	Peripheral vascular disease
Fatigue	Heavy work while diving

■ THERAPEUTIC INTERVENTIONS

Recompression
Oxygen at 10 L/min by mask
IV infusion
IV sodium bicarbonate
Transport in left lateral Trendelenburg's position to decrease the possibility of cerebral air embolization

■ SPECIAL NOTES

Any complaint of joint soreness 24 to 48 hours after a dive should be treated with decompression in a hyperbaric chamber.

Bends can occur at depths less than 33 feet (1 atmosphere).

*At a constant temperature, the solubility of any gas in a liquid is almost directly proportional to the pressure on the liquid.

OTHER MEDICAL PROBLEMS ENCOUNTERED IN DIVING

The "Squeeze"

The squeeze results from the compression of air trapped in hollow chambers, producing severe, sharp pain, when outside pressure is greater than inside pressure. It most frequently occurs in these areas:

Ears
Sinuses
Lungs and airways
Gastrointestinal tract

Thoracic cavity
Teeth
Added air spaces (face mask or wet suit)

■ SIGNS AND SYMPTOMS

Pain
Edema
Capillary dilation

Rupture
Bleeding

Hyperpnea Exhaustion Syndrome

Hyperpnea exhaustion syndrome results from diver fatigue.

■ SIGNS AND SYMPTOMS
Tachypnea
Anxiety
Feeling of impending doom
Difficulty floating
Exhaustion

■ THERAPEUTIC INTERVENTIONS
Ascent to the surface and rest aboard a flotation device or boat.

Ear Squeeze or Sinus Squeeze

The cause of the ear squeeze is a blocked eustachian tube; the cause of sinus squeeze is a blocked paranasal sinus and an inability to equalize the pressures (Table 17-2).

■ THERAPEUTIC INTERVENTIONS
Ascend to shallower water.

TABLE 17-2   Gas Toxicities in Diving

GAS	SIGNS AND SYMPTOMS	THERAPEUTIC INTERVENTIONS
Oxygen (from breathing 100% oxygen)	Twitching, nausea, dizziness, tunnel vision, restlessness, paresthesias, seizures, confusion, pulmonary edema, atelectasis, shock lung	ABCs, intubation, controlled ventilation to reduce Fio_2, decompression, PEEP
Carbon dioxide (from inhaling expired air; 8%-10% causes toxicity)	Dizziness, lethargy, heavy labored breathing, unconsciousness	Ascent to surface, ABCs, 100% oxygen
Carbon monoxide (from contaminated tank—filled too close to internal combustion engine)	Dizziness, pink or red lips and mouth, euphoria	Ascent to surface, ABCs (CPR if necessary), 100% oxygen in hyperbaric chamber at 3 atmospheres for 1 hour

NOTE: Occasionally gas toxicity will occur when the air in the scuba tank is not room air or has been contaminated.

EMERGENCY INFORMATION

The following information should be kept readily available when treating an injured diver:

Hyperbaric chamber location and telephone number*

Name and telephone number (24-hour number) of a physician trained in underwater emergencies

Environmental emergencies can prove devastating to the patient and challenging to the emergency care provider. An in-depth understanding of the scope and unique presentation of all patient care situations represented in this chapter is essential to competently evaluate and intervene effectively.

SUGGESTED READINGS

Auerbach PA: *Wilderness and environmental emergencies,* ed 3, St Louis, 1996, Mosby.

Clowers TD: Wound assessment of the Loxosceles reclusa (brown) spider bite, *J Emerg Nurs* 22: 283-287, 1996.

Dickey LS: Barotrauma. In Rosen P, Barkin RM, editors: *Emergency medicine concepts and clinical practice.* St Louis, 1997, Mosby.

Gardner J: Action STAT: rattlesnake bite, *Nurs 97* 27(6): 33, 1997.

Kol S, Weisz G, Melamed Y: Pulmonary barotrauma after a free dive—a possible mechanism, *Aviat Space Environ Med* 3:236, 1993.

Wilderness and environmental emergency issue, *J Emerg Nurs* 23: 507-656, 1997.

*If this information is unavailable, call the U.S. Navy Experimental Diving Unit in Washington, DC (202-433-2790, 24 hours a day, 7 days a week). Ask for the duty officer, who will give you the name, location, and telephone number of the nearest decompression chamber. A useful reference book is the *Directory of Worldwide Decompression Chambers,* available from the Superintendent of Diving, U.S. Navy, Naval Ships Systems Command, National Center Building #3, Washington, DC 20360.

Genitourinary Emergencies

Louise LeBlanc

TRAUMATIC GENITOURINARY EMERGENCIES

This chapter outlines signs and symptoms, diagnostic aids, and therapeutic interventions for traumatic and non-traumatic genitourinary emergencies, nonemergency genitourinary conditions, and emergencies in dialysis patients such as clotted access and cardiovascular and metabolic disorders.

Renal Trauma

Renal trauma (trauma to the kidneys) should be suspected in any injury that involves a blunt or penetrating blow to the anterior or posterior lower chest, a fracture of the 11th or 12th ribs or of the transverse process of L_1 to L_3 (Figure 18-1). It should also be suspected with fractures of the pelvis or in any patient who has sustained a multiple-systems injury. Of patients seen in the emergency department with abdominal trauma, it is estimated that 86% have injury to the kidney. Pedicle injuries are the most likely renal cause of poor outcome.[1]

■ **SIGNS AND SYMPTOMS**

History of trauma: *blunt*—motor vehicle crashes (MVC), falls, fights, contact sports; *penetrating*—associated with other intraabdominal and intrathoracic injuries (that is, liver, small bowel, colon)

Abdominal, flank, suprapubic, and/or back pain

Ecchymosis or hematoma in flank area

Microscopic or gross hematuria

Prior history of renal abnormality

■ **DIAGNOSTIC AIDS**

Check urine for hematuria (use reagent papers specifically designed to check for blood). Degree of hematuria may bear no relationship to the severity of the injury. Hematuria is absent in 10% to 25% of all renal injuries.[2]

Urinalysis: if catheterization is required for male patient, this must be preceded by a rectal exam by the physician. A "boggy" or "high riding" prostate may indicate urethral damage.

Chest x-ray film

Abdominal x-ray film of kidneys, ureters, bladder (KUB)

Intravenous pyelogram (IVP). If an IVP and cystogram need to be obtained, the IVP is done first (to avoid dye extravasation and obscuring of lower ureteral injury). If immediate surgery is indicated, a KUB with contrast is obtained quickly to check for the presence of both kidneys.

Renal angiogram

CT scan

CBC, electrolytes, BUN, serum creatinine, possible type and crossmatch

■ **THERAPEUTIC INTERVENTIONS**

Close monitoring of vital signs, urine output

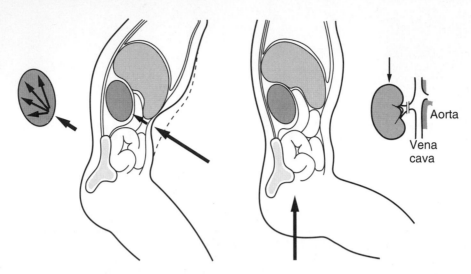

FIGURE 18-1. Mechanisms of renal injury. *Left,* Direct blow to abdomen. Smaller drawing shows force of blow radiating from the renal hilum. *Right,* Falling on buttocks from a height (contrecoup of kidney). Smaller drawing shows direction of force exerted upon the kidney from above. Tear of renal pedicle.
(From Tanagho EA, McAninch JW: *Smith's general urology,* ed 14, Stamford, Conn, 1995, Appleton & Lange.)

Penetrating injury: A culture of the site and tetanus and antibiotic prophylaxis are required in addition to previous interventions.
Possible
Abdominal rigidity
Swelling or mass in flank
Hypovolemic shock
Crepitus over lower rib cage or lumbar vertebrae

Renal Contusion

■ **SIGNS AND SYMPTOMS**
Flank ecchymosis
Subcapsular hematoma on x-ray film
Mild hematuria
Flank pain or pain upon palpation
Retroperitoneal hematoma (bruising at area of 11th and 12th ribs, Grey-Turner's sign (bruising around the umbilicus, and hematuria)
Perirenal hematoma (palpable flank mass)
■ **THERAPEUTIC INTERVENTIONS**
Blunt
Discharge to home
Bed rest until the hematuria resolves
Great volumes of fluids for a few days
Penetrating
There should be surgical exploration of all penetrating renal injuries because of a high incidence of associated intraabdominal injuries.

Renal Laceration

A laceration is an actual disruption of renal tissue:
>   Through the parenchyma
>   Through the renal pelvis
>   Through the capsule

■ SIGNS AND SYMPTOMS
Gross hematuria
Possible flank pain
Other signs of hypovolemia
Palpable flank mass
Possible shock

■ THERAPEUTIC INTERVENTIONS
Hospital admission
Observation
Bed rest
Possible surgical repair or partial/total nephrectomy

Renal Vascular Disruption

A renal vascular disruption involves the disruption of the renal arteries or veins. Renal artery thrombosis is commonly associated with falls and motor vehicle crashes and is usually unilateral.

■ SIGNS AND SYMPTOMS
Bruits auscultated at the first or second lumbar vertebra, near the midline

■ DIAGNOSTIC AIDS
No kidney visualization on IVP and extravasation of contrast during procedure

■ THERAPEUTIC INTERVENTIONS
Surgical intervention for reanastomosis of the artery or vein

Renal Fracture

A renal fracture is considered the most critical injury involving fragmentation of the kidney or fracture extension into the renal pedicle. Often seen with penetrating trauma due to gunshot and stab wounds.

■ SIGNS AND SYMPTOMS
Severe blood loss
Shock
Expanding flank mass

■ DIAGNOSTIC AIDS
Angiography

■ THERAPEUTIC INTERVENTIONS
Surgical exploration. A complete rupture of the kidney requires nephrectomy.

Ureteral Injury

Ureteral injury is caused by blunt or penetrating trauma such as a gunshot wound or an iatrogenic injury such as occurs during abdominal surgery and urologic procedures.

■ SIGNS AND SYMPTOMS
Delayed presentation of flank pain
Abdominal pain or tenderness
Urinary sepsis
Ileus

Soft palpable mass
Fever
Leukocytosis
■ **DIAGNOSTIC AIDS**
IVP
■ **THERAPEUTIC INTERVENTIONS**
Therapeutic intervention depends on the location of the injury. Surgical emergency treatment ranges from neoureteropyeloplasty, ureteroureterostomy with a stent or a neoureterocystostomy.

Bladder Trauma

Bladder trauma should be suspected with a fractured pelvis or direct suprapubic trauma. It also may be injured in penetrating trauma, where the bladder is in the path of the penetrating object.
■ **SIGNS AND SYMPTOMS**
Suprapubic pain
Urine extravasation
Possible hematuria
Possible shock
Possible anuria
Inability to void spontaneously
■ **DIAGNOSTIC AIDS**
Urinalysis
Retrograde cystogram
Abdominal x-ray film
■ **THERAPEUTIC INTERVENTIONS**
Surgical repair and drainage of the areas of extravasation
Urinary diversion from the injury

Penetrating Urethral Trauma

Penetrating urethral trauma is rare, but usually occurs as a result of a direct penetrating injury or pelvic injury (most commonly a straddle injury). The patient may have an iatrogenic injury or spontaneous rupture caused by urethral stricture.
■ **SIGNS AND SYMPTOMS**
Blood at meatus
Hematuria
Anuria
Flank pain
Urinary fistula
History of trauma
Prostate elevated above normal position
■ **DIAGNOSTIC AIDS**
Retrograde urethrogram
■ **THERAPEUTIC INTERVENTIONS**
Surgical repair to anastomose the urethra
Cystostomy with 3 to 6 month delayed closure

Obstructive Urethral Trauma

Obstructive urethral trauma may be caused either by a foreign body in the urethral tract or by constricting objects around external urethral structures. These types of injuries are commonly seen in young children, senile adults, victims of sexual assault, and those who practice unusual methods of sexual stimulation.

■ **SIGNS AND SYMPTOMS**

Blood at urethral meatus
Swelling or discoloration of the genitalia (butterfly-shaped hematoma in the perineal area)
Inability to void (In males, ensure attempt to void while standing.)
Hematuria
Anuria
Edema
Urethral tears
Possible infection with purulent discharge
Report of specific foreign body implantation
Urinary tract infection
Necrosis
Distended bladder
Abdominal pain

■ **DIAGNOSTIC AIDS**

Retrograde cystourethrogram

■ **THERAPEUTIC INTERVENTIONS**

Analgesia or sedation
Local anesthesia
Removal of foreign body
Suprapubic urine aspiration if the bladder is severely distended
Possible administration of antibiotics
Possible surgical intervention

Fracture of the Penile Shaft

A fracture of the penile shaft is a traumatic rupture of the corpus cavernosum. It may occur when an erect penis is bent forcibly during intercourse. It occurs exclusively during erection as a result of direct blunt trauma.[3] Penile fracture should be suspected in any male with multiple trauma involving the pelvic region, especially when the mechanism of injury was a straddle incident, such as would occur in an accident on a motorcycle or a bicycle with a crossbar. It is considered an urologic emergency.

■ **SIGNS AND SYMPTOMS**

A penile shaft fracture may be discovered when meeting obstruction/resistance when attempting to insert a urinary catheter during resuscitation in a multiple trauma situation.

Hematoma
Hemorrhage
Swelling, distortion of penis
Discoloration
Patient reports cracking sound and severe pain

■ **DIAGNOSTIC AIDS**

Retrograde urethrogram if there is blood at the meatus, hematuria, or with difficulty voiding

■ **THERAPEUTIC INTERVENTIONS**

Splint
Ice packs

Urologic consultation—immediate surgical repair and placement of a catheter
Evacuation of hematoma
Placement of suprapubic catheter by urologist if studies are positive or inconclusive

Soft-Tissue Zipper Injury

Soft-tissue zipper injury occurs when the soft tissue of the penis gets caught in the teeth of a metal or plastic zipper.
■ **THERAPEUTIC INTERVENTIONS**
Remove the bottom tab from the zipper (this usually involves prying the four sharp metal teeth of the tab at the bottom of the zipper), or
Cut the distal end of the zipper with strong scissors; the zipper should then easily separate.
If the soft tissue is caught in the moving mechanism of the zipper, it may be necessary to apply regional anesthesia to the penis before removal.
Control any bleeding.
Apply ice packs.

NONTRAUMATIC GENITOURINARY EMERGENCIES

Pyelonephritis

Pyelonephritis is an inflammation of the kidneys that involves the tubules, glomeruli, and renal pelvis. It is usually caused by a bacterial infection.
■ **SIGNS AND SYMPTOMS**

Severe flank or back pain at CVA (costal-vertebral angle)	Nocturia
	Dysuria
Fever	Tenderness over the affected flank area
Nausea/vomiting	
Chills	
Urinary frequency	
Urinary urgency	

Presence of pus in the urine
Presence of bacteria in the urine with a positive antibody on the surface of bacteria
Leukocytosis
Hematuria
■ **DIAGNOSTIC AIDS**
Urine and blood cultures
WBCs—leukocytosis
■ **THERAPEUTIC INTERVENTIONS**
Forced fluids
Bed rest
Broad-spectrum antibiotics
Possible hospital admission (especially in cases of abscess, gram-negative septicemia, or severe signs and symptoms) with drainage of abscess

Perinephric Abscess

Patients with perinephric abscess usually offer a history of a recent skin infection, usually within 1 month of the abscess, or a urinary tract infection that has lasted for a prolonged time, or pyelonephritis.

■ **SIGNS AND SYMPTOMS**
High-grade or low-grade fever
Exquisite tenderness in the flank area
Palpation of a mass in the flank area
Spinal scoliosis (concave on the affected side) that has recently occurred
■ **DIAGNOSTIC AIDS**
Visualizing an elevated diaphragm on the affected side on x-ray film
Visualizing a decreased psoas shadow on x-ray film
Ultrasound
CT
■ **THERAPEUTIC INTERVENTIONS**
Incision and drainage
Antibiotics

Renal Carbuncle

A renal carbuncle is a cortical abscess in the periphery of the kidney usually caused by *Staphylococcus aureus.*
■ **SIGNS AND SYMPTOMS**
Severe flank tenderness or pain
Fever
Chills
If these signs and symptoms are present and urinalysis is normal, renal carbuncle is suspected.
■ **THERAPEUTIC INTERVENTIONS**
Incision and drainage
Antibiotics

NOTE: A relapse is common if the carbuncle is incompletely treated.

Renal Colic/Renal Calculi

Pain from renal colic or calculi radiates from the flank to the left or right lower quadrant and occasionally to the leg. This pain results from ureteral distension caused by the passage of a renal stone (calculus) or from blood clots. The size of the stone or clot does not relate to the severity of the pain.
■ **SIGNS AND SYMPTOMS**
Restlessness
Severe flank pain that radiates to the right or left lower quadrant (sudden onset)
Urinary urgency and frequency
Diaphoresis
Low-grade fever
Hematuria
Dysuria
Decreased blood pressure
History of renal calculi, presence of an ileal conduit, hypercalcemia
■ **DIAGNOSTIC AIDS**
Straining urine for calculi
Intravenous pyelogram
Urinalysis
X-ray films of KUB
Ultrasound[4]

■ **THERAPEUTIC INTERVENTIONS**
Forced fluids
Analgesics
Pharmacologic dissolution of stone
Urologic consultation
Antiemetic if patient experiences nausea and vomiting
IV fluids at rapid rate to flush stone and provide rehydration
Possible hospital admission
Possible extracorporeal shock wave lithotripsy (ESWL), laser lithotripsy, or surgical intervention

Urinary Retention

Urinary retention is the inability to void. It may be caused by urethral strictures, an enlarged prostate, blood clots, renal stones, a reflex neurogenic bladder (usually associated with a CVA), multiple sclerosis, congenital stenosis, foreign bodies, bladder stones, hysteria, or as a side effect of parasympatholytics and certain other drugs. Rapid drainage avoids stretch injury to bladder.

■ **SIGNS AND SYMPTOMS**
Lower abdominal discomfort
Mass palpated just above symphysis pubis
Bladder distension

■ **THERAPEUTIC INTERVENTIONS**
Insertion of an indwelling catheter
Possible urologic consultation

Hematuria

Blood can appear in urine from trauma, renal calculi, anticoagulants, blood dyscrasias, ruptured scrotal varices, ruptured cysts, renal or bladder tumors, or recent urologic surgery manipulation. If bleeding occurs at the beginning of urination, bleeding from the anterior urethral region is suggested. If bleeding occurs at the end of the urinary stream, bleeding from the posterior urethra or the point at which the bladder connects to the urethra is suggested. If bleeding occurs throughout urination, it is most likely from the upper urinary tract or from the bladder itself.

The caregiver should be cautious not to assume that all red-colored urine indicates hematuria. Red-colored urine may be caused by food colorings, medications, and the ingestion of beets. If bleeding occurs in a female, check to see if the bleeding is from the vagina.

■ **DIAGNOSTIC AIDS**
History
Urinalysis (if during menstruation, obtain the sample via catheter)
CBC

■ **THERAPEUTIC INTERVENTIONS**
Depends on the cause of the bleeding.

Oliguria/Anuria

Oliguria is defined as the excretion of less than 500 ml of urine per day. Anuria is the complete absence of urine. A patient with one of these conditions may complain of inability to void, yet little or no urine may be obtained on catheterization. Oliguria and anuria may be caused by fluid and electrolyte imbalances, urinary tract obstructions, acute tubular necrosis, tumors, trauma, or accidental laceration of a ureter during abdominal surgery.

■ **SIGNS AND SYMPTOMS**
Dehydration
Complaint of inability to void
Weakness
Uremic frost
Distended abdomen
■ **THERAPEUTIC INTERVENTIONS**
Urologic consultation
IVP or CT scan to rule out obstruction
Specific treatment for the cause

Acute Cystitis

Acute cystitis is an infection of the bladder that occurs as a result of the migration of bacteria from the urethra (also known as "honeymoon cystitis") or occurring secondary to acute prostatitis.

■ **SIGNS AND SYMPTOMS**
Urinary urgency/frequency
Nocturia
WBCs, RBCs, bacteria on urinalysis
Fever
Suprapubic pain
Tender prostate
Urinary retention in males
■ **DIAGNOSTIC AIDS**
Urinalysis
Prostate examination in males
■ **THERAPEUTIC INTERVENTIONS**
Females
Nitrofurantoin or sulfonamides
Increased fluids
Warm baths
Males
Sulfa combination drugs (Septra) or tetracycline
Drainage of the abscess if one is present
Bed rest
Increased fluids

GENITOURINARY PROBLEMS UNIQUE TO MALES

Cryptorchidism

Cryptorchidism is an undescended testicle(s).
■ **SIGNS AND SYMPTOMS**
Mass in inguinal region
Absence of a testicle in scrotum
■ **THERAPEUTIC INTERVENTIONS**
Gonadotropins
Surgical intervention

Penile/Scrotal Edema

Penile/scrotal edema is often found in males with congestive heart failure or a recent abdominal surgery in which the pelvic lymph nodes were affected.

■ **SIGNS AND SYMPTOMS**
History of recent pelvic lymphadenectomy
Diffuse edema in penile and scrotal skin

■ **THERAPEUTIC INTERVENTIONS**
Treatment of the congestive heart failure
Elevation of the penis and scrotum on a towel
Taping the penis to the abdomen

Acute Epididymitis

Acute epididymitis is an infection of the epididymis (a portion of the male reproductive system). It may occur as the result of a physical strain, after cystoscopic examination, after prostate surgery with a history of urethral discharge, or after urinary bladder catheterization. Commonly caused by *Neisseria gonorrhoeae* or *Chlamydia trachomatis.*

■ **SIGNS AND SYMPTOMS**
Swelling/enlargement of scrotum, epididymis
Sudden tenderness in the scrotal area (unilateral), radiating up the spermatic cord
Elevated temperature
Sepsis

■ **DIAGNOSTIC AIDS**
Urethral smear for gram stain and culture
Urine culture

■ **THERAPEUTIC INTERVENTIONS**
Antibiotics—ceftriaxone and doxycycline
Bed rest
Elevation of scrotum
Forced fluids

Hemospermia

Hemospermia is a condition in which blood is present in semen. It may be caused by a rupture of varicosities.

■ **SIGNS AND SYMPTOMS**
Blood in the semen

■ **THERAPEUTIC INTERVENTIONS**
Reassurance
Urologic consultation if the condition recurs

Hydrocele

A hydrocele is a collection of fluid within the tunica vaginalis.

■ **SIGNS AND SYMPTOMS**
No pain or tenderness
Presence of a large scrotal mass

■ **DIAGNOSTIC AIDS**
Transillumination with a bright light
Scrotal ultrasound

■ **THERAPEUTIC INTERVENTIONS**
Drainage
Surgery, only if the mass is large and uncomfortable

Acute Orchitis

Acute orchitis is an inflammation of the testicle that may result from epidemic parotiditis (mumps) or other viral infection.

■ **SIGNS AND SYMPTOMS**
Unilateral testicular swelling
Unilateral tenderness
Elevated temperature

■ **THERAPEUTIC INTERVENTIONS**
Antibiotics
Bed rest
Scrotal support

Peyronie's Disease

Peyronie's disease is a syndrome in which a fibrous plaque forms on the corpora cavernosa of the penis. When the patient has an erection, he experiences considerable pain, and the penis curves.

■ **SIGNS AND SYMPTOMS**
Curved penis
Difficulty with intercourse

■ **THERAPEUTIC INTERVENTIONS**
There is no specific therapy for Peyronie's disease other than psychologic support and reassurance.

Priapism

Priapism is a prolonged erection that is not relieved by ejaculation. Physiological causes include spinal cord injury, sickle cell disease, tumors, or hematologic disorders. Pharmacologic treatment for impotence (papavarine/regitine, prostaglandin E_1 subcutaneously [SQ] given into corpus cavernosum) also may elicit priapism, which is considered an emergency state if erection lasts 4 hours.

■ **SIGNS AND SYMPTOMS**
Prolonged erection

■ **THERAPEUTIC INTERVENTIONS**
Analgesia/sedation
Possible surgical intervention if erection persists
Pharmacologic antidote: epinephrine 0.10 mg sq into corpus cavernosa if history of papavarine/regitine use.

Prostatitis

An inflamed prostate gland that is usually accompanied by cystitis.

■ **SIGNS AND SYMPTOMS**
Positive urine culture and analysis, positive urethral culture
Tenderness of the prostate
Pain in the lower abdomen and perineum
Elevated temperature
Possible urinary retention, irritative bladder symptoms
Hematospermia, hematuria

■ **DIAGNOSTIC AIDS**
Urine and urethral culture
Uroflowmetry
Prostate examination
■ **THERAPEUTIC INTERVENTIONS**
Antibiotics—if causative bacteria is identified, trimethoprim, doxycycline, acyclovir for herpes proctitis.[5]
Bed rest
Forced fluids
Possible incision and drainage if there is an abscess
Instruction to patient to increase ejaculation if possible

Testicular Torsion

Testicular torsion is the twisting of the testicle or the spermatic cord in the tunica vaginalis. It occurs most commonly in children and adolescents.

■ **SIGNS AND SYMPTOMS**
Severe scrotal pain and swelling (especially during physical activity) or testicular elevation
Swelling, especially during physical activity

Nausea and vomiting	Tense scrotal mass (epididymis cannot be palpated)
±High-riding testicle	Intense pain when the testicle is elevated

■ **DIAGNOSTIC AIDS**
Scrotal ultrasound
■ **THERAPEUTIC INTERVENTIONS**
Urologic consultation
Immediate surgical intervention is indicated for exploration

Testicular Tumor

Testicular tumor is most common in the 20- to 30-year age group. The chief complaint will be a scrotal mass with or without pain.

■ **SIGNS AND SYMPTOMS**
Swelling
A hard testicular mass with normal epididymis
Presence or absence of pain
■ **DIAGNOSTIC AIDS**
Scrotal ultrasound
■ **THERAPEUTIC INTERVENTIONS**
Surgical intervention

NONEMERGENCY GENITOURINARY CONDITIONS

Nonspecific Urethritis/Nongonococcal Urethritis

Patients with nonspecific urethritis will frequently come to the emergency department with a chief complaint of urethral discharge.

■ **SIGNS AND SYMPTOMS**
Burning on urination and urinary frequency
Dysuria
Urethral discharge

■ **DIAGNOSTIC AIDS**
Gram stain shows no gram-negative intracellular diplococci in cases of nonspecific urethritis; abundant polymorphonuclear leukocytes. *C. trachomatis* is implicated in about 50% of cases.[6]

■ **THERAPEUTIC INTERVENTIONS**
Doxycycline, Erythromycin base
Treatment of sex partners
Education/counseling

Varicocele

A dilation of the spermatic cord is known as a varicocele. It is caused by poor vascular drainage that results in dilation of the veins.

■ **SIGNS AND SYMPTOMS**
Scrotal mass above the testicle
Disappearance of the mass when the patient is supine

■ **THERAPEUTIC INTERVENTIONS**
Possible surgical intervention

VENEREAL DISEASES

Chancroid

A chancroid is a venereal disease that appears as an ulceration on the penis. Most patients with genital ulcers have genital herpes, syphilis, or chancroid. These patients may be at risk for HIV.

■ **SIGNS AND SYMPTOMS**
Genital lesions
Painful inguinal adenopathy 3 to 4 days after sexual intercourse
Positive culture of lesion
Positive skin test

■ **DIAGNOSTIC AIDS**
Exudate—dark field exam or direct immunofluorescence test for *Treponema pallidum:* serologic test for syphilis, culture for HSV, culture for *Haemophilis ducreyi*
Skin test

■ **THERAPEUTIC INTERVENTIONS**
Erythromycin base, Ceftriaxone, Trimethaprim/sulfamethoxazole, Amoxicillin
Treatment of sex partners
Follow-up with urologist
Education/counseling

Gonorrhea

Gonorrhea is a venereal disease that appears like urethritis. Caused by *N. gonorrhoeae.* A coexisting chlamydial infection exists in 45% of gonorrhea cases *(C. trachomatis).* Disseminated infection can lead to endocarditis or meningitis.[6]

■ **SIGNS AND SYMPTOMS**
Burning on urination
Positive gonococcus culture
White, creamy discharge 3 to 7 days after sexual intercourse

■ **DIAGNOSTIC AIDS**
Gram-negative diplococci on gram stain
Positive gonococcus culture, antibiotic sensitivity testing because of increased numbers of antibiotic resistant stains

■ **THERAPEUTIC INTERVENTIONS**
Antibiotics (penicillin or tetracycline), treatment for presumptive chlamydial infection
Follow-up care, counseling for HIV, HIV testing
Ceftriaxone plus doxycycline, spectinomycin, ciprofloxacin, tetracycline, erythromycin
Serologic testing for syphilis
Treatment of sex partners

Chlamydial Infections

Chlamydial infections are commonly found coexisting with gonorrheal infection; they may occur endocervically, rectally, or urethrally.

■ **SIGNS AND SYMPTOMS**
Same as gonorrhea
Positive *C. trachomatis* culture (available lab tests not sensitive enough)

■ **THERAPEUTIC INTERVENTIONS**
Doxycycline, tetracycline, erythromycin base
Treatment of sex partners
Education/counseling

Genital Herpes Simplex Virus Infections

Genital herpes is a viral disease that may be chronic and recurrent.

■ **SIGNS AND SYMPTOMS**
Genital ulcers

■ **THERAPEUTIC INTERVENTIONS**
Acyclovir first clinical episode and for recurrent treatment and early suppressive therapy
Counseling and treatment of sex partners

Syphilis

Syphilis is a type of venereal disease caused by the spirochete *T. pallidum.*

■ **SIGNS AND SYMPTOMS**
First stage early syphilis—primary and secondary
Painless ulcerations that appear several weeks after exposure through sexual intercourse, or painless red pustules.
Positive serologic skin testing
Second stage (occurs in 2 months), early latent <1 year duration
General malaise
Anorexia
Nausea
Fever
Headache
Alopecia
Bone/joint pain
White sores in mouth
Third stage (may take 3 to 15 years to develop), latent >1 year
Soft rubbery tumors attacking all areas of the body, including the central nervous system.
May also cause congenital syphilis.

■ **DIAGNOSTIC AIDS**
Serologic skin testing
HIV testing
Lumbar puncture and CSF examination dependent on stage

■ THERAPEUTIC INTERVENTIONS
Penicillin
Evaluation and treatment of sex partners
Counseling regarding risk of HIV
Follow-up

Granuloma Inguinale

Granuloma inguinale is a chronic venereal infection of the skin and subcutaneous tissue of the genitalia, the perineum, and the inguinal region.

■ SIGNS AND SYMPTOMS
Swelling
Ulceration
Pain

■ THERAPEUTIC INTERVENTIONS
Tetracycline
Education/counseling

Lymphogranuloma Venereum

Lymphogranuloma venereum is a venereal disease caused by a virus *(C. trachomatis)*.

■ SIGNS AND SYMPTOMS
Transient genital lesion
Inguinal lymphadenopathy 1 to 3 weeks after exposure through sexual intercourse
Rectal stricture (in females)
Painful nodes

■ THERAPEUTIC INTERVENTIONS
Doxycycline or tetracycline, erythromycin or sulfisoxazole, or equivalent sulfonamide course
Education/counseling

EMERGENCIES IN DIALYSIS PATIENTS

Dialysis patients often come to the emergency department with a variety of complaints. Some of the more common problem areas are discussed below.

Clotted Access

There are two common types of access used for hemodialysis. A Cimino-Brescia fistula is a surgically created fistula made from a native artery and vein. Many patients have a temporary subclavian or femoral catheter placed for hemodialysis in an acute situation, or if they are awaiting surgery for a new fistula. They may have a peritoneal catheter.

Bleeding

■ THERAPEUTIC INTERVENTIONS
Uremic patients may have a platelet defect. Also, postdialysis it is important to know that the patient has been heparinized. Because of the short half-life of heparin, bleeding tends to occur soon after the dialysis run.

Fistula infection

■ THERAPEUTIC INTERVENTIONS
If a Cimino-Brescia fistula is infected, there are usually signs of systemic infection.
Administer antibiotics.
Evaluate blood cultures for definitive therapy.

With peritoneal dialysis the patient may be seen with symptoms of peritonitis, complain of blood in their exchanges, or have peritoneal bleeding.

Cardiovascular Problems/Metabolic Imbalance

Pulmonary embolus

Patients with temporary arterial-venous access may form thrombi that become emboli. A patient presenting with shortness of breath and a temporary or endogenous fistula should be evaluated for a pulmonary embolus.

Uremic pericarditis

Assessment of patients with renal disease should involve close attention to heart sounds, because uremic-induced pericarditis is a common finding. Tamponade and worsening effusion is another complication.

Dialysis patients may develop dysrhythmias, hypotension, hypertension, and cardiac arrest. Sequelae from hypervolemia (pulmonary edema, CHF) and hypovolemia may be seen before and after dialysis. For the most part, these emergencies are treated as they are in any other patient. Dysrhythmias usually occur as a result of hyperkalemia. In the typical scenario, the patient begins to develop dysrhythmias just *before* a dialysis treatment. This usually results from hyperkalemia. The patient may even develop cardiac arrest because of an intolerably high potassium level. If a dialysis arrest occurs, chances are that it is caused by either hypovolemia, for which fluid replacement is the therapeutic intervention of choice, or hyperkalemia, for which the administration of calcium chloride in large doses and other advanced life support measures are indicated.

REFERENCES

1. Landis JS: Emergency department evaluation of genitourinary trauma: an overview, *J Urol Nurs* (3):285, 1989.
2. Bland CA, Hood IG, Mascitti-Mazur J: Genitourinary trauma, *J Urol Nurs* p. 11, 1991.
3. Mansi KM: Experience with penile fractures in Egypt: long term results of immediate surgical repair, *J Trauma* 1:67, 1993.
4. Haddard C et al: Renal colic: diagnosis and outcome, *Radiology* 184:83-88, 1997.
5. DeLa Rosette JJMCH: Diagnosis and treatment of 409 patients with prostatitis syndromes, *Urology* 41(4):301, 1993.
6. US Department of Health and Human Services: *Semin Urol,* IX (1):40-70, 1993.

SUGGESTED READINGS

Berg AO et al: Establishing the cause of genitourinary systems in women in a family practice, *JAMA* 251:620-625, 1984.

Carlson JJ, Mulley AG: Management of acute dysuria, *Ann Int Med* 102:244-249, 1985.

Durbin W, Peter G: Management of urinary tract infections in infants and children, *Ped Infect Dis* 3(6):564-574, 1984.

Harwood AL, Etheredge W, McKenna I: Urologic emergencies. In Rosen P, Barkin R, editors: *Emergency medicine: concepts and clinical practice,* ed 4, St Louis, 1998, Mosby.

Innerarity SA: Electrolyte emergencies in the critically ill patient, *Crit Care Nurs Clin North Am* 2(1):89, 1990.

Mariani P, Terndrup TE: Urinary tract infection in women. In Harwood-Nuss A: *The clinical practice of emergency medicine,* ed 2, Philadelphia, 1996, Lippincott.

Mears EM Jr, Barbabalis GA: Prostatistis: bacteria, non-bacterial and prostatodynia, *Semin Urol* 1(2):146-154, 1983.

Rapere JL: Priapism: cause and treatment, *Urol Nurs* 15(3):75-81, 1995.

Soud TE, Rogers JS: Testicular torsion. In *Manual of pediatric emergency nursing,* St Louis, 1998, Mosby.

Webster DC, Brennan T: Self care strategies used for acute attack of interstitial cystitis, *Urol Nurs* 15(3):86-94, 1995.

Weinman S: Straddle injury (with urethral disruption): a case study, *J Emerg Nurs* 20(1):76-78, 1994.

Wolfson AB: End-stage renal disease emergencies related to dialysis and transplantation. In Wolfson AB, Harwood-Nuss AH, editors: *Renal and urologic emergencies,* New York, 1986, Churchill Livingston.

Yoshikawa TT: Acute urethritis in males, *Dis Emerg Med Care* 4(4):1-8, 1984.

Zoller GW: Genitourinary trauma. In Rosen P, Barkin R, editors: *Emergency medicine: concepts and clinical practice,* ed 4, St Louis, 1998, Mosby.

Infectious Diseases

Susan Budassi Sheehy

An infection is the invasion and multiplication of an agent that causes a response in a host. Often therapeutic interventions must be initiated according to pertinent signs and symptoms without the benefit of confirming laboratory tests. Some of the more commonly seen infectious diseases are reviewed in this chapter (Box 19-1).

UNIVERSAL PRECAUTIONS

The approach to prevention of exposure when treating all blood and body fluids as potentially infectious is called *universal precautions*. The adoption of this practice is essential to the safe practice of all health care workers (Table 19-1). Universal precautions include the following:
- Gloves should be used when contact with mucous membranes, nonintact skin, blood, or body fluids is anticipated and must be changed and hands washed between patient contacts. Gloves can be made of vinyl, nitride, latex, or other appropriate material that is *intact*.
- Hand washing should occur after gloves are removed and whenever skin surfaces come into contact with blood or body fluids.
- Gowns should be worn during procedures that may generate splashes of blood or body fluids.
- Protective eyewear (goggles or glasses with solid side shields) and masks (or chin-length face shields) should be worn whenever there is a risk of splashing or spraying of blood or body fluids to prevent exposure to mucous membranes. All healthcare workers should take precautions to prevent injuries from needlesticks or other sharps (Figure 19-1).

ACQUIRED IMMUNE DEFICIENCY SYNDROME

Acquired Immune Deficiency Syndrome (AIDS) is caused by the human immunodeficiency virus (HIV). HIV infection interferes with the body's immune response, affecting both T-cell and B-cell immunity, thus allowing for opportunistic infections and diseases. HIV infection is chronic. The development of AIDS can range from 1 to 2 years after infection to more than a decade (Table 19-2). Transmission of HIV is known to occur through sexual intercourse, intravenous needle sharing, blood transfusions, open wound exposures from an infected source, and in utero transmission of the virus from mother to infant. Historically, persons considered at high risk to contract AIDS are homosexual and bisexual men, hemophiliacs, intravenous drug abusers, prostitutes, and recipients of blood transfusions. There has also been an increase in HIV among heterosexuals. The mortality rate remains 100% once the diagnosis of AIDS is confirmed.

■ SIGNS AND SYMPTOMS
Signs and symptoms of AIDS are highly variable and depend on the progression of the HIV infection and the amount of immunosuppression. Symptoms range from generalized and vague to diagnostic and fatal. The complex known as AIDS related complex (ARC) is generally recognized as a precursor of the life-threatening illness.

BOX 19-1   Classification of commonly used antibiotics

Penicillin
Penicillin G
Penicillin G benzathine
Penicillin G procaine
Penicillin V potassium (Pen-Vee K)
Broad-spectrum antibiotics
Amoxicillin
Ampicillin
Azlocillin
Carbenicillin (Geopen)
Mezlocillin
Piperacillin
Ticarcillin
Synthetic antibiotics
Cloxacillin
Dicloxacillin
Methicillin
Nafcillin (Unipen)
Oxacillin (Prostaphlin)
Cephalosporins
Cefaclor (Ceclor)
Cefadroxil (Duricef)
Cefamandol (Mandol)
Cefazolin (Kefzol, Ancef)
Cefotaxime (Cloforan)
Cefotentan (Cefotan)
Cefoxitin (Mefoxin)
Ceftazidime

Ceftriaxone (Rocephin)
Cefuroxime axetel (Ceftin)
Cephalexin (Keflex)
Cephalothin (Keflin)
Cephradine (Velosef)
Moxalactam (Moxam)
Macrolides
Clindamycin (Cleocin)
Erythromycin (Ilosone, Erythrocin)
Aminoglycosides
Amikacin
Gentamicin (Garamycin)
Kanamycin (Kantrex)
Polymixin B (Aerosporin)
Polymixin E (Colistin)
Streptomycin
Tobramycin
Others
Chloramphenicol (Chloromycetin)
Ciprofloxacin
Horfloxacin
Methenamine (Mandelamine)
Metronidazole
Nalidixic acid (NegGram)
Nitrofurantoin (Macrodantin, Furadantin)
Sulfonamides
Tetracycline
Vancomycin

Fever	Headache
Extreme fatigue	Unexplained weight loss
General malaise	Lymphadenopathy
General weakness	Diarrhea
Myalgias	Arthralgias

Clinical disease manifestations include:

Persistent unexplained fever	Weight loss
Persistent unexplained diarrhea	Encephalopathies
Aseptic meningitis	Peripheral neuropathies

Complications such as secondary infections and secondary cancers include:
Pneumocystis pneumonia
Fungal infections
Toxoplasmosis
Disseminated herpes zoster
Salmonella bacteremia
Tuberculosis
Oral hairy leukoplakia
Disseminated cytomegalovirus (CMV)

TABLE 19-1   Emergency Department Isolation Techniques*

TYPE OF ISOLATION	COMMON DISEASES	GOWN	GLOVES	MASK	ISOLATION ROOM	LINEN PRECAUTIONS	EATING UTENSILS
Strict	Varicella Herpes zoster AIDS	A	A	A	A	A	A
Modified strict	Group A streptococci Staphylococci Streptococcal pneumonia	B	B	A	A	A	A
Respiratory	Tuberculosis Rubella Mumps Pertussis Meningococcemia Meningococcal meningitis	C	C	A	A	C	C
Protective	Leukemia Lymphoma Patient taking immunosup- pressives	B	B	C	A	C	C
Enteric	Viral hepatitis Salmonella Shigella Gastroenteritis	B	B	B	C	A	A
Wound and skin†	Any draining wounds Skin infections Draining ulcers Abscesses	B	B	B	A	A	C

*A = always; B = only with direct contact with patient's secretions, excretions, urine, feces or blood; C = optional.
†Also, double-bag any waste materials or items that come into contact with drainage.

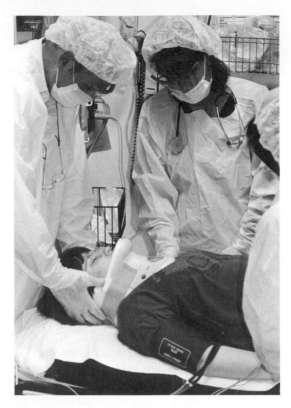

FIGURE 19-1. A gown, gloves, mask, and protective eye shields must be worn when there is a likelihood of contamination with blood or body fluids.
(Courtesy Emilie Goudey, Lenox, Mass.)

Kaposi's sarcoma (a malignant endothelial tumor that can involve the visceral organs, skin, mucous membranes, lung, and GI tract) or non-Hodgkin's lymphomas, as well as primary lymphomas of the brain.

■ **THERAPEUTIC INTERVENTIONS**

Therapeutic interventions for AIDS consist mainly of supportive care such as placement of an indwelling venous catheter for frequent blood drawing and hyperalimentation, along with much physical and psychological support. Prophylaxis and treatments for HIV infection with antiviral chemotherapy has recently become available because of intense international research efforts. These are not considered cures, although such agents help to prolong the person's life, decrease risk of opportunistic infections, and may prolong the HIV incubation period.

AIDS and Emergency Health Care Personnel

It remains essential that health care workers within the emergency department treat all patients as potentially infectious and thus follow universal precautions (Box 19-2). Other specific isolation procedures depend on other concurrent infections.

BACTEREMIA (GRAM-NEGATIVE)

The severity of bacteremia depends on the previous condition of the patient. The patient may have had an underlying disorder that precipitated the bacteremia, such as a gynecologic infection, a respiratory tract infection,

TABLE 19-2   Incubation Periods of Specific Diseases

DISEASE	DURATION OF INCUBATION
AIDS	More than 3 years
Bacillary dysentery (Shigella)	1 to 7 days; average 4 days
Botulism (food poisoning)	Fewer than 24 hours of food containing the toxin
Chickenpox (varicella)	14 to 16 days
Common cold	1 to 3 days
Diarrhea, viral	3 to 5 days
Diphtheria	2 to 6 days
Encephalitis	5 to 15 days; range of 4 to 21 days; varies as to the type
Hepatitis	
Infectious (virus A)	15 to 50 days
Serum (virus B)	2 to 6 months
Herpes simplex (cold sore, fever blister)	2 to 12 days; average 4 days
Herpes zoster (shingles)	4 to 24 days; average 4 days
Infectious mononucleosis (glandular fever)	Children, less than 14 days; adults, 33 to 49 days; average of 4 to 14 days
Influenza (haemophilus)	24 to 72 hours
Lyme disease	3 to 33 days; average 1 week
Malaria	Varies with particular species; 12 to 14 days or as long as 30 days; some strains from 8 to 10 months
Meningitis (bacterial)	2 to 7 days
Mumps (parotiditis)	14 to 28 days
Pertussis (whooping cough)	5 to 21 days
Plague *(Yersinia pestis)*	
Bubonic	2 to 6 days
Pneumonic	2 to 4 days
Pneumococcal pneumonia (bacterial)	1 to 3 days
Poliomyelitis (infantile paralysis)	7 to 14 days
Rabies (hydrophobia)	Dogs, 3 to 8 weeks; man, 10 days to 2 years with an average of 2 to 6 weeks.
Rocky Mountain spotted fever (tick fever)	2 to 12 days; may be as long as 14 days; average of 7 days
Rubella (German measles)	14 to 21 days; usually 18 days after exposure
Salmonella	7 to 72 hours
Scarlet fever (scarlatina)	24 hours to 10 days, but first clinical signs generally appear between 2 to 5 days
Smallpox (variola)	7 to 16 days; average of 12 days
Syphilis	3 weeks (primary); 6 to 20 weeks (secondary); 3 to 12 months (latent); more than 4 years (tertiary)
Tetanus	3 to 21 days; average of 10 days
Tuberculosis	Variable
Typhoid fever	10 to 14 days; may be as short as 7 days or as long as 21 days
Viral pneumonia (atypical pneumonia)	Varies widely, depending on specific virus; may be from a few days to a week or longer

---

BOX 19-2   The CDC's Recommendations for the Prevention of Occupational
Transmission of HIV

Use of protective gloves*
Gowns
Protective eyewear and masks or face shields
Safe, careful disposal of needles and other contaminated types of equipment and/or instruments

---

*NOTE: Use nonlatex gloves to prevent latex sensitivities.

a urinary tract infection, or a burn injury, or the condition may have been compromised by agents such as immunosuppressants or antibiotics.

■ **SIGNS AND SYMPTOMS**

Fever	Extremes of underlying condition
Chills	Decreased blood pressure
Shortness of breath	Petechiae
Tachypnea	Cool, clammy, moist skin
Weakness	Cyanosis
Syncope	

■ **THERAPEUTIC INTERVENTIONS**

Prevention (aseptic technique and decreasing source of infection)
Antimicrobial agents
Oxygen
Volume replacement
Possible use of steroids
Possible use of naloxone
Possible use of dopamine
Incision and drainage if abscess is present

BACTERIAL VAGINOSIS (NONSPECIFIC VAGINITIS)

The syndrome of bacterial vaginosis (BV) almost universally has the organism *Gardnerella vaginalis* present in the vagina of women, along with other infecting organisms. Recent studies suspect *G. vaginalis* to be the most common cause of vaginitis, more common among IUD users. Infection can lead to bacteremia and such conditions as postpartum endometritis and/or fever, chorioamnionitis, and postcesarean section infection.

■ **SIGNS AND SYMPTOMS**
Increased vaginal discharge
Pruritis

■ **THERAPEUTIC INTERVENTIONS**
Metronidazole
Antibiotics (for suspected *G. vaginalis* alone)

CELLULITIS

Cellulitis is an acute spreading disease of the skin that extends to the subcutaneous tissues, and in severe cases to the lymphatics and blood stream. Inciting causes include lacerations, crush injuries, and puncture wounds. Incubation period is within several days, generally 3 to 4. Common etiologic agents include Group A streptococcus and *S. aureus*.

- **SIGNS AND SYMPTOMS**
  Local tenderness/pain
  Local erythema
  Local edema
  Foul-smelling exudate
  Malaise, fever, chills may develop
- **THERAPEUTIC INTERVENTIONS**
  IV antibiotics
  Needle aspiration of exudate (for diagnostic purpose)
  Immobilization
  Elevation
  Cool compresses/moist heat
  Incision and drainage

CONDYLOMA ACUMINATA (GENITAL WARTS)

Condyloma acuminatum is a papilloma caused by the human papillomavirus (HPV). Condyloma acuminata is usually sexually transmitted and is most commonly seen in sexually active young adults. Genital warts have occasionally become malignant and have been associated with higher rates of HIV infection.

Condylomata acuminata are papillary or sessile, cauliflower-like, pink growths. They develop around the anus, anal canal, glans penis, urethra, vulva, vagina, or cervix.

- **THERAPEUTIC INTERVENTIONS**
  Tincture of benzoin mixed with 10% to 25% podophyllin (do *not* use on pregnant women)
  Cryotherapy
  Curettage
  Intralesional recombinant interferon alpha-2b (Interon A, Shering)
  C-section should be considered for cases of extensive papillomatosis in the genital tract.

DIPHTHERIA

Diphtheria is caused by the endotoxin *Corynebacterium diphtheria.* The usual sites of entry are the oropharynx, the nasopharynx, or via skin lesions.

- **SIGNS AND SYMPTOMS**
  If immunized:
    Low-grade fever and mild sore throat
  If not immunized:
    Fever
    Severe sore throat
    Cervical lymph node edema
    Nonproductive cough
    Respiratory stridor
    Respiratory embarrassment from edema
    Gray-black diphtheritic membrane
- **THERAPEUTIC INTERVENTIONS**
  ABCs
  Antitoxin
  Consider tracheostomy
  Antibiotics

EPIGLOTTITIS

Epiglottitis is a rapidly progressive cellulitis caused by a bacterial infection, usually *Haemophilus influenzae* type b. The epiglottis enlarges and causes airway obstruction. It may be a life-threatening condition. Epiglottitis most commonly appears in children aged 2 to 7 years, but may also occur in adults.

■ **SIGNS AND SYMPTOMS**

Sore throat   Muffled voice
Drooling   Stridor
Progressive dysphagia   Difficulty breathing
Low-grade temperature   Cyanosis
Upright sitting position, leaning forward

■ **THERAPEUTIC INTERVENTIONS**

Oxygen
Endotracheal intubation or cricothyrotomy
IV therapy
Antibiotics
Possible use of racemic epinephrine

GAS GANGRENE (CLOSTRIDIAL MYONECROSIS)

Gas gangrene is a soft-tissue infection caused by the organism *Clostridium perfringens*. It may occur after trauma, infection, or ischemia where an anaerobic environment exists. It is characterized by muscle necrosis and systemic toxicity. Clostridium infections are often accompanied by infections with other bacteria, such as *Streptococci* or *Staphylococci*. Many of these organisms produce gases that are secreted into soft tissues. Gas gangrene may develop within hours of bacterial invasion, although usually within 1 to 4 days.

■ **SIGNS AND SYMPTOMS**

Swelling
Local pain and pain when touched
Oozing serosanguinous material (initially brown or red and sweet smelling, then green or black)
Diaphoresis
Pallor
Low-grade fever
Delirium
Blebs
Inability of muscle to contract

■ **THERAPEUTIC INTERVENTIONS**

Antibiotics
Fasciotomy
Surgical intervention (debridement of necrotic tissue or amputation)
Possible use of hyperbaric oxygen therapy
Possible polyvalent antitoxin

GONORRHEA

Gonorrhea is the most common of the reportable sexually transmitted infectious diseases. It is caused by the organism *Neisseria gonorrhoeae*. Gonorrhea can infect any area of the genitourinary or reproductive system and may also infect the eyes or limb joints. The highest incidence is in persons 15 to 24 years old. Complications include meningitis, septicemia, epididymitis, pharyngitis, pelvic inflammatory disease, newborn conjunctivitis, sterility, polyarthralgias, skin lesions, and endocarditis.

- **SIGNS AND SYMPTOMS**
  Dysuria
  Urethritis
  Urinary frequency
  Purulent discharge from the urethra (especially in females)
  Vaginal discharge
  Cystitis
  Pruritis, tenesmus, and discharge in rectal infection
  Some patients are asymptomatic
- **THERAPEUTIC INTERVENTIONS**
  Antibiotics
  Probenecid
  Treatment of sexual partner(s)

GRANULOMA INGUINALE

Granuloma inguinale is caused by the gram-negative coccobacillus *Donovania granulomatis*. It is rarely seen in the United States. Complications include urethral strictures, engorged pelvic glands, and (rarely) elephantiasis.
- **SIGNS AND SYMPTOMS**
  Very red lesions that are granulating and painless
- **THERAPEUTIC INTERVENTIONS**
  Antibiotics

HEPATITIS A (INFECTIOUS HEPATITIS, HA)

Hepatitis A is an infectious disease of the liver that may be mild or disabling in severity, often seen as an acute self-limiting disease caused by the hepatitis A virus. It is frequently found among children and young adults, transmitted generally by the fecal-oral route (commonly via contaminated food/water). It often requires prolonged convalescence, although a complete recovery without sequelae is normal.
- **SIGNS AND SYMPTOMS**
  Abrupt onset
  Fever
  Malaise
  Abdominal pain
  Nausea
  Anorexia
  Jaundice
- **THERAPEUTIC INTERVENTIONS**
  Treat symptomatically.
  Take enteric precautions for 2 weeks from start of signs and symptoms (no longer than 1 week after development of jaundice).

VIRAL HEPATITIS B (SERUM HEPATITIS, HEPATITIS B, HB)

Hepatitis B is an inflammatory liver condition caused by the Hepatitis B virus. Infection can be transmitted via blood (and serum-derived fluids), semen, vaginal fluids, and saliva. Complications include cirrhosis and death. Vaccination is recommended for health care providers who are at high risk of contracting hepatitis B.

■ **SIGNS AND SYMPTOMS**

Abdominal pain	Jaundice
Nausea and vomiting	Erythema
Headache	Urticaria
Fever	Arthralgias
Anorexia	Hepatomegaly
Myalgias	Hepatic tenderness

■ **THERAPEUTIC INTERVENTIONS**
Treat symptomatically.

VIRAL HEPATITIS C (PARENTERALLY TRANSMITTED NON-A NON-B HEPATITIS, HC)

Hepatitis C results in an inflammatory liver condition. As yet the causative agent is unidentified, and the diagnosis is based on the exclusion of other causes. This form of serum hepatitis is the most common post-transfusion hepatitis and is frequently seen among IV drug users, dialysis patients, hemophiliacs, and health care workers. Transmission is also thought to occur through sexual, intimate, or intrafamilial exposure. This disease is frequently insidious and chronic in nature with death as a rare complication.

■ **SIGNS AND SYMPTOMS**
Anorexia
Vague abdominal discomfort
Nausea and vomiting
Jaundice (less frequently than with hepatitis B)
Cirrhosis (possibly)

■ **THERAPEUTIC INTERVENTIONS**
Treat symptomatically.

DELTA HEPATITIS (VIRAL HEPATITIS D)

Delta hepatitis is an inflammation of the liver caused by the delta hepatitis virus, which is always present in a coexistent state with hepatitis B. The disease may be self-limiting or chronic. Transmission is through blood, serous body fluids, or sexual contact.

■ **SIGNS AND SYMPTOMS**
Similar to HBV, abrupt onset

■ **THERAPEUTIC INTERVENTIONS**
Treat symptomatically.

VIRAL HEPATITIS E (ENTERICALLY TRANSMITTED NON-A NON-B HEPATITIS)

Viral hepatitis E is an inflammatory liver disease similar to hepatitis A, frequently linked to feces-contaminated water, considered to be caused by a hepatitis E virus. Outbreaks are generally self-limiting though they are associated with high mortality rates in pregnant women. Viral hepatitis E is thought to be the most common cause of jaundice and acute hepatitis in third world countries.

■ **SIGNS AND SYMPTOMS**
Fever
Malaise
Abdominal discomfort
Jaundice

■ **THERAPEUTIC INTERVENTIONS**

Treat symptomatically.

Enteric precautions for 2 weeks from start of signs and symptoms (but no longer than 1 week after the onset of jaundice).

HERPES SIMPLEX TYPE 1 (ORAL HERPES, HERPES LABIALIS)

Oral herpes simplex is caused by herpes virus type 1. In severe cases, usually in immunocompromised patients, it may present with CNS signs and symptoms. It is a common cause of meningoencephalitis.

■ **SIGNS AND SYMPTOMS**

Small fluid-filled blisters on facial area

Burning

Itching

Low-grade fever

Cervical lymphadenopathy

Headache

Leukocytosis

Meningeal irritation

Drowsiness

Stupor

Coma

■ **THERAPEUTIC INTERVENTIONS**

Wash hands with soap and water to avoid spreading

Contact isolation for disseminated or neonatal infections

Drainage/secretion precautions for recurrent lesions

Possible use of antiviral agents (such as Acyclovir)

HERPES SIMPLEX TYPE 2 (GENITAL HERPES)

Genital herpes is caused by herpes virus type 2. Complications include infection of the neonate (if herpes virus is present in the birth canal at the time of vaginal delivery), kernicterus, encephalitis, aseptic meningitis, and radiculitis.

■ **SIGNS AND SYMPTOMS**

Tender vesicles on penile shaft

Vesicles on prepuce or glans penis

Vesicles on scrotum or perineum

Grayish-colored lesions

Vulvular, perineal, vaginal, or cervical lesions

Dyspareunia (painful intercourse)

Erythema

Pain

Lymphadenopathy

Fever

Lethargy

Dysuria

Headache

Recurrent infection

Anorexia

■ **THERAPEUTIC INTERVENTIONS**

At this time there is no known absolute therapeutic intervention. Consider Acyclovir (currently considered antiviral drug of choice).

HERPES ZOSTER (SHINGLES)

Herpes zoster is caused by the organism varicella-zoster virus. Once lesions are crusted, virus is no longer present.

■ **SIGNS AND SYMPTOMS**

Skin eruptions that follow a cranial or spinal nerve tract

Severe pain along the nerve tract

Paresthesias

Fever

Headache

General malaise

■ **THERAPEUTIC INTERVENTIONS**

Topical antipruritics

Analgesics

Bed rest

Acyclovir currently considered the antiviral drug of choice

HISTOPLASMOSIS

Histoplasmosis is caused by the fungal organism *Histoplasma capsulatum*, which is found in the excrement of birds and bats. This disease has an appearance much like that of pulmonary tuberculosis.

■ **SIGNS AND SYMPTOMS**

Fever

Nocturnal diaphoresis

Ulcerations on mucosal surfaces

Anorexia

Weight loss

Lymphadenopathy

Hepatomegaly

■ **THERAPEUTIC INTERVENTIONS**

Amphotericin B for disseminated cases

Oral Ketoconazole

LYMPHOGRANULOMA VENEREUM

Lymphogranuloma venereum is caused by the parasite *Chlamydia trachomatis*. It most often occurs in warm tropical regions and is rarely seen in the United States.

■ **SIGNS AND SYMPTOMS**

Genital ulcer that is painless and not indurated

Regional lymphadenopathy

Fever

Chills

Headache

Joint pains

Anorexia

Arthritis

Meningitis (rare)

■ **THERAPEUTIC INTERVENTIONS**

Antibiotics

Possible aspiration of affected glands

MALARIA

Malaria is a parasitic infection caused by the one of four different species of *Plasmodium*. Transmission to humans is caused by the bite of an infected mosquito or occasionally by blood transfusion or in utero transmission from mother to fetus.

■ **SIGNS AND SYMPTOMS**

Fever
Flulike symptoms
Chills
Headache
Myalgias
Malaise
Anemia
Jaundice
Renal failure, coma, death with *P. falciparum* infection

■ **THERAPEUTIC INTERVENTIONS**

Supportive
Chloroquine/quinine/primaquine depending upon specific form of malaria

MENINGITIS (BACTERIAL)

The causative bacterial organisms of meningitis are *Neisseria meningitiditis, Haemophilus influenzae,* and *Streptococcus pneumoniae.* Children under the age of 5 are extremely susceptible. It is often preceded by a bout of influenza or a urinary tract infection.

■ **SIGNS AND SYMPTOMS**

Fever	Respiratory distress
Lethargy	Nuchal rigidity
Headache	Positive Kernig's sign
Projectile vomiting	Positive Brudzinski's sign
Anorexia	Papilledema
Febrile seizures	Petechiae over anterior trunk
Restlessness	

■ **THERAPEUTIC INTERVENTIONS**

ABCs	Antipyretics
Antibiotics	Diagnostic lumbar puncture
Anticonvulsants	

INFECTIOUS MONONUCLEOSIS

Infectious mononucleosis ("mono") is a mildly contagious disease caused by the Epstein-Barr herpetovirus. It is transmitted by droplet cross-infection. It most often affects young people. When it affects older people the symptoms are more severe. Once infected, a person is immune to further infection.

■ **SIGNS AND SYMPTOMS**

Fatigue
Fever
Sore throat
Lymphadenopathy (especially cervical)
Splenomegaly
Hepatomegaly

■ **THERAPEUTIC INTERVENTIONS**
Treat symptoms
Rest
Fluids
Analgesics
Warm saline solution gargles

MYCOPLASMA INFECTION

Mycoplasma are very small bacteria that can cause pneumonia, tracheobronchitis, pharyngitis, or myringitis. Mycoplasma pneumonia usually occurs in children and young adults. Complications include sinusitis, myocarditis, polyneuritis, and Stevens-Johnson syndrome.

■ **SIGNS AND SYMPTOMS**
Upper respiratory tract infection
Dry cough
Weakness
Fever
Decreased breath sounds
Inspiratory rales
Pulmonary infiltrates

■ **THERAPEUTIC INTERVENTIONS**
Antibiotics
Rest
Fluids
High-protein diet

NECROTIZING FASCIITIS

Necrotizing fasciitis is a severe infection of subcutaneous tissue and fasciae. This condition may be life-threatening. The most common sites of infection are the anterior abdominal wall and the perineal area. *Streptococci* and *Staphylococci* are the most common causative organisms.

■ **SIGNS AND SYMPTOMS**
Fever
Hyperesthesia
Decreased blood pressure
Edema
Crepitus
Blebs

■ **THERAPEUTIC INTERVENTIONS**
Surgical intervention
Antibiotics

PAROTIDITIS (MUMPS)

Parotiditis is edema of the parotid glands caused by the Paramyxovirus contracted from the saliva of an infected person. It usually affects children between 4 and 16 years old. When it occurs in adults, it may be critical. It is a seasonal disease, with its highest incidence in late winter and early spring. Complications include orchiditis (usually unilateral with testicular atrophy), arthritis, oophoritis, myocarditis, pancreatitis, nephritis, thyroiditis, sterility, and mumps meningitis. Incubation period is from 12 to 25 days and is contagious from 7 days before to 9 days after the parotid swelling is evident.

■ **SIGNS AND SYMPTOMS**

Headache	Painful chewing
Earache	Sore throat
Anorexia	General malaise
Swelling of parotid glands	Fever

■ **THERAPEUTIC INTERVENTIONS**

Airway management	Fluids
Analgesics	Consider IV fluid replacement
Antipyretics	Cool sponging

PEDICULOSIS PUBIS ("CRABS")

Pediculosis pubis is the infestation of the *pthirus pubis* louse, an insect that is initially gray in color and later turns red or brown when it has filled with blood. Complications are rare but include eczema, impetigo, or furunculosis. Pediculosis pubis can occur in any age group. It is contracted by direct contact with clothing, bedding, or a person who is infested with the louse.

■ **SIGNS AND SYMPTOMS**

Visualization of lice in pubic, anal, or abdominal hair

Itching

Erythema

■ **THERAPEUTIC INTERVENTIONS**

1% lindane and 25% benzyl benzoate lotion or shampoo (Kwell)

PERTUSSIS (WHOOPING COUGH)

Pertussis is caused by the gram-negative coccobacillus *Bordetella pertussis*. Infants and children up to 4 years old who have not been immunized are most commonly affected. The incidence of pertussis has increased in people age 10 and older, raising the question of the longevity of the childhood immunization. Complications include atelectasis, bronchiectasis, otitis media, seizures, intracranial hemorrhage, epistaxis, dehydration, asphyxia, hernia, pneumonia, and death.

■ **SIGNS AND SYMPTOMS**

Paroxysmal cough with loud end-cough whooping noise

Sneezing

Possible fever

Irritability

Weakness

Vomiting

Anorexia

Large amounts of viscous sputum

Vomiting

■ **THERAPEUTIC INTERVENTIONS**

Oxygen

Suction

Rest

IVs

Adequate diet

Antibiotics

Possible endotracheal intubation

Notification of Infection Control Department

PLAGUE

Plague is transmitted to humans by a bite from a flea that has been contaminated by a rat infested with the bacillus *Yersinia pestis*.

Bubonic Plague

Bubonic plague is also known as "black death."
■ **SIGNS AND SYMPTOMS**
Lymphadenopathy
Fever greater than 106° F (41.1° C)
Tachycardia
Hypotension
Hemorrhage into skin
Delirium
Buboes
■ **THERAPEUTIC INTERVENTIONS**
Antibiotics
Supportive care
Prevention by vaccination

Pneumonic Plague

Pneumonic plague has a high mortality rate. Primary pneumonic plague is defined as bubonic plague with lung involvement. Secondary pneumonic plague is contracted through inhalation of droplets from an infected person.

Septicemic Plague

Septicemic plague is the development of septicemia with meningitis from bubonic plague. It occurs before bubo formation.

POLIOMYELITIS

Poliomyelitis is caused by the virus *Poliovirus hominis*. The most severe complications are respiratory and muscular paralysis. Prevention is by immunization.
■ **SIGNS AND SYMPTOMS**
Nonparalytic
Fever
Malaise
Headache
Nausea and vomiting
Abdominal pain
Neck pain
Paralytic
Fever
Malaise
Headache
Generalized pain, weakness, and muscle spasm
Paralysis of limbs
Paralysis of muscles

■ **THERAPEUTIC INTERVENTIONS**
ABCs
Respiratory support
Rest
Range of motion exercises

RABIES

Rabies is an acute viral encephalitis caused by a rhabdovirus that can infect animals as well as humans. Transmission occurs through nonintact skin or mucous membranes. If the disease develops, it is usually fatal.

■ **SIGNS AND SYMPTOMS**
Sense of apprehension
Headache
Fever
Malaise
Paresis
Paralysis
Hydrophobia (caused by spasm of muscles of deglutition on trying to swallow)
Delirium
Convulsions

■ **THERAPEUTIC INTERVENTIONS**
Clean and flush wound immediately.
Seek prompt medical attention.
Consult public health official if animal escaped.
If bitten by known rabid domestic animal or by wild carnivore (skunk, fox, bat, coyote, bobcat, or raccoon), then proceed with:
Passive immunization with rabies immune globulin as soon as possible after exposure.
Active immunization with human diploid cells rabies vaccine (HDCV).
Consider tetanus prophylaxis.
Consider antibiotics.

RHEUMATIC FEVER

Rheumatic fever is infestation of the upper respiratory tract with the organism b-*Hemolytic streptococcus*. It most commonly occurs in young children. It affects the skin, joints, heart, and brain.

■ **SIGNS AND SYMPTOMS**
History of sore throat or scarlet fever within 5 weeks
Fever
Abdominal pain
Epistaxis
Nausea and vomiting
Polyarthritis
Carditis (chest pain, palpitations, heart failure)
Syndenham's chorea (awkwardness)
Erythema marginatum
Anemia
Leukocytosis

■ **THERAPEUTIC INTERVENTIONS**
Rest
Antibiotics
Analgesics
Fluids

ROCKY MOUNTAIN SPOTTED FEVER

Rocky Mountain spotted fever is a tick-borne disease for which the causative agent is *Rickettsia rickettsii*. Complications include renal failure and shock.

■ **SIGNS AND SYMPTOMS**
Chills
Fever
Severe headache
Myalgias
Hemorrhagic lesions, petechiae
Constipation
Abdominal distension
Decreased level of consciousness
Maculopapular rash (initially on wrists and ankles, then on extremities, trunk, face, palms, and soles of feet)

■ **THERAPEUTIC INTERVENTIONS**
Removing tick
Antibiotics

RUBELLA (GERMAN MEASLES)

Rubella is a viral illness that is contracted by droplet infection. There is a 10- to 12-day incubation period. It is contagious from the fifth day of incubation through the first few days of the rash. Once a patient has contracted rubella, he or she is immunized for life. Rubella is dangerous in the first trimester of pregnancy, because it may cause fetal injuries that lead to deafness, mental retardation, cataracts, and heart defects.

■ **SIGNS AND SYMPTOMS**
Fever
Possible cough and conjunctivitis
Upper respiratory infection
Red maculopapular rash (lasting 1 week to 10 days)
Lymphadenopathy
Arthralgias

■ **THERAPEUTIC INTERVENTIONS**
Antipyretics
Fluids
Cool compresses

SALPINGITIS AND OOPHORITIS

Salpingitis and oophoritis are bacterial infections of the fallopian tubes and ovaries, respectively. Usually these infections are recurrent, and they eventually cause scarring and contractures of the tubes. As the scarring becomes severe and adhesions form, the tubes become filled with exudate and eventually abscesses form. If rupture occurs, peritonitis will result.

■ **SIGNS AND SYMPTOMS**
Fever
Tachycardia

General malaise
Lower-quadrant abdominal pain (bilateral)
Palpated abdominal adnexal masses

■ **THERAPEUTIC INTERVENTIONS**
Cultures
Antibiotics
Possible surgical intervention

SCABIES

Scabies is caused by the mite *Sarcoptes scabiei* when it burrows into the skin in the area of the ankles, shins, elbows, wrists, fingers, and penis. The mite is transmitted via close body contact, particularly sexual intercourse, and via infested clothing and bedding. Complications include impetigo and pustular eczema.

■ **SIGNS AND SYMPTOMS**
Burrows 1 to 10 ml in length
Small red papule at end of burrow
Itching

■ **THERAPEUTIC INTERVENTIONS**
25% benzyl benzoate emulsion and lindane with crotamiton (Kwell lotion/shampoo)

SCARLET FEVER (SCARLETINA)

Scarlet fever is caused by group A hemolytic streptococcus.

■ **SIGNS AND SYMPTOMS**

Sore throat	Bright red, diffuse rash
Fever	Prostration
Cervical lymphadenopathy	

■ **THERAPEUTIC INTERVENTIONS**

Antipyretics	Fluids
Rest	Antibiotics

SYPHILIS

See Chapter 18 on genitourinary emergencies.

TETANUS

Tetanus is caused by the exotoxin *Clostridium tetani,* an anaerobic bacillus that is found in abundance in soil, human and animal excrement, and household dust. It forms hardy spores that can resist extremes of temperature and strong antiseptic solutions. Under proper conditions, the spores will germinate and infect the injured soft-tissue areas. The bacillus excretes a neurotoxin that is absorbed into the circulation and affects the central nervous system. The incubation period may vary from 3 days to several months, with 3 to 10 days after the invasion of the organism being most common. Cases of tetanus are rare in the United States because of the high immunization rate, but mortality is high, particularly in the elderly and infants. It may occur in individuals who have not been immunized or were only partially immunized.

■ **SIGNS AND SYMPTOMS**
History of penetrating injury or burn (regardless of size)
General malaise
Muscle rigidity

Low-grade fever
Headache
Trismus (lockjaw)
Inability to swallow
Distortion of facial muscles
Sardonic grin *(risus sardonicus)*
Opisthotonos
Seizures
Respiratory arrest
Clostridium tetani cultured from wound

■ **THERAPEUTIC INTERVENTIONS**
ABCs
Much supportive care
Darkened room with low stimulation
Possible tracheostomy
Diazepam (Valium)
Possible use of neuromuscular blocking agents
Careful fluid and electrolyte balance
Antibiotics
Tetanus immune globulin (preferably human)
Wound excision and debridement
Active tetanus immunization concurrent with therapy
Horse serum antitoxin
Consider sodium nitroprusside for severe hypertension
Consider propranolol for tachydysrhythmias

TRICHOMONIASIS

Trichomoniasis is caused by the protozoan organism *Trichomonas vaginalis.*

■ **SIGNS AND SYMPTOMS**
May be asymptomatic
Erythema of external genitalia
Edema of external genitalia
Vaginal discharge (greenish gray/frothy), foul smelling
Possible urethritis in males

■ **THERAPEUTIC INTERVENTIONS**
Metronidazole (contraindicated in first-trimester pregnancy)
No alcohol consumption while taking medication
Treatment of sex partners

TUBERCULOSIS

Tuberculosis is caused by the bacteria *Mycobacterium tuberculosis* and *Mycobacterium africanum* from humans, and *Mycobacterium bovis* from cattle. The bacteria typically locates itself in the lungs and spreads systemically. It is contracted by inhalation of tuberculosis-infested droplets. The infection has the appearance of a form of bacterial pneumonia. The organism may pass into the lymphatic vascular systems and then infect the entire body. Common sites for tuberculosis infection besides the lungs are the spine and other bony areas, the meninges, the kidneys, the liver, and the spleen. Susceptibility to disease is increased in those with HIV infection or other causes of immunocompromise.

■ **SIGNS AND SYMPTOMS**
Fever of undetermined origin
Pleuritic chest pain
Tachypnea
Productive cough
Abdominal pain
Nuchal rigidity
Delirium
Positive chest x-ray examination
Positive sputum test
Positive biopsy
Positive tuberculin skin test
Meningeal signs
Other signs and symptoms specific to areas of involvement
■ **THERAPEUTIC INTERVENTIONS**
Antituberculin medications (isoniazid, rifampin; consider addition of pyrazinamide)
Antibiotics
Oxygen
Possible BCG administration to tuberculin-negative household contacts

TYPHOID

Typhoid is an infection caused by the bacterium *Salmonella typhi,* which can be found in contaminated food, water, or milk. Typhoid has a high mortality. Complications include thrombophlebitis and intestinal hemorrhage.

■ **SIGNS AND SYMPTOMS**

Headache	Maculopapular rash on abdomen
Cough	Diarrhea
High fever	Splenomegaly

■ **THERAPEUTIC INTERVENTIONS**

Antibiotics	Cool sponging
Antipyretics	Prevention by vaccination
Consider steroids	

NONSPECIFIC URETHRITIS

Nonspecific urethritis may be caused by the organisms *C. trachomatis, Urea-plasma urealyticum, T. vaginalis,* or herpes virus. The most common age group affected is 15 to 24 years. Complications include cervicitis, salpingitis, prostatitis, epididymitis, proctitis, Reiter's syndrome, and ophthalmia neonatorum.

■ **SIGNS AND SYMPTOMS**
Urethral discharge
Dysuria
Some males may be asymptomatic
■ **THERAPEUTIC INTERVENTIONS**
Antibiotics

VAGINITIS (FROM *HAEMOPHILUS VAGINALIS*)

Vaginitis is usually caused by the gram-negative organism *Haemophilus vaginalis.* This particular organism is found in up to 96% of women with vaginitis. There are no known complications.

■ **SIGNS AND SYMPTOMS**
May be asymptomatic
Frothy, thin, grayish white vaginal discharge
Vulvar irritation

■ **THERAPEUTIC INTERVENTIONS**
Antibiotics

VARICELLA (CHICKENPOX)

Varicella is caused by the virus *Varicella zoster.* The incidence is highest in young children. It has a 14- to 16-day incubation period. It is contagious from 1 day before the appearance of the rash to 5 to 6 days after the initial appearance of the rash. Children with varicella appear mildly sick.

■ **SIGNS AND SYMPTOMS**
Purulent vesicular skin eruptions, initially on back and chest, then on head and limbs
Urticaria
Fever
Lymphadenopathy
Headache
Anorexia
General malaise

■ **THERAPEUTIC INTERVENTIONS**
Rest
Fluids
Topical antipruritics
Topical antibiotic ointment
Antihistamines
Cutting child's fingernails short to avoid bacterial infection when child scratches lesions
Possibly using Acyclovir as the antiviral drug of choice in treating varicella zoster infections

NOTE: There is an immunization available—Zoster immune globulin (ZIG)

VULVOVAGINITIS CANDIDIASIS

Vulvovaginitis candidiasis is caused by the gram-positive fungus *Candida albicans.* This organism can be found in approximately 20% of nonpregnant women. There are no known complications from candidiasis infections.

■ **SIGNS AND SYMPTOMS**
May be asymptomatic
Erythema of vulva
Edema of vulva
Vaginal discharge (normally whitish and thick, with the appearance of cottage cheese, but may also be thin and watery)
Groin lesions
Balanitis found in male sexual partners
Lesions on penis

■ **THERAPEUTIC INTERVENTIONS**
Nystatin vaginal suppositories or niconazole vaginal cream

LUMBAR PUNCTURE (SPINAL TAP)

A lumbar puncture is performed to measure cerebrospinal fluid pressure and/or to remove cerebrospinal fluid, to decrease pressure and for laboratory analysis. A lumbar puncture should *NOT* be done if there is suspicion of intracranial bleeding as removal of cerebrospinal fluid may produce a "vacuum effect" and lead to brainstem herniation.

■ **PROCEDURE**

1. Explain the procedure to the patient if possible.
2. Obtain a consent for the procedure.
3. Obtain baseline vital signs.
4. Empty the patient's bladder.
5. Position the patient on his or her side with neck flexed and knees drawn up to abdomen (Figure 19-2).
6. Prepare the tap site with antiseptic solution.
7. Drape the site with sterile towels.
8. Introduce 1% lidocaine into the space between L4 and L5.
9. Introduce a 20- or 22-gauge spinal needle with a stylet into the subdural space (Figure 19-3).
10. Rotate the needle to direct the bevel rostrally (to prevent obstruction).

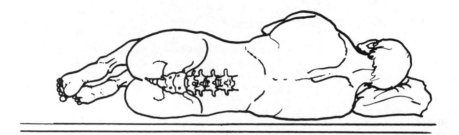

FIGURE 19-2. Position of patient for lumbar puncture.

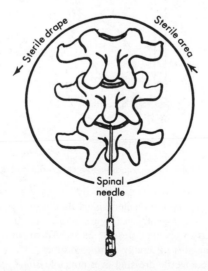

FIGURE 19-3. Introduction of spinal needle.

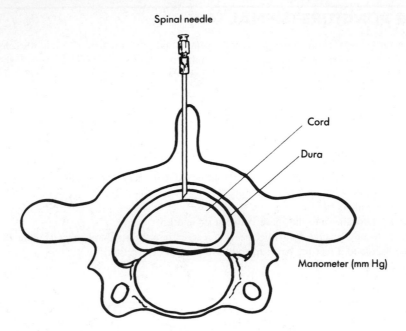

FIGURE 19-4. Spinal needle in subdural space.

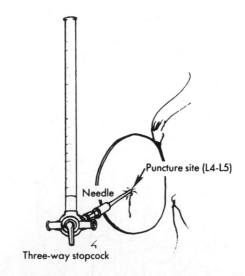

FIGURE 19-5. Spinal needle and manometer.

11. Remove the stylet after piercing the dura mater; spinal fluid will drip out at this point (Figure 19-4).
12. Attach a three-way stopcock with manometer (Figure 19-5).
13. Open the stopcock and record an opening pressure measurement (lowest level during fluctuations).
14. Collect cerebrospinal fluid samples in serially numbered tubes.
15. Remove the needle and place a sterile dressing over puncture site.
16. Keep the patient on bed rest for at least 1 hour after the procedure.

SUGGESTED READINGS

Abramowitz M, editor: Drugs for sexually transmitted diseases, *Medical Letter* 36(913): 1-6, 1994.

Centers for Disease Control and Prevention: Guidelines for preventing the transmission of mycobacterium tuberculosis in health-care facilities, *MMWR* 43(RR-13):1-132, 1994.

Centers for Disease Control and Prevention: Human rabies—West Virginia, *MMWR* 44:86-87, 93, 1995.

Danis DM: 15 years later: the changing face of the AIDS epidemic, *J Emerg Nurs* 22:343-346, 1996.

Infection control update '97, *Nurs 97* 27(6): 60-64, 1997.

Morton TA, Keler GD: Hepatitis C, *Ann Emerg Med* 31(3): 381-390, 1998.

Palmer S: *Infection control,* Aurora, Colo, 1996, Skidmore-Roth.

Polis MA: Viral infections. In Rosen P, Barkin R, editors: *Emergency medicine: concepts and clinical practice,* St Louis, 1998, Mosby.

Schaffer SD: *Pocket guide to infection prevention and safe practice,* St Louis, 1996, Mosby.

Turbiak TW, Riech JJ: Bacterial infections. In Rosen P, Barkin R, editors: *Emergency medicine: concepts and clinical practice,* St Louis, 1998, Mosby.

Allergies and Hypersensitivity

Faye P. Everson ■ Gail Pisarcik Lenehan

DEFINITIONS

allergy: An abnormal or hyper-response to antigens.

antigen: Substance that includes formation of antibodies. Examples include: drugs, foods, venom and pollens, and other inhalants introduced into the body by injection, ingestion, inhalation, or absorption.

allergen: A substance that *may* produce a hypersensitive reaction, but is not necessarily harmful.

anaphylaxis: An exaggerated hypersensitivity reaction to a previously encountered allergen.

antibody: A protective protein substance developed by the body upon exposure to antigens. Normally antibodies bind to the antigen that produced them and the antibodies are neutralized.

CELLS INVOLVED IN IMMUNE RESPONSE

monocyte: Circulating leukocyte that acts as a phagocyte and processes antigens so that antibodies are produced.

leukocyte: Blood component with the immune response.

lymphocyte: Two classes

1. T-cells: defend against foreign cells or viruses.
   Recognize and attach to antigens
   Produce cells with identical antigen receptors
   Some destroy invading pathogens and some stay as memory cells to respond if subsequent exposure occurs.
2. B-cells: have antigen-specific receptors
   Enhance work of phagocytic cells and retain memory

IMMUNOGLOBINS

These antibodies are molecules produced as a response to antigen response.

Types

There are five types of antibodies. These include:

1. IgG   Largest class
2. IgM   Dominant antibody in ABO incompatibilities
3. IgA   Second largest class. Combines with protein in mucosa and defends body surface against microorganisms.
4. IgE   Responsible for immediate hypersensitivity reactions.
5. IgD   Function unknown.

Allergic Reactions

Allergic reactions occur with increased physiologic response to an antigen *after* a previous exposure or sensitization to the same antigen.

TYPES OF ALLERGIC RESPONSE

TYPE I: Immediate Hypersensitivity

- Most important of the reactions
- Mediated through IgE
- Mast cells (or basophils) are disrupted and chemical mediators are released into extracellular spaces.
- Anaphylaxis is most extreme form of allergic reaction.
- 400 to 800 deaths per year
- 3% mortality

■ CAUSES: ANY SUBSTANCE
Drugs and biologic agents
- antibiotics
- anesthetics
- aspirin
- nonsteroidal anti-inflammatory drugs
- opiates
- vaccines
- chemotherapeutic agents
Insect bites and stings
- wasps/bees
Foods
- peanuts
- fish: cod, halibut
- shellfish
- egg whites
- strawberries
- food additives (MSG)
- wheat
- cottonseed
- milk

■ PATHOPHYSIOLOGY
The patient must have a previous exposure with an antigen entering the body. The immune system becomes activated. IgE is produced in large amounts and stays in the mast cells and basophils until there is a second exposure. With every subsequent exposure, mast cells and basophils are destroyed and a reaction occurs. Histamines and other chemical mediators are released and complex chemical processes occur.

■ SIGNS AND SYMPTOMS
Respiratory
- sneezing
- coughing
- wheezes
- throat tightness
- dyspnea
- stridor
- voice changes
- bronchospasm
- complete airway obstruction

Cardiovascular
- vasculature becomes more permeable and flaccid
- mild hypotension to vascular collapse and shock
- tachycardia
- dysrhythmias

Gastrointestinal
- nausea/vomiting/diarrhea
- abdominal cramping

Central nervous system
- agitation
- feeling of "impending doom"
- weakness
- headache
- syncope
- seizures
- coma

Cutaneous
- skin warmth
- itching
- urticaria, with wheals from 1 to 6 cm
  - raised margins and blanched center
- swelling of face, tongue or airway
- angioedema
- cyanosis (a late sign)

■ THERAPEUTIC INTERVENTIONS
Primary survey (ABCDs)

Airway maintenance
- watch for increasing edema, voice changes, increase in tongue size
- prepare for possible intubation
- prepare for possible needle cricothyroidotomy

Breathing
- assess rate, chest rise and fall, effort, breath sounds
- administer high concentration humidified oxygen at 10 to 15 lpm with a nonrebreather mask
- prepare for ventilatory assistance (BVM or ET)

Circulation
- assess rate, quality, location of pulses
- assess and reassess blood pressure
- vascular access with NS or LR
- apply cardiac monitor, pulse oximetry

Disability
- assessment of level of consciousness
- watch for change in level of consciousness
- anxiety, restlessness, lethargy
- may indicate early hypoxia

Drug interventions
- Epinephrine
- 0.1-0.5 ml of 1:1000 SC
- 0.1-0.5 ml of 1:10,000 IV
- May be repeated every 5 to 15 mins.
- Diphenhydramine (Benadryl)
- 25-50 mg IV or IM

- May give split dose in both routes (25 mg IV and 25 mg IM)
- Pediatrics 1-2 mg/kg
- Updrafts with Albuterol or Metaproteronal
- Steroids Methylprednisolone (Solumedrol)
- 40-125 mg IV
- Pediatrics 1-2 mg/kg
- Dexamethasone (Decadron) is not a first-line drug because of late onset
- Cimetadine (Tagamet) histamine blocker
- Glucagon 1 mg IV

TYPE II: Cytolytic or Cytotoxic Hypersensitivity

- Involves IgG or IgM antibodies and complement
- Antibodies attach to cells and cause lysis
- Usually caused by transfusion reactions

■ SIGNS AND SYMPTOMS
- headache and flank pain
- chest pain similar to angina
- nausea and vomiting
- increased heart rate and low blood pressure
- hematuria
- urticaria

■ THERAPEUTIC INTERVENTIONS
Stop the transfusion
Maintain patent IV access
Monitor vital signs
Treat life-threatening symptoms as described in Type I reactions
Obtain urine and blood samples as per hospital protocols

Type III: Immune Complex Hypersensitivity

- Are antigen-antibody mediated
- Known as serum sickness
- Antigen-antibody complexes are deposited in tissues
- Causes an acute or chronic disease in the organ involved.

■ SIGNS AND SYMPTOMS
- Depends on organ/system involved
  - Kidney = glomerulonephritis
  - Joints = rheumatoid arthritis
  - Vessels = arteritis

■ THERAPEUTIC INTERVENTIONS
Obtain history
Avoidance of allergen/discontinuation of offending medication

Type IV—Cell Mediated or Delayed Hypersensitivity

- Involves T-cells
- Occurs 24 to 72 hours after exposure
- Can be induced by chronic disease (TB) or contact dermatitis
- Occurs after PPD or TB antigen is injected
  - Edema and fibrin deposited leading to redness (TB Test)

- Graft vs host disease and transplant rejection are delayed reactions
- Contact dermatitis
  - Exposure to cosmetics, adhesives, topical medications, drug additives or plant toxins (poison ivy)
■ **SIGNS AND SYMPTOMS**
- Usually no reactions with first exposure
- Subsequently: itching, erythema, vesicular lesions
■ **THERAPEUTIC INTERVENTIONS**
Avoidance

DIAGNOSTIC TESTS FOR "ALLERGIES"

Assay of IgE levels
    radioallergosorbent test
    radioimmunosorbent test (RAST)
    eosinophil levels
Pulmonary function tests
Skin testing
    scratch, prick, or intradermal
Elimination diets and food diary
Challenge testing

LATEX ALLERGY

Definitions

latex: Can refer to a wide range of materials, (such as that found in carpet backing and paint), as well as natural rubber latex, but *latex* allergy is caused by natural rubber latex, which is commonly referred to as *latex.*

latex allergy: An IgE mediated allergy to proteins inherent in natural rubber latex.

Terms used with latex gloves:

hypoallergenic: Refers to the decreased chemical content of a product. Latex allergy (IgE mediated) involves the proteins in natural rubber latex, not chemicals. Thus, a glove could be called "hypoallergenic" and still be made of latex (and even have a high concentration of latex protein allergens). The FDA has mandated that manufacturers of medical products refrain from using this misleading term.

glove powder: Powder binds with latex particles, and can be a vehicle for latex to become airborne and come in contact with the eyes, respiratory tract, and lungs, with the potential for increased sensitization and reactions.

aerosolization: Process by which latex protein allergens become airborne. Latex protein allergens readily bind with cornstarch powder and become airborne with the donning of gloves. Even with "low-powder" or "powderless" latex gloves, latex protein allergens can still be propelled into the air, particularly when gloves are snapped on and off.

low-powder gloves: There is currently no definition of what constitutes a low-powder glove. They are thought to be less allergenic than high-powder gloves, although there is still the potential for sensitization and reactions to latex.

powderless gloves: The FDA allows gloves to be called "powderless," even when they contain up to 2 mgm of powder.

low allergen gloves: There is currently no standard definition of what constitutes a low allergen glove. Latex gloves, no matter what the powder or allergen level, have the potential for sensitizing and for causing allergic reactions.

sensitization: the process by which someone becomes allergic.

silicone coated latex catheters: Rubber catheters with a latex overlay. These products should not be used in the care of patients with an allergy to latex.

Screening for Latex Allergy

Emergency department patients at triage can be asked several questions to elicit need for latex precautions:
- History of surgeries or catheterizations or other procedures involving latex contacting mucosa
- History of allergic reactions to latex gloves, balloons, and condoms (hives, facial/mouth swelling, runny nose, itchy watering eyes, asthma, chest tightness, tachycardia, shock)
- Occupational exposure to latex
- Other allergies
   Cross-reactive foods: bananas, kiwi, avocado, tropical fruits, potato, cherry, chestnut, grape, tomato, papaya, apple, carrot, celery.

Latex products with potential for high allergenicity and/or contact with sensitive mucosa/vasculature

Latex gloves, particularly powdered, high allergen
Latex catheters or tubes which contact mucous membranes, airway, or blood vessels
Vial stoppers
Latex-tipped plungers of syringes
Rubber ports in IV tubing

Other products that contain latex

Some airway products, blood pressure cuffs, stethoscopes, tourniquets, cardiac monitor pads, adhesive tape, chux

Types of Latex Allergy

Type IV

Cell-mediated
- Caused by chemicals used in manufacturing
- Reactions—poison ivy–like rashes
- May occur 24 to 48 hours after contact
- Not life threatening, but may break down skin barrier giving latex protein allergens access to immune system

Type I

IgE mediated
- Reactions may occur immediately, or up to 2 hours after exposure
- Reactions run the gamut of systemic symptoms: watery eyes and/or nose, sneezing, urticaria (wheals), laryngeal edema (voice changes), abdominal cramping, diarrhea, nausea, wheezing, coughing, chest tightness, airway compromise, flushing, hypotension, tachycardia, shock
   Patients with latex allergy can go from asymptomatic to anaphylaxis. Treat severe reactions (latex-induced asthma, anaphylaxis) quickly. Patients can deteriorate rapidly.

Treatment for Anaphylaxis/Acute Latex-Induced Asthma

Same as for reactions to other allergens. The only difference is the need to treat in latex-safe environment with latex-free equipment by doing the following
- Move patient to area where no latex gloves have been used in the immediate vicinity for 12 hours or more and where no powdered latex gloves are used in areas that share the same ventilation system.
- Make sure that no latex gloves are used in vicinity of patient

- Do use synthetic, nonlatex gloves (for example, nitrile, vinyl, tactylon), synthetic (nonlatex) syringes or glass syringes, single-dose glass vials of medication or remove the rubber vial stopper, synthetic tourniquets
- Do *not* use prepackaged kits that include latex gloves (danger from glove, and from protein allergen contaminated products in the kit), latex ports in IV tubing (tape them over to prevent anyone else from using them), latex vial stoppers of multidose vials, and latex endotracheal tubes

Discharge Instructions

Patient teaching

Seriousness of allergy (acute reactions can be as severe as reactions to penicillin or bee venom)
Recognition of signs and symptoms of reactions
Need to carry epinephrine injection system
Potential for "rebound reactions," 4 to 10 hours after acute reaction
Food cross-sensitivities

Medications:

Diphenhydramine or hydroxyzine for 3 days
Steroids, tapered course

INFORMATION REGARDING EDUCATION AND SUPPORT

- Latex Allergy News: 860-482-6869
- Web sites: http://www.netcom.com/~nam1/latex__allergy.html http://www.latexallergyhelp.com
- Medic-Alert (209-668-3333)

"Latex" is used throughout this section to refer to natural rubber latex.

SUGGESTED READINGS

Brown AFT: Anaphylactic shock: mechanisms and treatment, *J Accid Emerg Med* 12:89-100, 1995.
Compton J: Use of glucagon in intractable allergic reactions and as an alternative to epinephrine: an interesting case review, *J Emerg Nurs* 23(1):45-47, 1997.
Kellner R, Warner D, Murray G: Severe latex allergy: three first person accounts, *J Emerg Nurs* 23:130-134, 1997.
Kelly KJ, Sussman G, Fink JN: Stop the sensitization, *J Allergy Clin Immunol* 98(5):857-858, 1996.
Luckman J, Sorenson K: *Luckman and Sorenson's medical-surgical nursing: a psychophysical approach,* ed 4, Philadelphia, 1993, Saunders.
Miller K: The latex allergy triage or admission tool: an algorithm to identify which patients would benefit from "latex safe" precautions, *J Emerg Nurs* 24(2):1-8, 1998.
Muelleman RL, Lindzon RD, Silvers WS: Allergy, hypersensitivity, and anaphylaxis. In Rosen P, Brakin R, editors: *Emergency medicine: concepts and clinical practice,* St Louis, 1998, Mosby.
National Institute for Occupational Safety and Health: *Alert: preventing allergic reactions to natural rubber latex in the workplace,* Publication No 97-135, July, 1997.
Safadi GS et al: Latex hypersensitivity in emergency medical service providers, *Ann Allergy, Asthma, Immunol* 77:39-42, 1996.
Sanders MJ: *Mosby's paramedic textbook,* St Louis, 1994, Mosby.
Schwartz JF: Anaphylaxis: a potentially fatal, avoidable and often ignored clinical problem, *Mayo Clin Proc* 69-93, 1994.
Newbury L, Emergency Nurses Association: *Sheehy's Emergency nursing: principles and practice,* ed 4, St Louis, 1998, Mosby.
Vassallo SA et al: Allergic reaction to latex from stopper of a medication vial, *Anesth Analg* 80:1057-1058, 1995.

Trauma Emergencies

PART THREE

Treating
Emergencies

Wound Management

Robert D. Herr ■ Polly Gerber Zimmermann

GENERAL

General Principles and Concerns

The aim of wound care is:
- to identify underlying injury to bone, nerve, or artery
- to decrease the likelihood of infection/promote optimal wound healing
- to minimize scarring.

Important factors to consider in wound management are:
- What caused the injury?
- How did the injury happen?
- What were the circumstances surrounding the injury?
- When did the injury occur?
- On what part of the body is the wound?
- In what condition is the tissue surrounding the wound?
- Can the edges of the wound be approximated?
- What is the patient's age?
- What is the patient's occupation?
- What is the patient's physical condition?
- Is the patient taking any medications?
- Does the patient have any other pertinent medical history?
- What is the condition of the patient's skin?
- Was any care given to the wound before arrival in the emergency department?
- Is there movement and sensation distal to the wound?
- Is vascular status intact distal to the wound?

THE PROCESS OF WOUND HEALING

Tissue injury causes immediate vasocontriction of the affected vessels followed by vasodilation. This causes erythema and edema in the subepithelial layer of skin. In open wounds, epithelial cells begin to migrate within 24 hours of the injury. Fibrin begins to form, followed in days by collagen formation. The process of epithelialization will cause wound closure in two to three days, if the skin edges can be approximated and no infection occurs.

Epithelialization is slower for those with:

Poor nutritional state

Compromised vascular supply (those with diabetes, severe atherosclerosis, smokers)

Patients taking medications that slow collagen formation (such as corticosteroids or phenytoin)

Wounds on the lower legs, feet, and toes

Advanced age

Lower oxygen tension in tissues (especially those with COPD or on home oxygen therapy)

General Principles of Wound Management

Treat the patient

Ensure there is an airway and breathing

Apply direct pressure over bleeding wounds to prevent further blood loss

Identify and treat shock

Complete the primary survey by assessing the level of alertness, the pupil size and reactivity, and exposing the patient to determine if there are other wounds that also warrant treatment.

Treat the extremity

Assess distal pulses, capillary refill, and extremity warmth and color

Assess the extremity sensation and ability to move the digits

Splint any fractures; notify the physician immediately if there could be an open fracture. An open fracture is defined as any skin disruption near the fracture site. Open fractures require irrigation, intravenous antibiotics, and sometimes operative debridement.

Treat the wound

Remove old dressings

Get a soft tissue x-ray if a foreign body is suspected (for example, in a missile injury or if the weapon could have fragmented in the wound).

Notify the physician for copious or pulsatile bleeding.

Cleanse the wound with jet irrigation (if a puncture or laceration) or by scrubbing the wound (if an abrasion or there is much foreign material present).

Explore the wound to search for foreign bodies and injury to vessel, nerve, or bone.

Debride devitalized tissue.

Either approximate the wound edges or, if unsuitable for closure, dress it appropriately.

Identify need to alert authorities.

TERMINOLOGY AND APPROACH TO WOUND CARE

There are six basic types of wounds: abrasion, abscess, avulsion, contusion, laceration, and puncture. Each is distinct and warrants different treatment.

Abrasion ("brush burn")

Rubbing the skin against a hard surface causes an abrasion by removing at least the epithelial layer of skin, exposing the dermal or subcutaneous layer. The wound base may appear yellow, white, or pink depending upon the exposed tissue. Foreign bodies are typically granular and, in the case of gravel or asphalt ("road rash"), may cause permanent tattooing of the skin if not removed. Large abrasions may cause significant fluid loss and hypothermia because of evaporation.

■ **THERAPEUTIC INTERVENTIONS**

Cleanse the wound by irrigating it and scrubbing it.

Remove all foreign material

Abscess

An abscess results from localized infection that has not drained through the skin. Underlying infection arises from inoculation by an insect, a puncture wound, an infected hair follicle, or a wound that has been surgically closed (and skin allowed to epithelialize) before it has properly drained away infection. Abscess typically comes to someone's attention when it enlarges to the point of distending the skin and causing pain. The overlying skin may be tense and discolored because of underlying pus. When the pus tents the skin, the abscess is said to "point" and be ready for drainage. Abscesses that point will eventually drain spontaneously. However, draining them at the time of the emergency department visit will decrease pain, allow for wound packing, and prevent cellulitis from developing.

■ THERAPEUTIC INTERVENTIONS

Abscesses in the perirectal area are much deeper than they appear and should be drained under general anesthesia in the operating room.

A pointing abscess should be drained by making an incision in the overlying, tense skin using a scalpel blade. Needle drainage is not adequate to prevent a rapid recurrence of the abscess. Local anesthetic may be injected around the abscess to dull pain. Inhaled nitrous oxide may be used to blunt the pain, but this technique has not been very successful. After pus is allowed to drain, further pus should be expressed by pressing on the wound edges.

To prevent premature closure of the skin and facilitate further drainage of infection, the abscess cavity should be packed with iodinated gauze. Packing should be directed to the edges of the abscess cavity, making sure to break up all loculated pus in the corners. The packing should be changed in 1 to 2 days. Abscess drainage and packing is inherently uncomfortable, even painful, but adequate packing and drainage is the only way to prevent recurrence. Pain medication should be avoided. Antibiotics are unnecessary unless there is a coexisting cellulitis.

Avulsion

An avulsion is a peeling of the skin from the underlying tissue where the skin is either completely separated (also called an amputation) or is connected by a bridge of tissue. Avulsion can compromise the blood supply and lead to further devitalized tissue. Such avulsions are described as proximal-based or distal-based avulsions, with the proximal-based avulsions, in general, having a better blood supply. Nonetheless, the edges of the wound may look gray or dusky, indicating the tenuous nature of the blood supply.

■ THERAPEUTIC INTERVENTIONS

The wound should be cleansed, irrigated, and debrided of devitalized tissue just as in lacerations.

In contrast to other wounds, epinephrine should be avoided because its vasoconstriction properties can further compromise the blood supply of the avulsed fragment. Avulsed skin that is crinkled or folded can usually be extended to cover the entire wound and sutured in place.

Even skin that appears gray or dusky will heal surprisingly well. Such skin edges should not be debrided, but approximated. The edges can be debrided the following day when the wound is rechecked.

Avulsions are common in patients with thin skin because they are elderly or taking long-term corticosteroids. Such skin may be too thin to suture; instead, approximate the skin edges using adhesive strips such as steristrips®.

Contusion

Contusions result from blunt injuries that cause extravasation of blood. When viewed through the skin, such blood looks "black and blue." After two days, the breakdown of blood pigments changes color to yellow. Although most contusions are minor and resolve with local treatment, some contusions can cause large painful hematomas or cause tissue swelling in fascial compartments that can threaten blood supply to tissues or nerves resulting in compartment syndrome.

■ **THERAPEUTIC INTERVENTIONS**

Ice, elevation, systemic analgesia with narcotics of nonsteroidal, antiinflammatory agents (NSAIDs)

No dressing is necessary

Laceration

A superficial laceration involves the epidermis and dermis. A deep laceration extends beyond the dermis. Lacerations can be linear or stellate, have jagged or smooth edges, and have edges that are either vertical or beveled. A linear laceration is relatively resistant to infection.

■ **THERAPEUTIC INTERVENTION**

Anesthetize the wound.

Cleanse the wound using scrubbing and irrigation.

Explore the wound for damage to underlying structures and for bone exposure.

Remove any foreign bodies.

Excise any necrotic tissue.

Approximate the wound edges.

Apply antibiotic ointment.

Apply a sterile dressing.

Puncture

A puncture results from a sharp object that leaves a hole rather than a laceration. Exploration of the wound is limited; therefore, a high index of suspicion is needed to predict underlying injury. Although missiles can cause extensive underlying tissue damage, punctures from nails, glass, pins, and other foreign bodies usually move aside vessels or nerves rather than sever them. Punctures are also difficult to clean, cause inoculation of bacteria into the wounds, and tend to close early. Infection occurs in 11 to 15% of puncture wounds.

Punctures into joint spaces can lead to septic arthritis. Punctures into cartilage, bone, and periosteum can lead to osteomyelitis. Such punctures warrant exploration in the operating room. Evaluation should include obtaining an x-ray if the puncture has occurred near a bone or joint.

In addition, any infected puncture wound should be suspected of harboring a retained foreign body that serves as a nidus of infection. The propensity for a retained foreign body can be ascertained by asking the patient who removed the object whether the object appeared to be intact. The presence of wound contaminants such as clothing, rust, or dirt should also be assessed.

Specific types of punctures warranting separate discussion are bite and gunshot wounds and punctures of the plantar area of the foot.

■ **THERAPEUTIC INTERVENTION**

A plain x-ray is indicated for all infected puncture wounds and all those with the possibility of a foreign body.

Uncomplicated, clean puncture wounds less than 6 hours old can be irrigated and cleansed.

The entrance site should be inspected for foreign bodies.

Probing the wound with a sound can help to locate a foreign body but cannot be used to rule out its presence.

Avoid extensive debridement or "coring" of the wound.

When there is an uncomplicated puncture wound in a healthy individual, prophylactic antibiotics have not proven to be helpful and can predispose to secondary infections with *Pseudomonas*.

Prophylactic antibiotics such as intravenous first-generation cephalosporins (that is, cephalothin/"Ancef" or "Kefzol") should be used for puncture wounds that are contaminated, or on the plantar area of the foot, or in patients with immunocompromised conditions such as diabetes mellitus, peripheral vascular disease, or systemic immunodeficiency.

Tetanus prophylaxis should be updated; all puncture wounds are considered tetanus prone and require current prophylaxis status tetanus immunization.

Observe for complications such as cellulitis, abscess, joint infection, or osteomyelitis.

Gunshot wounds

In contrast to other puncture wounds, gunshot wounds may cause extensive damage to underlying tissues and organs. The amount of damage has no relationship to the size of the entrance wound or exit wounds. Bullets can shatter bone and cause injury from these secondary projectiles. Bullets can create a wound cavity with negative pressure that sucks in overlying clothing and debris. Bullets fired from rifles have a high velocity that causes shock waves in tissues that can shear and crush nerves, vessels, muscle, bone, and organs several centimeters or more from the path of the missile. Finally, shotgun wounds at close range can embed the shotgun wadding in the tissues.

Forensic concerns include notifying police of gunshot wounds, documenting the exact location of the wound, distinguishing entrance from exit wounds, and protecting evidence on the patient's hands such as gunpowder and blood by placing paper bags over the hands. Clothing should be cut off in such a way as to preserve bullet holes and given to the police.

WOUND PREPARATION

Anesthetic Use

Adequate cleansing, irrigation, and debridement can be best accomplished in the cooperative, well anesthetized patient.

Conscious sedation is a medically controlled state of depressed consciousness that maintains protective reflexes, airway, and response to command. Although some authors extol the benefits of conscious sedation for relieving anxiety and controlling pain, its use at hospital emergency departments is best reserved for the pediatric patient. Its routine use in adult patients may be humane, but compliance with requirements for monitoring and documenting required by JCAHO (and often abetted by the department of anesthesia) require one-on-one nursing care that may be impossible to carry out in a busy emergency department.

The anesthesia of choice is a digital block or other regional nerve block because it does not distort the wound and allows better approximation of the wound edges. These types of blocks can be used whenever the nerve supply to the wound is superficial. They are especially superior to infiltration anesthesia in regions where the skin is sensitive, such as the digits, palms, soles, and face. Locations for injecting anesthetic for these areas can be found in other texts.

Infiltration anesthesia anesthetizes the subcutaneous nerves by injecting lidocaine into the edges of the wound. Some authorities recommend injecting through the intact, antiseptically-cleansed skin at the periphery of the wound because it does not introduce contamination that occurs inside the wound. Others recommend injecting through the cut edge of the wound because it is less painful.

The discomfort of infiltration anesthesia can be reduced by the following:

Use the thinnest possible needle; 30 gauge or smaller is best.

Minimize the number of injections; a longer needle inserted to its hub can cover much of a wound edge.

Inject subsequent needles through already anesthetized skin.

Inject into the subdermal area rather than into the dermis; raising a wheal is very painful.

Injecting slowly over 10 seconds is more comfortable than injecting in under 2 seconds.

Lidocaine injection can be made more comfortable by either warming the lidocaine to 37° (place it in the blanket warmer) or by buffering it with sodium bicarbonate as a 10:1 solution of 10 ml 1% lidocaine and 1 mEq/ml (3 ml of 4.2%) sodium bicarbonate. This buffering reduces the shelf life of lidocaine from 3 years to a few days, after which the solution precipitates out in the bottle.

Topical anesthesia

The advantages of topical anesthetics includes no pain of injection, no tissue swelling, and achieving vasoconstriction that prevents bleeding. The traditional agent is TAC, or a solution of 0.5% tetracaine, 0.5% epinephrine (adrenalin), and 11.8% cocaine. TAC is effective at controlling pain when applied 20 minutes before wound repair, after the skin becomes blanched.

Significant disadvantages mar the success of TAC. These include toxic reactions if applied to mucous membranes, the danger of ischemia when applied to the ear, digits, and penis because of its vasoconstriction properties, the need to prepare it at the hospital pharmacy and store it in the emergency department as a narcotic and, most important, its propensity to cause wound infection and necrosis of the wound edges. TAC is being supplanted by newer agents.

The topical solution of 4% lidocaine, 0.1% epinephrine, and 0.5% tetracaine "LET" is equal to TAC when anesthetizing the scalp, forehead, and eyebrow in adult patients. Children over age 6 had incomplete anesthesia using LET.

Topical anesthesia can be achieved by applying a mixture of 5% lidocaine and prilocaine (EMLA) under occlusion for 60 minutes. This is supplied as a cream that has been used on intact skin for split-thickness skin graft donor sites, venipuncture, curettage, and cautery of certain skin lesions. Its use on lacerations is not recommended because it excites inflammation that increases the rate of infection.

Types of anesthetics

Lidocaine is the most common anesthetic for infiltration or regional use. It has minimal toxic tissue effects. Whereas multiple-dose vials of lidocaine contain an antimicrobial preservative, single-use vials do not and should therefore be used only once. Lidocaine's short duration of anesthesia is desirable when repairing areas such as the mouth or lip as the recovery of sensation can prevent the patient from biting the tongue or lip. Likewise, prompt return of sensation in a finger is desirable if the patient wants to avoid injuring it again.

Bupivacaine (Marcaine, Sensorcaine) has four times the duration of anesthesia of lidocaine. It should be used if wound closure is expected to require longer than 2 hours or where prolonged anesthesia is desirable.

Epinephrine is a vasoconstrictor that increases the duration of anesthesia and decreases bleeding. Its benefits must be weighed against its drawbacks. Epinephrine increases the rate of infection and can cause ischemia when injected into the ear, tip of the nose, digit, or penis. It is therefore contraindicated in heavily contaminated wounds or wounds with tentative blood supply such as avulsions.

Wound Assessment

The size of the scar depends directly upon the tension at the edges of the wound when they are approximated. The amount of tension, and the resultant scar, can be predicted by how much the wound gapes. Wounds that gape by more than 5 mm will heal with a wide scar.

It is surprising but true that the jagged edges of a gaping wound actually leave less of a scar if these edges can be approximated. This jaggedness distributes the tension over a wider perimeter than the linear laceration, reducing tension and leaving a narrow scar. It is therefore a mistake to trim the jagged edges unless there is contamination.

Plain x-rays will detect 90% of foreign bodies such as glass and metal. They will not detect objects with a density close to that of soft tissue, including wood splinters, thorns, cactus spines, and pieces of plastic. Other imaging modalities for wood and plastic include ultrasound, CT, and MRI.

Skin Antisepsis

The skin around the wound harbors bacteria in the outer layer of dead skin that can migrate into the wound. Fortunately, these bacteria can be killed by using either chlorhexidine (Hebiclens) or iodophor (Betadine). However, both chlorhexidine and 10% iodophor antiseptics injure wound defenses, so avoid spilling them into the wound itself. A 1% iodophor solution is not toxic to tissues and has been shown as effective as 10% iodophor at killing *S. aureus*. Hydrogen peroxide in the 3% concentration commonly stocked in the emergency department also damages tissues through hemolyzing erythrocytes, occluding local microvasculature, and releasing gas that causes crepitus and tissue distortion.

Hair Removal

Wounds in hairy areas heal best without hair in the approximated edges. However, shaving hair with a razor abrades the skin, can increase the rate of wound infection, and is cosmetically irritating. Rather than shaving hair, it should be snipped with scissors or removed with an electric clipper. Better yet, attempt to move hair out of the way with either a lubricant, ointment such as bacitracin, or tape.

Eyebrows may not grow back and should not be shaved. In addition, they provide landmarks for approximating the skin edges.

Mechanical Irrigation

Irrigation remains the best, sometimes the only, way to decrease the chance of wound infection. It has been shown that infection results when the edges of a wound contain more than 10 to the sixth power of bacteria per gram of tissue, when there is a retained foreign body, or when the wound contains certain kinds of clay found in dirt. This clay, commonly found in wounds from industrial or farming accidents, has been found to contain charged particles that inhibit the action of antibiotics and leukocyte activity.

Mechanical removal of bacteria is essential in wounds that result from bites and those with fecal contamination. This is because both the gingival crevices of teeth and fecal matter harbor concentrations of bacteria of up to 10 to the 11th power per gram.

Large particles of contamination such as sand and dirt can be removed by low-pressure irrigation using a bulb syringe. However, small particles such as clay and bacteria require high-pressure irrigation. Animal studies show a higher-pressure irrigation is more effective than the low-pressure high-volume method. Higher-pressure irrigation of at least 7 psi can be supplied by forcing fluid through a narrow catheter or needle. Examples are using a 19-gauge needle with a 35-mL syringe or 12-mL syringe. Another example is a disposable irrigation assembly of a 19-gauge syringe attached to a 35-mL syringe that attaches directly to IV tubing. The nurse then pushes a sterile solution, such as 1000 mL of 0.9% sodium chloride solution, through the one-way valve attached to the syringe barrel.

There is no evidence that any one fluid is superior to another. Regardless of the solution or type of apparatus, mechanical irrigation is accomplished by placing the needle perpendicular to the wound as close as possible to the surface, and then forcefully depressing the plunger of the syringe.

The proper irrigation technique may cause a splatter of fluid that can spread hepatitis and human immunodeficiency viruses. Therefore, proper protective equipment must be used by the caregiver.

Mechanical Cleansing

Animal studies show that scrubbing with a saline-soaked gauze can prolong the effective period for antibiotics, presumable by removing bacteria. The type of sponge is important. A coarse, bristle-laden brush will injure tissue. A fine-pore sponge minimizes tissue damage when it is combined with a nonionic surfactant. Some authors recommend Poloxamer 188 (Calgon, St. Louis, MO) because it is nontoxic to tissue. Pluronic F-68 is also non-toxic, but like Poloxamer it exerts no antibacterial activity. Avoid scrubbing with Hibiclens or Betadine Surgical Scrub Solution because they are painful and damage tissue defense, increasing the likelihood of infection.

Prophylactic Antibiotics

Simple lacerations less than 8 hours old will become infected at a rate of 6% both with or without antibiotic prophylaxis. Therefore, prophylaxis is recommended only for other types of lacerations. Even then, antibiotics are an adjunct to debridement and irrigation rather than a substitute for it. Specific antibiotics depend on many factors, including the location of the wound, the pathogens usually encountered in the particular type of injury, and the fact that most wounds are contaminated by a wide variety of organisms.

WOUND CLOSURE

Primary closure is the goal for lacerations when the patient presents within 8 to 10 hours after injury. Patients with lacerations who present after 8 hours have a higher rate of infection because of high bacterial counts in the wound edges that resist irrigation and debridement.

Wounds that will remain contaminated following irrigation are not closed but are left open for about 4 days. Doing this allows the wound to increase resistance to infection. The wound may then be closed on the fourth day without developing infection.

An important exception to the above rule is a facial laceration. Blood supply and infection resistance is so good in the face that primary closure may be attempted no matter how old the wound. Even bites on the face may be closed following copious irrigation. Although infection may occur, it is thought that the need for good cosmetic repair from primary closure outweighs the relatively smaller risk of infection that can usually be readily resolved. Drains are not recommended because they have been shown to increase the rate of infection.

Wound Closure Material

Choices for wound closure are sutures, staples, tape, and adhesive bonding material. The choice of material and technique depends on the preference of the care provider, the tension at the wound edge, the likelihood of wound infection, and the closure material that is available.

Absorbable suture is degraded in the tissues and loses tensile strength within 60 days. So-called nonabsorbable suture retains strength for 60 days but is nonetheless slowly absorbed over months to years. Nonabsorbable sutures should be removed as soon as epithelialization occurs to minimize the scar from the suture itself. This process takes the shortest time in facial lacerations and the longest time in legs and feet. Figure 21-1 illustrates the optimal time for suture removal in various body areas. Because the wound itself does not regain full tensile strength for a considerable period, the provider should apply tape across the wound to reduce tension on the wound. In addition, sutures should be left in longer on patients with delayed healing from debilitation or from taking the medications phenytoin or corticosteroids such as prednisone.

Suturing Technique

For a thorough discussion, the reader is directed to Ira Dushoff's classic article "A stitch in time." The most important points are summarized here.

Taping with sterile, microporous tape (such as Steristrips®) is appropriate for well approximated wound edges in areas that are subjected to weak skin tensions. Areas in children are transverse lacerations over the brow, under the chin, or across the malar prominence. Taping avoids the pain of anesthesia and later suture removal. Tape adheres poorly to wet skin. Adherence can be increased by applying tincture of benzoin to the skin edges.

Stapling is faster than suturing, has a lower level of tissue reactivity and a higher resistance to infection. Unfortunately, stapling cannot align wound edges as well as sutures because the edges must be prepositioned and held in place while the staple is being applied. Almost inevitably, the edges are malpositioned slightly. Therefore, stapling is most appropriate where scarring can be tolerated, such as on the scalp.

Adhesive bonding is the newest approach to wound repair. One such bonding agent is n-butyl cyanoacrylate monomer 2.0 ml (Nexaband Liquid, Veterinary Product Laboratories, Phoenix AZ 85013). It has been used extensively in the United Kingdom. Upon contact with an alkaline pH, it polymerizes to form a thin, waterproof bandage. This requires 1 second on moist skin and several seconds on dry skin. It is most effective on wounds that have little tension.

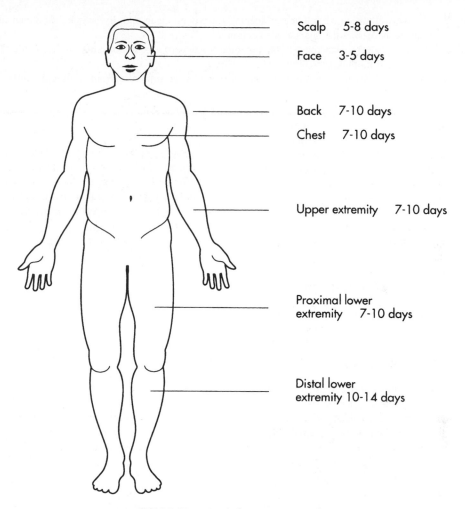

Scalp   5-8 days

Face   3-5 days

Back   7-10 days

Chest   7-10 days

Upper extremity   7-10 days

Proximal lower
extremity   7-10 days

Distal lower
extremity 10-14 days

FIGURE 21-1. Guide for suture removal.

WOUND DRESSING AND AFTERCARE

One 1995 study showed that topical bacitracin zinc and the combination of bacitracin zinc, neomycin sulfate, and polymyxin B sulfate (Neosporin) each reduced infection to 5% from 12% as compared to petrolatum alone. Other studies show conflicting results, leaving room for a variety of practices.

Pending definitive answers, it is reasonable to apply an antibiotic ointment over a wound as a adjunct to preventing infection. It is also important to keep the wound free from contamination with pathogenic bacteria until it becomes resistant, usually in 2 to 3 days. The sutured wound should be dressed with a sterile, dry dressing for 2 days unless the area is either a gingival surface or too hairy to accommodate a dressing. If the dressing prevents evaporation of water from the healing wound to create a moist scab, it will promote healing by allowing the epidermal cells to migrate more easily than they would if the dressing is porous to water and the scab becomes dry.

Wounds closed only with tape are more infection resistant than those sutured closed. No topical antibiotic is indicated for taped wounds.

In contrast to the well-accepted practice of keeping the wound clean and dry, studies show that the patient may shower without increasing the chance of infection.

Any skin that is abraded is sensitized to the potential for hyperpigmentation after sun exposure. Therefore advise a sunscreen for 6 months after the injury.

Because immobilized wounds are more immune to infection, an injured extremity should be elevated to limit edema.

TETANUS

Tetanus is caused by the organism *Clostridium tetani,* a gram-positive spore-forming, anaerobic bacillus. It is highly resistant to any measure taken against it, including sterilization, because of its tendency to form spores when conditions for its survival are not favorable. The incubation period is from 2 days to 2 weeks or more. The organism is present in soil and garden moss, on farms, and anywhere else animal and human excreta can be found. It enters the human circulation through an open wound and attaches itself to cells within the central nervous system. Tetanus causes depression of the respiratory center in the medulla.

■ **SIGNS AND SYMPTOMS**

Mild tetanus

Local joint stiffness

Mild trismus (inability to open jaw)

Moderate tetanus

Generalized body stiffness	Difficulty swallowing
Moderate trismus	Decreased vital capacity

Tetanus Immunization

Every year in the United States approximately 100 individuals contract the disease tetanus, most after having an acute injury. Tetanus is 100% avoidable if immunizations (tetanus prophylaxis) are current. At the same time, tetanus immunization should be given only when needed. Injection causes pain, expense, and the need for additional documentation. Also, some individuals become hyperimmune to tetanus from too frequent immunizations. Subsequent tetanus immunization causes the arm to become painfully swollen for several days. This type of reaction is the usual source of a "tetanus allergy" reported by patients.

Recommendations for tetanus immunization are based on the guidelines recommended by the Centers for Disease Control and Prevention.

The adult tetanus vaccine also contains diphtheria toxin on the recommendation of the CDC, because many adults lack circulating antitoxin against diphtheria. The resultant dT is a combined preparation of 0.5 mL to be given IM.

Tetanus immunization is normally given along with diphtheria and pertussis at ages 2 mos, 4 mos, 6 mos, 18 months, 4 to 6 years, and then as a booster at 16 years. A fully immunized individual has had a tetanus vaccine within the last 10 years. Typically, the teenager or young adult will not recall the booster. However, they probably received it in high school. Let them call their parent or find their records at home before giving them a potentially unnecessary booster. If no record of a vaccine exists, they typically have several days in which to get the vaccine.

Patients with a tetanus-prone wound should be given a dT unless they have had a booster in the last 5 years. Tetanus-prone wounds are those that are infected, result from bites of humans or animals, are greater than 6 hours old, are punctures, or have been caused by a crush mechanism.

Patients who have had 1 or no previous injections should begin their immunization regimen with 0.5 mL of dT and, if the wound is prone to tetanus, simultaneously should be given tetanus antitoxin 250 Units IM.

Patients with partial immunity from 2 or more previous tetanus injections have enough immunity. The CDC recommends giving them only a booster of 0.5 mL dT, even with a tetanus-prone wound.

The patient over age 6 years who needs to complete the primary series of immunizations should be referred for a second dT .05 mL in 4 to 6 weeks, then again at 6 to 12 mos.

BITES

All bites from humans or animals involve inoculation of bacteria into a wound. This predisposes to infection, is considered tetanus prone, and may require prophylaxis for viral infections such as hepatitis or rabies. In addition, the care provider should document for legal purposes the circumstances of the bite, the bite number, type, locations, depth, and presence of any infection.

All bites require assessment for damage to underlying bone, muscle, tendon, and nerves, and should be irrigated and debrided to minimize bacterial contamination. Practice patterns differ about wound closure. Most clinicians will immediately close lacerations from bites on the face but not those on the hand, which instead are closed after 3 to 5 days or are packed open. Bites to the torso, arms, and legs are managed in a variety of different ways to minimize infection and scarring. All puncture wounds from bites close by secondary intent.

Rabies Prophylaxis

Rabies can be inoculated only into bites from those animals that carry it. The local animal control office is the expert on your community's animals and their likelihood of carrying rabies. Call them both to report the bite (mandatory in some locations) and to get advice on the need to administer rabies prophylaxis.

Rabies prophylaxis must be begun before symptoms of rabies begin or it is useless. Rabies incubation is at least 2 weeks as the virus migrates up the nerve to the brain. Consequently, extremity bites having a longer incubation that face or head bites.

Theoretically any animal can be a carrier of rabies, but herbivores such as rodents could only contract it from being bitten by a rabid animal before then biting a human. This is an unlikely scenario. On the other hand, animals such as bats can be heavily infected with rabies. Bites from bats routinely require rabies prophylaxis.

Victims of bites from dogs that are vaccinated against rabies, or that can be observed for signs of developing rabies for 2 weeks, usually do not need to get rabies prophylaxis. However, if the dog dies within these 2 weeks, even from injuries, then the dog's brain must be autopsied to look for signs of rabies infection and prompt prophylaxis given to the victim if rabies is detected.

Dog Bites

Dog bites can be grouped into those that are provoked or unprovoked. *Provoked* means the bite was incurred while petting, teasing, or reaching for the dog, when the dog was in great pain (from injury, for example), or when the victim entered the dog's yard or territory. Unprovoked attacks are more suspicious as being motivated by rabies.

Dog bites become infected from 5 to 15 percent of the time, most commonly from a variety of pathogens in dog saliva. These include *Staphylococcus aureus* and *Pasteurella multocida.* Prophylactic antibiotics are often given to prevent infection.

Infected wounds should be cultured and antibiotics should be initiated. Infection that occurs within 24 hours of injury is almost always from *Pasteurella multocida.* This can be treated with penicillin VK. When infection occurs more than 24 hours after the injury the likely organism is *Staphylococcus aureus* or Streptococcus. This should be treated with dicloxicillin or cephalexin. Progressive infection and sepsis can occur, and warrant intravenous antibiotics, hospital admission, and sometimes operative debridement.

Cat Bites

Cats have long, slender fangs that cause puncture wounds rather than lacerations. The major infecting organism is *Pasteurella multocida*. The patient will present with a rapidly progressive painful and swollen infection around the cat bite. The antibiotic of choice for these infections is penicillin. If there is doubt about the cause of infection, the coverage should be broadened to dicloxicillin or cephalexin similar to treatment of dog bites.

Prophylactic antibiotics are also given, especially for bites on the hand, and wounds are left open unless located on the face.

PLANTAR PUNCTURE WOUNDS

Wounds over the metatarsal-phalangeal joints warrant special attention, because the injury is usually from weight bearing on a sharp object that has penetrated deeply. Penetration to bone is frequent, and results in osteomyelitis in adults or osteochondritis in children for an overall rate of 0.4 to 0.6% of all punctures. Suspect these when the patient reports pain and redness 4 days to 1 week after injury and the wound is red or swollen. Because *Pseudomonas aeruginosa* has been cultured from the inner soles of tennis shoes and sneakers, the occurrence of Pseudomonas osteomyelitis after plantar puncture wound can be attributed to inculcation of Pseudomonas by the sharp object when it penetrates the shoe, the sole, the skin, and contacts the bone or cartilage.

An infected plantar puncture wound will contain a foreign body—usually a piece of fabric—about half the time. For this reason, careful inspection of any puncture wound for foreign body whenever the patient presents for care is essential. It is controversial whether probing under regional anesthesia or irrigation is useful, and giving prophylactic antibiotics is also controversial.

SUMMARY

The primary goal in wound repair is rapid healing without infection. Healing is more rapid through primary closure, so wound edges are approximated with sutures, staples, tape, or cyanoacrylate glue. Bites, other punctures, and contaminated wounds are so prone to infection that precedence is given to wound irrigation, debridement, and prophylactic antibiotic therapy.

With any type of wound, patients must be given careful aftercare instructions in an attempt to prevent complications or detect early signs of complications. Instructions should include:

Elevation of the injured part, if possible

Cleansing or dressing change instructions

Signs of infection: redness, pain, increasing swelling, red streak, pus discharge (thicker drainage after 3 days), fever

SUGGESTED READINGS

Cummings P: Antibiotics to prevent infection in patients with dog bite wounds: a meta-analysis of randomized trials, *Ann Emerg Med* 23(3):535-540, 1994.

Dire DJ et al: Prospective evaluation of topical antibiotics for preventing infections in uncomplicated soft tissue wounds repaired in the ED, *Acad Emerg Med* 2(1):4-10, 1995.

Dushoff IM: A stitch in time, *Emerg Med* October 15:22-28, 31-32, 45-50, 53-57, 1988.

Edlich RF, Rodeheaver GT, Thacker JG: The evaluation of wounds in the emergency department. In Tintinalli JE, Ruiz E, Krome RL, editors: *Emergency medicine: a comprehensive study guide,* ed 4, New York, 1996, McGraw-Hill.

Edlich RF, Rodeheaver GT, Thacker JG: Wound preparation. In Tintinalli JE, Ruiz E, Krome RL, editors: *Emergency medicine: a comprehensive study guide,* ed 4, New York, 1996, McGraw-Hill.

Edlich RF, Rodeheaver GT, Thacker JG: Methods for wound closure. In Tintinalli JE, Ruiz E, Krome RL, editors: *Emergency medicine: a comprehensive study guide,* ed 4, New York, 1996, McGraw-Hill.

Mehta PH et al: Contaminated wounds: infection rates with subcutaneous sutures, *Ann Emerg Med* 27(1): 43-48, 1996.

Quinn JV et al: A randomized controlled trial comparing tissue adhesive with suturing in the repair of pediatric facial lacerations, *Ann Emerg Med* 22(7): 1130, 1993.

Simon B: Principles of wound management. In Rose P et al, Editors: *Emergency Medicine,* ed 4, St Louis, 1998, Mosby.

Wahl RP, Eggleston J, Edlich RF: Puncture wounds and animal bites. In Tintinalli JE, Ruiz E, Krome RL, editors: *Emergency medicine: a comprehensive study guide,* ed 4, New York, 1996, McGraw-Hill.

Head Trauma

Debra DeLorenzo and Stephen H. Johnson

In 1994 motor vehicle crashes (both car and light truck) on public roads injured on estimated 4.78 million people. Of the injured, 118,000 suffered head injuries.[1]

Over one half of all trauma deaths in the United States each year are caused by head trauma. More than 4000 victims of head trauma are children.[2] More than 80,000 people sustain head or spinal cord injuries that result in disabilities. Of these people, 2000 remain in a vegetative state.[3] The most severe head injuries occur to those people who are riding in the front passenger's seat.[4] Of children with multiple trauma, 75% have a head injury.[4] The etiology of head injury is as follows:[4]

1. Motor vehicle crashes
2. Falls
3. Recreation injuries
4. Gunshot wounds
5. Stab wounds

ANATOMY

The brain is protected by hair, the scalp, the skull, the meningeal layers, and cerebrospinal fluid. The scalp has five layers: Skin, Connective tissue, Aponeurotica, Ligaments, and Periosteum. Because the scalp is very vascular, disruption causes profuse bleeding (Figure 22-1).

The skull is the bony structure that protects the brain. It is composed of the frontal, parietal, occipital, and temporal regions. It is divided into two major parts: the calvarium (the cranial vault) and the base.

The three meningeal layers provide protection for the brain and spinal cord. The layers are the pia mater, the arachnoid, and the dura mater (forming the mnemonic PAD, because they "pad" the brain). The pia mater is very thin and adheres to the cortex of the brain. The arachnoid layer is also very thin. Major arteries are located in the subarachnoid space. The dura mater adheres to the internal skull surface. The meningeal arteries are between the internal surface of the skull and the dura in the area known as the epidural space.

Cerebrospinal fluid (CSF) is produced in the ventricles of the brain and acts as a cushion for the brain and spinal cord. CSF is located in the subarachnoid space. The brain comprises 80% to 85% of the intracranial mass. It is composed of a collection of very delicate tissues and water. The main part of the brain, the cerebrum, is divided into two hemispheres and each hemisphere is subdivided into four lobes—frontal, parietal, temporal, and occipital.

The frontal lobe's function is primarily to conceptualize, abstract, and form judgments. Injury to this area may result in impaired judgment and reasoning, and the patient may frequently use foul language.

The parietal lobe is the area of highest integration and coordination of perception and interpretation of sensory phenomena. If a patient's parietal lobe suffers an injury, the patient will have difficulty with receptive communication.

The occipital lobe is the area responsible for vision. If there is injury to this area, the patient may develop blurred vision, diplopia, or even blindness.

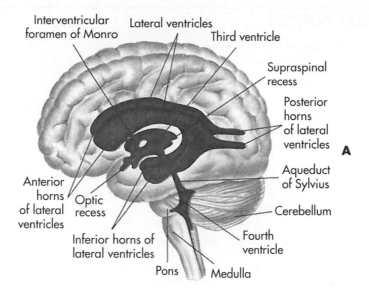

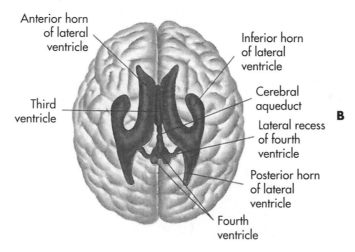

FIGURE 22-1. Cerebral ventricles. **A,** Lateral view. **B,** Superior view.
(From Thompson JM et al: *Mosby's clinical nursing*, ed 4, St Louis, 1997, Mosby.)

The temporal lobe (the lobe that looks like the thumb of a boxing glove) is thought to be responsible for memory. Injury to this area may affect recent memory.

The brainstem, which contains the reticular activating system, is responsible for consciousness. The lower part of the brainstem, the medulla, contains the cardiorespiratory center.

The cerebellum, located under the cerebrum and next to the brainstem, is responsible for movement and coordination. The tentorial notch, often the site of herniation, is located where the cerebrum and the midbrain meet.

THE CRANIAL NERVES

There are twelve pairs of cranial nerves. A description of each pair follows.

Olfactory (I)

This nerve is responsible for smell. It is tested by checking the patient's ability to smell. Injury to the olfactory nerve, common in head injury, will result in the ability to discern sweet and bitter taste only, because of loss of sense of smell.

Optic (II)

The optic nerve controls sight. If the optic nerve is intact, the patient will be able to count fingers, perceive light, or blink when the eyes are threatened.

Oculomotor (III), Trochlear (IV), Abducens (VI)

Check the patient's pupil size, shape and reactivity, and extraocular movement to assess the function of these nerves. The third cranial nerve passes through the tentorium. Brain herniation through the tentorium will produce pressure on the third nerve, causing the pupil to dilate and fix on the ipsilateral (same) side as the herniation. One millimeter difference in pupil size may be significant; however, 10% of the population normally have unequal pupils (anisocoria).

Trigeminal (V)

The trigeminal nerve controls facial sensation and jaw movement. Check for facial sensation, strength of mastication muscles, and jaw movement.

Facial (VII)

The facial nerve controls facial expression and taste in the anterior two thirds of the tongue. Have the patient raise the eyebrows, close the eyelids tightly to resistance, show the teeth, smile, frown, and puff the cheeks. If there is a peripheral ipsilateral injury, both the upper and lower face will be involved. If there is a central injury, the brow of the contralateral (opposite) side will be spared.

Acoustic and Auditory (VIII)

The eighth nerve is responsible for hearing and balance. It has two branches—the acoustic branch, which controls balance, and the auditory branch, which controls hearing. Assess the auditory branch by having the patient respond to a loud voice or clap. The eighth nerve can also be tested by using ice water calorics.

Glossopharyngeal (IX), Vagus (X)

These nerves are evaluated together because they are closely related anatomically and functionally. The glossopharyngeal nerve controls taste in the posterior two thirds of the tongue and sensation in the pharynx and nostrils. The vagus nerve controls the soft palate, pharynx and larynx, the heart, the lungs, and the stomach. Both nerves are tested by checking the gag and swallow reflexes and by assessing the patient's ability to discriminate between a salty taste and a sweet taste.

Spinal Accessory (XI)

The spinal accessory nerve controls movement of the sternocleidomastoid and trapezius muscles. To test this nerve, have the patient turn the head against resistance or shrug the shoulders. Do not test this nerve until the likelihood of cervical spine injury has been ruled out.

Hypoglossal (XII)

The hypoglossal nerve controls tongue movement. It can be tested by having the patient stick out the tongue. If, when the patient sticks out the tongue, the tongue is in midline, the nerve is considered intact.

THE BRIEF NEUROLOGICAL EXAMINATION

It is essential to obtain an initial neurological evaluation as soon as possible in the care and evaluation of the head-injured patient. The evaluation should then be repeated frequently. Using the DERM neurologic evaluation and the Glasgow Coma Scale, the caregiver can perform a brief neurologic examination in a consistent, precise manner, both observing clinical changes and measuring calculated improvements or deteriorations.

DERM

D = Depth of Coma
Use a stimulus/describe the response:

STIMULUS	RESPONSE (DESCRIBE)
Voice	Appropriate (Inappropriate)
Touch	Appropriate (Inappropriate)
Pain	Appropriate (Inappropriate)

E = Eyes
Note pupillary response to light and accommodation. If the corpus callosum is intact, there will be simultaneous consensual reaction of the unstimulated pupil with light stimulation. (Note that 10% of the population have unequal pupils [anisocoria] with no disease.)

R = Respirations
Note regular or irregular rate, rhythm, and depth.

M = Motor/Movement
Does the patient move extremities? All?

Glasgow Coma Scale*

The Glasgow Coma Scale has been designed to quantitatively relate consciousness to motor response, verbal response, and eye opening. Coma is defined as no response and no eye opening. Scores of 7 or less on the Glasgow Scale qualify as coma; scores of 9 or more do not qualify as coma. The examiner determines the best response the patient can make to a set of standardized stimuli. Higher points are assigned to responses that indicate increasing degrees of arousal.

1. **Best motor response.** (Examiner determines the best response with either arm.)
   a. *6 points.* Obeys simple commands. Raises arms on request or holds up specified number of fingers. Releasing a grip (not grasping, which can be reflexive) is also an appropriate test.
   b. *5 points.* Localizes noxious stimuli, fails to obey commands, but can move either arm toward a noxious cutaneous stimulus and eventually contacts it with the hand. The stimulus should be maximal and applied in various locations, for example, sternal pressure or trapezius pinch.

*Modified from Teasdale G, Jennett B: *Lancet* 2:81, 1974.

    c. *4 points.* Flexion withdrawal. Responds to noxious stimulus with arm flexion, but does not localize it with the hand.

    d. *3 points.* Abnormal flexion. Adducts shoulder, flexes and pronates arm, flexes wrist and makes a fist in response to a noxious stimulus. Previously known as decorticate posturing.

    e. *2 points.* Abnormal extension. Adducts and internally rotates shoulders, extends forearm, flexes wrist and makes a fist in response to a noxious stimulus. Previously known as decerebrate posturing.

    f. *1 point.* No motor response.

A problem with the Glasgow Coma Scale is that it scores "best motor response." How should we interpret the findings if we see flexion in one arm and extension in the other?

2. **Best verbal response.** (Examiner determines the best response after arousal. Noxious stimuli are employed if necessary.) Omit this test if the patient is dysphasic, has oral injuries, or is intubated. Place a check mark after the other two test category scores after totaling to indicate omission of the verbal response section.

    a. *5 points.* Oriented patient. Can converse and relate who he is, where he is, the year, and the month.

    b. *4 points.* Confused patient. Is not fully oriented or demonstrates confusion.

    c. *3 points.* Verbalizes. Does not engage in sustained conversation, but uses intelligible words in an exclamation (curse) or in a disorganized manner that is nonsensical.

    d. *2 points.* Vocalizes. Makes moaning or groaning sounds that are not recognizable words.

    e. *1 point.* No vocalization. Does not make any sound, even in response to noxious stimulus.

3. **Eye opening.** (Examiner determines the minimum stimulus that evokes opening one or both eyes.) If the patient cannot realistically open the eyes because of bandages or lid edema, write "E" after the total test score to indicate omission of this component.

    a. *4 points.* Eyes open spontaneously.

    b. *3 points.* Eyes open to speech. Patient opens eyes in response to command or on being called by name.

    c. *2 points.* Eyes open to noxious stimuli.

    d. *1 point.* No eye opening in response to noxious stimuli.

The examiner should remember that the Glasgow Coma Scale may not be valid in patients who have used alcohol or other mind-altering drugs, are hypoglycemic, in shock (with systemic blood pressure less than 80 mm Hg), or who are hypothermic (below 34° C).[4]

DIAGNOSTIC EXAMINATION TECHNIQUES/DEVICES USED IN HEAD INJURY

Cross-Table Lateral Cervical Spine X-ray

Of all patients with significant head trauma, approximately 10% have concurrent spinal cord trauma. The caregiver must ensure that the C-spine is immobilized and protected while radiographic studies are obtained to rule out fracture. If a cross-table lateral film cannot adequately visualize the entire C-spine, to include T1, a "swimmer's view" should be obtained. (Figure 22-2).

Skull X-rays

Skull x-rays offer the least amount of clinically useful information in terms of treatment intervention. The patient should be treated systematically and not on the basis of the x-ray film. If, however, CT is not available, a skull x-ray may confirm the diagnosis of skull fracture.

Computerized Axial Tomography (CT Scan, CAT Scan, EMI Scan)

CT scans detect 90% of head trauma accurately. The test should be done quickly if the patient has an altered level of consciousness, hemiparesis, or any kind of aphasia.

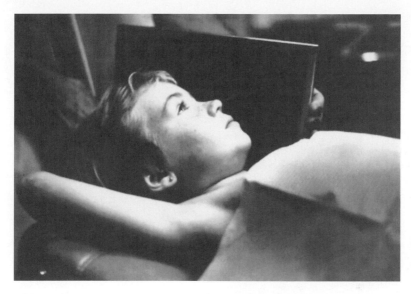

FIGURE 22-2. X-ray film; swimmer's view.

Magnetic Resonance Imaging (MRI, NMR)

The atoms of the body broadcast signals from which images may be created. These broadcasts can be tracked through nuclear magnetic resonance, using ionizing radiation or sound waves as a noninvasive method to obtain a visual image. By using NMR, the caregiver can also chemically analyze cellular content by measuring phosphorus emissions. NMR is not generally used in trauma because it cannot be used if the patient is unstable, uncooperative, and unable to remain still.

Pupillary Responses
Normal reactions

Pupils constrict when exposed directly to light.
Light shined into one pupil causes the other pupil to constrict as well.

Abnormal reactions

Fixed pinpoint pupils indicate pons involvement or use of opiates.
Ptosis may indicate third cranial nerve involvement.
Dilated fixed pupil (unilateral) indicates third cranial nerve involvement (early).
Bilateral, fixed pupils indicate severe brainstem injury and may represent brain death.

Reflexes
Corneal

Touch the cornea with a wisp of cotton from a swab.
Normal reaction—blinks eye
Abnormal reaction—no response

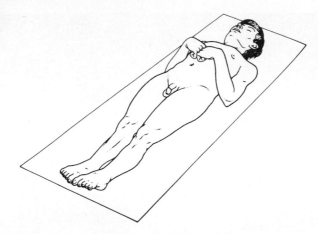

FIGURE 22-3. Abnormal flexion.

Gag

(Cranial nerves IX and X)
Normal reaction—intact
Abnormal reaction—loss of gag reflex

Deep tendon

Scored from 0 to 4.
0 = Absent
1 = Decreased
2 = Normal
3 = Increased
4 = Hyperactive
Normal reaction—normal reflexes
Abnormal reaction—hypoactivity or absence of reaction indicates cerebellar lesions or intricate peripheral nerve or anterior horn cell disease; hyperactivity indicates pyramidal tract lesions and sometimes psychogenic disorders.

Babinski

Checked by applying cutaneous stimulation to the plantar surface of the foot.
Normal reaction—Great toe and other toes flex.
Abnormal (positive) reaction—Great toe extends upward and other toes fan out toward the head ("it points to where the problem is"). This is a normal reaction in children under age 2. No response at all is also considered an abnormal reaction.

Posturing

Elicited by verbal or painful stimulation.
Abnormal flexion (Figure 22-3)—arms flex, wrists flex, legs and feet extend. Indicates a lesion *above* midbrain. This is also known as decorticate posturing.
Abnormal extension (Figure 22-4)—arms extend, wrists flex, legs and feet extend. Indicates brainstem herniation. This is also known as decerebrate posturing.

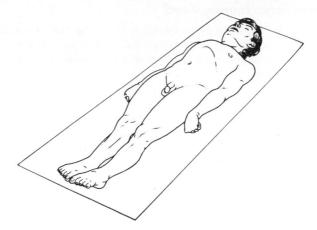

FIGURE 22-4. Abnormal extension.

SPECIFIC HEAD INJURY CONDITIONS

Scalp Lacerations

A scalp laceration is one of the most frequently seen types of head injuries. If the scalp is lacerated, it may bleed profusely because of its ample vascular supply. A scalp laceration may be caused by any blunt or penetrating trauma to the head. When the head hits the car windshield, the scalp will absorb the first 33% of the force.[4]

■ **SIGNS AND SYMPTOMS**
Direct observation of the laceration
Bleeding

■ **DIAGNOSIS**
Clinical observation of the laceration

■ **THERAPEUTIC INTERVENTIONS**
Apply direct or peripheral pressure to control bleeding.
Palpate underlying skull for fractures.
Protect cervical spine. (It is imperative to rule out cervical spine injury with any head injury.)
Cleanse laceration area with surgical prep solution.
Debride devitalized tissue.
Sutures or staples may be used to close wound as indicated.
Apply small sterile dressing or open to air and Bacitracin ointment.
Ensure tetanus prophylaxis.
Give aftercare instructions for both wound management and head trauma.

Skull Fracture

Examine the patient's skull for bumps, defects, bruises, or lacerations. The presence of a skull fracture does not necessarily indicate that a cerebral injury has occurred. There are three types of skull fractures:
Simple
Depressed
Basilar

Simple skull fractures (linear/nondisplaced)

A simple skull fracture is a linear crack in the surface of the skull. The bone is not displaced, and therapeutic intervention involves observation of the patient for other associated injuries. If there are no other obvious findings and a good support system (family or friends) is present, the patient may be discharged to home with careful head trauma aftercare instructions.

Depressed skull fracture

A depressed skull fracture is a depression of a segment of the bony skull. If the fragment is depressed beneath the table of the adjacent bone by more than 5 mm, surgery must be performed to elevate the depression and decrease the possibility of intracranial infection. If the depression overlies the sinuses (sagittal or lateral), there may be profuse bleeding, underlying brain contusion, or tears of the cerebral tissue.

■ **SIGNS AND SYMPTOMS**
Observation/palpation of the deformity
Bleeding
Altered level of consciousness

■ **DIAGNOSIS**
Observation/palpation of the deformity
X-ray
CT scan

■ **THERAPEUTIC INTERVENTIONS**
Ensure airway management, cervical spine protection.
Control external bleeding.
Place sterile dressing over wound.
Surgical intervention to:
    Elevate the depressed segment.
    Remove fragments.
    Debride necrotic brain tissue.
    Remove hematomas.
    Repair lacerations.
Consider antibiotics.
Ensure tetanus prophylaxis.

Basilar skull fracture

A basilar skull fracture is a fracture at the base of the skull. On impact, all forces go to two bones: the sphenoid (causing periorbital ecchymosis), or the petrous temple (causing Battle's sign). The danger of a basilar skull fracture is that it may cross the course of the middle meningeal artery, disrupting it and causing:
    A hematoma of the scalp
    An epidural hematoma (cause of 90% of epidurals)
    A subarachnoid hemorrhage
    An intracerebral bleed
    In addition, a cerebrospinal fistula may occur. The mechanism of injury is usually a significant blow to the head.

■ **SIGNS AND SYMPTOMS**
Headache
Nausea and/or vomiting
Scalp laceration
Periorbital ecchymosis ("raccoon eyes") (Figure 22-5)
    Unilateral or bilateral periorbital ecchymosis that occurs as a result of intraorbital bleeding from an intraorbital root fracture or a cribiform plate fracture

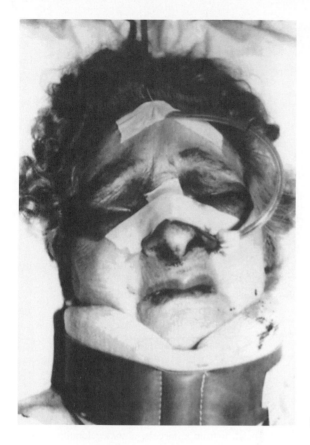

FIGURE 22-5. Periorbital ecchymosis (raccoon eyes).

Battle's sign (Figure 22-6)
    Formation of an ecchymosis behind the ear in the mastoid region. It usually occurs 12 to 24 hours after
        injury.
Hematotympanum
    Blood behind the eardrum caused by temporal bone fracture near the tympanic membrane
Cerebrospinal fluid leak (CSF rhinorrhea, CSF otorrhea)
    Caused by a fracture of part of the cranial vault that creates an opening between the cranium and the
        outside of the cranium. CSF otorrhea is caused by a crack in the petrous temple bone. If the tympanic
        membrane is intact, CSF may exit via the eustachian tube. The patient may complain of a salty taste in
        the mouth. CSF contains 15.9 mEq of sodium chloride. A scar formation from an old basilar skull frac-
        ture may dislodge, forming an open fistula into the cranium and a CSF leak. Blood and CSF separate to
        form two distinct rings, known as a "target sign," "ring sign," or "halo sign" on filter paper or bed
        clothing.
■ **THERAPEUTIC INTERVENTIONS**
Protect cervical spine.
Do *not* attempt to stop CSF leak.
Do *not* put nasogastric tube or endotracheal tube through the nose—use the oral route.
Do a baseline neurologic exam.
Obtain an x-ray film (basilar skull fractures are not seen on 25% of routine skull films).
Consider antibiotics.

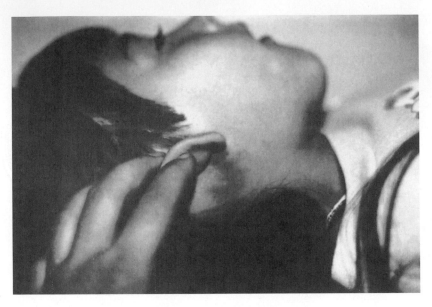

FIGURE 22-6. Battle's sign.

Ensure tetanus prophylaxis.
Admit patient to hospital for observation.

Concussion

A concussion usually occurs as a result of a direct blow to the head or from an acceleration/deceleration injury where brain tissue impacts with the inside of the bony skull. A brief interruption of the reticular activating system occurs, causing a short period of amnesia. This is a transient, limited process that usually requires no therapeutic intervention, but the patient may take up to 3 months to fully recover. Concussion is often accompanied by a coup/contrecoup injury (Figure 22-7).

■ **SIGNS AND SYMPTOMS**
Nausea and vomiting
Possible brief loss of sight or "seeing stars" (precipitated by occipital lobe involvement)
Uncontrolled use of foul language (caused by frontal lobe involvement)
Headache
Loss of consciousness
Flaccid paralysis
Hypertension or hypotension
Apnea

■ **THERAPEUTIC INTERVENTIONS**
Protect cervical spine.
If nausea and vomiting are severe and dehydration results, admit to hospital for rehydration.
If loss of consciousness is more than 2 to 3 minutes, admit to hospital for observation.
If the skull is fractured, admit to hospital for observation.
Administer *non*narcotic analgesics for headache to observe level of consciousness.
If family member and/or friend is reliable, patient may be discharged to home with careful verbal and written aftercare instructions.

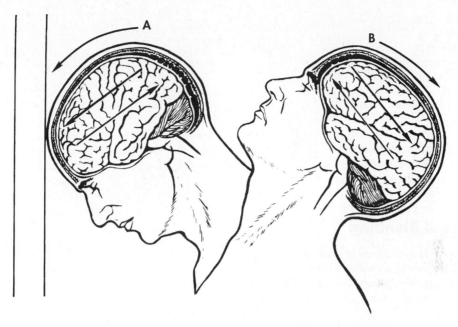

FIGURE 22-7. **A,** Coup: the brain impacts with the skull, during the point of impact of the skull with another force. **B,** Contrecoup: the brain accelerates forward after the initial impact, thereby causing an additional injury as the interior brain impacts with the skull.

Postconcussion syndrome

Late sequelae of concussion may include:

Headache   Syncopal episodes
Nausea   Loss of coordination
Memory loss   Numbness
Decreased concentration   Tinnitus ("ringing" in ears)
Decreased organizational skills   Diplopia (double vision)
Difficulty handling more than one task at   Loss of menstrual periods
    once   Breast secretions

■ **DIAGNOSIS**
Reevaluation
CT scan (may be normal, but will be evident on MRI)
MRI
■ **THERAPEUTIC INTERVENTIONS**
Treat in accordance with findings.

Contusion

A contusion is an actual bruise on the surface of the brain causing a structural alteration of the brain.
■ **SIGNS AND SYMPTOMS**
Altered level of consciousness for more than 6 hours
Nausea and vomiting
Vision disturbances
Neurologic dysfunction
    Weakness

  Ataxia
  Hemiparesis
  Confusion
  Speech problems
 Seizures (5% of patients)
■ **DIAGNOSIS**
 Clinical signs and symptoms
 CT scan
 MRI
■ **THERAPEUTIC INTERVENTIONS**
 Protect cervical spine.
 Admit to hospital for observation.
 Give antiemetics.

Intracranial Bleeding

The three meningeal layers of the brain are the pia, the arachnoid, and the dura. Lesions or bleeding sites in the head are named according to their location in respect to these meningeal layers (Figure 22-8).

 One compensatory mechanism for increasing edema or blood in the cranial vault is for fluid to be squeezed out of the cerebral sinuses and the cerebral sinuses to compress. This mechanism can accommodate approximately 75 ml of edema or fluid before more serious consequences occur.

Epidural (extradural) hematoma

An epidural hematoma is a collection of blood between the skull and the dura mater (Figure 22-9) in the epidural space. This bleeding may be venous, but is usually arterial. Venous bleeding is rare and may be manageable medically. Epidural bleeds occur in 1% to 2% of all head injuries.[5] The usual etiology is a middle meningeal artery rupture or a tear of a dural sinus. Death is often rapid because the bleed is usually arterial,

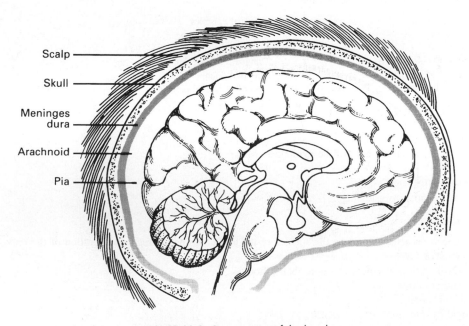

Scalp
Skull
Meninges dura
Arachnoid
Pia

FIGURE 22-8. Cross-section of the head.

causing much pressure and uncal herniation. It is most commonly seen with a temporal or parietal skull fracture near the middle meningeal artery. Of patients with epidural bleeds, however, 50% will show no evidence of skull fracture. Mortality rate is between 25% and 50%, and morbidity rate is equally high.[5]

■ **SIGNS AND SYMPTOMS**

Short period of loss of consciousness, caused by a concussion, followed by a lucid period, followed by a loss
   of consciousness, caused by the bleed. There may be loss of consciousness without a lucid period.

Before unconsciousness, complaint of severe headache

Hemiparesis

Ipsilateral (same side) dilated pupil

Bradycardia

Increased blood pressure

■ **DIAGNOSIS**

CT scan

■ **THERAPEUTIC INTERVENTIONS**

Airway management

Protecting cervical spine

Ventilation with 100% oxygen

   Positive pressure to maintain P_{CO_2} at 26 to 28 torr. (deliberate hypocapnia).

   When P_{CO_2} rises, vasodilation occurs and blood volume in the brain is increased. When this occurs, intracranial pressure increases and heightens the possibility of brainstem herniation. If P_{CO_2} level is reduced, intracranial pressure will be decreased. Hyperventilation is usually only effective to decrease intracranial pressure the first 48 hours following injury.

Oral intubation

   Administer 25 mg lidocaine before endotracheal intubation. Lidocaine causes a very transient (2 to 3 minutes) decrease in intracranial pressure that may prevent the possibility of increased intracranial pressure as a result of the process of endotracheal intubation.[4]

Diuretic agent

   Mannitol 1 to 1.5 mg/kg bolus, an osmotic diuretic

Head of bed elevated to 30 degrees

IVs at a maintenance rate (100 to 125 cc of normal saline or 0.45 of normal saline)

Possible surgical intervention

Subdural hematoma

A subdural hemorrhage is bleeding between the dura mater and the arachnoid membrane in the subdural space (Figure 22-10). It is usually caused by severe blunt trauma, such as an acceleration/deceleration incident, where a venous bridge (where it crosses the subdural space) or cortical artery is torn. It is the most frequently seen type of intracranial bleed and carries a 73% mortality rate and a 90% morbidity rate.[4]

   It may occur rapidly (acute) or develop over a period of days, weeks, or months (chronic). If a subdural

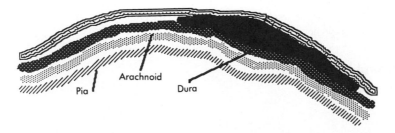

FIGURE 22-9. An acute epidural hematoma.

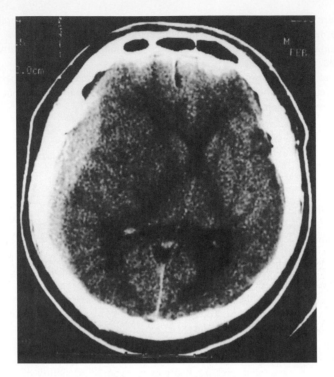

FIGURE 22-10. Subdural hematoma.

hemorrhage is seen in a child less than 1 year of age, the etiology should be considered child abuse until proven otherwise.

If a subdural hemorrhage is not rapidly surgically controlled, transtentorial herniation and death may ensue (Figure 22-11). If there is an operative delay of 4 or more hours on operable subdural hemorrhages, mortality rate increases to 94%.[4] If the bleeding is bilateral, the diagnostic "ventricular shift" may not be seen on computerized tomography. Chronic subdural hemorrhage may occur nontraumatically in the elderly and in chronic alcoholics.

■ SIGNS AND SYMPTOMS
Loss of consciousness
Positive Babinski reflex
Fixed dilated pupil(s)
Hemiparesis
Hyperreflexia to abnormal flexion to abnormal extension to flaccidity
Abnormal respirations (type depends on level of herniation)
Elevated temperature

Chronic subdural hematoma

■ SIGNS AND SYMPTOMS
Headache
Ataxia
Incontinence
Increasing dementia
Decreasing level of consciousness

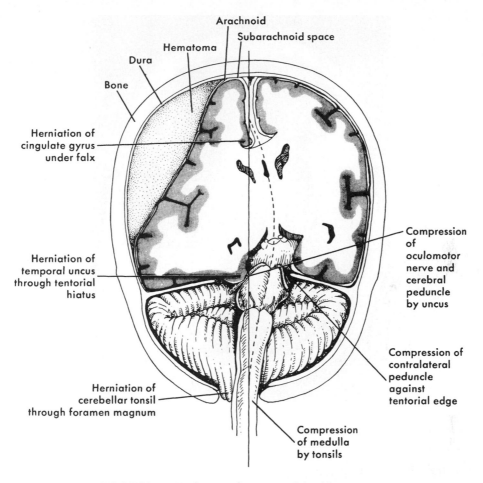

FIGURE 22-11. Mechanism of injury in subdural hematoma.

■ **DIAGNOSIS**
Clinical findings
CT scan
MRI
■ **THERAPEUTIC INTERVENTIONS**
Airway management
Protecting cervical spine
    Oral intubation
Ventilation with 100% oxygen
Diuretic agents
    Mannitol
IVs at maintenance rate (100 to 125 ml/hr of normal saline or 0.45 of normal saline per hour)
Nonaspirin antipyretics
Surgical intervention
    If the patient is an infant with retinal hemorrhage and abnormal flexion, consider the option of subdural tap
        in the emergency department.

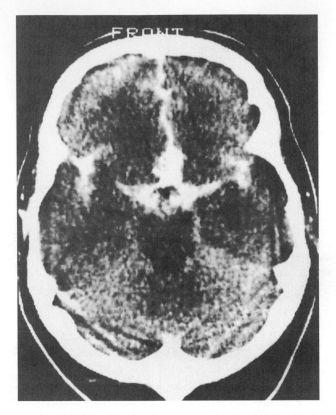

FIGURE 22-12. Subarachnoid hemorrhage.

Subarachnoid hemorrhage

A subarachnoid hemorrhage occurs between the arachnoid membrane and the pia mater (Figure 22-12). It may result from severe head trauma, severe hypertension, aneurysm, or an arteriovenous malformation rupture. The most common cause is trauma.

■ **SIGNS AND SYMPTOMS**
Severe, "piercing" headache
Meningismus
Nausea and vomiting
Delirium, obtundation, syncope, coma
Photophobia
Respiratory abnormalities
  Type depends on level of herniation
Fixed dilated pupils
Papilledema, retinal hemorrhage
Focal motor signs
Seizures

■ **DIAGNOSIS**
Clinical signs and symptoms
CT scan
MRI

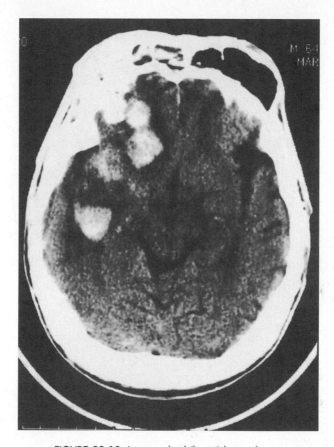

FIGURE 22-13. Intracerebral (brain) hemorrhage.

■ **THERAPEUTIC INTERVENTIONS**
Airway management.
Protecting cervical spine if suspected trauma
Ventilation with 100% oxygen
Surgical intervention
IVs at a maintenance rate (100 to 125 ml/hr of normal saline or 0.45 of normal saline)

Intracerebral (brain) hemorrhage

An intracerebral hemorrhage (Figure 22-13) is a hemorrhage into the brain tissue or the cerebral/ventricular sinuses. It may result from a penetrating injury, a diffuse injury, or a laceration, particularly in the basilar area of the skull where there are bony prominences. In addition to the hemorrhage, there is usually an additional area of edema. Overall prognosis is poor.

■ **SIGNS AND SYMPTOMS**
Loss of consciousness
Fixed dilated pupils
Abnormal respirations
   Type in accordance with level of herniation
Abnormal motor function
   Type in accordance with level of herniation

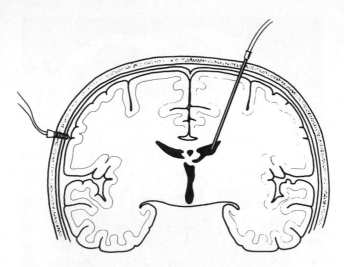

FIGURE 22-14. Intracranial pressure monitoring.
(From Budassi SA: *J Emerg Nurs*, May, 1979.)

■ **DIAGNOSIS**
Clinical observation
CT scan
MRI
■ **THERAPEUTIC INTERVENTIONS**
Airway management
Ventilation with 100% oxygen
Diuretics
    Mannitol
Surgical intervention
IVs at a maintenance rate (100 to 125 ml/hr)

Brainstem Herniation

Brainstem herniation occurs when the brainstem herniates through the tentorial notch or the foramen magnum or the cerebellar tonsils jam into the foramen magnum causing severe permanent neurologic deficits. It occurs as a result of an expanding hematoma in a meningeal space or in cerebral tissue or cerebral/vascular sinuses, cerebral edema or a mass that propels brain and brainstem tissue toward the path of least resistance, which is usually the tentorial notch or the foramen magnum.

Transtentorial (uncal) herniation

A transtentorial herniation occurs when lesions or bleeds at the lateral middle fossa or the temporal lobe cause the inner edge (basal edge) of the uncus and the hippocampal gyrus to be pushed toward the midline and into the lateral edge of the tentorial notch. Pressure builds at the tentorial notch, causing the midbrain to be pushed into the opposite side of the tentorial notch. At this point, the third cranial nerve (oculomotor) and posterior cerebral artery may become caught between the part of the uncus that has herniated and the edge of the tentorial notch.

■ **EARLY SIGNS OF TRANSTENTORIAL HERNIATION**
Decreased level of consciousness
Ipsilateral or bilateral dilated pupils
Cheyne-Stokes breathing

Contralateral hemiparesis
Positive Babinski sign
■ **LATE SIGNS OF TRANSTENTORIAL HERNIATION**
Unconsciousness
Bilateral fixed dilated pupils
Central neurogenic breathing
Abnormal extension

Central herniation (rostral-caudal deterioration)

When intracranial pressure increases and is uniformly distributed throughout the brain, the cerebral tissue is forced downward, causing the cerebellar tonsils to herniate through the foramen magnum, compressing the medulla.

The brain, cerebrospinal fluid, and blood are contained in the skull, which allows very little space for expansion of these substances. When one of these substances increases in volume, the others compensate by decreasing their volume, thereby maintaining a constant intracranial pressure. This compensation can only occur when there is a slight increase in volume. If volume increase is excessive, intracranial pressure will rise.

When intracranial pressure increases beyond mean arterial pressure, the brain cells become anoxic because of inadequate perfusion of brain tissue and eventually suffer irreparable damage. The brain tissue itself begins to shift, compressing the ventricles and forcing brain tissue into the tentorial notch. This compresses the brainstem and the third cranial nerve.

It is therefore necessary to avoid, or at least moderate, those activities that cause an increase in intracranial pressure in those patients who are already at risk of increased pressure.

Signs and symptoms of supratentorial herniation are: coma from impairment of the reticular activating system; changes in pupil size and reaction to light, including the dilated, fixed pupil; decreased motor response, decerebrate posturing if the herniation is at the midbrain level or decorticate posturing if the herniation is at the thalamic level, and flaccidity if the herniation has reached the level of the lower pons; and Cheyne-Stokes, central neurogenic, or ataxic respirations.

Intracranial pressure monitoring is appropriate in patients with severe head injury and an abnormal CT scan (Figure 22-14). Severe head injury is defined as a Glasgow coma scale of 3 to 8 after resuscitation. Abnormal findings on a CT scan may include hematoma, contusion, edema or severe brain swelling with absence of basal cisterns.

Normal intracranial pressure (ICP) is 0 to 10 mmHG (0 to 136mm H_2O). More important is cerebral perfusion pressure (CPP). CPP = mean blood pressure ICP. CPP should be maintained greater than 70 in head injury.

ICP is most commonly monitored using a fiber optic transducer system. The fiber optic cable is inside either a parenchymal or intraventricular catheter. The parenchymal catheter is inserted into brain substance and can also be used to monitor brain temperature. The intraventricular catheter serves as both a drainage and pressure monitoring system. Both systems are extremely accurate and are closed systems that require little nursing attention. Digital readouts can be incorporated on most ICU transducer monitoring systems.

ICP monitoring is useful as a guide to the administration of osmotic diuretics, hyperventilation and sedative analgesics. ICP monitoring improves prognostic accuracy and may improve outcome. Familiarity with monitoring is essential.

■ **EARLY SIGNS OF CENTRAL HERNIATION**
Restlessness to lethargy
Pupils constricted, but equal and reactive
Cheyne-Stokes breathing with yawns and sighs that deteriorate to central neurogenic breathing
■ **LATE SIGNS OF CENTRAL HERNIATION**
Unconsciousness
Midpoint to dilated fixed pupils

■ **DIAGNOSIS**
Clinical observation
CT scan
Increased intracranial pressure
■ **THERAPEUTIC INTERVENTIONS**
Airway management. Protect cervical spine
　　Oral tracheal intubation
　　Consider lidocaine IV just before intubation
Hyperventilation using 100% oxygen with positive pressure
Diuretics
　　Mannitol
Surgical intervention

SPECIAL CONSIDERATIONS

Impaled Objects

An object that is impaled into the skull and cranial vault may or may not produce a severe injury. The extent of trauma depends on the location of the wound and the caliber and velocity of the impaled object.

■ **DIAGNOSIS**
Observation
X-ray
CT scan
■ **THERAPEUTIC INTERVENTIONS**
Airway management.
Protect cervical spine.
Provide oxygen.
Do *not* remove impaled object!
Secure impaled object.
Control bleeding.
Apply sterile dressing around impaled object.
Give psychological support.
Treat for other associated findings.
Ensure tetanus prophylaxis.

Seizures After Head Trauma

Patients often develop seizures after a head trauma incident. The seizures may result from a direct injury to the brain or increased intracranial pressure. Seizure activity will cause P_{CO_2} to rise and P_{O_2} to fall, resulting in cerebral edema and cerebral hypoxia.

■ **SIGNS AND SYMPTOMS**
Seizure activity
Other neurologic findings
■ **DIAGNOSIS**
Clinical observation
Clinical history
■ **THERAPEUTIC INTERVENTIONS**
Airway management
Oxygen

Diazepam (Valium) IV as prescribed to control seizure activity (usually 2.5 to 5 mg IV, titrated to effect)

If the seizure continues, administer 1 g phenytoin IV.

Consider phenobarbital and/or general anesthesia (a neuromuscular blocking agent) if seizures remain uncontrolled.

SUMMARY OF THERAPEUTIC INTERVENTIONS FOR ALL PATIENTS WITH SEVERE HEAD INJURIES

Maintain airway.

Protect cervical spine.

Give 100% oxygen with positive pressure.

Maintaining Pco_2 at 26 to 28 torr in the first 48 hours after injury is controversial among neurosurgeons.

Provide diuretics

Mannitol

Obtain cervical spine x-ray film.

Maintain IV fluids at 100 to 125 mL/hr of normal saline or 0.45 of normal saline.

Monitor and record baseline and serial neurologic exams.

Maintain head in midline position.

Keep head elevated at 30 degrees unless contraindicated by spinal injury.

Foley and hourly urine output

Monitor temperature.

Keep patient normothermic (use cooling blanket or alpha blockade [2.5 to 3 mg thorazine] if necessary).

Consider neurosurgery consult.

Assess for other injuries.

Consider transfer to appropriate facility.

Minimize external stimulation.

Consider dextrose 50% and naloxone 0.8 mg IV if unsure if unconscious state is caused by trauma.

Draw toxicology or alcohol screen if indicated.

Victims of head trauma often have serious to life-threatening injuries. The patient's prognosis and outcome will depend upon how quickly the patient is diagnosed and treated. It is imperative, therefore, for emergency nurses to be familiar and comfortable with identification and treatment of head trauma.

REFERENCES

1. National Highway Traffic Safety Administration, 1992-1994.
2. Kraus JF et al: The incidence of acute brain injury and serious impairment in a defined population, *Am J Epidemiol* 119:186, 1984.
3. Kraus JF: Epidemiology of brain injury. In Cooper PR, editor: *Head injury,* ed 2, Baltimore, 1986, Williams and Wilkins.
4. Newbury L, Emergency Nurses Association: *Sheehy's emergency nursing,* ed 5, St Louis, 1998, Mosby.
5. Rosen P et al: *Emergency medicine: concepts and clinical practice,* ed 4, St Louis, 1997, Mosby.

Spinal Cord and Neck Trauma

Mary Dahlgren Gunnels

It is estimated that there are 10,000 new cases of spinal cord injury each year in the United States, which represents an incidence of approximately 40 persons per million population. Motor vehicle crashes cause approximately 35% of all spinal cord injuries, followed by acts of violence, falls, and recreational sports.[1,2] Alcohol and substance abuse, coupled with high-risk behaviors (for example, extreme sports), result in spinal cord injuries being most common to the young adult male between the ages of 15 and 30 years.[2,3,4]

The spinal cord and vertebrae can be injured as a result of fractures, dislocations, or subluxations that produce abnormal anatomic movements:

Hypertension	The head is forced back and the neck is placed in an overextended position.
Hyperflexion	The head is forced forward and the neck is placed in an overflexed position.
Axial loading	A severe blow to the top of the head results in a blunt force that transmits into the spinal column.
Compression	A force from above and a concurrent force or nongiving surface from below.
Lateral bend	The head and neck are bent to one side, beyond normal limits.
Overrotation	The head and neck turn beyond normal limits.
Distraction	The vertebrae are pulled out of alignment.

THE SPINAL CORD

A weight as little as 400 mg (approximately the weight of a Kennedy half-dollar) dropped onto the spinal cord from a 7 inch height can cause permanent injury.[5] Intramedullary hemorrhage and edema, not severing or transection, cause the majority of spinal cord injuries.[5]

The spinal cord is an integral part of the central nervous system. It controls consciousness, regulates body movement and function, and transmits nerve impulses. It has both voluntary and involuntary functions. The spinal cord is enclosed in a canal that extends the length of the vertebral column. Spinal nerves extend through openings in the vertebrae. The anterior part of the spinal cord contains motor tracts. The posterior part of the spinal cord contains sensory tracts. It is possible to have an incomplete lesion, where motor function below the level of the lesion is gone and sensation remains intact.

The spinal cord transmits nerve impulses to and from the brain and the body to regulate function and movement. It is, like the brain, protected by the three layers of meninges—the pia, the arachnoid and the dura, the vertebrae, and the paravertebral muscles. The openings in the vertebrae form the canal through which the spinal cord passes. The spinal cord itself may be concussed, contused, or transected. A concussed cord produces transient changes that can resolve within minutes or hours. A contused spinal cord may result in a structural defect and permanent disability. Spinal cord transection causes permanent disability or death. The disability causes loss of motor and sensory functions below the level of the injury. An acute transection can cause spinal shock (see Chapter 9).

The immediate problems with cervical spine injury are to ensure airway maintenance and adequate breathing. Cervical vertebrae 3, 4, and 5 contain the phrenic nerve. Injury at or above this level causes loss of control of the diaphragm (the main muscle of respiration). Survival from such an injury is rare—lesions above C3 or

C4 level can result in death. Recent advances in resuscitation have enabled more persons with quadriplegia to survive despite the dramatic nature of this type of spinal cord injury.

Innervations at the level of the vertebrae include the following:

C2 to C4	diaphragm, neck muscles
C5, C6	biceps brachii, deltoid, triceps brachii, wrist extensors
C6 to T1	latissimus dorsi, hand muscles
T2 to T7	intercostal muscles
T6 to L1	abdominal muscles
T12 to L2	quadratus lumborum
L1 to L5	leg muscles
L2 to L3	psoas muscles
L2 to L4	quadriceps
L4 to L5	tibialis anterior
S1	bowel and bladder

LESIONS OF	PRODUCE
C3, C4, or above	Respiratory arrest; flaccid paralysis; quadriplegia
C5, C6	Reduced respiratory effort; near total dependence; flaccid paralysis; quadriplegia
C7	Reduced respiratory effort; near total dependence; splints necessary for forearms to function; quadriplegia
T1	Reduced respiratory effort; partial dependence; paraplegia
T1, T2	Reduced respiratory effort; complete independence; paraplegia
T7	Complete independence; walk with long leg braces; paraplegia
L4	Complete independence; walk with foot braces; paraplegia

INCOMPLETE CORD LESIONS

Central Cord Syndrome

The most common cause of central cord syndrome (Figure 23-1) is hyperextension. It is commonly seen in the elderly following a fall. This type of injury produces loss of function (lower motor neuron disease) in the upper extremities; bowel and bladder function are maintained.

Anterior Cord Syndrome

Anterior cord syndrome (Figure 23-2) is usually seen in flexion injuries. It results from an occlusion of the anterior spinal artery, a herniated nucleus pulposus (ruptured disc), or a transection of the anterior portion of the cord. The patient experiences hyperesthesia, hypoalgesia, and either incomplete or complete paralysis. The patient is able to feel vibrations and maintain proprioception because of preserved posterior column function.

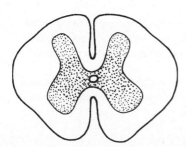

FIGURE 23-1. Central cord syndrome.

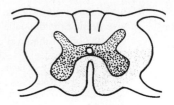

FIGURE 23-2. Anterior cord syndrome.

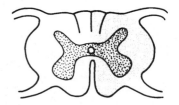

FIGURE 23-3. Brown-Séquard syndrome.

Brown-Séquard Syndrome

Involvement of the hemisection of the cord in the anterior-posterior plane is known as Brown-Séquard syndrome (Figure 23-3). It is most often caused by penetrating trauma, such as those that occur with gunshot or stab wounds. Hallmarks are ipsilateral (same side) paresis or hemiplegia and contralateral (opposite side) reduced sensation to pain and temperature. A person with Brown-Séquard syndrome can feel on one side but not the other, and can move on the opposite side but not on the side with sensation loss.

Root Injuries

Injuries to the nerve roots (Figure 23-4) often occur with spinal cord trauma. Most common findings are hypoalgesia, pain, or referred pain.

Posterior Cord Syndrome

This less common finding is usually related to extension injury. Below the level of injury there will be decreased sensations of vibration, light touch, and limited ability to maintain proprioception.

THE VERTEBRAE

The human body has seven cervical, twelve thoracic, and five lumbar vertebrae; the sacrum, five fused sacral vertebrae, and one or two coccygeal segments (Figure 23-5). Vertebrae may become subluxed, fractured, compressed, or dislocated; the mechanism of injury significantly impacts the severity of the injury and its impact on spinal nerves and blood supply.

A Jefferson fracture is a fracture of the first cervical (atlas) vertebral arch. Initially, there may be no neurologic deficit. This patient will require traction and surgical fixation. A hangman's fracture is a bilateral arch

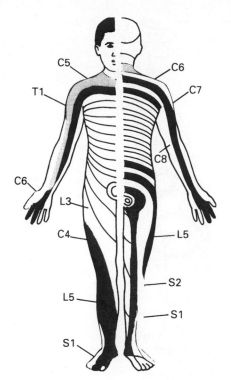

FIGURE 23-4. Nerve roots and the muscles they innervate.

fracture of the second cervical vertebrae (axis). Fractures of the spinal cord vary in severity according to the mechanism of injury.

There are three major types of spinal injury: injury to the cord itself, fracture of the vertebrae, and injury to the spinal nerves.[2,6] Document all clinical findings and changes associated with a type or specific level of injury.

Assessment

Spinal immobilization must be maintained throughout assessment to ensure minimal movement and decrease the possibility of further harm to the spinal cord.[2,6]

Before assessment immobilize the patient's spine completely and ensure that there will be minimal movement.

Assess for patent airway.

Assess respiratory rate, rhythm, and depth. Pay particular attention to the use of accessory muscles of respiration, especially the diaphragm.

Evaluate blood pressure, pulse, and skin vitals (color, temperature, and texture).

Observe patient's level of consciousness; check for neurologic deficits.

Inspect for a cerebrospinal fluid leak from the nose or the ears.

Palpate the spine.

    Assess for the presence of pain, tenderness, step-off deformity, and/or edema.

Assess motor strength or weakness and document.

Assess sensory levels (Figure 23-6) and document

    to touch, pain

    for paresthesias and paralysis

Inspect for ecchymosis.

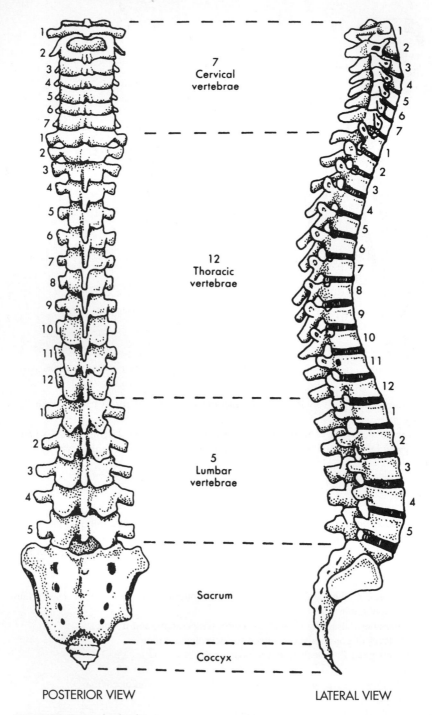

7
Cervical
vertebrae

12
Thoracic
vertebrae

5
Lumbar
vertebrae

Sacrum

Coccyx

POSTERIOR VIEW

LATERAL VIEW

FIGURE 23-5. Vertebral column.

(From Rosen P et al: *Emergency medicine: concepts and clinical practice*, ed 2, St Louis, 1988, Mosby.)

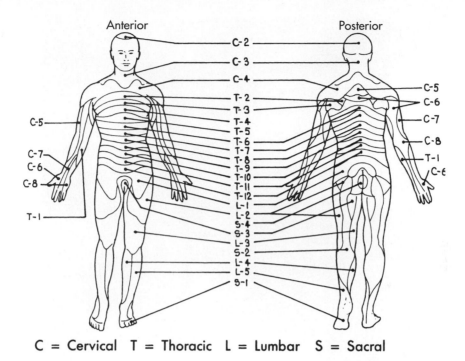

Anterior | Posterior

C = Cervical   T = Thoracic   L = Lumbar   S = Sacral

FIGURE 23-6. Dermatome chart demonstrating sensory and motor levels.

Inspect for tracheal deviation.

Inspect for a hematoma in the posterior pharyngeal area.

Assess sphincter tone.

Inspect for priapism.

Inspect for diaphoresis.

> Injuries above T4 usually cause sympathetic nervous system disruption. When this occurs, vasodilation occurs below the level of the injury because of inability to vasoconstrict. If the patient is diaphoretic, this is apparent above the level of the injury and not below.

Assess for other associated injuries, especially:

> Head injuries
>
> Chest, abdominal, and pelvic injuries

■ SIGNS AND SYMPTOMS OF SPINAL CORD INJURY

Guarding, pain or tenderness over the spine

Weakness of extremities

Numbness and tingling or paralysis

Decreased motor activity distal to the level of the injury

Unexplained hypotension (or neurogenic shock)

Altered level of consciousness

Localized edema or deformity

Priapism

Cough tenderness (coughing induces neck pain)

Feeling of "electric shock" or "hot water" running down the patient's back

Mouth breathing (Gautman's position)

> The patient laps air because of loss of diaphragm control

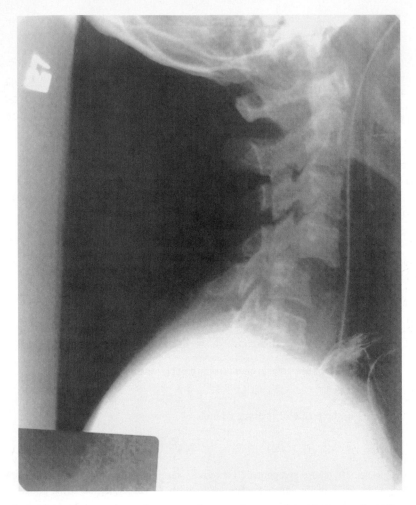

FIGURE 23-7. Visualizing only six cervical vertebrae is inadequate. One must be able to visualize all seven cervical vertebrae on a cross-table cervical spine film.

"Cock Robin" appearance of head and neck
    Can indicate C1-C2 injury
Arms folded across chest
    Can indicate C5-C6 injury

■ **DIAGNOSIS**

Diagnosis is performed by clinical assessment and tests such as x-rays, CT scan, or MRI examinations

X-rays. Obtain a cervical spine series that includes a cross-table lateral cervical spine film. One must be able to visualize all seven cervical vertebrae and the level of T-1. X-rays may illustrate subluxations, fractures, dislocations, and narrowing of paravertebral spaces (Figure 23-7). MRI examination is particularly useful to view compression injury.

To clear the cervical spine, four x-ray views are necessary: cross-table lateral, anterior-posterior, oblique, and open-mouth odontoid. If T1 cannot be visualized on the cross-table lateral view, obtain a swimmer's view (with the x-ray being shot through the axilla). If there is a high probability of injury, one should also include flexion-extension views (if the patient is conscious and can tell you if she or he is having pain when the procedure is stopped) to check for soft-tissue injury that would compromise ability to maintain vertebral column alignment.

The patient's arms may need to be pulled downward to cause the shoulders to drop to ensure adequate visualization of the C-spine. Ensure adequate C-spine immobilization during this procedure. Assess the films for:

Anterior-posterior column alignment

Anterior/posterior diameter of the spinal canal

Presence of bone fragments or bone displacement

Presence of linear fractures or comminuted fractures

Soft-tissue edema at or below C-3

Presence of a retropharyngeal hematoma

Vertebral inclination

An angle that is greater than 11 degrees or one that exceeds one fourth of the vertebral body is considered "unstable."

NOTE: If a patient has an associated head injury, alcohol or drug ingestion, even if cervical spine radiographs are read as negative for fracture, it is very important for the patient to remain in a collar until flexion/extension views are completed to rule out ligamentous injury.

Bulbocavernosus reflex. Place a finger in the patient's rectum and compress the glans or the clitoris or tug on the Foley catheter. With a normal finding the anal sphincter contracts. If this reflex is absent initially and then returns within 24 hours, it is indicative of a total lesion.

Anal "wink" or contraction. The anal sphincter should contract when a pin prick is applied in close proximity. When there is spinal cord injury, there is no response.

MEASURES TO PREVENT FURTHER INJURIES

Ensure that sufficient personnel are available to move the patient carefully and maintain alignment of the spine at all times.

Immobilize the cervical, thoracic, and lumbar spine in accordance with trauma protocol.

■ THERAPEUTIC INTERVENTIONS

Ensure airway, breathing, and circulation.

The airway is always at risk secondary to edema associated with spinal cord injury.

(Ninety-six percent of persons with neck fractures can be safely orally intubated.)[7]

Consider cricothyrotomy or tracheostomy.

Monitor circulation closely with ongoing assessment for neurogenic or spinal shock.

Immobilize the cervical, thoracic, and lumbar spine.

Consider placement of tongs (Figure 23-8) and cervical traction.

Perform closed reduction for injuries (below C_3)—begin with No. 15 then increase by No. 5 until reduction is accomplished.

Initiate two large-bore IV lines with Ringer's lactate solution, and run at a keep-open rate unless hemodynamic signs require fluid resuscitation.

Place a urinary catheter to gravity drainage and monitor urinary output hourly. Prevent urinary retention.

Consider steroids to reduce edema; prevent posttraumatic ischemia by increasing blood flow. Give methylprednisolone, initially 30 mg/kg bolus with 5.4 mg/kg/hr for 24 hours within 12 hours of acute spinal cord injury.[6,8]

Place a nasogastric tube; consider oral gastric when there is a head or facial injury present.

If patient demonstrates poikilothermy, then use caution to correct. Patient's temperature/normal regulatory mechanisms may not be functioning.[6,9]

Pad pressure points.

One hour on an unpadded backboard provides an 80% chance of significant skin problems later.[10]

Administer tetanus prophylaxis and antibiotics as appropriate.

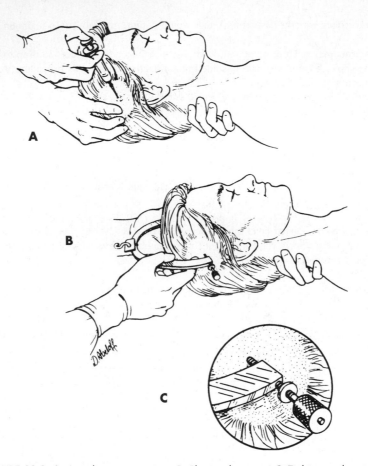

FIGURE 23-8. **A,** Anesthetizing pin sites. **B,** Placing the tongs. **C,** Tightening the pins.

Facilitate early neurosurgical consultation.

Consider transfer to facility with neurosurgical and rehabilitation capabilities.

If transferring a patient in tongs and traction, do *not* tape the hanging weights to anything.

Give hopeful and honest psychological support. Do not reinforce denial.

CERVICAL SPINE IMMOBILIZATION

Cervical spine immobilization should be considered simultaneously with airway management as one of the first priorities of care of a patient with multiple injuries, known or suspected trauma to the cervical spine, or whose mechanism of injury suggests the possibility of cervical spine injury. This needs to be done regardless of subjective cervical spine pain. The responsibility of "doing no further harm" cannot be overemphasized. Extreme caution and a high index of suspicion are recommended when handling trauma patients before a cervical spine injury has been ruled out.

Equipment List

Semirigid cervical collar
Kedrick extrication device

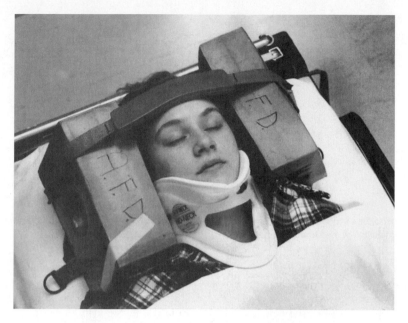

FIGURE 23-9. Full cervical spine immobilization, utilizing long board, C-blocks, straps, and stiffneck collar.

Short spine board with straps
Long spine board with straps
Sandbags
Blankets, towels for padding
2- or 3-inch adhesive tape
Cervical extrication device

Equipment used to immobilize the neck may be as varied as the situation in which it is being utilized (Figure 23-9). If it is being applied in the hospital or in the field by prehospital rescue personnel, many commercial devices are available. However, if cervical spine immobilization is indicated in the absence of this equipment, everyday materials on hand are adequate for achieving the necessary stabilization.

Procedure

1. Assess airway; maintain patency by using jaw thrust maneuver (Figure 23-10); do not hyperextend neck; if endotracheal intubation is necessary and not possible without hyperextension, consider nasotracheal or digital intubation or cricothyrotomy to ensure airway patency.
2. Evaluate cervical spine by observation; palpate each spinous process; note deformity, crepitus, pain, and instability. (Talk to the patient; remember to inform the patient of each step of the procedure to alleviate anxiety and movement and elicit the patient's cooperation.)
3. Gently apply manual stabilization by placing the hands on either side of the head and stabilizing the head and neck in a neutral, vertical position; in children this is defined as the "sniffing" position. (Once this stabilization is applied, it must be maintained until a comparable alternative has been implemented or until cervical spine injury has been ruled out clinically.)
4. Have other members of the team assist by gently placing a spine board under the patient while one caregiver continues to maintain stabilization. (Synchronized logroll with absolute cervical spine protection by manual stabilization is preferred; adequate personnel is essential to avoid further harm.)

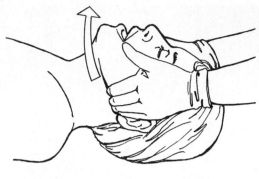

Jaw thrust

FIGURE 23-10. Maintenance of airway may involve jaw thrust technique, allowing the examiner to monitor the airway closely and ensure protection of the cervical spine.

5. Secure the patient to the board by:
   Using chest, hip, and leg straps across the patient, snugly attached to handles or cutouts in board (remember to undress patient completely if possible, or at least remove any sharp or bulky items that may cause soft-tissue pressure areas; pad bony prominences liberally).
   Securing straps diagonally from legs to chest.
   Padding behind the head and neck to support the cervical spine (always manually maintaining the neutral position of the spinal stabilization).
   Securing the patient's head to the spine board using 2- or 3-inch tape applied across the eyebrows and across the chin; this tape must be secured snugly to both sides of the spine board. Exercise caution to prevent any of the securing devices from interfering with the patient airway.
6. When satisfied with the absolute immobility of the patient's cervical spine, release manual stabilization.
7. Be prepared to logroll the patient using the backboard if vomiting occurs; have suction on hand.
8. If a short spine board or other short device is used, use a long board or scoop stretcher for extrication and further movement.
9. If the patient has a helmet on (for example, motorcycle, football), leave it in place if the airway is not compromised until the condition of the cervical spine is confirmed and measures can be taken to remove the helmet safely.

Helmet Removal

A variety of helmets are available for those sports that recommend head protection—motorcycling, bicycling, kayaking, ice hockey, football, auto racing, skating, and horseback riding, to name a few. The careful removal of this gear is imperative for protection of the cervical spine.

Procedure

1. *Never* attempt to remove a helmet alone: airway protection can be achieved with most helmets in place and the potential for complicating an injury with a difficult removal is great.
2. One person should apply inline traction by placing hands on each side of the helmet with fingers on the patient's mandible, exerting careful pulling; remember to loosen or cut the chin strap (Figure 23-11).
3. A second person should then receive the weight of the patient's head by placing one hand behind the head, resting on the occiput, and placing the front hand on the angles of the mandible, thumb on one side, fingers on the other *(the second person is now in control of the head and neck)*.
4. The first person should then remove the helmet by pulling laterally on the sides and sliding it off. If the helmet has full face protection, special consideration must be given to the eye covering, which must be

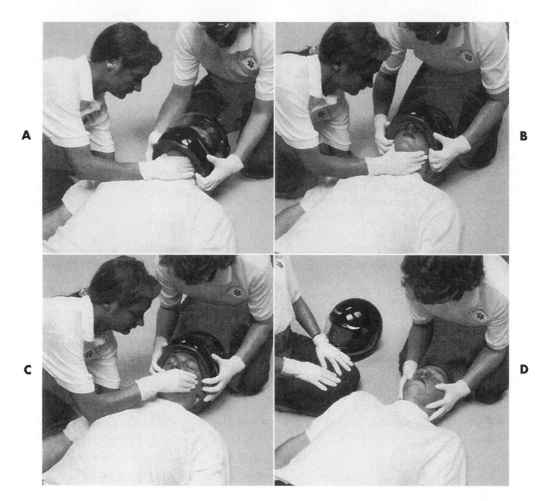

FIGURE 23-11. Demonstration: helmet removal should be done with manual control of the cervical spine by one individual while the other person spreads the helmet laterally and removes it. **A,** Rescuer 1 immobilizes the helmet and head in an in-line position. Rescuer 2 grasps the patient's mandible by placing the thumb at the angle of the mandible on one side and two fingers at the angle on the other side. Rescuer 2's other hand is placed under the neck at the base of the skull, producing in-line immobilization of the patient's head. **B,** Rescuer 1 carefully spreads the sides of the helmet away from the patient's head and ears. **C,** The helmet is then rotated toward the rescuer to clear the nose and removed from the patient's head in a straight line. **D,** After removal of the helmet, Rescuer 1 applies in-line immobilization. A rigid cervical collar is applied.

(From Sanders MJ: *Mosby's paramedic textbook,* St Louis, 1994, Mosby.)

removed first; if it cannot be removed, tilt the helmet (not the head) back to pass the face protector over the patient's nose.

SOFT-TISSUE INJURIES OF THE NECK

Fractured Larynx

The most common cause of a fractured larynx is blunt trauma from sudden impact with steering wheel or from a deceleration caused by a rope, wire, or assault (for example, karate chop by a human hand).

■ **SIGNS AND SYMPTOMS**
Hoarse voice
Cough with hemoptysis
Difficulty breathing/respiratory distress
Subcutaneous emphysema
Changes in voice characteristics

■ **DIAGNOSIS**
Clinical observation
Ecchymoses and abrasions
Auscultation of progressive inspiratory stridor
Displacement of landmarks

■ **THERAPEUTIC INTERVENTIONS**
Emergency cricothyrotomy or tracheostomy. (See Chapter 5.)
High-flow oxygen therapy
Broad-spectrum antibiotics

Penetrating Neck Wounds

Penetrating objects, such as bullets and knife blades, can cause trauma to the tissues of the neck. The extent of injury depends on the type of penetrating object, the force of the object, and the location and angle of the penetration.

■ **SIGNS AND SYMPTOMS**
Obvious penetrating wound
Airway obstruction or stridor
Signs of hypovolemia, hemothorax, or shock
Presence of a large or expanding hematoma

■ **DIAGNOSIS**
Clinical observation
Arteriography
Exploratory surgery

■ **THERAPEUTIC INTERVENTIONS**
Airway management
    Consider surgical procedure.
Breathing
    Ensure adequate oxygenation.
Circulation
    Control bleeding.
    Replace volume (2 large-bore, 16-gauge or larger IVs with Ringer's Lactate).
Prepare for surgery if indicated.

REFERENCES

1. DeVivo MJ et al: Trends in spinal cord injury demographics and treatment outcomes between 1973 and 1986, *Arch Phys Med Rehab* 73:424, 1992.
2. Walleck CA: Central nervous system II: spinal cord injury. In Cardona VD et al, editors: *Trauma nursing: from resuscitation through rehabilitation,* ed 2, Philadelphia, 1994, Saunders.
3. Domzalski F: Spinal cord injury and injury syndromes. In Hamilton G, editor: *Presenting signs and symptoms in the emergency department: evaluation and treatment,* Baltimore, 1993, Williams & Wilkins.
4. Walleck CA: Peripheral nerve and spinal cord problems. In Lewis S, Collier I, editors: *Medical-surgical nursing and management of clinical problems,* St Louis, 1992, Mosby.
5. Shea J: Lecture presented at Emergency Nurses Association Annual Meeting, Orlando, Fla, Sept 1992.
6. Lower JS: Neurological emergencies. In Emergency Nurses Association: *Emergency nursing core curriculum,* ed 4, Philadelphia, 1994, Saunders.
7. Bauer D, Errico T: Cervical spine injuries. In Errico T, Bauer D, Waugh T, editors: *Spinal trauma,* Philadelphia, 1991, Lippincott.
8. Bauer D, Errico T: Pharmacologic therapy of acute spinal cord injury. In Errico T, Bauer D, Waugh T, editors: *Spinal trauma,* Philadelphia, 1991, Lippincott.
9. Mangiardi JR et al: Spinal injuries. In Schwartz G, Cayten CG, Mangelsen MA et al, editors: *Principles and practice of emergency medicine,* Philadelphia, 1992, Lea and Febiger.
10. American College of Surgeons, Committee on Trauma: *ATLS manual,* Chicago, 1992, ACS.

SUGGESTED READINGS

Burchiel KJ: Emergency management of stable and unstable injuries. In Tollison CD, Satterthwaite JR, editors: *Painful cervical trauma: diagnosis and rehabilitative treatment of neuromusculoskeletal injuries,* Baltimore, 1992, Williams & Wilkins.

Committee on trauma: Neurotrauma care, In *Resources for the optimal care of the injured patient,* USA, 1993, ACS.

Danis DM, Cullen MM: Cervical spine immobilization: unanswered questions, *Int J Tr Nsg* 1:47, 1995.

Orenstein JB et al: Delayed diagnosis of pediatric cervical spine injury, *Pediatrics* 89:1185, 1992.

Sweeney TA, Marz JA: Blunt neck injury, *Emerg Med Clin North Am* 11:71, 1993.

Wright S et al: Cervical spine injuries in blunt trauma in patients requiring emergent endotracheal intubation, *Am J Emerg Med* 10:104, 1992.

WEBSITES

www.accessunlimited.com/spinal_cord_injury.html

This wonderful site provides statistics and links to organizations that serve people with spinal cord injuries and health care professionals.

www.sci.rehabm.uab.edu

This site gives spinal cord injury statistics and provides a link to the National Spinal Cord Injury Center in Washington DC.

Facial Trauma

Anne Marie E. Lewis

Facial trauma may cause severe complications, such as airway obstruction and respiratory distress, and may mask other problems, such as spinal cord injury or intracranial bleed. Most cases of facial trauma result from motor vehicle collisions (Figure 24-1) but they may also be the result of domestic violence or physical assault, falls, contact sports, or a blow by any mechanism that can cause blunt or penetrating trauma to the face.

ASSESSMENT

Always begin assessment and therapeutic intervention of facial trauma with the following:

Airway and Cervical Spine

Ensure that there is an open airway. Avoid tilting the head; assume that there is a concurrent cervical spine injury until proven otherwise. If one must manually control the airway, first use the jaw thrust maneuver and consider using airway adjuncts (see Chapters 4 and 5).

Always remember that noisy breathing means an obstructed airway. Broken teeth, dentures, other foreign materials, vomitus, blood, avulsed soft tissues, edema, or a posteriorly displaced fractured mandible all may cause obstructions.

While ensuring a patent airway, simultaneously stabilize the cervical spine. Check for a laryngeal fracture.

Breathing

Administer supplemental oxygen.

Circulation

Control any obvious bleeding by direct pressure, if possible. Consider initiating an IV line.

(NOTE: Although facial trauma can cause severe bleeding, it is seldom the sole cause of hypovolemic shock in a patient with multiple injuries.)

Level of Consciousness

Evaluate level of consciousness, pupillary reaction, and movement.

ation by a foreign body.

Complaint of a salty taste
It is important to remember that facial injuries are diagnosed through astute clinical assessment and confirmed via appropriate radiographs.

GENERAL TREATMENT RECOMMENDATIONS FOR ALL FACIAL TRAUMA

- Elevate head of bed at least 30° *if* the C-spine is cleared to reduce facial swelling and to assist with airway clearance.
- Have suction available.
- Do *not* insert airways, suction catheters, gastric tubes, or endotracheal tubes via the intranasal route. Intranasal balloons and packing should be avoided if there is a possibility of basal skull fracture.
- Apply cold packs. (Care must be taken to keep the patient warm.)
- Administer prophylactic antibiotics.
- Administer tetanus prophylaxis.
- Provide emotional support and explain all procedures and instructions.

NOTE: Facial fractures with minimal or no displacement or malocclusion may not require surgical intervention.

NOTE: Use of rigid fixation for repair of facial trauma in children is controversial because of the possibility of impairment of facial growth.

FACIAL LACERATIONS/AVULSIONS

Facial lacerations can bleed profusely and may cause severe disfigurement. They may be caused by penetrating objects such as glass, metal, or knives, by animal or human bites or by blunt or crushing trauma.
■ THERAPEUTIC INTERVENTIONS
Cold pack
Assist with local anesthesia (with epinephrine to control bleeding unless injury is to the nose) or regional anesthesia.
Copiously irrigate the wound with normal saline and/or cleanse with an antibacterial solution.
Assist with debridement of the wound and removal of foreign bodies, if necessary.
Assist with suturing of the wound.
■ SPECIAL NOTES
A plastic surgery consultation may be appropriate because of the extent or type of injury, or when requested by patient/family.
When there is a lip laceration, the vermilion border must be carefully approximated.
Eyebrows should be carefully approximated. (Never shave eyebrows!)
An opthalmologic consult is needed for all injuries to the eyelid or medial canthus. Eye injuries should be treated before eyelid injuries.

ABRASIONS AND CONTUSIONS

(See Chapter 21.)
■ THERAPEUTIC INTERVENTIONS
Anesthetize.
Cleanse wound with normal saline and/or an antibacterial solution. Carefully remove foreign bodies to avoid tattooing.
Assist with conservative debridement of devitalized or grossly contaminated tissue.
Dress with a topical antibiotic.
Provide antibiotics for severely contaminated wounds or wounds more than 24 hours old.

FACIAL FRACTURES

When a patient suffers multiple trauma injuries, facial fractures do not usually receive a high priority until other, more life-threatening injuries can be treated. Unlike treatment of a laceration, treatment of a facial fracture often is delayed for 4 to 10 days to allow the facial edema to subside.

Nasal Fractures

The mechanism of injury for a nasal fracture is usually blunt trauma to the front or side of the nose. Treat any fracture of the nose as an open fracture. Also check and treat for a septal hematoma, because a septal hematoma that is not excised and packed may become infected or necrotic.

■ **SIGNS AND SYMPTOMS**
Deformity
Nasal and periorbital edema and ecchymosis
Crepitus
Point tenderness
Internal and external bleeding
Subconjunctival hemorrhage
Flattening or broadening of the nose

■ **DIAGNOSIS**
X-ray (Water's view)

■ **THERAPEUTIC INTERVENTIONS**
Cold pack
Control bleeding.
Assist with anesthetic administration.
Assist with nasal packing.
Splint PRN.
Antibiotics
Tetanus prophylaxis
Reduction, if fracture is displaced.
Nasal decongestant
Oral analgesics

Zygomatic Fracture

The zygomatic bone will often be fractured in three places: at the arch itself, at the zygomatic suture line, and at the posterior half of the infraorbital rim (Figure 24-2). This injury is caused by a blunt force to the front and side of the face. Fractures of the zygomatic bone frequently are associated with fractures of the orbit.

■ **SIGNS AND SYMPTOMS**

NOTE: Use the mnemonic TIDES.

Trismus
Infraorbital hyperesthesia
Diplopia with impaired upward gaze
Epistaxis
Symmetry, absence of
Possible CSF rhinorrhea
Periorbital and facial edema and ecchymosis

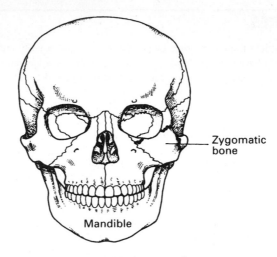

FIGURE 24-2. Zygomatic fracture.

Subconjunctival hemorrhage
Palpable step defect and point tenderness
Facial flattening
Anesthesia of the cheek, upper lip, side of the nose, teeth, and/or gum
■ **DIAGNOSIS**
Clinical exam
X-ray (Water's and Caldwell's views, modified basal view of the skull)
CT scan
■ **THERAPEUTIC INTERVENTIONS**
Airway management
Cervical spine precautions
Cold pack
Surgery for reduction and fixation PRN
Ophthalmologic consult

Orbital Blow-out Fractures

A fracture of the orbital floor occurs when the globe of the eye is struck by a blunt force, forcing the globe inward and causing a fracture of the very thin orbital floor bone.
■ **SIGNS AND SYMPTOMS**
Impairment of upward gaze
Diplopia
Enophthalmos
Epistaxis
Infraorbital paresthesia
Periorbital edema and ecchymosis
Subconjunctival hemorrhage
■ **DIAGNOSIS**
Good history of mechanism of injury
Clinical exam
X-ray (Water's view)
CT scan

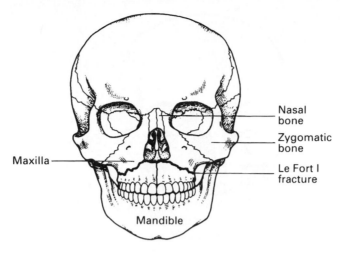

FIGURE 24-3. LeFort I facial fracture.

■ **THERAPEUTIC INTERVENTIONS**
Cold pack
Ophthalmologic consultation
Surgery for reduction and fixation, PRN
IV antibiotics

Maxillary Mid-Face Fracture

French pathologist René LeFort observed in 1901 that facial bones often fracture in specific patterns when blunt trauma occurs. The most common cause is severe blunt trauma to the face, with the most common etiology being motor vehicle collisions involving unrestrained occupants.

These fractures are categorized into three levels, LeFort I, LeFort II, and LeFort III, depending on the pattern of fracture. Patients may have unilateral or bilateral LeFort fractures or may have combinations of these fractures (for example, LeFort II fracture on the right and LeFort III fracture on the left). Associated head injuries are common with LeFort fractures and should be treated first.

LeFort I fracture

A LeFort I fracture (Figure 24-3) is a fracture of the transverse alveolar process at the nasal floor. It extends from the upper teeth into the nose.

■ **SIGNS AND SYMPTOMS**
Malocclusion of teeth, anterior open bite
Moveable maxilla
Epistaxis
Facial edema and ecchymosis
Elongated midface

■ **DIAGNOSIS**
History of mechanism of injury
Clinical exam
X-ray
CT scan

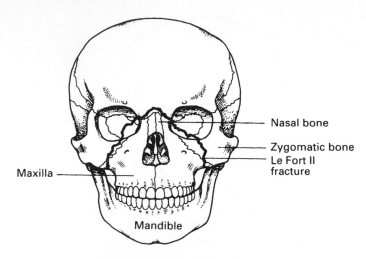

FIGURE 24-4. LeFort II facial fracture.

■ **THERAPEUTIC INTERVENTIONS**
Airway management
Cervical spine precautions
Cold pack
Surgery for reduction and fixation
Check for other associated injuries.
IV antibiotics for open fractures

LeFort II fracture

A LeFort II fracture (Figure 24-4) is a pyramidal fracture that extends through the central part of the maxilla up through the superior nasal area. It also usually involves the orbits.

■ **SIGNS AND SYMPTOMS**
Nose and dental arch move together when manipulated.
Epistaxis
Periorbital and facial edema and ecchymosis
Subconjunctival hemorrhage
Infraorbital paresthesia
Point tenderness
Malocclusion of teeth
CSF rhinorrhea
Concave look to the midface

■ **DIAGNOSIS**
History of mechanism of injury
Nose and dental arch move together when manipulated.
Clinical exam
Extraocular muscle entrapment
X-ray (Water's view)
CT scan

■ **THERAPEUTIC INTERVENTIONS**
Airway management; consider oral endotracheal intubation.
Cold pack
Surgery for reduction and fixation

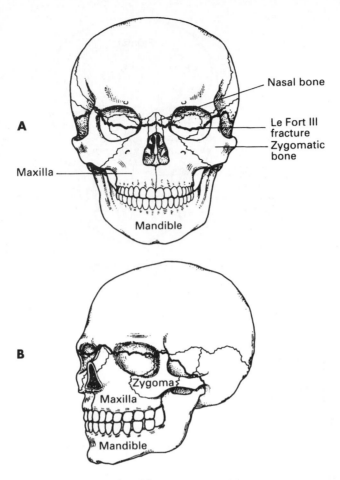

FIGURE 24-5. LeFort III facial fracture. **A,** Frontal view. **B,** Lateral view.

IV antibiotics
Check for other associated injuries.
Ophthalmologic consult
Neurosurgical consult in presence of CSF leak

LeFort III fracture

A LeFort III fracture (Figure 24-5) is a major fracture that is usually caused by a major blunt trauma to the face. When fracture occurs, a total craniofacial separation results. It may involve the maxilla, zygoma, mandible, nasal bones, ethmoids, vomer, orbits, and all lesser bones of the base of the cranium.

■ **SIGNS AND SYMPTOMS**

Massive bleeding
Loss of consciousness (usually)
Facial bones move without frontal bone movement when manipulated.
CSF rhinorrhea
Epistaxis
Periorbital and facial edema and ecchymosis
Subconjunctival hemorrhage

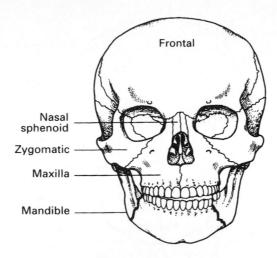

FIGURE 24-6. Mandibular fracture.

Infraorbital paresthesia
Malocclusion of teeth; anterior open bite
■ **DIAGNOSIS**
History of mechanism of injury
Facial bones move without frontal bone movement when manipulated.
Extraocular muscle entrapment
Clinical exam
X-ray (Water's view)
CT scan
■ **THERAPEUTIC INTERVENTIONS**
Airway management; consider oral endotracheal intubation.
Cervical spine precautions
Cold pack
Surgery for reduction and fixation
IV antibiotics
Check for other associated injuries.
Ophthalmologic consult
Neurosurgical consult if there is CSF leak

Mandibular fracture

The most common causes of mandible fractures (Figure 24-6) are domestic violence altercations, motor vehicle collisions, and contact sports. Because the mandible is arch-shaped, in most cases, when it is fractured, it will fracture in two places. Often these are open fractures as evidenced by obvious intraoral bony fragments or simply bleeding around the teeth.
■ **SIGNS AND SYMPTOMS**
Palpation of the fracture(s)
Malocclusion of the teeth
Point tenderness, especially with movement
Trismus
Edema and ecchymosis

■ **DIAGNOSIS**

Palpation of the fracture(s)

Clinical exam

X-ray (Towne's view, Panorex films)

■ **THERAPEUTIC INTERVENTIONS**

Airway management

Cold pack

Surgery for reduction and fixation

IV antibiotics for open fractures

Facial trauma is frequently associated with complications that may prove life threatening. Airway occlusion, respiratory distress, and associated C-spine injuries can prove devastating. Astute, systematic, thorough patient assessment and rapid, effective intervention are critical to positive patient outcome.

SUGGESTED READINGS

Cardona VD et al: *Trauma nursing: from resuscitation through rehabilitation,* ed 2, Philadelphia, 1994, Saunders.

Carithers JS, Koch BB: Evaluation and management of facial fractures, *Amer Fam Physician* 55(8):2675, 1997.

Chu L, Gussack GS, Muller T: A treatment protocol for mandible fractures, *J Trauma* 36(1):48, 1994.

Emergency Nurses Association: *Trauma nursing core course: instructor manual,* ed 4, Park Ridge, Ill, 1995, ENA.

Hussain K et al: A comprehensive analysis of craniofacial trauma, *J Trauma* 36(1):34, 1994.

Klein AR et al: *Emergency nursing core curriculum,* Philadelphia, 1994, Saunders.

Koltai PJ, Rabkin D: Management of facial trauma in children, *Pediatr Clin North Amer* 43(6):1253, 1996.

Moncada GA: Traumatic injuries of the face and hands, *Nurs Clin North Amer* 29(4):777, 1994.

Reisdorff EJ et al: *Pediatric emergency medicine,* Philadelphia, 1993, Saunders.

Rickelmann MP, Marsh EE: Stabilizing a patient with massive facial injuries, *Nurs 95* 25(7):32FF, 1995.

Selfridge-Thomas J: *Emergency nursing: an essential guide for patient care,* Philadelphia, 1997, Saunders.

Tintinalli JE, Ruiz E, Krome RL: *Emergency medicine,* ed 4, New York, 1996, McGraw-Hill.

Eye, Ear, Nose, Throat, and Dental Emergencies

Kathy Sciabica Robinson

Eye Emergencies

There are many occasions when rapid, careful assessment and intervention can prevent permanent or temporary loss of vision.

BASIC ANATOMY AND PHYSIOLOGY OF THE EYE (Figure 25-1)

body rim   The bony process that protects the eyeball.

eyelid   The covering that closes to protect the eyeball, distribute tears, and regulate light.

eyelashes   Hairs that minimize the number of dirt particles that enter the eye area.

sclera   The tough protective coating of the eyeball.

cornea   The convex, transparent anterior portion of the eye.

retina   The inner lining of the posterior eyeball that collects and focuses light rays.

choroid   The middle layer of the eyeball that supplies the retina with blood, oxygen, and other nutrients.

macula   The area of the retina most sensitive to light and color.

lens   The normally transparent disc through which light is refracted. Light passes through the cornea, the anterior chamber, the lens, and the vitreous humor to the retina.

iris   Colored diaphragm that controls the amount of light entering the posterior chamber by means of expanding and contracting its opening (the pupil).

oculomotor muscles   The six muscles that control eyeball movement.

lacrimal glands   Glands that secrete fluid (tears) to soothe the eyeball and reduce friction.

tears   Fluid that coats the eyeball; tears are distributed by blinking of the eyelids. Tears are secreted by the lacrimal glands and through the lacrimal puncta into the lacrimal and nasolacrimal ducts

meibomian glands   Glands that secrete the oil that lines the eyelid margins and prevents tears from running out of the conjunctival sac.

visual acuity   Central vision; stimuli on macula; a measure of the resolving power of the eye.

peripheral vision   Vision in which stimuli are on an area of the retina other than the macula.

Certain conditions should be given priority treatment in the emergency department. They are the following:

- Loss of vision without pain (may be caused by central artery occlusion or central vein occlusion, intraocular hemorrhage, or retinal detachment).
- Chemical burns
- Foreign bodies
- Painful eyes (may be caused by conjunctivitis, iritis, or keratitis).

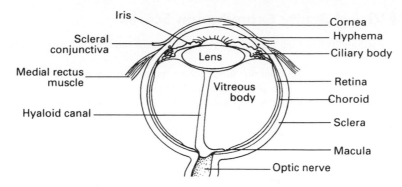

FIGURE 25-1. Horizontal section of left eye seen from above.

- Laceration of the globe
- Hyphema

EXAMINATION OF THE EYE

Visual acuity should be performed on both eyes for all patients presenting with opthalmologic complaint.
If there is much pain, a topical anesthetic agent, such as proparacaine (Ophthaine) or tetracaine, may assist in examination of the eye.
Be gentle and explain the procedure to the patient.
Assess for potentially life-threatening conditions of vital organ systems related to illness or trauma.
Evaluate the anatomy of the angle (anterior chamber) before use of mydriatic agents, which can precipitate acute glaucoma.
NPO until possibility of surgery is ruled out.

VISUAL ACUITY EXAMINATION

Whenever possible, perform a visual acuity examination before examination of the eye, because manipulation may increase blurring and decrease acuity.
If the patient wears glasses, test vision first with glasses, then without.
If the patient's glasses are not available, have him or her read the chart through a pinhole poked in a piece of cardboard.
Check each eye separately, then both eyes together.
Follow specific instructions on how to conduct the examination according to the chart to be used:
  The Snellen chart is read at 20 feet.
  The Rosenbaum Pocket Vision Screener is read 14 inches from the tip of the nose.
If a Snellen or other vision chart is not available, have the patient read newsprint, and record the distance from the eye the paper must be held for the patient to read it.
If the patient cannot see newsprint, hold up a specific number of fingers and record the distance at which the patient can see the fingers (and be able to tell how many are being held up).
If the patient cannot see fingers, record the distance at which he can perceive hand motion.
If the patient cannot see hand motion, record the distance at which he or she can perceive light.
If the patient cannot perceive light, record this on the chart.

Examples of Visual Acuity Examination Scores

20/20   When standing 20 feet from the Snellen chart, the patient can read what the normal eye can read at 20 feet.

20/40—2   When standing 20 feet from the Snellen chart, the patient can read what the normal eye can read at 40 feet (and, in this example, has also missed two letters).

20/200   When standing 20 feet from the Snellen chart, the patient can read what the normal eye can read at 200 feet.

10/200   If the patient cannot read any of the letters on the Snellen chart, have him or her stand half the distance (10 feet) and read what he or she can; record this as the distance the patient actually is standing from the chart over the smallest line he or she can read.

CF/3 feet   The patient can count fingers at a maximum distance of 3 feet.

HM/4 feet   The patient can see hand motion at a maximum distance of 4 feet.

LP/position   The patient can perceive light and determine from which direction it came.

LP/no position   The patient can perceive light, but cannot determine from which direction it came.

NLP   The patient cannot perceive light.

When recording information about the eyes, use the following abbreviations:

ABBREVIATION	LATIN WORD	ENGLISH TRANSLATION
OD	oculus dexter	right eye
OS	oculus sinister	left eye
OU	oculus uterque	each eyes
gt	guttae	drops

Otherwise simply write Ⓡ or Ⓛ or both eyes.

EYE TRAUMA

In addition to obvious eye trauma, search for associated eye trauma when there is head or facial trauma. If there is great pain, sometimes it will help to patch both eyes. This minimizes movement and may decrease pain.

If the patient is unconscious, be sure to check for contact lenses and be sure to protect the cornea from drying by instilling an ophthalmic ointment and taping the eyelids shut or frequently instilling artificial tears.

When dealing with a patient with eye trauma, it is important to obtain a good history:

- What happened?
- How did it happen?
- Is there something in the eye? What?
- Were chemicals involved? What chemicals?
- Where did it happen?
- Did anyone see it happen? Who?
- Was care given at the scene? By whom?
- Was patient wearing safety glasses?
- Is patient on any medication?
- Does the patient wear corrective lenses?
- Was the patient wearing contact lenses at the time of the injury? Are they in now?
- Does the patient have a history of glaucoma, diabetes, hypertension, or previous eye problems?

Lacerated Eyelid

The care provider will be able to diagnose a lacerated eyelid simply by observing it.

■ **THERAPEUTIC INTERVENTIONS**

Irrigation

Wound approximation and suturing

If a section of tissue is missing, consulting a plastic surgeon to reconstruct the section so the cornea will be protected

Checking for laceration of the lacrimal duct

Orbital Rim Trauma

This type of injury may occur as a result of blunt or penetrating injury to the face. The main sign of orbital rim trauma is periorbital ecchymosis.

■ **THERAPEUTIC INTERVENTIONS**

Ice pack

Examination for fracture and eyeball trauma

Visual acuity examination

Assess ocular motility for possible muscle entrapment

If there is a fracture of the prominent supraorbital rim and frontal sinus, checking for cerebrospinal fluid leak in the form of CSF rhinorrhea.

If there is a visual disturbance, checking for a fracture of the orbital roof resulting in entrapment of the optic nerve

Hyphema

Blunt trauma to the eye may cause aqueous humor to depress the diaphragm of the iris or the ciliary bodies, causing a tear in the iris vasculature. When this occurs, hyphema results (a hemorrhage into the anterior chamber of the eye). This condition requires immediate ophthalmologic consultation.

■ **SIGNS AND SYMPTOMS**

Visible blood in the anterior chamber

Decrease in vision

Pain

Photophobia

Nausea

■ **THERAPEUTIC INTERVENTIONS**

Head of bed up at least 45 degrees

Quiet activity or bedrest

Antiemetic, analgesics

Patch affected eye.

Avoid ASA and nonsteroidals.

Consider beta adrenergic drops; mydriatics, acetazolamide or other carbonic anhydrase inhibitor.

Massive hemorrhage can occur at any time up to 2 weeks after blunt trauma. It can cause corneal blood staining, secondary glaucoma, loss of vision, and maybe even loss of the eye.

An 8-ball hemorrhage is a condition in which old, clotted blood is found in the anterior chamber. Therapeutic intervention for this condition is to remove the clot surgically. Retrobulbar hemorrhage may occur as a result of ruptured intraorbital vessels. It can be diagnosed by the presence of a protruding eyeball (exophthalmos) and diplopia (double vision).

Subconjunctival Hemorrhage

A subconjunctival hemorrhage is common after trauma to the eye. It is usually left untreated and will resolve in about 2 weeks.

Blow-out Fracture

Blow-out fracture results from direct blunt trauma to the eyeball, which causes an increased intraocular pressure that fractures the orbit floor.

■ **SIGNS AND SYMPTOMS**
Periorbital hematoma
Subconjunctival hemorrhage
Periorbital edema
Enophthalmos/exophthalmos
Restricted extraocular movement
Diplopia
Anesthesia of infraorbital nerve
Crepitus (from orbital and lid subcutaneous emphysema)
Possible epistaxis

■ **THERAPEUTIC INTERVENTIONS**
Ice packs
Reduction of fracture (if there is bony displacement)
Packing of maxillary sinus
Possible surgery
Analgesia
Antibiotic ointment
Patch

Foreign Bodies

Foreign bodies in the conjunctiva

The foreign body most commonly found in the conjunctiva is an eyelash.

■ **THERAPEUTIC INTERVENTIONS**
Give topical anesthesia, visual acuity examination.
Evert the eyelid (Figure 25-2).
Irrigate with normal saline.
Gently remove the foreign body with a moist cotton swab.
Administer local antibiotics 4 times a day for 5 days.
An eye patch may be applied, depending on the nature of the injury and the amount of damage.
The patient should return for follow-up care in 1 day if no improvement.

Foreign bodies in the cornea

The presence of a foreign body in the cornea is very painful. As the eyelid moves up and down over the foreign body, pain increases.

■ **THERAPEUTIC INTERVENTIONS**
Topical anesthesia, visual acuity exam
Irrigation of eye with normal saline
Removal of foreign body with moistened swab
Checking for more than one foreign body
Slit lamp examination to look for corneal abrasion
If the foreign body is metal, it will form a rust ring that must be removed, usually by an ophthalmologist.

Intraocular foreign bodies

Intraocular foreign bodies are usually caused by a small object moving at a high speed that penetrates the eyeball and comes to rest somewhere within the posterior chamber. Pain may be minimal. The entrance wound

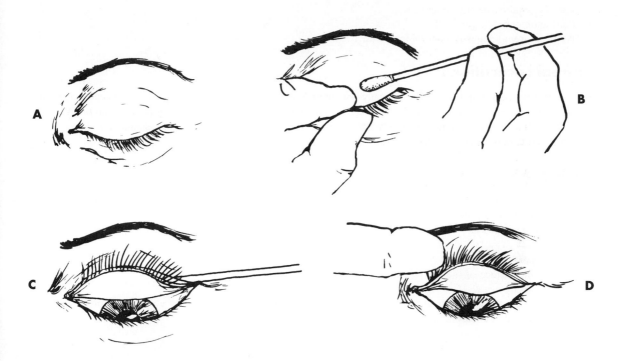

FIGURE 25-2. Steps in everting eyelid. **A,** Eyelid, **B,** Placement of cotton swab, pulling eyelashes down and over swab. **C,** Eyelid everted over swab. **D,** Examination of inside of eyelid and eye.
(From Newbury L, Emergency Nurses Association: *Sheehy's emergency nursing: principles and practice,* ed 4, St Louis, 1998, Mosby.)

may be very small and difficult to locate. Finding the wound requires a high index of suspicion. This condition constitutes an extreme emergency.

■ **THERAPEUTIC INTERVENTIONS**

Surgical intervention to prevent further injury.

All foreign bodies should be considered contaminated, and antibiotics should be considered.

Assess current tetanus immunization status.

Obtain x-ray film of the eye to inspect for the foreign body.

Cover both eyes to decrease movement.

Perforating and Penetrating Injuries to the Eyeball or Ruptured Globe

Therapeutic intervention is essential in the early stages of the injury, and will decrease the likelihood of further injury. This condition constitutes an ophthalmologic emergency.

■ **THERAPEUTIC INTERVENTIONS**

Consider parenteral analgesia and sedation.

Avoid manipulation of eye for evaluation or medications.

Secure the impaling object, if present.

NPO Fox shield recommended (without underlying pressure patch).

Cover both eyes to decrease eye movement.

Reserve detailed examination for an ophthalmologist.

Usually requires surgical intervention.
Start antibiotics—parenterally.
Assess current tetanus immunization status.

Corneal Lacerations

If a corneal laceration is small, it is usually not sutured. Therapeutic intervention for small corneal lacerations is antibiotic ointment and eye patch. If the laceration is large, it is usually sutured by an ophthalmologist with 8-0 silk or 7-0 chromic suture on a very fine needle prior to a dressing application. Assessment is done to rule out possible corneal perforation (using fluorescein).

Corneal Abrasions

Corneal abrasion occurs when the epithelium is denuded by a foreign object, such as a contact lens. It is important to obtain a history from the patient as to what caused the injury.

■ **SIGNS AND SYMPTOMS**
Tearing
Eyelid spasm
Pain on the surface of the eye (sensation of a foreign body)
Photophobia
Corneal abrasions can be diagnosed by staining the surface of the eye with fluorescein dye and observing the cornea with a cobalt lamp and magnification.

How to use fluorescein strips to stain the cornea (Figure 25-3)
1. Explain the procedure to the patient.
2. Use local anesthesia before exam.
3. Use individually wrapped sterile fluorescein strips (fluorescein is easily contaminated by *Pseudomonas*).
4. Moisten the end of the sterile strip with normal saline.
5. Pull down on the lower eyelid.
6. Touch the strip to the inner edge of the lower eyelid.
7. Ask the patient to blink to distribute the dye.
8. Examine the cornea using a cobalt lamp (an abrasion will be highlighted by the fluorescein).

■ **THERAPEUTIC INTERVENTIONS**
Local anesthesia during examination
Visual acuity examination
Local antibiotics
Patching of injured eye(s) for 24 hours

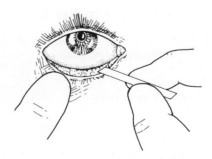

FIGURE 25-3. Fluorescein staining. Touch moistened fluorescein strip to inner canthus of lower eyelid.
(From Emergency Nurses Association: *Sheehy's emergency nursing: principles and practice*, ed 4, St Louis, 1998, Mosby.)

Follow-up visit in 1 day if no improvement

Instructing the patient not to use local anesthetic agents at home because they will delay healing

Assess current tetanus immunization status

Conjunctival Lacerations

The main symptom of conjunctival laceration is swelling and bleeding from the conjunctiva.

■ **THERAPEUTIC INTERVENTIONS**

Local antibiotics

Application of an eye patch

Close observation

If the laceration is longer than 1 cm, an ophthalmologic consultation is needed for suturing (less than 1-cm lacerations are not usually repaired).

Corneal Ulcer or Bacterial/Fungal Keratitis

Corneal ulcer can be found in the unconscious patient or the patient who has left contact lenses in place for an inordinately long period.

■ **SIGNS AND SYMPTOMS**

Whitish spot on the cornea

Pain

Photophobia

Profuse tearing

Vascular congestion

Blue-green cast on fluorescein staining

NOTE: If *Pseudomonas* is present, the patient may lose the eye within 48 hours.

■ **THERAPEUTIC INTERVENTIONS**

Antibiotics

Warm compresses

Eye patch

Optic Nerve Avulsion

Optic nerve avulsion usually results from severe trauma to the eye. The nerve avulses at the level where the optic nerve enters the eyeball. A partial tear will result in partial blindness; a total tear will result in total blindness. An immediate ophthalmologic consultation is indicated.

Iris Injury

Traumatic iridocyclitis is an inflammation of the iris and ciliary body following contusion of the eye. The main sign is the presence of uveal pigment and lens tissue in the anterior chamber.

■ **THERAPEUTIC INTERVENTIONS**

Treatment with topical cycloplegics

Topical systemic steroids

Ophthalmology consultation

Lens Injury

Injuries that can occur to the lens include partial dislocations (subluxations), total dislocations (luxations), and opacifications (cataracts). Surgical intervention is indicated for all of these conditions. There is potential for developing closed angle glaucoma.

Retina and Choroid Injury

Trauma to the retina and choroid may produce a white ellipse where the sclera is visible through the rupture. If the macula is injured, a decrease in visual acuity will result. Surgical intervention is indicated for these injuries.

Problems with Contact Lenses

The most common problem experienced by the wearer of contact lenses is the presence of dirt particles or chemical irritants under the lenses, causing irritation, abrasion, or erosions of the cornea. The second most common problem results when the lenses are worn too long. This causes redness, swelling, pain, and corneal abrasions (Figure 25-4). Therapeutic intervention is removal of the lens and cleansing of lens and the eye.

■ **THERAPEUTIC INTERVENTION FOR PROLONGED CONTACT LENS USE**
Instruct the patient to refrain from wearing the lenses for 24 to 48 hours.
Check for and treat corneal abrasions.
If a contact lens is lost in the eye, it is usually in the cul-de-sac of the upper eyelid. Evert the eyelid, and
remove the lens.
Look at the eye tangentially with a flashlight.
Check for a Medic-Alert bracelet.
Check for an identification card.

To remove a contact lens
Corneal hard lens. Use removal technique as demonstrated in Figure 25-4 or use a suction tip designed especially for removing contact lenses.
Soft lens. Locate the lens, slide the lens laterally onto the sclera, grasp it between the thumb and forefinger, and lift it off the cornea. If the lens does not remove easily, place a few drops of irrigating solution onto the eye to moisten it. Place soft lenses in an isotonic solution without preservatives.

Burns of the Eye

Chemical burns

■ **THERAPEUTIC INTERVENTIONS**
Immediate therapeutic intervention for any type of chemical burn to the eye is irrigation with copious amounts of saline solution or water, followed by careful examination.

Acid burns

Tissue denatures from acid and denatured tissue neutralizes acid.

■ **THERAPEUTIC INTERVENTIONS**
Topical anesthetic
Irrigation with copious amounts of normal saline solution or water
Topical antibiotics and cycloplegics
Analgesics may be indicated

Alkali burns

An alkali burn is a *serious emergency* situation, because alkalis cause great tissue destruction. Initially the burn may appear as white spots in the eye, and severe damage may not be evident until 3 to 4 days after the initial injury.

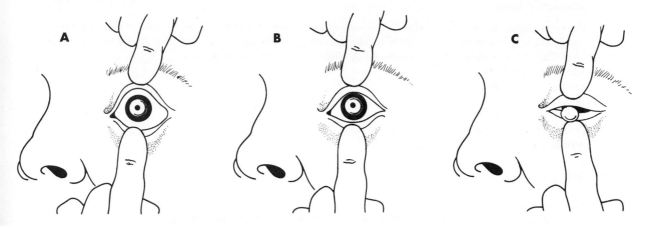

FIGURE 25-4. Technique for removing hard corneal contact lenses from an individual's eye. **A,** Spread eyelids apart. **B,** Push lids toward center of eye under contact lens. **C,** Remove lens.
(From Newbury L, Emergency Nurses Association: *Sheehy's emergency nursing: principles and practice,* ed 4, St Louis, 1998, Mosby.)

■ **THERAPEUTIC INTERVENTIONS**
Irrigate with copious amounts of normal saline solution or water for 30 minutes, then check pH; continue irrigation until pH is 7.0.
Antibiotics
Cycloplegics
Analgesics may be indicated
Ophthalmology consultation
■ **COMPLICATIONS OF ACID AND ALKALI BURNS**
Adhesion of globe to eyelid
Corneal ulceration
Entropion (eyelashes that turn in toward the eyeball)
Iridocyclitis
Glaucoma

Thermal burns

When facial burns are present, it is rather common to find associated burns of the eyelids. It is not common, however, to see burns of the eyeballs unless the burning agent was steam, metal, or gasoline.
■ **THERAPEUTIC INTERVENTIONS**
Topical anesthetic before exam
Analgesia
Sedation
Eye irrigation
Antibiotics
Cycloplegics
Bilateral eye patches
Ophthalmology consultation

Radiation burns

There are two types of radiation burns—ultraviolet and infrared.

Ultraviolet burn

Ultraviolet burns are seen with welder's flash and in snow skiers, ice climbers, people who read on the beach, and people who use sunlamps. The burn is caused when ultraviolet radiation is absorbed by the cornea. Keratitis or conjunctivitis or both result. Symptoms develop 3 to 6 hours after exposure.

■ **SIGNS AND SYMPTOMS**

Feeling of a foreign body

Tearing

Excessive blinking

Possible associated facial and eyelid burns

■ **THERAPEUTIC INTERVENTIONS**

Topical antibiotics

Analgesics

Cycloplegics

Bilateral eye patches

Signs and symptoms should be relieved within 24 hours after these measures are taken.

Infrared burn

An infrared burn is a severe type of burn. It may cause permanent loss of vision, because infrared rays are absorbed by the iris. This results in an increase of the temperature of the lens, which produces cataracts. When the lens is damaged, the repair process is very slow, and the lens remains much more vulnerable to injury during the healing process.

Common types of infrared burns

Glassblower's cataracts. Result from prolonged exposure to intense heat.

Focal retinitis. Caused by eclipse blindness or exposure to nuclear energy; the lens condenses heat, causing retinal scarring and blindness.

X-ray burns. Proportional to the amount of exposure and penetration of the x-rays; grenz rays are soft rays that produce superficial keratoconjunctivitis and dermatitis; gamma rays are hard rays that produce retinal damage and cataracts.

Irrigating the Eye

Instill topical anesthetic.

Cleanse the external area around the eye and eyelid.

Have the patient lie down or adjust the treatment chair so that the patient is in a supine position.

Have the patient turn the head with the affected side down.

Pull down on the lower eyelid of the affected side.

Run irrigation fluid directly over the globe of the eye and into the cul-de-sac of the lower eyelid from the inner to the outer canthus.

Have the patient blink occasionally to distribute the irrigation solution over the globe.

Irrigate for about 30 minutes (more if pH indicates).

Irrigation Using the Morgan Therapeutic Lens

The Morgan Therapeutic Lens (Figure 25-5) is a specially designed lens that is placed on the eye and used to provide continuous ocular lavage or medication. It is a scleral lens made of hard plastic (polymethyl methacrylate). The tubing is made of soft silicone plastic and has a female adapter at the distal end.

1. Explain the procedure to the patient.
2. Instill anesthetic ocular medication.
3. Ask the patient to look down.
4. Retract the upper eyelid.
5. Grasp the lens by the tubing and the small finlike projections.
6. Slip the superior border of the lens up under the upper eyelid.

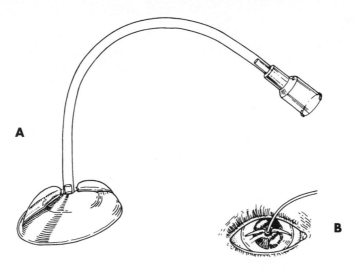

FIGURE 25-5. **A,** Morgan therapeutic lens. **B,** Lens in place for continuous irrigation.

7. Have the patient look up.
8. Retract the lower eyelid and place the lower border of the lens beneath it.
9. Have the patient turn the head toward the affected side, and place a folded towel under the head to collect irrigation solution.
10. Attach the female adapter at the end of the lens tubing to:
    a. A syringe filled with the solution of choice, and instill the solution at the desired rate, or
    b. Intravenous tubing that is connected to the solution of choice in an IV bottle or bag instilled at the selected drip rate.
11. To remove the lens, follow steps 3 through 8 in reverse order.
12. Dry the patient's face and eye area with a dry towel.
13. Dispose of the lens.

NOTE: The Morgan lens should be used for chemical burns of the eye. It should not be used for foreign bodies, because the foreign body may become entrapped under the Morgan lens.

MEDICAL PROBLEMS INVOLVING THE EYE

Blepharitis

Anterior blepharitis is an inflammation of the lid margin, usually caused by *Staphylococcus aureus.* The condition is frequently ulcerative.
■ **THERAPEUTIC INTERVENTIONS**
Cool, moist compresses
Antibiotic ophthalmic ointment

Hordeolum

A hordeolum or "sty" is an infection of the upper or lower eyelid at the accessory gland. It is caused by *Staphylococcus aureus.*

■ **SIGNS AND SYMPTOMS**

Small external abscess

Pain

Redness

Swelling

■ **THERAPEUTIC INTERVENTIONS**

Warm compresses four times a day until the abscess points

Antibiotic ophthalmic ointment

Abscess may be incised by a physician when it points.

Chalazion

A chalazion is a cyst that forms on the inside surface of the eyelid. It results from congestion of the meibomian gland.

■ **SIGNS AND SYMPTOMS**

Small mass beneath the conjunctiva of the lid

Redness

Swelling

Extreme pain

■ **THERAPEUTIC INTERVENTIONS**

Antibiotic ophthalmic ointment

Incision and drainage by a physician

Keratitis

Keratitis is an inflammation of the cornea.

■ **SIGNS AND SYMPTOMS**

Light sensitivity

Redness of the cornea

Pain

Profuse tearing

■ **THERAPEUTIC INTERVENTIONS**

Culture and sensitivity

Warm compresses

Antibiotic ophthalmic ointment

Herpetic keratitis

    Debridement

    Antiviral eye drops

Cycloplegics indicated.

Narcotic analgesics

Uveitis

Uveitis is a uveal tract inflammation that usually includes the iris, ciliary body, and choroid.

■ **SIGNS AND SYMPTOMS**

Signs and symptoms of uveitis appear unilaterally.

Photophobia

Tearing

Pain

Blurred vision

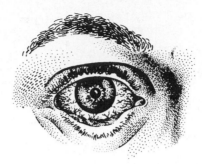

FIGURE 25-6. Conjunctivitis.

Constricted pupil
Headache
■ **THERAPEUTIC INTERVENTIONS**
Warm compresses
Systemic analgesics
Antibiotic ophthalmic ointment
Topical steroids
Mydriatics to dilate the pupil
Carbonic anhydrase inhibitors

Acute Conjunctivitis (Pinkeye)

Acute conjunctivitis (Figure 25-6) is most commonly a bacterial infection of the conjunctiva. It may be caused by *Staphylococcus, Gonococcus, Pneumococcus, Haemophilus,* or *Pseudomonas.* Other causes may include: chlamydia, chemical irritation, allergies, and systemic disease (Kawasaki disease, Stevens-Johnson syndrome).
■ **SIGNS AND SYMPTOMS**
Eyelids "stick together" on waking
Scratchy sensation, purulent discharge, infected conjunctiva
■ **THERAPEUTIC INTERVENTIONS**
Application of antibiotic ophthalmic ointment after a culture is obtained.
If chlamydia is suspected, tetracycline or erythromycin should be given topically and systemically.
Acute conjunctivitis is a *contagious* condition. Careful aftercare instructions should be given to the patient about how to avoid spreading the infection.

Acute Iritis

Acute iritis is an inflammatory condition of the iris. It is not an infectious process.
■ **SIGNS AND SYMPTOMS**
Acute pain
Constricted pupil
Photophobia
Tenderness of the globe
Can have blurred vision.
■ **THERAPEUTIC INTERVENTIONS**
Cold compresses
Mydriatics, cycloplegics

Analgesics

Dark glasses

Consider topical steroids.

Central Retinal Artery Occlusion

Central retinal artery occlusion produces painless sudden blindness. It is usually embolic in origin. Prognosis for regaining sight is very poor if the occlusion has lasted longer than 1 hour.

■ **THERAPEUTIC INTERVENTIONS**

Anticoagulants may be indicated.

tPA may be given IV within 60 minutes of onset.

Gentle ocular massage or intermittent digital pressure

Rebreathing CO_2 from a paper bag may decrease the blood pH and dilate the artery.

Surgical intervention by ophthalmologist

Cavernous Sinus Thrombosis (Orbital Cellulitis)

Cavernous sinus thrombosis is a pneumococcal, staphylococcal, or streptococcal infection that spreads from an infected sinus or throat to the orbital area. It usually begins unilaterally and can spread to the other cavernous sinus. There is a strong association with bacteremias, septicemia, and meningitis in infants and toddlers.

■ **SIGNS AND SYMPTOMS**

Facial and globe edema

Vascular congestion in eyelids

Aching pain

Pain in globe

Exophthalmos

Conjunctival chemosis

Fever

Decreased visual acuity

Decreased pupil reflexes

Papilledema

Paralysis of extraocular muscles

■ **THERAPEUTIC INTERVENTIONS**

Antibiotic ophthalmic ointment

Parenteral antibiotics

Bed rest, hospitalization

Warm compresses

Ophthalmology consultation

Retinal Detachment

When the retina is torn, vitreous humor seeps between it and the choroid, resulting in the separation of the retina from the choroid, which decreases blood and oxygen supply to the retina. This decreased blood and oxygen supply renders the retina unable to perceive light.

■ **SIGNS AND SYMPTOMS**

Flashes of light

A "veil" or "curtain" effect in the visual field

A dark spot or particles in the visual field

■ **THERAPEUTIC INTERVENTIONS**

Strict bed rest

Bilateral eye patches

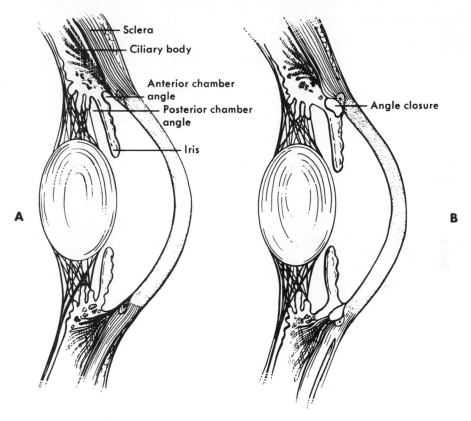

FIGURE 25-7. **A,** Normal eye. **B,** Closed-angle glaucoma.

Consider sedation
Possible surgical intervention

Glaucoma

Glaucoma occurs when aqueous humor cannot escape from the anterior chamber, causing a rise in anterior chamber pressure (Figure 25-7). This increase in pressure causes a decrease in circulation to the retina and an increase in pressure on the optic nerve. Blindness may eventually result.

Acute glaucoma

Acute (closed-angle) glaucoma results when there is blockage in the anterior chamber angle near the root of the iris. ACUTE GLAUCOMA IS AN EMERGENCY SITUATION! It may cause blindness in just a few hours.

■ **SIGNS AND SYMPTOMS**

Acute eye pain
Fixed and slightly dilated pupil
Hard globe
Foggy-appearing cornea
Severe headache
Halos around lights

Decreased peripheral vision
Nausea and vomiting

■ **THERAPEUTIC INTERVENTIONS**

Therapeutic intervention for acute glaucoma is aimed at decreasing pupil size to allow for aqueous humor drainage.

Frequent (every 15 minutes) instillation of miotic eyedrops (usually 1% or 4% pilocarpine)—the strength of the solution is not as important as frequent instillation

Topical beta adrenergic antagonists (such as timolol 0.5% and betaxolol) to decrease aqueous production

Systemic analgesia (usually morphine sulfate)

Sedation

Drugs such as acetazolamide (Diamox, mannitol, or glycerin) in an attempt to decrease intraocular pressure

Possible surgery

Chronic glaucoma

Chronic (open-angle or wide-angle) glaucoma occurs gradually and is caused by an obstruction of Schlemm's canal. Because it comes on very slowly, the patient may be unaware of its development.

■ **THERAPEUTIC INTERVENTIONS**

Instillation of miotic eyedrops
Possible surgery

Secondary glaucoma

Secondary glaucoma is an increase in intraocular pressure resulting from surgery, trauma, hemorrhage, inflammation, tumor, or various other conditions that may interfere with aqueous humor drainage. Therapeutic intervention will vary with the cause.

■ **HOW TO MEASURE INTRAOCULAR PRESSURE WITH A TONOMETER**

Tonometric examination is used to measure intraocular pressure. The Schiötz tonometer is one of the most commonly used type in the emergency department. It has a plunger that, when placed on the eye, measures the amount of indentation pressure on the cornea.

To properly use the tonometer, anesthetize the globe with an ophthalmic anesthetic agent.

Explain the procedure to the patient.

Have the patient lie down.

Have the patient stare upward at a spot on the ceiling.

Place a sterile (previously calibrated) tonometer on the globe.

Be careful not to put pressure on the globe while retracting the lids.

Position the footplate on the cornea and allow the plunger to indent the surface. This technique is correct when the gauge point pulsates with the pulse. Convert the tonometer reading to the pressure readings found in Table 25-1.

A normal indentation tonometer reading is 12 to 20 mm Hg. (Readings commonly reach 40 to 65 mmHg with angle closure glaucoma.)

Applanation tonometry—more accurate than Schiötz. Goldmann tonometer attached to slit 1 amp. Pressure measured as force needed to flatten area of cornea.

Tonopen—handheld, battery-operated applanator preferred by some for portability.

Amaurosis Fugax

Transient ischemic attack of an ocular nature. Occurs from a temporary obstruction of the retinal artery/arteriole from cholesterol or fibrin platelet emboli. Usually lasts 5 to 30 minutes.

■ **SIGNS AND SYMPTOMS**

Painless monocular vision loss

TABLE 25-1   Schiötz Tonometry

TONOMETER SCALE READING (UNITS)	TONOMETER WEIGHTS (G)		
	5.5 (mm Hg)	7.5 (mm Hg)	10 (mm Hg)
2.50	27	39	55
3.00	24	36	51
3.50	22	33	47
4.00	21	30	43
4.50	19	28	40
5.00	17	26	37
5.50	16	24	34
6.00	15	22	32
6.50	13	20	29
7.00	12	18	27
7.50	11	17	25
8.00	10	16	23
8.50	9	14	21
9.00	8	13	20
9.50	8	12	18
10.00	7	11	16

The table provides estimates of the intraocular pressure to the nearest mm Hg for the different weight of the Schiötz tonometer.
From Barr DH, Samples JR, Hedges JR: Ophthalmologic, Otolaryngologic, and Dental Procedures. In Roberts JR, Hedges JR, editors: *Clinical Procedures in Emergency Medicine,* ed 2, Philadelphia, 1991, WB Saunders.

■ **THERAPEUTIC INTERVENTIONS**
Usually resolves without treatment
Patient needs systemic evaluation to determine the cause.

Cyanacrylate Exposure

(i.e., Crazy or Super Glue)
Inadvertent instillation because glue container resembles eyedrop bottles. Quickly adheres to surfaces. Can cause corneal abrasion and/or chemical conjunctivitis.

■ **SIGNS AND SYMPTOMS**
Pain
Lids may or may not be sealed

■ **THERAPEUTIC INTERVENTIONS**
Copious irrigation with warm water or saline (most effective within 15 min of splash)
Do not pry lids apart (will usually loosen on their own in a day or two).
Can attempt to soften glue with mineral oil.
Opthalmology consult recommended
Patch with antibiotic ointment.

Eyedrops and Ophthalmic Ointments

Eyedrops are used to decrease pain, provide antibiotic therapy, increase or decrease the size of the pupil, decrease allergic reactions of the eye, or cleanse the eye.

Procedure for instilling eyedrops

1. Explain the procedure to the patient.
2. Pull the lower eyelid downward.
3. Have patient look upward.
4. Instill one or two drops of solution into the cul-de-sac (the center of the lower lid).
5. Have the patient blink to distribute the solution.
6. Instruct the patient not to squeeze the eyelids shut tightly, because this will cause the solution to leak out.

Procedure for instilling ophthalmic ointment

1. Explain the procedure to the patient.
2. Pull the lower eyelid downward.
3. Have the patient look upward.
4. Apply ointment in a thin line into the inner aspect of the lid from the inner to the outer canthus.
5. Have the patient blink to distribute the ointment.
6. Instruct the patient not to squeeze the eyelids shut tightly, as this will expel the ointment.

Ear Emergencies

There are three requirements for proper ear care:
- Good illumination
- Magnification
- Adequate physical control of the patient, including proper positioning and sedation, if necessary

Simple Lacerations

Simple lacerations of the outer ear are commonly seen in the emergency department.

■ **THERAPEUTIC INTERVENTIONS**

Cleanse the wound (scrub and irrigate).

Debride the wound.

Rejoin cartilage edges.

Cover the cartilage with skin.

Auriculectomy

An auriculectomy (Figure 25-8) is an amputation of the outer structures of the ear. Good results can be obtained if strict attention is paid to detail when reanastomosing the ear.

■ **THERAPEUTIC INTERVENTIONS (USUALLY PERFORMED BY A PLASTIC SURGEON)**

Reanastomose cartilage and skin.

Give IV antibiotics.

Hematoma of Pinna

Hematoma of the pinna usually results from blunt trauma.

■ **THERAPEUTIC INTERVENTIONS**

Anesthetize the area.

Aspirate the hematoma with an 18-gauge or larger needle.

Place a drain if necessary.

Apply a pressure dressing (cotton soaked in mineral oil or petrolatum gauze).

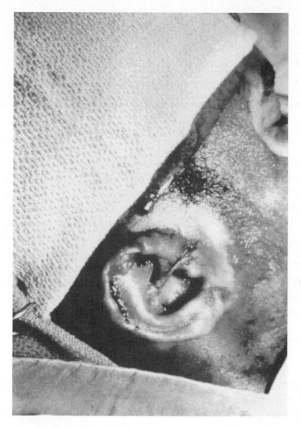

FIGURE 25-8. Repair of partial traumatic amputation of the pinna.
(Courtesy Dr Daniel Cheney.)

Bleeding from External Ear

Bleeding from the external ear is usually a result of a ruptured eardrum, a foreign body, or a canal laceration. Other sources of bleeding are basilar skull fracture or temporal bone fracture. Canal lacerations result from the ear being probed by sharp items. If the temporal bone is fractured, there may be cerebrospinal fluid otorrhea, a ruptured tympanic membrane, or a lacerated facial nerve.

■ **THERAPEUTIC INTERVENTIONS (FOR LACERATIONS ONLY)**

Cleanse the wound.

Apply antibiotic ointment.

Otolaryngologic consultation may be indicated.

If there is any question of CSF leakage, a neurosurgeon should be consulted and nothing should be placed in or over the ear.

Ruptured Tympanic Membrane

Ruptured tympanic membrane (eardrum) occurs as a result of positive pressure over the tympanic membrane or a penetrating foreign body. It may be caused by a slap over the ears (pressure from the outside), a diving injury (vacuum from the inside), an aircraft or altitude injury (expanding air inside), or self-instrumentation.

■ **SIGNS AND SYMPTOMS**

Sharp pain

Bleeding

Slight hearing impairment

May be asymptomatic

(NOTE: Presence of vertigo and tinnitus strongly suggest inner ear damage and are generally not considered symptoms for ruptured membrane.)

■ **THERAPEUTIC INTERVENTIONS**

Leave the area alone (do not probe it). Instruct the patient to do so as well.

Most small perforations will heal spontaneously; large perforations should be repaired by reapproximating the fragments with a suction apparatus; anesthesia is needed.

Antibiotics should be given if there is history of seawater or other contaminated water in the ear.

Note that diving injuries may cause a permanent loss of hearing and associated infection.

If associated with severe tinnitus or complete hearing loss, obtain an otolaryngologic consultation.

Foreign Body

Cerumen is a natural foreign body of the ear. Other common foreign bodies include beans, beads, and bugs. Children are especially prone to putting foreign bodies in their ears. Bleeding may occur when the patient attempts to remove the foreign body.

■ **THERAPEUTIC INTERVENTIONS**

If there is no perforation, remove the foreign body (visualize it first).

It may be necessary to administer general anesthetic to a child.

Remove round objects with an ear hook or rubber-tipped suction.

Do not push the object deeper in the ear canal.

If the foreign body is an insect, shine a flashlight into the ear. The insect will usually go toward the light. (Do not try to remove it while it is alive; the insect may struggle and cause more damage.) Live insects may be immobilized by instilling a few drops of lidocaine, mineral oil, or ether.

If there is a perforation, make sure that the object is clearly visualized, and remove the object with suction.

Do not instill anything into the ear if it is draining any type of fluid.

Acute External Otitis

Acute external otitis, or swimmer's ear, is an infection of the external ear caused by bacteria or fungus. It is a common finding in children.

■ **SIGNS AND SYMPTOMS**

Severe pain

Ear tender to touch

Swelling to the canal

Cellulitis of the pinna and other structures possible

Occasionally, purulent discharge

■ **THERAPEUTIC INTERVENTIONS**

Culture.

Give analgesics.

Drain the abscess, if present.

Insert a wick soaked in antibiotic solution or ointment.

Apply hot compresses.

Acute Otitis Media

Otitis media is an inflammation of the middle ear lining. As fluid builds up in the middle ear, pain becomes severe.

■ **SIGNS AND SYMPTOMS**
Sharp pain
Sensation of fullness in the ear
Difficulty hearing
Bulging of tympanic membrane
Elevated temperature
Nausea and vomiting
History of upper respiratory infection

■ **THERAPEUTIC INTERVENTIONS**
Decongestants
Antibiotics
Analgesics
Myringotomy

■ **COMPLICATIONS**
Tympanic membrane rupture
Acute mastoiditis

Acute Mastoiditis

Acute mastoiditis is the most common middle ear infection.

■ **SIGNS AND SYMPTOMS**
Pain in the mastoid area
Elevated temperature
Tenderness in the mastoid area
Difficulty hearing
Local swelling
Vertigo
Possible history of acute external or internal otitis
Thick, purulent drainage in ear canal

■ **THERAPEUTIC INTERVENTIONS**
Heat packs
Analgesia
Antibiotics
Otolaryngologic consultation (in case surgical drainage is required)

Labyrinthitis

An inflammation of the labyrinth of the inner ear. Thought to be associated with a viral illness, the condition has a commonly intense presentation. Symptoms can last one to many hours, even days in some cases, with gradual offset.

■ **SIGNS AND SYMPTOMS**
Intense vertigo
Nystagmus
Nausea and vomiting
Increased vagal stimulation
Hearing loss
Difficulty in standing or walking

■ **THERAPEUTIC INTERVENTIONS**
Bed rest
IV hydration
Antiemetics
IV diazepam

Cerumen Impaction

Persons with narrow, tortuous ear canals are more prone to this condition. It is complicated by continued use of cotton-tipped swabs.

■ **SIGNS AND SYMPTOMS**
Progressive hearing loss

■ **THERAPEUTIC INTERVENTIONS**
Cerumenolytics to soften and loosen debris
Removal via currettage
Warm water irrigation (unless suspicion of TM perforation)
Patient education to avoid causes

Nose Emergencies

Foreign Bodies

Foreign bodies in the nose are common in children and often are discovered only after a purulent discharge is seen draining from one of the nostrils.

■ **THERAPEUTIC INTERVENTIONS**
Decongestant nose drops
Topical anesthetic
Place the patient in Trendelenburg's position
Remove the object with a ring curette or alligator forceps

Epistaxis (Nosebleed)

Epistaxis can be a relatively minor problem, or it can turn into a life-threatening emergency. It commonly occurs in the following groups:

Children
Adults 50 to 70 years old
Patients with blood dyscrasias, hypertension, or arteriosclerotic heart disease
Patients on anticoagulant therapy
Alcoholics
Patients with allergies
Patients with hereditary hemorrhagic telangiectasia (Rendu-Osler-Weber disease)

Nasal Fractures

■ **SIGNS AND SYMPTOMS**
Pain
Epistaxis
Deformity
Swelling
Crepitance

Ecchymosis
Rhinorrhea
■ **THERAPEUTIC INTERVENTIONS**
Ice
Analgesia
Manual pressure as tolerated for bleeding
ENT referral recommended

Anterior epistaxis

Anterior epistaxis is common at Kiesselbach's area or in the anterior and inferior turbinates.
■ **THERAPEUTIC INTERVENTIONS**
Give much reassurance.
Place the neck in slight hyperextension.
Suction clots.
Check for bleeding site.
Soak cotton pledgets in a vasoconstrictor agent (usually 10% cocaine solution).
Insert pledgets into the nostril.
Apply pressure for 5 to 10 minutes.
Cauterize bleeding sites with silver nitrate.

NOTE: In patients with blood dyscrasias or immunosuppression, use a wedge of salt pork in place of the cotton pledgets; this is much more comfortable and appears much more effective.

Posterior epistaxis

Posterior epistaxis is a more serious problem. It usually results from hypertension, arteriosclerotic heart disease, a blood dyscrasia, or a tumor.
■ **THERAPEUTIC INTERVENTIONS**
Check blood pressure.
Give volume replacement if necessary.
Ask about the medical history.
Check coagulation studies.
Anesthetize the nose (10% cocaine).
Check the bleeding site, if possible.
Pack as described below.
If bleeding continues, ligation of the internal maxillary or anterior ethmoid artery may be necessary (usually done by otolaryngologist).
■ **PACKING FOR POSTERIOR NOSEBLEED**
Analgesia and/or sedation is usually required during packing for posterior nosebleed. The patient should be given antibiotics and admitted to the hospital for 3 to 5 days following packing.
Equipment
No. 18 or 20 Foley catheter with balloon or specially designed nasal balloon catheter or tampon (tonsil or vaginal) with three ties or rolled 4 × 4-inch sponge with three ties
Antibiotic ointment
Rubber catheter
Half-inch selvage-edge petrolatum gauze
Bayonet forceps
Gauze pad
Eye pad

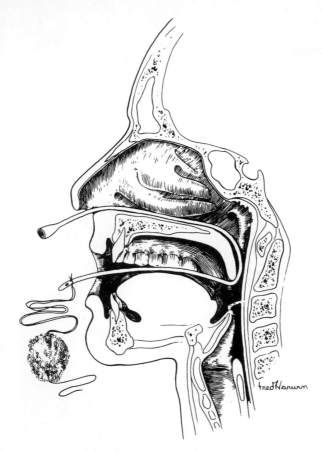

FIGURE 25-9. Steps used in passing a postnasal pack.
(From DeWeese DD, Saunders WH: *Textbook of otolaryngology*, ed 6, St Louis, 1982, Mosby.)

Procedure with tampon

1. Pass the rubber catheter through the nostril to the back of the palate and forward out of the mouth.
2. Tie two of the ties of the tampon to the catheter (Figure 25-9).
3. Pull the catheter out of the nose; the tampon will seat near the choana.
4. With the fingers, push the tampon into place (Figure 25-10).
5. Bring the other tie, which is dangling in the back of the mouth, forward and secure it to the outside of the face with tape.
6. Pack the nasal cavity bilaterally from the anterior openings through a nasal speculum with bayonet forceps with ½-inch selvage-edged petrolatum gauze, layering front to back. (Be sure to count and record the number of packs used.)
7. Tie the ties from the tampon around a gauze pad outside of the nostril. (Make sure both strings are coming out of the same nostril; never have one string coming out of each nostril, because this will cause necrosis.)

Procedure with catheter

1. Pass the Foley catheter into the nostril and to the palate area.
2. Inflate the Foley balloon (with 10 ml saline).
3. Pull the catheter forward until the balloon seats near the choana.
4. Hold the catheter firmly and pack the anterior chambers with ½-inch selvage-edged petrolatum gauze, layering front to back. (Be sure to count and record the number of packs used.)

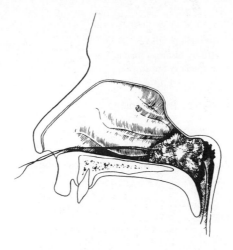

FIGURE 25-10. Postnasal pack in place.
(From DeWeese DD, Saunders WH: *Textbook of otolaryngology*, ed 6, St Louis, 1982, Mosby.)

5. Place an eye pad or 4 × 4-inch sponge around the Foley catheter.
6. Clamp the Foley catheter distal to the eye pad with an umbilical clamp.
   Epistaxis nasal balloon. This is a short (5-inch) catheter designed for control of epistaxis, and employs two separately inflatable balloons.
1. Insert the catheter into the nose until the posterior balloon is located in the nasopharynx.
2. Fill the posterior balloon with 10 cc sterile saline or water.
3. Pull the catheter gently forward until the balloon is set.
4. Inflate the anterior balloon with 30 cc sterile saline or sterile water.
5. To remove, deflate both balloons and withdraw the catheter gently.

Throat Emergencies

Foreign Bodies

Foreign bodies in the throat may be penetrating, obstructing, or aspirated.

■ **THERAPEUTIC INTERVENTIONS**
Visualize the foreign body.
Remove it with the appropriate instrument.
If the foreign body is totally obstructing the airway:
    Give four abdominal thrusts (Heimlich maneuver).
    Attempt to breathe for the victim.
    If this is unsuccessful, do an emergency cricothyrotomy.

Fractured Larynx

A fractured larynx is usually caused by a direct blow to the neck. Often the patient comes to the emergency department with multiple injuries, making this injury easy to overlook. A fracture of the larynx produces edema and consequently blocks the upper airway. Fracture of the larynx is a surgical emergency.

■ **SIGNS AND SYMPTOMS**

Shortness of breath	Respiratory stridor
Vocal changes	History of throat trauma
Subcutaneous emphysema	Respiratory arrest

■ **THERAPEUTIC INTERVENTIONS**

Perform cricothyrotomy or tracheostomy (see Chapter 5).

Epiglottitis

A potentially life-threatening condition, epiglottitis consists of swelling of the epiglottis with the ability to partially or completely obstruct the airway.

■ **SIGNS AND SYMPTOMS**

Patient sitting in an upright position	Fever
Muffled speech	Respiratory distress; can progress to complete airway obstruction
Stridor	Drooling

■ **THERAPEUTIC INTERVENTIONS**

Hospital admission and close observation in an ICU is indicated

Direct laryngoscopy, intubation, or tracheostomy occasionally necessary

IV antibiotics

IV hydration

Corticosteroids controversial

Supplemental oxygen

Cool mist

Esophageal Foreign Bodies

The most common type of esophageal foreign body seen in the ED is comprised of a food bolus that is unable to pass beyond anatomical strictures in the esophagus, and occasionally a sharp object such as a piece of bone the patient inadvertently swallowed. Children also sometimes swallow small toys, pieces of toys, coins, batteries, and other objects, which can lodge at the esophagogastric junction.

■ **SIGNS AND SYMPTOMS**

Feeling of object or sense of "fullness" in the throat

Pain with swallowing or inability to swallow even water

Patient usually able to locate point of obstruction.

Drooling

(Can cause perforation of the esophagus.)

■ **THERAPEUTIC INTERVENTIONS**

IV Glucagon

Laryngoscopy or endoscopy

There has also been some degree of success in the case of a partial obstruction by passing a Foley catheter into the esophagus under fluoroscopy and once past the food bolus inflating the balloon with barium and slowly withdrawing the catheter to disimpact the obstruction.

ENT or GI consult sometimes indicated, with potential removal under general anesthesia.

Upper Respiratory Tract Infection or Pharyngitis ("The Common Cold")

■ SIGNS AND SYMPTOMS

Sore throat	Malaise
Difficulty swallowing	Foul breath odor
Pain referred to the ears	Enlarged tonsils
Elevated temperature	Enlarged cervical nodes
Feeling of fullness in the head	

■ THERAPEUTIC INTERVENTIONS

Throat culture
Warm saline gargles
Aspirin or acetaminophen
Antibiotics
Antihistamines
Decongestants

Peritonsillar Abscess

A peritonsillar abscess is a collection of pus in the peritonsillar fascial planes and most commonly follows an episode of pharyngitis or tonsillitis.

■ SIGNS AND SYMPTOMS

Initially, pharyngitis
Difficulty speaking
Trismus
Difficulty swallowing
Drooling
Possible airway difficulties
Soft palate swollen on affected side
Deviation of uvula toward unaffected side

■ THERAPEUTIC INTERVENTIONS

Parenteral antibiotics
Otolaryngology consult
Possible irrigation and debridement

Dental Emergencies

Dental Pain

The most common cause of dental pain is tooth decay or pulpal disease. Pulpal disease has three phases:
Hyperemic—the vascular system responds to an external stimulus, such as dental caries (cavity) or dental trauma; this is a reversible condition.
Pulpitis—the pulp becomes infected.
Pulpal necrosis—the pulp dies; fluid and pressure build, causing pain.
Therapeutic intervention for these conditions consists of analgesia, antibiotics, and referral to a dentist.

Other causes of dental pain

Exposed root surfaces as a result of receding gums
Fractured teeth

Periodontal disease (in the supporting tissues)
Foreign bodies (such as a toothbrush bristle embedded in tissues)
Dry socket
Pressure from a prosthetic device
Mandibular fractures
Vincent's angina, or "trench mouth" or necrotizing ulcerative gingivitis (ulcers of the gingiva)
Pericoronitis (pain of wisdom teeth erupting)
Sinusitis
Trigeminal neuralgia
Glossodynia (a burning pain in the tongue)
Fractured styloid process
Hematomas (usually resulting from trauma, which may include injections of anesthetic)
Coronary artery disease (referred pain to jaw)
Carcinoma (hemostomatitis and radiation therapy)
Teeth in process of eruption
TMJ dysfunction

Toothaches

The most common cause of toothaches is pulpal disease or dental caries. This type of pain is paroxysmal and usually begins with a heat or cold stimulus. The pain usually occurs spontaneously and continues to worsen, especially at night when intracranial pressure increases.

■ **THERAPEUTIC INTERVENTIONS**
Topical oil of clove or other analgesia
Referral to a dentist

Dental Abscess

Abscesses in the periapical areas usually result from pulpal necrosis secondary to caries or trauma. Periodontal abscesses usually result from bony destruction at the periodontal membrane, which can form a pocket resulting in abscess formation.

■ **THERAPEUTIC INTERVENTIONS**
Drainage of the abscess
Antibiotics
Analgesics
Hot packs on the area
Warm saline rinses every 2 hours
Aspirin or other antipyretic for fever above 101° F (38.3° C)
Referral to a dentist

Periodontal Emergencies Requiring Dental Referral

gingivitis   Inflammation of the gums characterized by redness, swelling, pain, and bleeding.
periodontal disease   Loss of periodontal bone; symptoms more severe than gingivitis; definitive diagnosis is made on x-ray films.
necrotizing ulcerative gingivitis (Vincent's angina or "trench mouth")   Painful bleeding, foul-smelling breath, lymphadenopathy, chills, fever, and malaise.
pericoronitis   Painful eruption of wisdom teeth accompanied by swelling, lymphadenopathy, and trismus; therapeutic intervention is by removal of tissue over the tooth, warm saline rinses, antibiotics, and dental referral for possible tooth extraction.

Postoperative Bleeding

Often a patient comes to the emergency department bleeding from the mouth, with a history of recent tooth extraction or other oral surgery. Usually all that is needed is to apply a pressure pack over the area of hemorrhage. If the bleeding persists, a hemostatic dressing such as absorbable gelatin sponge (Gelfoam), oxidized cellulose (Surgicel), or thrombin should be packed into the socket. A home remedy that may also be effective is to place a wet teabag over the socket. (The tannic acid may help produce hemostasis.) If the packing is unsuccessful, sutures may be placed or the bleeding vessels may be cauterized. Caution the patient to avoid mouth rinses until the bleeding has completely stopped, to eat a soft diet, to use intermittent ice packs, to avoid hot liquids, and not to drink through a straw.

Dry Socket (Postextraction Alveolitis)

Dry socket usually occurs 3 to 5 days after surgery, when a blood clot is lost and bone is exposed.
■ THERAPEUTIC INTERVENTIONS
A pledget soaked in oil of clove packed into the socket
Analgesia
Dental referral

Chipped (Broken) Teeth

Chipped or broken teeth are the most frequently seen dental emergencies in the emergency department. The four center upper teeth are the teeth most frequently injured.

Check for bleeding from gums and from pulp. Bleeding from pulp requires emergency dental consultation. Because these injuries are frequently associated with head injuries, be sure to check the mouth and pharynx area for pieces of teeth and debris that may obstruct the airway.

Avulsed Teeth

Avulsed teeth are teeth that have been totally dislodged from the socket by trauma. If found, these teeth may be reimplanted.
■ THERAPEUTIC INTERVENTIONS
Place the tooth in saline solution, milk, or water. If the patient is conscious, the tooth may be placed between the gum and lip in the patient's mouth.
Refer patient to a dentist or oral surgeon.
Irrigate the wound.
Anesthetize the wound area.
Reimplant the tooth as soon as possible.

NOTE: Blood supply to the tooth comes via the pulp, so the viability of the tooth depends on the patency of the pulp.

Teeth that have been driven into the gums, especially in children, should be left alone. Patient should be referred to dentist.

NOTE: Remember to look for teeth and foreign bodies such as prostheses and bridges in the mouths of trauma patients and to remove these objects to avoid airway obstruction.

SUGGESTED READINGS

Barbarito C: Emergency! Hypertension-induced epistaxis, *Am J Nurs* 98(2): 48, 1998.

Bruckenthal P: A guide to the diagnosis and management of migraine headaches for the nurse practitioner, *Am J Nurs Pract* 1(3): 12-18, 1997.

Centor RM: The diagnosis of strep throat in an emergency room, *Med Decis Making* 1: 239, 1981.

Cohen EL: Epiglottitis in adults, *Ann Emerg Med* 13: 620, 1984.

Janda AM: Ocular trauma: triage and treatment, *Postgrad Med* 90:51, 1991.

Janda AM: Ophthalmic disorders in primary care, *Hosp Physician* 29:44, 1993.

Kearny KM: Emergency! Retinal detachment, *Ann J Nurs* 97(8): 50, 1997.

Moreland LW, Corey J, McKenzie R: Ludwig's angina: report of a case and review of the literature, *Arch Intern Med* 148: 461, 1988.

Rosen P et al: *Emergency medicine concepts and clinical practice,* ed 4, St Louis, 1997, Mosby.

26

Chest Trauma

Mary Dahlgren Gunnels

Patients who suffer blunt or penetrating trauma to the chest can have severe, life-threatening injuries. Of all trauma deaths in the United States, approximately 25% result from injuries to the chest.[1] It is essential that the patient's condition be assessed rapidly and life-saving therapeutic interventions applied concurrent with findings to reduce morbidity and mortality. Many life-threatening conditions can be reversed if they are identified early and interventions are rapid.

THORACIC CAVITY ANATOMY

The thoracic cavity (Figure 26-1) extends from the first rib under the clavicle to the diaphragm. The diaphragm can elevate as high as the fourth intercostal space anteriorly upon exhalation and as low as the tenth intercostal space upon inhalation (Figure 26-2). Injuries between the fourth and tenth intercostal spaces should be considered both chest and abdominal until one or both are ruled out, because the diaphragm is mobile and separates the thoracic cavity from the abdominal cavity. A gunshot or stab wound just below the right nipple may involve the skin, connective tissue, muscle, ribs, pleura, lungs, *and* liver.

The thoracic cavity contains the lower airway: the mainstem and right and left bronchi, the lungs, and the heart, the great vessels, and the esophagus. It is surrounded by twelve pairs of ribs that provide protection and structure. At the inferior border of each rib run the intercostal vein, artery, and nerve. It is important to note that chest procedures should be performed at the superior border of the ribs or at the sternum or subxiphoid, because intercostal arteries bleed profusely when disrupted.

The Angle of Louis is the most constant landmark on the anterior chest wall. The second intercostal space is at the Angle of Louis in the midclavicular line just below the clavicle (Figure 26-3).

The lungs are elastic in nature and have a natural tendency to collapse. Normally, with the presence of negative pressure (a "vacuum") in the intrathoracic space, the lungs do not collapse. When there is an inspiratory effort, the intercostal muscles pull the ribs upward, the diaphragm drops downward, and negative pressure increases. The lungs respond to this negative pressure by filling with air. If negative pressure (the vacuum) is lost, the lungs collapse because of their elasticity. The normal tidal volume of the lungs is 5 to 7 ml per pound of body weight.

The intrathoracic space expands when the intercostal muscles lift the ribs and the diaphragm drops down. This process is assisted by the accessory muscles of respiration: the abdominal wall muscles, the pectoralis muscles, and the sternocleidomastoid muscles.

The phrenic nerve runs through the diaphragm. Irritation of the phrenic nerve by blood or other sources may cause hiccoughs or referred pain to the shoulder.

When assessing and treating a patient with chest trauma, *always* assume that the injury is serious until it is proven otherwise. Of people with chest trauma, 85% require nonsurgical intervention to improve their condition. There is usually a problem with hypoxia, circulation, or obstruction.[2] Hypoxia is a major cause of death in chest trauma. It is associated with one of four states: perfusion (blood circulating) of an unventilated lung; ventilation of an unperfused lung; an abnormal airway/lung relationship, which may be due to a mechanical or physiological obstruction; or hypovolemia (and therefore decreased oxygenation).

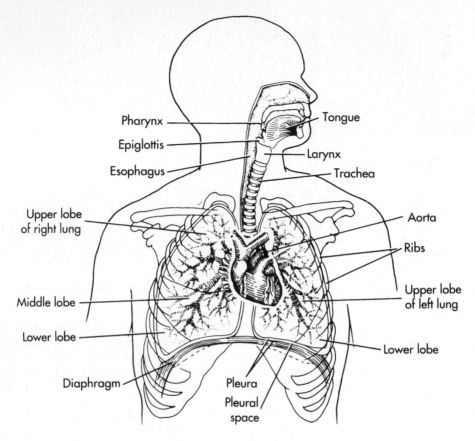

FIGURE 26-1. Anatomy of the thoracic cavity.

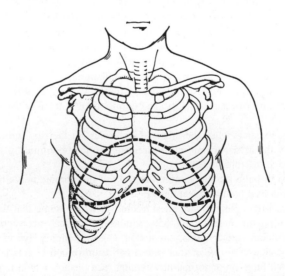

FIGURE 26-2. Level of diaphragm on inspiration and expiration.

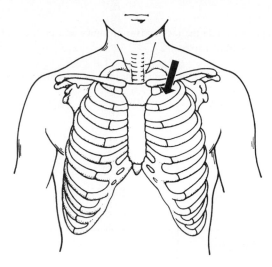

FIGURE 26-3. The Angle of Louis and the second intercostal space.

PRIORITIES IN THE TREATMENT OF PATIENTS WITH CHEST INJURIES

- To maintain an adequate airway
  Assure that there are no obstructions.
- To ensure good ventilation
  Administer supplemental O_2 via nonrebreather mask or endotracheal tube.
  Visualize the chest rise and fall.
  Listen for bilateral breath sounds. When air enters the lungs, it enters the bases first. Listen at the fifth or sixth intercostal space at the midaxillary line. Breath sounds only on the right side may indicate the presence of an endotracheal tube in the right mainstem bronchus or a pneumothorax.
  Check SaO_2 and end-tidal CO_2 (when available).
  Estimate tidal volume. Place your hands on the patient's chest with fingers spread and thumb tips touching on exhalation. If the thumbs spread apart on inspiration, the patient is breathing a tidal volume of at least 78% of normal. With loss of intercostal muscles 50% of tidal volume is lost.[3]
  If the ribs do not move on inspiration, there may be a spinal cord injury with diaphragmatic breathing.
- To ensure adequate circulation
  Check skin vitals (color, temperature, moisture).
  Check capillary refill (greater than 2 seconds—the time it takes to say "capillary refill"—is abnormal).
  Check vital signs.
  Start two large-bore IV lines—16 gauge or larger; run warmed lactated Ringer's normal saline solution.
- To protect the cervical and thoracic spines
  Assume spinal cord injury until proven otherwise.
  Immobilize from the top of the head to the hips.
- To perform a rapid assessment for life-threatening injuries of the chest
  These include flail chest, tension pneumothorax, pericardial tamponade, massive hemothorax, open pneumothorax, and dissecting or ruptured aorta.
  Potentially life-threatening conditions include pulmonary contusion, tracheobronchial rupture, esophageal rupture, diaphragmatic rupture, myocardial contusion, and dissecting aorta.

In addition:
    Obtain a medical history and include the mechanism of injury and prehospital events.
    Obtain an upright chest x-ray film (if possible)

NOTE: If the chest x-ray film is done in a supine position, the mediastinum will appear widened.

    Check for entrance and exit wounds.
    Consider chest tube(s) placement.
    Consider autotransfusion.
    Obtain arterial blood gases.
    Place the patient on a cardiac monitor and obtain a 12-lead ECG.
    Consider emergency thoracotomy.
    Consider any therapeutic intervention specific to the injury.
    Measure urinary output.

TYPES OF CHEST INJURIES

Rib Fractures

Rib fractures are the most common type of chest injuries. A rib consists of the head, where it attaches to the vertebrae, the tubercle, the angles, and the body. Ribs fracture most commonly at the angle junctures. The third through ninth ribs are most commonly injured. If there is a first rib fracture, a flail chest, or multiple rib fractures, suspect a severe injury. Rib fractures may cause decreased ventilation, increased secretions, atelectasis, and pneumonia.

A first rib fracture is often associated with a clavicle fracture and sometimes a scapular fracture. First, second, and third rib fractures should be considered serious. Fractures of these ribs carry a 15% to 30% mortality rate caused by the proximity of those ribs to the subclavian artery, subclavian vein, aorta, and the tracheobronchial tree.[4]

When there are lower rib fractures, consider the possibility of damage to underlying structures. Fractures of ribs 5 through 9 on the right are dangerous because they overlie the liver. Ribs 9 through 11 on the left overlie the spleen and may cause it to rupture when the ribs are fractured.

■ **SIGNS AND SYMPTOMS**
Mechanism of injury that could cause chest trauma
Pain that increases with inspiration (bone spicules irritate the parietal pleura.)
Splinting of the chest
Crepitus or subcutaneous emphysema at the fracture site
Possible palpation of the fracture
■ **DIAGNOSIS**
Chest x-ray film
■ **THERAPEUTIC INTERVENTIONS**
    For simple fractures
Rest
Intermittent ice for first 24 hours, then heat
Simple analgesia or regional anesthesia
    For displaced rib fractures or any rib fractures in the elderly
Hospital admission
Regional anesthesia for severe pain
    Local infiltration
    Intercostal nerve block

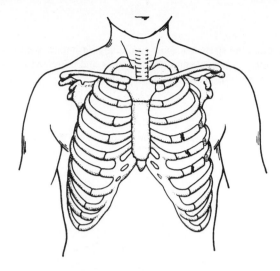

FIGURE 26-4. Flail chest. Two or more ribs fractured in consecutive places.

Flail Chest

When two or more adjacent ribs are fractured in two or more places or the sternum is detached, the segment becomes flail (Figure 26-4). This segment loses continuity with the rest of the chest wall and responds directly to intrathoracic pressure changes; paradoxical chest wall motion results. When negative pressure increases (on inhalation), the flail segment is drawn inward (Figure 26-5, *A*). When negative pressure decreases (on exhalation), the segment is pushed outward (Figure 26-5, *B*). The flail segment moves in the opposite direction from the rest of the chest wall (paradoxical motion). This injury is usually caused by a massive blunt force to the chest. A major danger of a flail chest is that complications will arise, particularly hypoxia, from the underlying pulmonary contusion that is caused by the great force that caused the ribs to fracture. Therefore flail chest is life-threatening and indicates high potential for serious, associated injuries.

■ **SIGNS AND SYMPTOMS**
Observed paradoxical motion of the chest wall
Respiratory distress (tachypnea to respiratory failure)
Palpation of subcutaneous emphysema
Pain

■ **DIAGNOSIS**
Clinical observation
Chest x-ray
Arterial blood gases/SaO_2

■ **THERAPEUTIC INTERVENTIONS**
The goal of therapeutic intervention is to provide good ventilation; treat the pulmonary contusion.
Selective endotracheal intubation
Oxygen with positive pressure
    Consider positive end expiratory pressure (PEEP).
Consider stabilizing the flail segment.
IVs
    Carefully administering crystalloids
    Consider using arterial pressure or pulmonary wedge pressure valves to guide fluid replacement.
Pain control
Admission to ICU for close observation and pulmonary stabilization

Sternal Fracture

It takes a great force to fracture the sternum—most commonly an impact with a steering wheel or following CPR. A totally detached sternum is considered a flail segment and is treated accordingly. With sternal fractures, the most common underlying injury is a myocardial contusion.

■ **SIGNS AND SYMPTOMS**

Chest pain

Dysrhythmias/ECG changes

    Especially premature ventricular contractions, arterial fibrillation, right bundle branch block, and ST segment elevation

Pain on inspiration

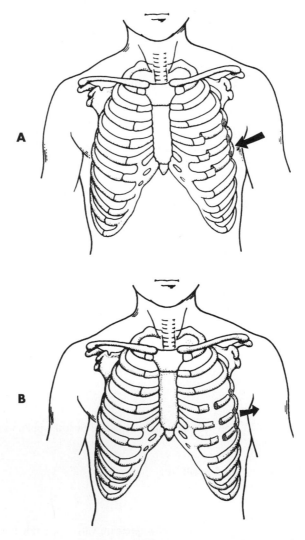

FIGURE 26-5. **A,** Flail chest; when diaphragm is drawn down and respiratory effort is made, flail segment pulls in. **B,** Flail chest; when diaphragm rises and exhalation occurs, flail segment moves outward.

■ **DIAGNOSIS**
Palpation of the fracture
ECG/cardiac monitor
Chest x-ray film
■ **THERAPEUTIC INTERVENTIONS**
Close observation
Pain control
Treat dysrhythmias
Consider surgery for fixation

Fractured Clavicle

A fractured clavicle is usually not a serious injury. However, a jagged fracture may lacerate the subclavian artery or vein. This injury is usually caused by a blunt force and is commonly seen as an athletic injury, where the blunt force is received laterally (for example, a football injury).

■ **SIGNS AND SYMPTOMS**
Pain (especially on palpation)
■ **DIAGNOSIS**
Clinical observation of the deformity
Chest x-ray film
Consider arteriogram to rule out vascular damage.
■ **THERAPEUTIC INTERVENTIONS**
Figure-of-eight (splint)
Pain control

PNEUMOTHORAX

Simple Pneumothorax

A simple pneumothorax (Figure 26-6) is a condition that causes a ventilation defect when air enters the chest cavity, causing a loss of negative pressure (the vacuum) and a partial or total collapse of the lung. It may be

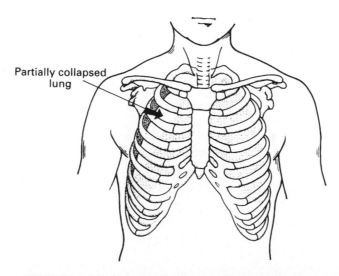

Partially collapsed
lung

FIGURE 26-6. Simple pneumothorax; partial collapse of a lung.

caused by a hole in the chest wall or a hole in the lung tissue, the bronchus, or the trachea. A spontaneous pneumothorax is the occurrence of a pneumothorax without evidence of trauma. It is thought to be caused by a ruptured bleb or a ruptured cyst.

■ **SIGNS AND SYMPTOMS**
History of blunt or penetrating trauma to the chest
Sudden onset of sharp pleuritic chest pain
Diminished breath sounds on the affected side
Shortness of breath
Tachypnea
Syncope
Hamman's sign (a crunching sound with each heartbeat, caused by mediastinal air accumulation)
Hyperresonance on percussion

■ **DIAGNOSIS**
Clinical observation
Chest x-ray film

■ **THERAPEUTIC INTERVENTIONS**
Close observation
Oxygen by nonrebreather mask
Semi-Fowler's position
Consider placement of a large-bore needle through the anterior chest wall in the second intercostal space.
Consider placement of a chest tube.

Tension Pneumothorax

When air enters the pleural space during inspiration and is trapped during exhalation, pressure in the intrathoracic space begins to build, forming what is known as a *tension pneumothorax*. This usually occurs as the result of a penetrating injury, but may also be caused by blunt trauma, use of mechanical ventilation with positive end expiratory pressure (PEEP), a nonsealing puncture, or a ruptured bleb. A tension pneumothorax (Figure 26-7) is a life-threatening condition. Usually there is good perfusion, but inadequate ventilation can eventually lead to poor perfusion.

Pressure forces the heart and great vessels to be pushed toward the opposite side (Figure 26-8). This event is known as mediastinal shift. This shift causes the great vessels to kink, which results in a backup of blood into the venous system. This is demonstrated by distension of the neck veins and a decreased blood return to the heart, causing a decreased cardiac output. The trachea will also be pushed toward the uninjured side, causing tracheal deviation.

■ **SIGNS AND SYMPTOMS**
Severe respiratory distress
Deviated trachea (toward the unaffected side)
Mediastinal shift
Jugular vein distension
Cyanosis
Decreased blood pressure and other hemodynamic deterioration signs
Increased pulse
Restlessness
Paradoxical movement of the chest
Distant heart sounds
Hyperresonance on percussion

■ **DIAGNOSIS**
Clinical observation
Chest x-ray film

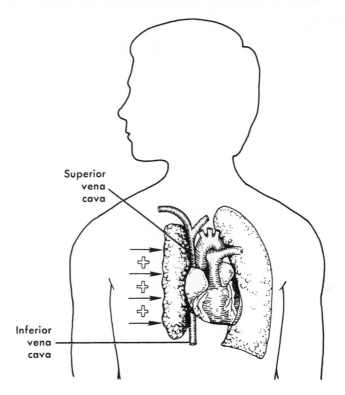

Superior
vena
cava

Inferior
vena
cava

FIGURE 26-7. Tension pneumothorax.

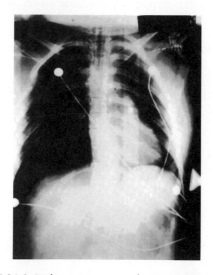

FIGURE 26-8. Right tension pneumothorax as seen on x-ray.

■ **THERAPEUTIC INTERVENTIONS**

NOTE: If the patient is severely symptomatic, do not wait for chest x-ray film results before providing therapeutic intervention.

Airway

Oxygen at high-flow rate (be careful not to administer oxygen under positive pressure until the chest tube is placed because this may increase the tension)

Needle thoracotomy (Heimlich valve)

Chest tube placement

IV Ringer's lactate or normal saline

Needle thoracotomy. The definitive therapy for tension pneumothorax is the placement of a chest tube. If a patient is in the field or it will be a while before a chest tube can be placed, consider placing a needle into the anterior chest wall of the affected side to partially relieve the tension until a chest tube is placed. This procedure may buy some time, but must be followed by chest tube insertion.

The procedure

1. Rapidly prepare the area in which the needle will be placed with alcohol or Betadine; use the second intercostal space at the midclavicular line.
2. Insert a needle (at least a 16 gauge, preferably metal) over the superior portion of the rib (the vein, artery, and nerve, and located behind the inferior border) and through the tissue covering the pleural cavity.
3. When the needle has entered the pleural cavity, there will be a hissing sound.
4. If desired, the needle may be attached to a flutter valve or a syringe filled with saline.
5. Leave the needle in place until the chest tube is placed.
6. Continue to ventilate the patient or provide supplemental oxygen.

Sucking Chest Wound (Open Pneumothorax)

A sucking chest wound (Figure 26-9) is a chest wall defect that results in an open pneumothorax. It is usually caused by a penetrating force, such as a high-velocity missile. If there is a two-way flap, air will pass into the pleural space and back out again with inspiration and expiration. If the diameter of the hole in the chest wall is greater than two thirds the diameter of the trachea, there will be preferential flow of air through the chest wall

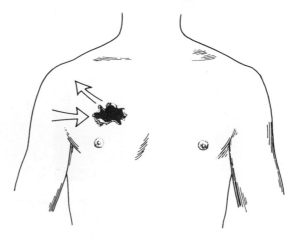

FIGURE 26-9. Sucking chest wound—open pneumothorax.

defect (the path of least resistance).[5] This causes a simple pneumothorax as negative pressure is lost, which may be overcome with positive pressure ventilation. If there is a one-way flap, air can enter the pleural space but cannot escape. Pressure will build with each inspiratory effort until a tension pneumothorax has formed.

■ **SIGNS AND SYMPTOMS**
Dyspnea
Chest pain
Visualization of the defect
Sucking sound
Possible signs of tension pneumothorax

■ **DIAGNOSIS**
Clinical findings

■ **THERAPEUTIC INTERVENTIONS**
Ensure ABCs.
Oxygen under positive pressure
It is not necessary to cover the wound if the defect is less than two thirds the diameter of the trachea and the patient is intubated and being ventilated with positive pressures.
Consider covering the wound with an occlusive dressing (per EMS or hospital policy), sealed on three sides.
    Leave one side open for flutter valve effect.
        Observe for the development of a tension pneumothorax. If a tension pneumothorax develops:
            Remove the occlusive dressing. This should convert the tension pneumothorax to a simple pneumothorax.
            If this does not relieve the tension pneumothorax, follow the steps for therapeutic intervention for tension pneumothorax.
    Consider chest tube placement.
    Consider autotransfusion.

Chest tube placement

Chest tubes are placed so that air and blood can be removed from the intrathoracic cavity. The procedure involves placing the chest tube in the appropriate space so that air is removed and the tension pneumothorax is relieved, or to drain blood and/or fluids by gravity drainage or with the assistance of suction.

■ **INDICATIONS**
Hemothorax
Pneumothorax
Empyema

■ **EQUIPMENT NEEDED** (Figure 26-10)
Betadine or other prep solution
Prep sponges
2 large curved Kelly clamps
6 × 10 ml syringes with 18- and 25-gauge needles
Scalpel and blade
1% lidocaine
Suture to secure chest tube
Suture for wound approximation
Needle holder
Appropriate size chest tube
Chest drainage collection device
Sterile surgical gloves
Occlusive dressing material
Sterile drape
Wide adhesive tape
Benzoin

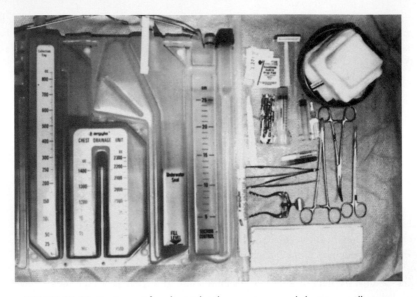

FIGURE 26-10. Equipment for chest tube thoracostomy and drainage collection.

■ **PROCEDURE**

1. Monitor the patient throughout procedure.
2. Determine chest tube placement site—usually the second intercostal space, midclavicular line for a pneumothorax, or fifth intercostal space, slightly anterior to the midaxillary line for a hemothorax.
3. Prep and drape the site.
4. Infiltrate the skin and rib periosteum with lidocaine.
5. Using a scalpel and blade, make a 2 to 3 cm transverse incision through the skin.
6. Using a Kelly clamp, bluntly dissect and spread through the subcutaneous tissue over the superior edge of the rib.
7. Puncture the tip of the Kelly clamp (carefully) through the pleura (if there is a pneumothorax, air will rush out of the puncture hole).
8. Explore the intrathoracic area with the sterile gloved index finger of the dominant hand to free adhesions or clots.
9. Place half of the tip of a Kelly clamp through a perforation on the distal end of the chest tube, so that the tip of the tube is firm.
10. Advance the distal tip of the tube into the intrathoracic cavity, ensuring that it is situated well past the most proximal fenestration.
11. Once the tube is determined to be in the proper place, secure it using silk suture attached to the tube and to the skin.
12. Close the skin edges with nonabsorbable suture.
13. Apply Benzoin to the skin surrounding the chest tube.
14. Apply an occlusive dressing (for example, Vaseline® gauze)
15. Secure the dressing and the chest tube with adhesive tape.
16. Attach the tube to a closed chest drainage system and confirm that suction equipment is in working order (Figure 26-11).
17. Note the amount of the initial drainage and any subsequent drainage directly on the collection chamber and on nurses' notes/flow chart.
18. Obtain a chest x-ray film to ensure proper placement of the tube.

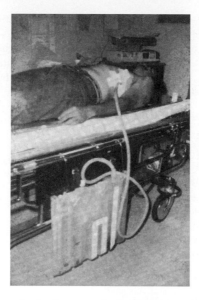

FIGURE 26-11. Chest tube in place, attached to a water seal chest drainage unit.

Hemothorax

A hemothorax is a collection of blood in the intrathoracic space. It generally occurs when a lung or vessel is lacerated as the result of a blunt or penetrating trauma. Because hemothorax will cause a hypovolemic state, observe the patient carefully for signs and symptoms of shock. Hemothorax is often seen in conjunction with a simple or tension pneumothorax. Greater than 1500 ml of blood in the intrathoracic cavity is considered a *massive hemothorax.*

■ **SIGNS AND SYMPTOMS**

Similar to those of simple or tension pneumothorax

Signs of shock (including cool clammy skin, decreased capillary refill, decreased blood pressure, tachycardia, tachypnea, dullness to percussion of affected side, restlessness, anxiety, agitation, confusion, or unconsciousness)

■ **DIAGNOSIS**

Clinical observation

Laboratory—check hematocrit

Chest x-ray film

■ **THERAPEUTIC INTERVENTIONS**

Treat shock condition

ABCs

IVs (bilateral, large bore, 16 gauge or greater)

Chest tube placement

Consider autotransfusion.

Consider emergency thoracotomy or surgery.

  If initial drainage is 1000 ml or greater, followed by at least 200 ml of blood for each of four consecutive hours, or if there is an initial drainage of 1500 ml of blood or greater, this may indicate the need for emergency thoracotomy.[6]

  Autotransfusion. Autotransfusion is a technique that is used to collect blood from an exsanguinating chest wound through a chest tube. The blood is filtered, anticoagulated, and reinfused into the patient. There are several types of autotransfuser set-ups. Caregivers should be familiar with the particular type of autotransfusion equipment used at their own facility.

In the emergency setting only blood from the chest can be used because it is considered relatively uncontaminated. This procedure has the advantage of having immediately available blood that is warm, perfectly cross-matched, and free from infectious diseases other than those the patient may already be carrying.

Autotransfusion may be indicated with the following conditions:

Massive hemothorax

Myocardial rupture

Great vessel rupture

Other chest trauma when there is:

  Nonavailability of banked blood

  A history of transfusion reactions

  Refusal of blood for religious reasons

Autotransfusion is contraindicated:

When wounds are more than 4 hours old

When the patient has inadequate kidney or liver function

When there is contamination of blood by:

  Outside sources

  Abdominal/intestinal contents

  Cancer cells

LUNG INJURIES

Pulmonary Contusion

Pulmonary contusion is the most common potentially life-threatening problem that occurs with chest trauma.[4,7] It is also one of the most common injuries in major trauma. It is often seen with flail chest and associated with severe blunt trauma to the chest, and can cause respiratory failure.

With pulmonary contusion, blood extravasates into the parenchyma of the lung because of an injury to the lung tissue. That causes the lung tissue to become anoxic and more permeable. Occasionally pulmonary contusion can cause tracheal obstruction.

■ SIGNS AND SYMPTOMS

The diagnosis of pulmonary contusion is usually made by suspecting it based on the mechanism of injury and looking for specific signs and symptoms to confirm one's suspicions.

 Hemoptysis

 Increasing hyperpnea

 Dyspnea

 Ineffective cough

 Restlessness and agitation

 Presence of other severe chest injuries

NOTE: Pulmonary contusion may be slow to develop (1 to several hours).[4,8]

■ DIAGNOSIS

High index of suspicion

Clinical observation

Chest x-ray film

Arterial blood gases

O_2 saturations

■ **THERAPEUTIC INTERVENTIONS**

Airway management; selective endotracheal intubation

Oxygen at high flow (humidified)

Consider ventilatory support.

Limit fluids during resuscitation, unless there is associated injury causing hypovolemic shock.

   Use whole blood products to replace lost blood, maintain oncotic pressure, and decrease pulmonary edema.

Consider diuretics.

Consider steroids.

Pain control

   Morphine sulfate may be given incrementally via IV; however, monitor for bradycardia and hypoxia.

Laceration of Lung Parenchyma

Lacerations of the parenchyma are usually caused by penetrating trauma or jagged rib fractures. They are usually self-limiting and rarely require surgical intervention.

■ **SIGNS AND SYMPTOMS**

Small hemothorax or pneumothorax

Hemoptysis

Subcutaneous emphysema

■ **DIAGNOSIS**

Clinical observation

Chest x-ray (showing hemothorax, pneumothorax, or subcutaneous emphysema)

Arterial blood gases

■ **THERAPEUTIC INTERVENTIONS**

Usually none necessary

Consider surgery if signs and symptoms are severe.

Injury to Tracheobronchial Tree

Injury to the tracheobronchial tree usually involves the trachea or mainstem bronchus, most commonly near the bifurcation of the mainstem bronchus, 1 inch from the carina. This injury is usually caused by blunt or penetrating trauma. *Signs and symptoms may not appear for up to 5 days following injury, and they may be subtle.* There is a 50% mortality rate in the first hour.[4,9]

■ **SIGNS AND SYMPTOMS**

Airway obstruction

Atelectasis

Hemoptysis (massive)

Mediasternal and subcutaneous emphysema (progressive)

Air leak "somewhere in the chest"

Possible signs and symptoms of tension pneumothorax

■ **DIAGNOSIS**

Clinical findings

If the disruption is below the carina, chest x-ray film will demonstrate mediastinal air

Bronchoscopy

■ **THERAPEUTIC INTERVENTIONS**

Maintaining airway

Oxygen at high flow

Chest tube

Semi-Fowler's position

Surgical repair

Diaphragmatic Rupture

Diaphragmatic rupture may be a life-threatening injury. Disruption of the diaphragm, the main muscle of respiration, causes major interference with ventilation.[10] Consider the possibility of diaphragmatic injury when there is an injury below the level of the nipples caused by a forceful blow to the left side of the abdomen or by increased intraabdominal pressure (for example, a motor vehicle crash where the victim was using a lap seat belt only). Blunt trauma usually causes large tears. A ruptured diaphragm is usually associated with other major injuries, and is often diagnosed late or during surgery.[7]

■ SIGNS AND SYMPTOMS

Bowel sounds in the thoracic cavity
Chest pain referred to the shoulder
Severe shortness of breath
Difficulty breathing
Decreased breath sounds
Undigested food or fecal material in chest tube

■ DIAGNOSIS

Chest x-ray film (supine—demonstrating bowel that herniated into the thoracic cavity and an elevated left hemidiaphragm) (Figure 26-12), or the presence of the nasogastric tube in the thoracic cavity, or loss of the costophrenic angle on the side opposite the injury.[11]

GI series demonstrating stomach and/or intestines in the thoracic cavity

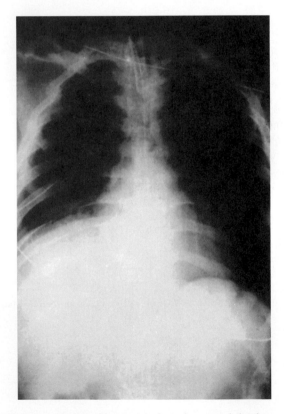

FIGURE 26-12. Bowel herniating through ruptured diaphragm.

■ THERAPEUTIC INTERVENTIONS
Placement of a gastric tube
Surgery

CARDIAC INJURIES

Myocardial Contusion

Myocardial contusion probably occurs more frequently than it is diagnosed. It may be overlooked because of other, more obvious, severe injuries. Always suspect myocardial contusion in any patient who gives a history of blunt trauma to the chest or a severe acceleration/deceleration force, in any motor vehicle crash where a bent steering wheel has occurred, and in any patient who has recently had cardiopulmonary resuscitation/chest compressions.

■ SIGNS AND SYMPTOMS
Suspicion of myocardial contusion because of mechanism of injury
Severe chest pain
Chest wall contusion and ecchymosis (Figure 26-13)
Dysrhythmias/ECG changes
    Usually within the first hour, but up to 24 hours
    Usually premature ventricular contractions, atrial fibrillation, right bundle branch block, or elevated ST segment
Tachycardia
Hypotension
Dyspnea
Other associated signs of cardiogenic shock

■ DIAGNOSIS
High index of suspicion
Signs of injury on ECG
Elevated ST segment in V1, V2, V3 if injury is on the left

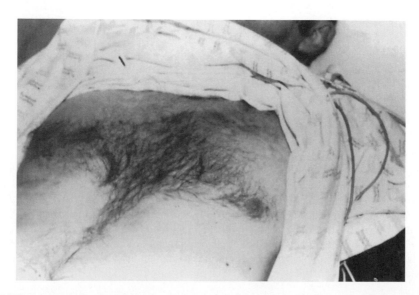

FIGURE 26-13. Mechanism of injury and chest abrasion suggest potential myocardial contusion.

Elevated cardiac isoenzymes
Echocardiography
■ **THERAPEUTIC INTERVENTIONS**
Therapeutic interventions for myocardial contusion are similar to those for an acute myocardial infarction. The patient should be treated symptomatically.
Oxygen
Semi-Fowler's position (complete bed rest)
Pain control
Treatment of dysrhythmias
Admission to monitored intensive care unit bed for at least 48 hours

Penetrating Cardiac Injuries

Penetrating injuries to the heart carry a high mortality rate. If the patient survives the prehospital phase of care and arrives at the emergency department, immediate thoracotomy and surgical repair are indicated.[12]
■ **SIGNS AND SYMPTOMS OF MYOCARDIAL DISRUPTION**
Severe hypotension
Elevated central venous pressure
Distended jugular veins
Decreased ECG voltage
Decreased heart sounds
■ **SIGNS AND SYMPTOMS OF AORTIC OR MITRAL VALVE DISRUPTION**
Sudden onset of severe chest pain
Severe dyspnea
Hemoptysis
Loud "roaring" murmur
Other associated signs of severe congestive heart failure and/or pulmonary edema
■ **DIAGNOSIS**
High index of suspicion
Chest x-ray film
Direct visualization
■ **THERAPEUTIC INTERVENTIONS**
Oxygen
Immediate surgery
To repair rupture
To replace valve

Pericardial Tamponade

Pericardial tamponade occurs when a wound of the heart, such as a pericardial laceration or a ruptured coronary artery, bleeds into the pericardial sac. Blood accumulates in the sac, causing pressure within the sac to rise. This interferes with ventricular filling and consequently with cardiac output. The heart attempts to compensate by activating the sympathetic nervous system, which causes the heart rate to increase. Because this compensation cannot continue for very long, the efficiency of the heart begins to deteriorate. As the heart rate increases, venous pressure increases, blood pressure falls, and heart sounds diminish.

A pericardial tamponade is usually caused by severe blunt trauma to the chest. It is often confused with tension pneumothorax. Consider the possibility of pericardial tamponade when there is unexplained pump failure that is not responsive to volume replacement. Pericardial tamponade is an immediate life-threatening injury.

■ **SIGNS AND SYMPTOMS**

Decreased blood pressure ⎫
Distended jugular veins   ⎬   Beck's triad—the hallmark of pericardial tamponade
Muffled heart sounds   ⎭
Increased heart rate
Dyspnea
Pulsus paradoxus
Cyanosis
Other associated signs of shock

■ **DIAGNOSIS**

High index of suspicion
Clinical observation
Chest x-ray film (demonstrating a widened mediastinum)
Pericardiocentesis
Echocardiography

■ **THERAPEUTIC INTERVENTIONS**

Oxygen at high flow
IVs
High Fowler's position
Pericardiocentesis and/or pericardial window

AORTIC DISRUPTION

Tears of the aorta are usually the result of a blunt force such as occurs in motor vehicle accidents or falls from great heights. The aorta usually tears at the points of attachment, particularly at the ligamentum arteriosum and the aortic root. Patients who sustain aortic tears are usually in quite critical condition and rarely survive. There is a 90% at-the-scene mortality rate.[13] Of the remaining 10% of survivors, there is a 50% mortality rate with each day of treatment delayed. The cause of death from aortic disruption is usually the result of a pericardial tamponade or massive exsanguination.

■ **SIGNS AND SYMPTOMS**

Signs of hypovolemic shock
Signs of pericardial tamponade
Chest wall bruise
First or second rib fracture
Sternal fracture
Scapula or multiple rib fractures
Large murmur heard best at the left parascapular region
Upper extremity blood pressure higher than lower extremities
Tracheal deviation to the right
Paraplegia
Trauma arrest

■ **DIAGNOSIS**

High index of suspicion
Chest x-ray film
    Widened mediastinum
    Obliteration of aortic knob
    Presence of a pleural cap
    Hemothorax
    Esophageal deviation (by N/G tube on x-ray film)
    Elevated right mainstem bronchus/lower left mainstem bronchus

Thoracic aortogram

CT scan

Transesophageal echo cardiogram (TEE)

■ **THERAPEUTIC INTERVENTIONS**

CPR

Oxygen at high flow

IVs (with whole blood as soon as possible)

Thoracotomy and surgical repair

RUPTURED ESOPHAGUS

A ruptured esophagus is a rare event, but when it does occur, the mortality rate is high if the diagnosis is missed.[13] It usually occurs as a result of penetrating trauma or a severe blunt epigastric blow. When the cause is blunt trauma, the rupture often occurs just above the diaphragm. Consider esophageal rupture whenever there is evidence of a first or second rib fracture. It may be seen in conjunction with a pneumothorax or a hemothorax without evidence of fracture. It also may occur iatrogenically, during esophagoscopy.

■ **SIGNS AND SYMPTOMS**

Sudden onset of severe chest pain or upper abdominal pain following trauma

Signs and symptoms of pneumothorax

Pain on swallowing

Mediastinitis

Subcutaneous emphysema

Mediastinal "crunch" sound (Hamman's sign)

Increased respiratory effort

Pleural effusion

Gastric contents or bile in chest tube

Shock without associated pain

Elevated temperature

■ **DIAGNOSIS**

Clinical observation

Upper GI series

Endoscopy

■ **THERAPEUTIC INTERVENTIONS**

Oxygen at high flow

IVs

Immediate surgical intervention

SUMMARY

Chest trauma is potentially life-threatening; the primary focus of therapeutic intervention should be on maintenance of an airway, adequate breathing/ventilation, and adequate circulation. All injuries to the chest should be considered severe until proven otherwise.

REFERENCES

1. American College of Surgeons/Committee on Trauma: *Advanced trauma life support manual,* ed 2, Chicago, 1998, ACS.
2. Lawrence P: *Essentials of general surgery,* ed 3, Baltimore, 1998, Williams & Wilkins.
3. Shea J: Lecture presented at The Emergency Nurses Association Annual Meeting, Orlando, FL, Sept 1992.
4. Cardona VD et al: *Trauma nursing: from resuscitation through rehabilitation,* Philadelphia, 1994, WB Saunders.
5. American College of Surgeons/Committee on Trauma: *Advanced trauma life support manual,* ed 2, Chicago 1998, ACS.
6. Sheehy SB et al: *Manual of clinical trauma care: the first hour,* ed 3, St Louis, 1999, Mosby.
7. Jachimczyk K: Blunt chest trauma, *Emerg Med Clin North Am* 11(1):81, 1993.

8. Lawrence P: *Essentials of general surgery,* ed 3, Baltimore, 1998, Williams & Wilkins.
9. American College of Surgeons/Committee on Trauma: *Advanced trauma life support manual,* ed 2, Chicago, 1998, ACS.
10. Lawrence P: *Essentials of general surgery,* ed 3, Baltimore, 1998, Williams and Wilkins.
11. American College of Surgeons/Committee on Trauma: *Advanced trauma life support instructor manual,* ed 2, Chicago, 1998, ACS.
12. Galliard M et al: Mortality prognostic factors in chest injury, *J Trauma* 30(1):93, 1990.
13. Mattox K, Moore EE, Feliciano DV: *Trauma,* San Mateo, CA, 1991, Appleton & Lange.

SUGGESTED READINGS

Baker P, Bennett B, editors: *Trauma nurse core curriculum provider manual,* Chicago, Ill, 1995, Emergency Nurses Association.

Emergency Nurses Association: *Cases in advanced trauma nursing: a conceptual approach,* Park Ridge, Ill, 1995, the Association.

Kaytal D, Mclellan BA, Brenneman FD et al: Lateral impact motor vehicle collisions: significant cause of blunt traumatic ruptiure of the thoracic aorta, *J Trauma* (42)5:769-772, 1997.

Klein A: *Emergency nursing core curriculum,* Philadelphia, 1994, Saunders.

Selfridge-Thomas J: *Manual of emergency nursing,* Philadelphia, 1995, Saunders.

Emergency Nurses Association: *Sheehy's Emergency nursing: principles and practice,* ed 4, St Louis, 1998, Mosby.

Trupka A, Waydhas C, Hallfeldt KKJ et al: Value of thoracic computed tomography in the first assessment of severely injured patients with blunt chest trauma: Results of a prospective study, *J Trauma* (43)3:405-412, 1997.

Abdominal Trauma

Kathy Sciabica Robinson

There are two mechanisms of injury for abdominal trauma: *blunt* and *penetrating*. Blunt trauma results from a force to the abdominal wall that causes energy to diffuse into the abdominal cavity without causing an open injury. The abdominal organs are injured either by compression (squeezing the organ between the vertebral column and the impacting object) or deceleration (abdominal organs move forward with gravitational force until impacting an object, rupturing, or tearing away from supporting structures). The organs most commonly injured are the liver, spleen, and kidneys, because they are solid organs and more likely to rupture when struck by a force. "Seatbelt syndrome," caused by use of a lap belt only, may cause rupture of viscera or compression injuries.

Penetrating trauma results when an object such as a bullet, knife blade, or metal fragment pierces the abdominal wall and enters the abdominal cavity. Stab wounds often do not penetrate the peritoneal cavity and have a surprisingly low mortality rate (1% to 2%). Gunshot wounds, however, usually cause significant injury to abdominal organs and require surgical intervention.

Knowledge of the mechanism of injury, diligent physical exam, and maintaining a high degree of suspicion of injury are essential to reduce the morbidity and mortality related to abdominal trauma.

BLUNT TRAUMA

Blunt trauma most frequently occurs as a result of a motor vehicle crash, contact sports, falls, and child maltreatment. In the emergency care setting it is most important to determine whether the patient requires surgery and/or hospital admission for observation; it is not as important to determine which structures have been injured. Keeping this concept in mind, care is directed at frequent assessment and diagnostic tests in addition to keeping the patient stabilized through the use of emergency care adjuncts such as airway management and fluid replacement.

Give special consideration to those patients who are not reliable for diagnostic information, such as patients with spinal cord injuries, those who are unconscious or who have used mind-altering drugs or alcohol, and small children. The absence of signs and symptoms does not rule out abdominal injury. Further diagnostic studies are essential to reduce morbidity and mortality.

■ SIGNS AND SYMPTOMS

Bruises or abrasions
Distension (not a reliable sign)
Pain
Involuntary guarding
Rigidity
Crepitus
Masses
Signs of shock
    Decreased level of consciousness
    Cool, clammy skin

Poor capillary refill
Tachycardia
Tachypnea
Hypotension
Other associated severe injuries

■ **DIAGNOSIS**

Diagnosis may be difficult in the patient with blunt abdominal trauma. The importance of obtaining a good history of the mechanism of injury cannot be stressed enough. All potential and actual injuries require prioritization to assure that life- or limb-threatening injuries are stabilized first.

The diagnostic examination should include:

Clinical observation with special attention to pain, rigidity, guarding, bruising
Peritoneal lavage to rule out intraabdominal injury; or
Abdominal CT to rule out intraabdominal or peritoneal bleeding
Abdominal and pelvic ultrasound
Arteriogram to rule out vascular injury
Cystogram to rule out bladder injury
Intravenous pyelogram (IVP) to rule out kidney and ureter injury
Retrograde urethrogram to rule out penile shaft injury
Rectal exam to rule out rectal injury
Nasogastric tube to rule out gastric injury and to decompress the stomach
Urinalysis to rule out renal and urinary tract injury
Laboratory studies (CBC, serum amylase, liver enzymes, renal function studies)
Surgery (indicated when involuntary guarding, abdominal expansion, hemodynamic instability, or gastrointestinal blood is present)

■ **THERAPEUTIC INTERVENTIONS**

Provide airway management and 100% supplemental oxygen.
Start IVs (two large bore with crystalloids).
Stabilize cervical, thoracic, and lumbar spine.
Consider PASG (very controversial at the time of this printing).
Place nasogastric or orogastric tube.
Place Foley catheter.
Prepare patient for surgery.

Diagnostic Peritoneal Lavage

Indications for diagnostic peritoneal lavage (DPL) include:

- Evidence of blunt trauma to the abdomen in which shock ensues *but immediate CT scan is not possible.* It may also be done in the operating room if there is an urgency to take the patient to surgery for a severe head or chest injury and abdominal trauma has not yet been ruled out.
- Cases in which the patient is not conscious and cannot tell of abdominal tenderness, and signs of abdominal guarding and so on cannot be elicited.
- Patients who are inebriated or have spinal cord injury, from who it would be almost impossible to elicit signs and symptoms of blunt abdominal trauma.
- Diagnostic peritoneal lavage is not recommended for children.

The only absolute contraindication to the procedure is a distended bladder (Figure 27-1). The bladder must be emptied and the stomach decompressed prior to diagnostic peritoneal lavage.

■ **RELATIVE CONTRAINDICATIONS**

A gravid uterus
An abdominal wall hematoma
Abdominal scars from previous surgery

In all of these instances, the location of the incision should be changed, but the procedure may still be per-

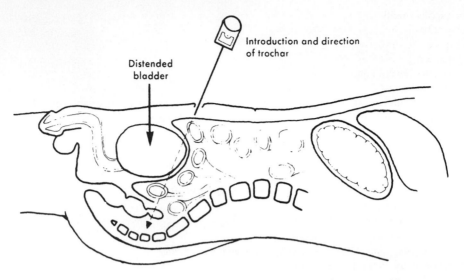

FIGURE 27-1. Distended bladder may be perforated by trochar for peritoneal lavage.

formed. If there is evidence of penetrating injury, diagnostic peritoneal lavage should not be performed; the wound should be explored surgically.

■ **EQUIPMENT**

Surgical antiseptic solution
Sterile drapes
Sterile gloves
1% lidocaine with epinephrine
No. 11 scalpel
No. 15 peritoneal dialysis catheter (with or without trocar)
Syringe with small-gauge needle
Ringer's lactate (1000 ml, warmed) and IV tubing
Nasogastric tube
Foley catheter
Skin retractors
4-0 nylon suture and needle
Antibiotic ointment
Small dressing for covering stab wounds

■ **PREPARATION OF PATIENT**

Explain the procedure to the conscious patient and give instruction about how to cooperate with the procedure.
Empty the bladder with a Foley catheter.
Empty the stomach with a nasogastric or orogastric tube.

■ **PROCEDURE**

1. Prepare the anterior abdominal wall by cleansing with a surgical solution such as 1% povidone-iodine (Betadine) and draping with sterile towels.
2. Inject 5 ml of 1% lidocaine with epinephrine in a subcutaneous wheal to 2 to 3 cm below the umbilicus.
3. Make a 2 cm or larger incision through the skin and subcutaneous adipose tissue to the linea retractor. Provide *absolute* hemostasis. If blood from the incision is allowed to escape, it can give a false indication to the lavage.

4. Engage the trochar into the linea alba at a 30° to 45° angle. (Instruct the patient to tense the abdomen if possible.) Apply rotary motion and pressure until the peritoneum is perforated or place the trochar through a surgical incision.
5. Direct the trochar tip toward the caudad pelvis and slide off the catheter 15 to 20 cm into the peritoneal cavity.
6. Attach a 20-ml syringe and aspirate the catheter. If aspiration yields 20 ml of blood, the tap is considered positive, and the procedure is terminated. If little or no blood is obtained, attach the IV line of 1000 ml Ringer's lactate and infuse over 15 minutes. Manually manipulate the abdomen to permit the solution to mix with abdominal cavity fluids.
7. Place the IV solution flask on the floor to siphon off the infused fluid.
8. When the majority of the fluid is returned, remove the catheter.
9. Close the skin with a 4-0 nylon suture.
10. Dress stab wounds with antibiotic ointment and a small sterile dressing.

Analysis of Findings

■ LABORATORY METHOD

The laboratory method requires three samples for analysis.

Hematocrit and red blood cell (RBC) count.	The level of hematocrit and RBCs that is considered significant for surgery will depend on institutional policy.
White blood cell count	500/cu mm or more
Amylase	200 Somogyi units or more
Bile	Any free bile
Culture and Gram's stain	Any significant quantity of bacteria indicates perforation of the intestine.

Indications for Exploratory Laparotomy

Unexplained hemorrhagic shock
Peritoneal perforation
Increasing abdominal tenderness or rigidity
Evidence of peritonitis
Visualized free air in the abdomen
Definitive diagnostic peritoneal lavage or CT scan
Enlarging abdominal mass in the absence of pelvic or vertebral fractures
Progressive drop in hemoglobin and hematocrit in the absence of hypotension, especially in the second 24 hours after injury
Blunt abdominal trauma is rarely a singular event. Head and chest trauma or other life-threatening injuries may complicate assessment. Abdominal injuries account for 10% of all trauma-related deaths in the U.S.; hemorrhage is the most common cause of death.

PENETRATING TRAUMA

Civilian violence, particularly in urban settings, accounts for most penetrating abdominal trauma, with gunshot wounds being the most lethal. A thorough inspection of the patient's front and back should allow for examination and documentation of all entrance and exit wounds. Surgical exploration is recommended, because 96% to 98% of penetrating abdominal gunshot wounds produce significant intraabdominal injury. Stab wounds cause less significant injury, most often to the intestine, and require surgical intervention less frequently.

As with all major trauma patients, treat the patient with the standards of:
Airway management
Supplemental oxygen
Control of bleeding

Initiation of two large-bore IVs

Protection of the cervical, thoracic, and lumbar spine

Saline-to-dry dressings on eviscerated tissue

Consideration of PASG (in accordance with institutional protocol)

Preparation for surgery

In the prehospital setting, most of these therapeutic interventions should be accomplished en route to the hospital. While therapeutic interventions are ongoing, someone should be trying to ascertain the type and size of weapon used, the amount of elapsed time since the injury, and the amount of estimated external blood loss.

THE ORGANS IN ABDOMINAL TRAUMA

The Stomach

Because the stomach is a hollow organ and can readily be displaced, it is rarely injured in blunt trauma to the abdomen. It is, however, often injured when trauma to the abdomen is penetrating. To check for stomach damage, insert a nasogastric tube and examine the aspirate. An abdominal x-ray might also prove useful if free air is seen, which is indicative of stomach or intestinal injury.

The Liver

The liver is the largest solid organ in the body. It is often injured in both blunt and abdominal trauma because it is located anteriorly, is large, very dense, and part of it is relatively unprotected. Be particularly suspicious of a liver injury when the eighth through twelfth ribs on the right are damaged and when trauma has involved the upper central abdomen.

Liver injury is diagnosed definitively on CT scan and at surgery. Large stellate lacerations must be surgically repaired, but small lacerations may be self-healing.

The Spleen

The spleen is the intraabdominal organ most frequently injured by blunt force. It is a very dense, encapsulated organ located behind the eighth through tenth ribs in the left upper abdominal quadrant, and injury should be suspected following any blow to the left upper quadrant. Pain and tenderness in the left upper quadrant that radiates to the left shoulder (Kehr's sign), along with peritoneal irritation and hypotension, aid in the diagnosis. Definitive diagnosis is made by CT scan or surgery. On occasion it may be advisable to observe a patient with a splenic injury, provided that the patient is hemodynamically stable. Close observation and repeated CT scans are in order. Splenic preservation may prevent immune response problems in the future.

The Pancreas

The pancreas is rarely injured in blunt abdominal trauma, but may be injured in penetrating trauma. The pancreas is a solid organ that is well protected by the stomach and the liver. It is located retroperitoneally, so that damage will not be evidenced on peritoneal lavage. Pancreatitis, a main concern of pancreatic injury, exhibits the delayed symptoms of pain, nausea/vomiting, abdominal distension, and altered vital signs. Serum amylase will elevate over 24 to 48 hours.

The Kidneys

The kidneys are located retroperitoneally in the flank area. They may be contused, which is usually self-limiting, or lacerated (fractured), which may require surgery. Contusion is usually treated with forced fluids and bed rest. A lacerated kidney may cause hemorrhage or may cause urine to extravasate, depending on the location and extent of the laceration. Diagnosis of the laceration is made by IVP or CT scan and urinalysis. Surgery may range from repair to nephrectomy.

The Ureters

Because the ureters are hollow and quite flexible, they are not usually injured in blunt trauma to the abdomen. They may, however, be disrupted in penetrating trauma. Diagnosis is made by IVP. If disruption occurs, surgery for reanastomosis is indicated.

The Bladder

The bladder, although a hollow organ, often contains urine, which essentially converts it to a solid organ, making it more vulnerable to injury in blunt trauma to the abdomen. It is also at great risk for injury when pelvic fractures occur. Bladder rupture is diagnosed by cystogram. If there is a laceration or rupture, surgical repair is indicated.

The Urethra

Urethral disruptions are more common in males than in females because of the external location of the urethra in males. It usually results from a straddle injury, such as occurs with impact of the crossbar on a bicycle or a motorcycle. Diagnosis is made by retrograde urethrogram. If disruption is present, urology consult is indicated.

The Intestines

The large and small intestines are hollow organs, but they are frequently injured in both blunt and penetrating trauma because of their size, anterior and relatively unprotected position, points of fixation, and vascularity. Intestinal disruptions must be repaired to control hemorrhage and to cleanse the abdominal cavity of abdominal contents that may later cause peritonitis and severe infections. Although abdominal x-rays, peritoneal lavage, and abdominal CT scan are used in diagnosis, definitive diagnosis is made by exploratory laparotomy.

The Diaphragm

Diaphragmatic ruptures may cause severe complications and even death because abdominal contents may herniate into the chest cavity, causing severe respiratory difficulty. In addition, the diaphragm is the main muscle of respiration and is required in order for respiration to occur. Diagnosis is made by observing bowel in the chest cavity or the distal end of the nasogastric or orogastric tube in the chest on chest x-ray.

The Abdominal Aorta, Inferior Vena Cava, and Hepatic Veins

These are the major blood vessels of the abdomen. If disrupted, hemorrhage will occur; and death will ensue if the injury is not corrected. They can be diagnosed by diagnostic peritoneal lavage, CT scan, and aortography. If disruption is present, immediate surgery is indicated.

SOME CONSIDERATION FOR THE PREGNANT PATIENT WITH ABDOMINAL TRAUMA

- A fetus may cause compression of abdominal vasculature and result in obstructive hypovolemia. Whenever possible, elevate the woman's right hip or manually displace the uterus to allow for venous return to the right side of the heart.
- If the woman is hypovolemic and requires volume replacement, administer blood products as soon as possible. Both the woman and the fetus require the oxygen-carrying capacity of the blood.

• Remember to shield the uterus with a lead shield as much as possible during x-ray procedures.
• Continue to monitor the fetus throughout the resuscitation and treatment period.
• Consider inflating only the leg chambers of the PASG, if PASG is local protocol for abdominal trauma.
Abdominal trauma is a frequent finding, especially following motor vehicle crashes. Careful attention to physical examination and diagnostic findings is essential.

SUGGESTED READINGS

Feeman LM, Newberry L: Gastrointestinal trauma. In Emergency Nurses Association: *Sheehy's emergency nursing: principles and practice,* ed 4, St Louis, 1998, Mosby.

American College of Surgeons Committee on Trauma: *Advanced trauma life support course, manual,* Chicago, 1996, ACS.

Emergency Nurses Association: *Trauma nursing core course,* ed 4, Park Ridge, Ill, 1995, the Association.

McGinty P: Helpful websites, *Intl J Trauma Nurs* 4:27, 1998.

Rothlin M, Naf R, Amgwerd M et al: Ultrasound in blunt abdominal and thoracic trauma, *J Trauma* 34(3), 1993.

Musculoskeletal Emergencies

Susan F. Strauss

Orthopedic trauma and nontraumatic musculoskeletal injuries are found in a large portion of the patients seen in the emergency department. These injuries are seldom life threatening but many result in long term disability, loss of income, disfigurement and pain. Orthopedic injuries remain the leading cause of impairment and loss of years of productive life.[1]

These complaints can be associated with fractures, sprains, ligament tears, tendon lacerations, arterial lacerations, and joint dislocations. In any orthopedic injury or complaint neurovascular compromise must be suspected.

Skeleton

The skeleton is made up of 206 bones. It provides the following:
- Support and protection for vital organs
- Leverage and movement of various body parts and for the body as a whole

Ligament

Ligaments are fibrous connective tissue that connect bone to bone. They provide joint stabilization and facilitate movement.

Tendon

Tendons are fibrous connective tissue that connect muscle to bone. They permit flexion and extension of muscle groups.

DEFINITIONS

Skeleton

The skeleton forms the framework of the body; it provides both support and protection.

Bone

There are two types of bone: (1) cancellous (spongy) bone, which can be found in the skull, vertebrae, pelvis, and long-bone ends; and (2) cortical (dense) bone, which is found in the long bones. Bone has its own blood and nerve supply and is usually capable of healing itself. Bones serve to protect vital organs and serve as levers for movement.

Ligament

Ligament is fibrous connective tissue that connects bone to bone.

Tendon

Tendon is fibrous connective tissue that connects muscle to bone.

Cartilage

Cartilage is dense connective tissue found between the ribs; in the nasal septum, ear, larynx, trachea, and bronchi; between vertebrae; and on the articulating surfaces of bones. Cartilage has no neurovascular supply.

Joints

A joint is the connection of two bones for mobility and stability; it may provide flexion and extension, medial and lateral rotation, and abduction and adduction. A joint consists of articulating bone surfaces that are covered with cartilage, a two-layered sac containing synovial membranes (to lubricate), and a capsule that thickens and becomes a ligament. Muscles that overlie joints attach the bone surfaces to one another and provide movement.

INITIAL EMERGENCY MANAGEMENT

Because of the disfiguring nature of some orthopedic injuries, there is a tendency to evaluate the specific injury and not the patient as a whole. As with all patients presenting to the emergency department, initial management begins with airway and C-spine, breathing, and circulation.

General emergency management of acute musculoskeletal injuries include the following:

Primary assessment and appropriate interventions

Evaluation of neurovascular status of the extremity

Securing of impaled objects

Immobilization of the extremity above and below the site of suspected fractures

Reevaluation of neurovascular status after immobilization

Covering of any wounds with a sterile dressing

Application of cold

Elevation of extremity

Radiography as indicated

Evaluation of immunization status

Pain management

Repeat radiography after any manipulation

Unless otherwise indicated with specific injuries, these guidelines should be followed with all patients presenting with a musculoskeletal complaint.

Neurovascular Status is Assessed for the Presence of the Five Ps

Pain A description of the pain is helpful. Is it diffuse or point tender? Ischemic pain is usually described as burning or throbbing. Did the pain occur immediately upon injury or later? Pain should be rated on a scale of 1 to 10 so that the effectiveness of interventions can be evaluated.

Pallor What is the color of the injured extremity, the capillary refill, the temperature of the extremity, is there mottling?

Pulses What are the strength of proximal and distal pulses? How are these pulses compared to the pulses on the unaffected side?

Paresthesia Does the patient have two-point discrimination of the toes or fingers on the affected and unaffected side? Is there tingling, numbness, or other abnormal sensation?

Paralysis What is the general mobility of the limb? Was there loss of movement after the initial injury?

Inspection

Inspection should include the following:
Integrity and color of the extremity
Position of extremity
Presence of edema/swelling/ecchymosis
Range of motion
Symmetry/alignment/deformity

Palpation of the Injury

Palpation of the injury for the following:
Temperature
Pain/point tenderness
Crepitus, joint stability
Peripheral nerve assessment

AGE-RELATED DIFFERENCES

Pediatric

Injuries in this age category are frequently related to recreational activities. They often increase as the child's environment expands to include bicycles, skateboards, trampolines, and automobiles. Specific pathophysiology related to pediatric injuries include:

The epiphyseal "growth" plate does not close until after adolescence. Injury to the growth plate may arrest bone growth and healing.

Incomplete bone calcification renders the bone more pliable. Fractures in children are commonly greenstick fractures and do not extend throughout the cortex.

Fractures, lacerations, abrasions, or other trauma not consistent with the mechanism of injury should be evaluated for child maltreatment. Approximately 25% of fractures in children younger than 3 years old are caused by nonaccidental trauma.[2]

The elasticity of ligaments rarely produces dislocations. Most dislocations are associated with fractures.

Geriatric

Falls are a frequent mechanism of injury in the elderly. The risk of fractures, especially to the hip and wrist, increase with age. Physiologic changes in the elderly population include:

The presence of chronic conditions such as diabetes or Paget's disease
The presence of osteoporosis
The loss of muscle mass and strength because of atrophy of muscle cells
The presence of arthritis that may limit mobility and joint flexibility.
The decrease in the subcutaneous layer of skin and fat, providing less protection to underlying structures.
The decrease in bone density
The decrease in skin elasticity and delayed healing time
The presence of gait and balance disturbances

Evaluation for elderly abuse

SPLINTING ORTHOPEDIC INJURIES

Splinting is done to prevent further damage to bone or tissue, prevent damage to nerves, arteries, and veins, and decrease pain. Always splint above and below the injury site.
Splints are divided into four basic types:
Soft splint—soft, not rigid, such as a pillow
Hard splint—firm, rigid surface; such as a board
Air splint—inflatable; provides rigidity without being hard
Traction splint—provides support, decreased angulation, traction

There are a variety of splint materials.

General Principles of Splinting

Assess neurovascular status.
Remove all jewelry.
Assemble all equipment and padding before moving the injured part.
Elicit adequate personnel to apply the splinting device.
Immobilize the parts proximal and distal to the injury.
Correct severe angulation only if it is impossible to apply splint or neurovascular compromise is present.
Reassess neurovascular status after any change or movement of the injured site.
Secure the injured part to the splint.
Avoid impairing circulation by adhering the device too tightly.

Patient Education/Discharge Instructions

Return to the emergency department, the orthopedic clinic, or your private physician in 24 hours for follow-up
   care.
Keep the cast dry.
Keep the limb elevated above the level of the heart for 24 hours after the injury.
Do not place sharp objects (for example, coat hangers, knitting needles) down the cast.
   If skin itches, blow cool air (hairdryer) down the cast or scratch the other extremity.
If any of the following abnormalities are present, return to the follow-up clinic immediately:
   Check the temperature of the digits; it is abnormal if they are very cold or very hot.
   Check the color of the digits; it is abnormal if they are blue.
   Check if there is feeling in the digits; it is abnormal if there is no feeling, a tingling, or decrease in sensa-
      tion.
Wiggle the digits at least once each hour.
If a foreign object is dropped into the cast, call the follow-up care facility immediately.
Return to the follow-up clinic if the cast becomes too tight or if a foul odor is present.

SOFT-TISSUE INJURIES

Soft-tissue injuries may include injuries to the skin and underlying tissues, muscles, tendons, cartilage, ligaments, veins, arteries, or nerves.

Abrasion

An abrasion is caused by the rubbing of skin against a hard surface, thereby scraping the epithelial layer away and exposing the epidermal or dermal layer. An abrasion is similar to a partial-thickness burn. Debris embedded in the skin can cause permanent disfigurement, poxing, or scarring.

■ **THERAPEUTIC INTERVENTIONS**
General emergency orthopedic management
Wound cleansing—this may require anesthetics for adequate scrubbing and irrigation
Removal of foreign bodies on the extremities within 4 to 6 hours and those on the face within 8 hours.
Topical antibodic ointment
Nonadherent dressing
Leave facial abrasions uncovered.
Change dressings daily until an eschar has formed.
Avoid sunlight to the damaged area for 6 months because of hypopigmentation.

Avulsion

An avulsion is a full-thickness loss of skin in which the edges can not be approximated. Small avulsions occur frequently at the tip of the fingers and bleed profusely. Large avulsions are commonly caused by machinery, and can result in "degloving" injuries.

■ **THERAPEUTIC INTERVENTIONS**
General emergency management for orthopedic emergencies
Control of bleeding
Wound cleansing
Bulky nonadherent pressure dressing
Metal protectors may be indicated over sensitive fingertips
Large avulsions or degloving injuries will require:
    Split thickness skin graft or flap replacement
Antibiotics

Contusion

A contusion is extravasation of blood into tissues where vessels are damaged but skin is not disrupted.

■ **THERAPEUTIC INTERVENTIONS**
General emergency orthopedic management
Wrapped cold pack for 20 to 30 minutes 4 times a day
Compressive dressings may be required to decrease swelling/hemorrhage.
Splinting at joints may be required.

Laceration

A laceration is an open wound or cut through the dermal layer that varies in depth, length, and width. Attention to the penetrating implement, mechanism of injury, and age of injury will clue the emergency nurse to the severity of the laceration.

■ **THERAPEUTIC INTERVENTIONS**
General emergency management of orthopedic injuries
Culture if contaminated or more than 8 to 12 hours old
Cleansing (copious irrigation and scrubbing)
Control of bleeding (pressure and elevation)
Anesthesia
Inspection
Removal of foreign bodies
Excision of necrotic margins
Approximation
Closing (steri-strip or suture)
Dressing

Puncture

Puncture is the penetration of the skin by a pointed or sharp object. It may appear innocent but may have damaged underlying structures, or may be grossly contaminated. Puncture wounds bleed minimally and tend to seal off, thereby creating a high potential for infection.

■ **THERAPEUTIC INTERVENTIONS**

Depends on depth of penetration and amount of contamination

Generally:

Soaking in surgical soap solution twice a day for 2 to 4 days. Soaking should not be done for wood foreign bodies, because they will partially dissolve and make removal difficult.

Removal of foreign bodies (taped to chart)

Soft-tissue x-ray examination if a foreign body is suspected.

If contaminated:

Soaking

Anesthesia

Cleansing (scrub and irrigate)

Inspection

Removal of foreign bodies

Excision of necrotic tissue

Drain placement

Packing

If the object is impaled, leave it in place until it can be thoroughly evaluated.

Abscess

An abscess is a localized collection of pus.

■ **THERAPEUTIC INTERVENTIONS**

Anesthesia

Drain in dependent position

Removal of elliptical area

Loose packing to allow for drainage

Loose dressing

Antibiotics if patient is febrile

■ **SPECIAL NOTES**

Do not wait until an abscess "points." If an abscess is suspected, drain with a needle if assessment reveals a fluctuant mass.

Strains

Strains are caused by the stretching or tearing of the muscle. First-degree strains are usually the result of stretching of the muscle by excessive force. A second-degree strain involves a disruption of more fibers. In third-degree strain, there is complete disruption of the muscle fibers and the overlying fascia may be ruptured. Common areas include the gastrocnemius, biceps, hamstrings, and quadriceps.

■ **SIGNS AND SYMPTOMS**

First-degree strains

Local pain aggravated by movement

Point tenderness

Spasm

Ecchymosis

Second-degree strains
Signs and symptoms are the same as for first-degree strain.
Third-degree strains
Point tenderness
Severe pain
Swelling
Discoloration
Hematoma formation
Snapping noise at the time of injury
Loss of muscle function at the time of injury
■ THERAPEUTIC INTERVENTIONS (FIRST- AND SECOND-DEGREE STRAINS)
General emergency orthopedic management
Compression bandage
Elevation for 48 hours
Cold pack for 48 hours
Heat after 72 hours
Immobilize injured muscle as needed
Avoid active or passive stretching
Light weight bearing when pain is resolved
■ THERAPEUTIC INTERVENTIONS (THIRD-DEGREE STRAINS)
General emergency orthopedic management
Splint
Elevation for 48 hours
Cold for 48 hours
No weight bearing
Surgical orthopedic referral

Sprains

Sprains are the most common injury to a joint presenting to the emergency department and the most commonly mistreated orthopedic emergency.[3] Sprains are the result of stretching or tearing of the supporting ligaments. Ankle sprains are most commonly caused by inversion stress. The average disability from ankle sprains is from 4.5 to 26 weeks.[4]

Categories

First degree—a few fibers are disrupted; there is no joint instability and minimal swelling and discoloration
Second degree—partial tear, intact joint, increased swelling and ecchymosis
Third degree—complete disruption/rupture; joint will be unstable when stressed; significant swelling
■ SIGNS AND SYMPTOMS
First-degree sprains
Slight pain
Patient may not complain of pain until 24 hours after injury
Slight swelling
Second-degree sprains
Point tenderness
Local pain
Swelling
Discoloration
Inability to use for a short time

Third-degree sprains

Pain

May be painless with complete rupture

Point tenderness

Diffuse swelling

Discoloration

Joint instability

Egg-shaped swelling within 2 hours of the injury

■ **THERAPEUTIC INTERVENTIONS**

General emergency orthopedic management

Posterior splint

Unna boot or cast

Orthopedic surgical referral

PERIPHERAL NERVE INJURIES

Peripheral nerve injuries (Table 28-1) can be caused by trauma (mechanical, chemical, or thermal), toxins, malignancy, metabolic disorders, or collagen disease. In the emergency situation they are usually associated with lacerations, fractures, dislocations, and penetrating wounds.

Accurate assessment requires an understanding of the distribution of nerves, the origin of motor branches, and the muscles they supply.

Diagnostic tests such as electromyography, nerve conduction tests, and electrical stimulation are of little or no value in the emergency evaluation of peripheral nerve injury.

Repair of peripheral nerves should not be undertaken as an emergency department surgical intervention.

FRACTURES

Fractures are divided into two general categories.

Categories

1. Closed (simple)—the skin is not disrupted.
2. Open (compound)—the skin is disrupted by
   A bone puncturing from the inside out
   An object puncturing from the outside in, with resultant fracture

TABLE 28-1   Modes for Assessing Common Peripheral Nerve Injuries

NERVE	FREQUENTLY ASSOCIATED INJURIES	ASSESSMENT TECHNIQUE*
Radial	Fracture of humerus, especially middle and distal thirds	Inability to extend thumb in "hitchhiker's sign"
Ulnar	Fracture of medial humeral epicondyle	Loss of pain perception in tip of little finger
Median	Elbow dislocation or wrist or forearm injury	Loss of pain perception in tip of index finger
Peroneal	Tibia or fibula fracture, dislocation of knee	Inability to extend great toe or foot; may also be associated with sciatic nerve injury
Sciatic and tibial	Infrequent with fractures or dislocations	Loss of pain perception in sole of foot

*Test is invalid if extension tendons are severed or if severe muscle damage is present.

Types of Fractures

Transverse

Results from angulation force or direct trauma.

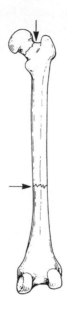

Oblique

Results from twisting force.

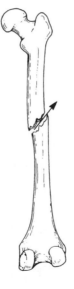

Spiral

Results from twisting force with firmly planted foot.

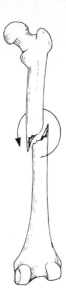

Comminuted

Results from severe direct trauma, such as crush injuries and high-velocity bullets; has more than two fragments.

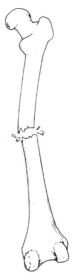

Impacted

Results from severe trauma causing fracture ends to jam together.

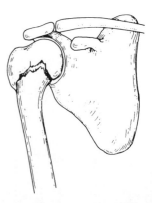

Compressed

Results from severe force to top of head or os calcis or from acceleration/deceleration injury.

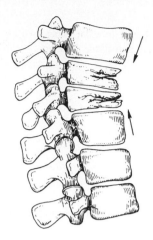

Greenstick

Results from compression force; usually occurs in children under 10 years of age.

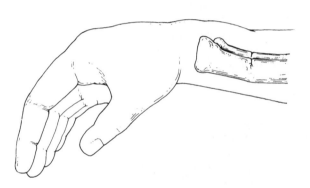

Avulsion

Results from muscle mass contracting forcefully, causing bone fragment to tear off at insertion. Ligament can tear fragment from bone rather than rupturing.

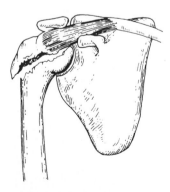

Depression

Results from blunt trauma to a flat bone;
usually involves much soft-tissue damage.

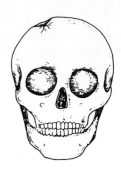

Specific Upper Extremity Fractures/Injuries

Clavicular Fractures

Clavicular fractures are the most common of all childhood fractures. Eighty percent of clavicular fractures occur in the middle one third of the clavicle.

- ■ **MECHANISM OF INJURY**
  Fall on arm or shoulder
  Direct trauma to shoulder laterally
- ■ **SIGNS AND SYMPTOMS**
  Pain in clavicular area
  Point tenderness
  Refusal to raise arm
  Swelling
  Deformity
  Crepitus
- ■ **THERAPEUTIC INTERVENTIONS**
  General emergency management of orthopedic injuries
  Sling, figure-eight bandage, or both
- ■ **COMPLICATIONS**
  Injury to adjacent neuromuscular tissue (rare)
  Subclavian vascular injury
  Ligament damage
  Malunion

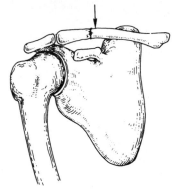

■ **SPECIAL NOTES**
    Pad the axillary area well to
        avoid damage to the
        brachial plexus and artery.

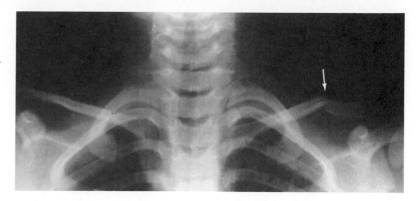

Shoulder injuries (humeral head, proximal humeral, and humeral neck)

Anatomically, proximal humeral fractures include all humeral fractures proximal to the surgical neck. Shoulder fractures occur more commonly in the elderly because of weaker bone structure and a weaken muscular structure.

■ **MECHANISM OF INJURY**
    Fall on outstretched arm
    Direct trauma to shoulder from
        blunt instrument or fall

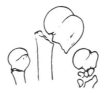

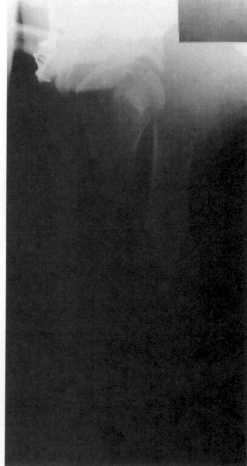

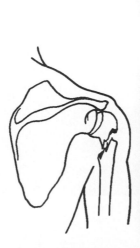

■ **SIGNS AND SYMPTOMS**
Pain in shoulder area
Point tenderness
Inability to move arm
Posterior rotation
Adduction of humerus
Abduction of humerus (this carries a higher incidence of neurovascular compromise)
Gross swelling and discoloration may extend to chest wall.

■ **THERAPEUTIC INTERVENTIONS**
General emergency orthopedic management
Sling and swath
Surgery may be required for impacted comminuted or displaced fractures, especially of the humeral neck

■ **COMPLICATIONS**
Humeral neck fractures (also called surgical neck fractures) may cause axillary nerve or brachial plexus injuries. Laceration of the axillary artery is also seen.

Scapular fractures

Scapular fractures are a relatively uncommon injury. A great deal of force is required to cause fractures of the scapula. Because of the intensity of the trauma, these fractures may be associated with life-threatening injuries.

■ **MECHANISM OF INJURY**
Direct trauma

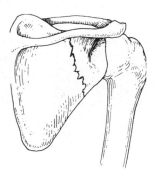
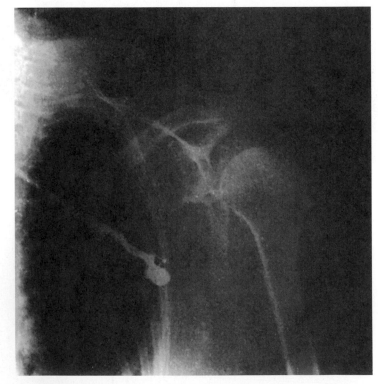

■ **SIGNS AND SYMPTOMS**
  Point tenderness
  Swelling and ecchymosis
  Usually held in adduction with resistance to abduction.
  Bony displacement
  Pain on shoulder movement
■ **THERAPEUTIC INTERVENTIONS**
  General emergency management of orthopedic injuries
  Sling and swath
  Axillary care
■ **COMPLICATIONS**
  Underlying injury to the ribs
  Pneumothorax
  Compression fractures of the spine

Upper arm fractures (humeral shaft)

■ **MECHANISM OF INJURY**
  Fall on arm or direct trauma
  Twisting of the arm
■ **SIGNS AND SYMPTOMS**
  Pain
  Point tenderness
  Swelling
  Inability or hesitance to move arm
  Severe deformity or angulation
  Crepitus

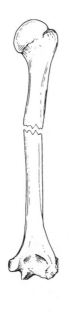
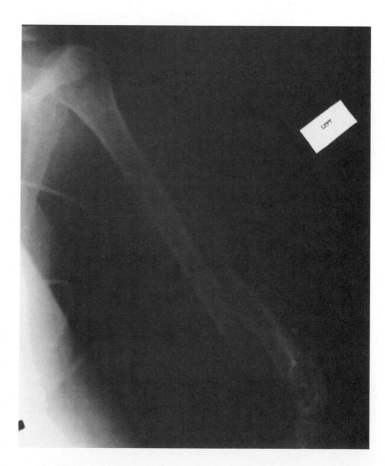

■ **THERAPEUTIC INTERVENTIONS**
General emergency management of orthopedic injuries
Sling and swath
Supportive splint
Surgical intervention for:
    shaft fracture with vascular compromise
    spiral fracture of distal third with radial nerve palsy
    fractures extending into the elbow
■ **COMPLICATIONS**
The delayed development of radial nerve palsies occur in 5% to 10% of humeral shaft fractures.[5]

Elbow fractures (supracondylar, epicondylar, and intercondylar)

■ **MECHANISM OF INJURY**
Fall on extended arm
Fall on flexed elbow

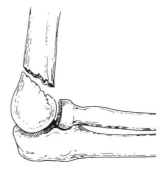

■ **SIGNS AND SYMPTOMS**
Severe pain
Point tenderness
Rapid swelling
Shortening of the arm/deformity
Delayed capillary refill
■ **THERAPEUTIC INTERVENTIONS**
General emergency orthopedic management
Splint in presenting position—"as it lies"
Flexing of arm to greater degree if there is neurovascular
    compromise
Admit for observation of neurovascular status
Arteriogram

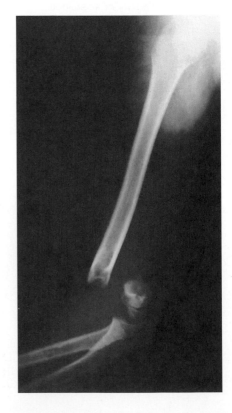

■ **COMPLICATIONS**
Brachial artery laceration
Median and/or radial nerve damage
Volkmann's contracture

Forearm fractures (radius or ulna)

Although radial fractures alone are not rare, injuries severe enough to fracture the radius usually fracture the ulna also. Monteggia fractures account for 60% of ulna fractures; they are characterized by a fracture of the proximal third of the ulna and an anterior dislocation of the radial head.[6]

■ **MECHANISM OF INJURY**
Fall on extended arm
Direct blow. Fractures of the ulna are frequently called "nightstick fractures."
Forced pronation of the forearm

■ **SIGNS AND SYMPTOMS**
Pain
Point tenderness
Swelling
Deformity or angulation
Shortening

■ **THERAPEUTIC INTERVENTIONS**
General management of orthopedic injuries
Closed reduction
Casting
Possible open reduction and internal fixation

■ **COMPLICATIONS**
Paralysis of the radial nerve
Malunion
Volkmann's contracture

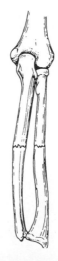

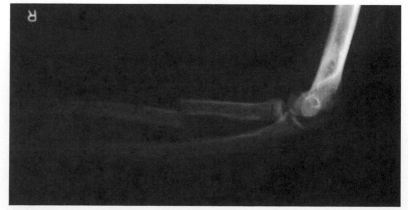

Wrist fractures (distal radius, distal ulna, and carpal bone)

■ **MECHANISM OF INJURY**
Dorsiflexion—usually because of a fall on an extended arm and open hand

■ **SIGNS AND SYMPTOMS**
Pain
"Snuff box" tenderness in navicular (scaphoid) fracture
Swelling
Deformity (may be severe with Colles' fractures)
Limited range of motion
Numbness
Weakness

■ **THERAPEUTIC INTERVENTIONS**
General emergency management of orthopedic injuries
Closed reduction of displaced fractures
Rigid splinting or casting
Referral to orthopedic surgeon

■ **COMPLICATIONS**
Rare aseptic necrosis

■ **SPECIAL NOTES**
Navicular (scaphoid) bone fractures may not be apparent on radiography for 4 to 6 weeks. Patients presenting with pain in the "snuff box" after trauma should be splinted and referred to a orthopedic surgeon for evaluation.

Fracture of the distal radius and ulna is known as a Colles' fracture or silver fork deformity.

Check the mechanism of injury. The patient may have had a fall from a height that originally resulted in a heel (os calcis) fracture, a lumbodorsal compression fracture, and a fall forward onto the open hand, resulting in a Colles' fracture.

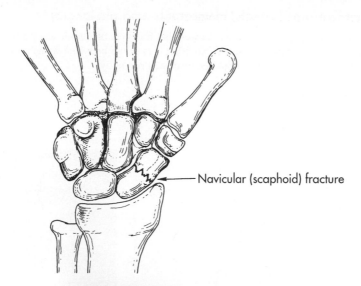

Navicular (scaphoid) fracture

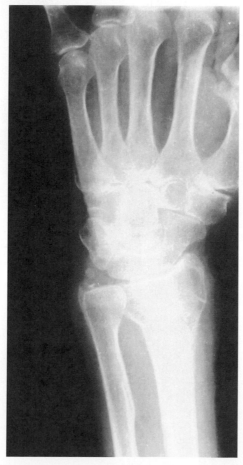

Hand and finger fractures (carpals, metacarpals, and phalanges)

A review of workman's compensation injuries showed that fractures of the metacarpal and phalanges are the most common fractures in the skeletal system.[7] No other part of the body plays such a major role in the activities of daily life, therefore these injuries should be evaluated promptly.

■ **MECHANISM OF INJURY**
Forceful hyperextension
Direct trauma
Crush injury

■ **SIGNS AND SYMPTOMS**
Pain
Severe swelling
Deformity
Inability to use hand
Often open fracture

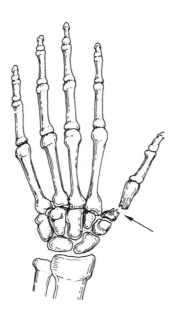

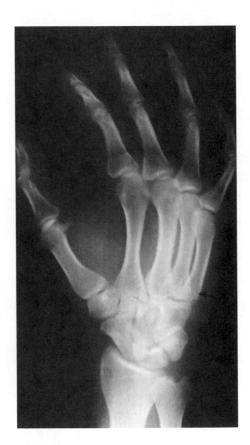

■ **THERAPEUTIC INTERVENTIONS**
General emergency management of orthopedic injuries
Closed reduction in displaced fractures
Finger traction
Splinting with padded aluminum guard for distal phalanges
"Buddy" taping
Antibodies for open fractures
Internal fixation is rarely required.

■ **COMPLICATIONS**
Malunion
Osteomyelitis
Subungual hematoma

■ **SPECIAL NOTES**
Fracture of the fifth metacarpal is commonly referred to as a "boxer's" fracture. These fractures are commonly caused by a punch and result in an open fracture and wound contamination.

It is important to determine the patient's hand dominance, occupation, and other factors that may influence recovery.

High-pressure injection injuries

Injection injuries may involve extensive loss of tissue and are associated with a high rate of infection. Toxins such as paint, grease, or other industrial toxins require surgical debridement immediately.

■ **MECHANISM OF INJURY**
Injection of a stream of paint into the fingertip and up into the hand, wrist, and arm.
The injury appears only as a small pinhole in the tip of the finger.

■ **SIGNS AND SYMPTOMS**
Pain
Numbness
Coolness of the digit
Hot sensation in the hand
Leaded paint may appear on radiograph

■ **THERAPEUTIC INTERVENTIONS**
Depending on the agent, the patient may be treated conservatively or require open debridement.
Immobilization
If gas injected, elevate the limb, for other toxins, lower the limb.
Fasciotomy and extensive irrigation
Antibiotics
Steroids

Subungual hematoma

Fractures of the distal phalanx are frequently associated with significant soft-tissue injury. Evacuation of the hematoma will give noticeable relief of pain.

■ **MECHANISM OF INJURY**
This injury is caused by a crushing force on the distal phalanx.

■ **THERAPEUTIC INTERVENTIONS**
Nail removal or trephination
Nail trephination
Equipment
Nail drill, scalpel, or paper clip
Alcohol lamp if paper clip is used
Procedure
1. Prepare the nail with antiseptic solution.
2. Penetrate the nail:
   a. With nail drill
   b. With scalpel, using rotation motion
   c. With paper clip after it is heated red hot
3. Release the pressure caused by the hematoma.
4. Dress with an adhesive bandage.
5. Elevate the fingernail.

■ **COMPLICATIONS**

Reaccumulation of hematoma

Deformity of the nail occurs frequently; the extent will not be known until the nail has fully regrown in 4 to 5 months.

Pelvic fractures

Pelvic fractures are one of the most life-threatening of all orthopedic traumas with a mortality rate of from 5% to 20%.[8] Early resuscitation and management of these patients is crucial to decrease morbidity and death.

■ **MECHANISM OF INJURY**

Crush injury

Automobile or motorcycle accident

Direct trauma

Fall from height

Sudden contraction of muscle against resistance

■ **SIGNS AND SYMPTOMS**

Tenderness over pubis or when iliac wings are compressed

Paraspinous muscle spasm

Sacroiliac joint tenderness

Paresis or hemiparesis

Pelvic ecchymosis

Hematuria

Groin pain

Inability to bear weight

Inability to void

Blood at the urethral meatus

Prostate displacement or lack of sphincter tone

■ **THERAPEUTIC INTERVENTIONS**

General emergency management of orthopedic injuries

Immobilization of spine and legs (long board)

Flexing knees to decrease pain

Frequent (every 5 minutes) monitoring of vital signs

PASG if indicated

Peritoneal lavage

Type and cross-match

Stable pelvic fractures (does not transect the pelvic ring)

If pelvic fracture is suspected, primary survey and attention to ABCs should be initiated until pelvic stability is established.

General emergency management of orthopedic injuries

Can be treated symptomatically.

Bed rest for 2 to 3 weeks

Pelvic belt, strap, or traction

Crutches or walker

Laxatives

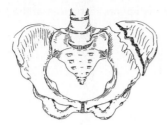

Stable fracture not
involving the ring

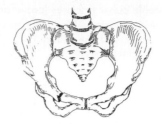

Stable fracture; minimal
displaced fracture of the ring

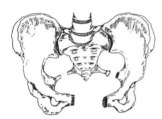

Rotationally unstable,
vertically stable open
book fracture

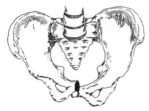

Rotationally unstable,
vertically stable lateral
compression (ipsilateral)

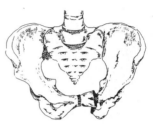

Rotationally unstable,
vertically stable lateral
compression (contralateral
bucket handle)

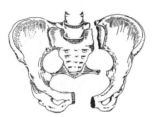

Rotationally and vertically
unstable bilateral

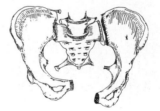

Rotationally and vertically
unstable associated with
acetabular fracture (not shown)

(From Kozin S, Berlet A: Pelvis and acetabulum. In *Handbook of common orthopaedic fractures*, ed 2, Chester, PA, 1992,
Medical Surveillance.)

Open or unstable pelvic fractures (posterior element disruption, disruption of the pelvic ring)

Trauma management and aggressive resuscitation
  Oxygen, fluids, type, and cross match
Diagnostic peritoneal lavage
PASG
Possible laparotomy
Antibiotics
Angiography
Surgical fixation

■ **COMPLICATIONS**

Hemorrhage (average blood loss, 2 units)
Bladder trauma
Genital trauma
Lumbosacral trauma
Ruptured internal organs
Pulmonary or fat emboli
Gastrointestinal injury
Chronic pain
Compartment syndrome
Osteomyelitis
Shock
Death

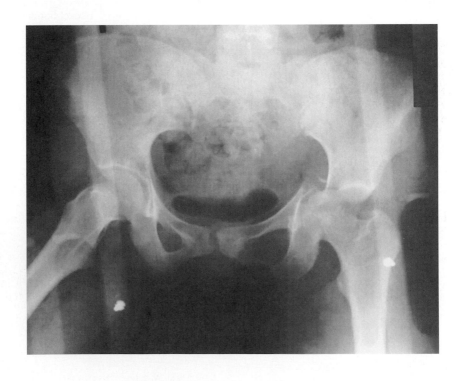

Hip fractures (acetabulum, greater trochanter, and femoral head)

■ **MECHANISM OF INJURY**

Frequently seen in pedestrian trauma

Direct blow or fall (common mechanism in the elderly)

Axial transmission of force from the knees (vehicular trauma)

■ **SIGNS AND SYMPTOMS**

Pain in hip or groin area

Severe pain with movement

Inability to bear weight

External rotation of hip and leg

Minimal shortening of limb

If injury is extracapsular and associated with trochanteric
  fracture:

  Pain in lateral area of hip

  Increased shortening

  Greater external rotation

■ **THERAPEUTIC INTERVENTIONS**

Will depend on the mechanism of injury.

General emergency management of orthopedic injuries

Immobilize in a position of comfort. Backboard and other
  splinting will require padding, especially in the elderly.

Traction

Surgical intervention

■ **COMPLICATIONS**

Avascular necrosis of femoral head

Phlebitis of femoral vein

Osteoarthritis

Sciatic nerve injury

Fat emboli syndrome

Hypovolemic shock

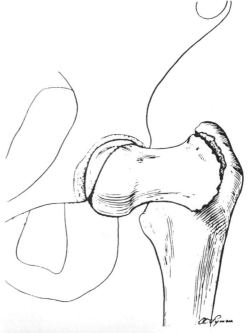

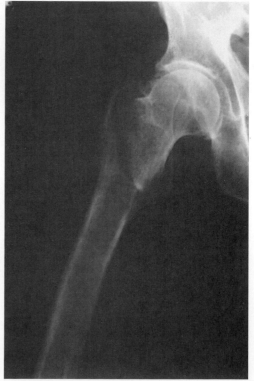

Femoral shaft fractures

■ **MECHANISM OF INJURY**
Indirect force transmitted through flexed knee
Direct trauma

■ **SIGNS AND SYMPTOMS**
Angulation
Shortening of limb and severe muscle spasm
Crepitus
Severe pain
Swelling of the thigh
Hematoma formation in the thigh
Inability to bear weight on leg
Deformity

■ **THERAPEUTIC INTERVENTIONS**
Trauma management
    Airway, fluids, type and cross-match, frequent reassessment
General emergency management of orthopedic injuries
Immobilization in skin traction splint, (that is, Sager, Thomas, or Hare traction)
Open reduction with In-
    ternal fixation
Severe muscle damage
Knee trauma (overlooked
    at time of injury)

■ **COMPLICATIONS**
Hemorrhage—average
    blood loss 1000 cc

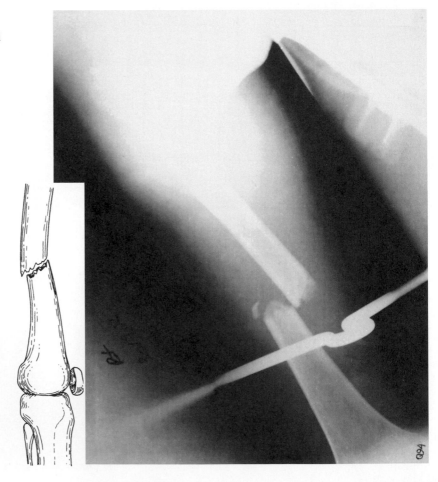

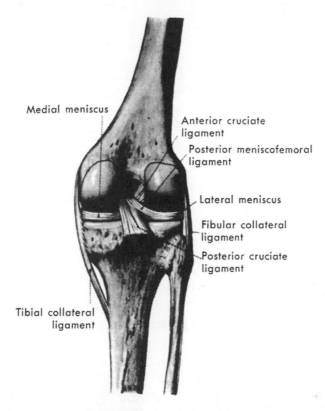

Medial meniscus

Anterior cruciate
ligament

Posterior meniscofemoral
ligament

Lateral meniscus

Fibular collateral
ligament

Posterior cruciate
ligament

Tibial collateral
ligament

FIGURE 28-1. Anterior knee joint.

Knee injuries

Figure 28-1 shows the anterior knee joint. Figure 28-2 depicts mechanisms of knee sprains.

■ **MECHANISM OF INJURY**

Knee injuries are caused by rotational or hyperflexion trauma.

■ **COMMON TYPES**

Medial meniscus injury from rotational trauma

Collateral ligament injury: medial from valgus stress, lateral from varus stress

Anterior and posterior cruciate ligament injury from hyperextension trauma

■ **SIGNS AND SYMPTOMS**

Swelling

Ecchymosis

Effusion

Pain

Tenderness—instability of the joint

■ **THERAPEUTIC INTERVENTIONS**

General management of orthopedic injuries

Compression bandage

Knee immobilizer

Crutches

No weight bearing

Orthopedic consult for possible surgical repair

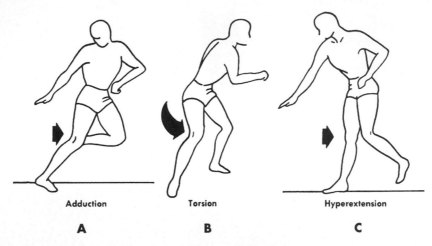

Adduction   **Torsion**   **Hyperextension**

A   **B**   **C**

FIGURE 28-2. Mechanisms of knee sprains. **A,** Direct lateral force on knee causes torn medial collateral ligament. **B,** Knee rotation injury may cause lateral, collateral, and medial collateral ligament injury. **C,** Posterior cruciate ligament mechanisms of injury.

Knee fractures (supracondylar fracture of femur, intraarticular fracture of femur or tibia)

■ **MECHANISM OF INJURY**
High velocity vehicular trauma
Pedestrian trauma—"bumper" or
"fender" fractures
Fall from heights onto flexed knee
Hyperabduction

■ **SIGNS AND SYMPTOMS**
Crepitus
Tense swelling in the popliteal area
Hemarthrosis
Knee pain
Inability to bend or straighten knee
Swelling
Tenderness

■ **THERAPEUTIC INTERVENTIONS**
General management of orthopedic
injuries
Nonweight-bearing cast
Open reduction and internal fixation
Traction
Crutches

■ **COMPLICATIONS**
Popliteal nerve or artery injury
Fat emboli
Rotational deformities/impairment
Traumatic arthritis

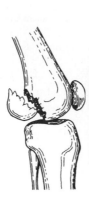

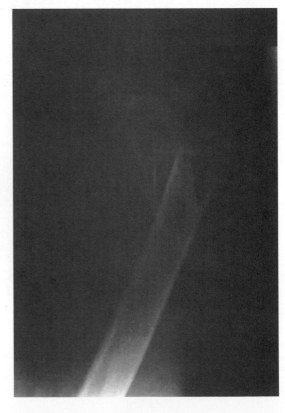

Patellar fractures

■ **MECHANISM OF INJURY**
Usually direct trauma (fall or impact with dashboard)
Indirect trauma secondary to quadriceps muscle pull or contraction

■ **THERAPEUTIC INTERVENTIONS**
General emergency management of orthopedic injuries
May require surgery for repair of quadriceps.
If open fracture, antibiotics and inpatient care

■ **SIGNS AND SYMPTOMS**
Pain in knee
Frequently opened fracture
Hemarthrosis
Inability to actively extend knee

■ **COMPLICATIONS**
Avascular necrosis

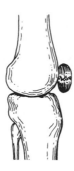

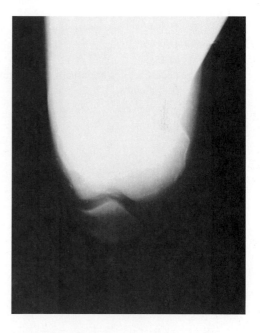

Tibial/fibular fractures

Tibial fractures are not only the most common long-bone fracture but the most common open fracture seen. Fibula shaft fractures are uncommon alone. The fibula is a nonweight-bearing bone, but distally is essential for ankle stability.

■ **MECHANISM OF INJURY**
Rotational or twisting forces
Direct trauma
Fall with compression forces or a fixed foot

■ **SIGNS AND SYMPTOMS**
Pain
Point tenderness
Swelling
Deformity
Crepitus

■ **THERAPEUTIC INTERVENTIONS**
General emergency management of orthopedic injuries
Check for any puncture site cause by the tibial fracture.
Wound debridement and irrigation
Casting
Crutches
Open reduction internal fixation may be indicated for displaced fractures.

■ **COMPLICATIONS**
Compartment syndrome is usually present within 24 to 48 hours
Infection
Osteomyelitis
Nonunion

■ **SPECIAL NOTES**
Tibial plateau fractures are usually nonweight-
bearing for 6 months.

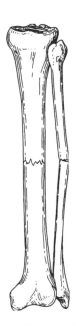

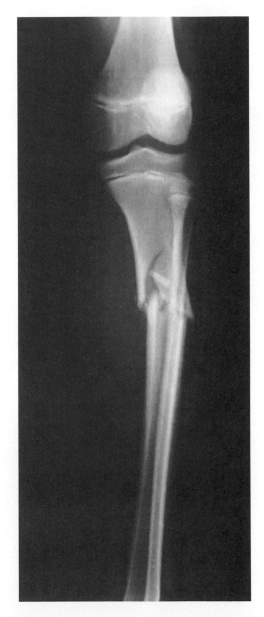

Ankle fractures

The ankle bears more weight then any other joint in the body.

■ **MECHANISM OF INJURY**

Injury can vary greatly depending on the position of the foot (fixed, supination, pronation, or inversion) and the type of force exerted (eversion, inversion or rotation); 60% of fractures occur because of external rotation on a fixed foot[9]

Direct trauma

Indirect trauma

Torsion/inversion/eversion

■ **SIGNS AND SYMPTOMS**

Popping sound with tearing of the ligaments

Ecchymosis

Crepitus

Inability to bear weight in unstable injury

Pain upon ambulation, or altered gait

■ **THERAPEUTIC INTERVENTIONS**

General emergency orthopedic management

Closed reduction

Posterior splint

Possible open reduction and internal fixation

Casting

Crutches

■ **COMPLICATIONS**

Nonunion—primarily with closed reductions

Infection

Post-traumatic arthritis

Sudeck's atrophy—a form of sympathetic dystrophy, characterized by rapidly developing osteoporosis, burning pain and trophic changes in the foot.

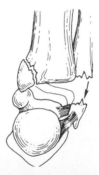

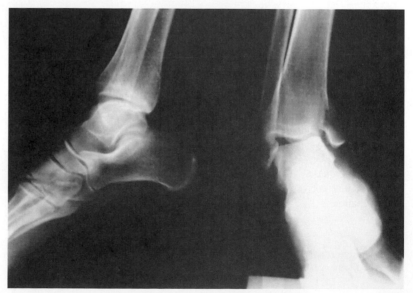

Achilles tendon ruptures

■ **MECHANISM OF INJURY**
This injury usually occurs in stop-and-start sports (such as tennis or racquetball) in which one steps off abruptly on the forefoot with the knee forced into extension.

■ **SIGNS AND SYMPTOMS**
Deformity along Achilles tendon (palpable deficit)
Severe sharp pain in lower calf with complete tear
Inability to walk
Inability to plantar flex
Positive Thompson's sign*

■ **THERAPEUTIC INTERVENTIONS**
General emergency management of orthopedic injuries
Compression dressing
Orthopedic surgery referral
Possible walking cast
Possible surgical repair
Crutches

Foot fractures (metatarsal)

The foot contains 28 bones and 57 articulating surfaces. Foot injuries are often associated with ankle injuries. The foot and ankle should always be assessed together. Certain systemic disorders, such as diabetes and peripheral vascular disease, may influence the treatment and severity of foot injuries.

■ **MECHANISM OF INJURY**
Similar to that of ankle injuries
Athletic injury
Direct trauma

■ **SIGNS AND SYMPTOMS**
Deep pain
Ecchymosis
Subungual hematoma
Hesitance to bear weight
Point tenderness
Deformity
Swelling

■ **THERAPEUTIC INTERVENTIONS**
General emergency orthopedic management
Bulky dressing
Wooden shoe
Posterior splint
Cane or crutches
Early weight bearing in most cases
Orthopedic referral

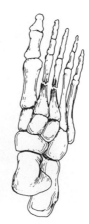

■ **COMPLICATIONS**
Avascular necrosis
Malunion
Gait abnormalities

*Positive Thompson's sign: With the leg extended and the foot over the end of a table, squeeze the calf muscle; no heel pull or upward movement will be seen.

Heel fractures (calcaneal)

- **MECHANISM OF INJURY**
  Fall from a height
- **SIGNS AND SYMPTOMS**
  Increase in pain with hyperflexion
  Point tenderness
  Superficial skin blistering
  Deformity
- **THERAPEUTIC INTERVENTIONS**
  Special attention to the mechanism of injury
  General emergency management of orthopedic injuries
  Bulky compressive dressing
  No weight or partial weight bearing
  Crutches
  Casting is usually not performed for 2 days to 2 weeks
  Closed reduction for displaced fractures
- **COMPLICATIONS**
  Chronic pain
  Nerve entrapment
- **SPECIAL NOTES**
  Twenty-six percent of calcaneal fractures are associated with other injuries to the lower extremities. Ten percent of calcaneal fractures are bilateral. Compression fractures of the dorsolumbar spine are associated with 10% of calcaneal fractures.[10]

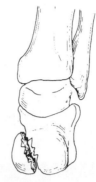

Toe fractures (phalange)

- **MECHANISM OF INJURY**
  Direct trauma—such as kicking, stubbing of toe
  Athletic injury
- **SIGNS AND SYMPTOMS**
  Subungual hematoma
  Deformity
  Pain
  Discoloration
- **THERAPEUTIC INTERVENTIONS**
  General emergency management of orthopedic injuries
  Compression dressing
  Buddy taping
  Wooden shoe or other foot support
  Cane as needed

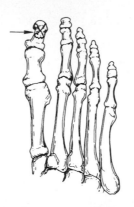

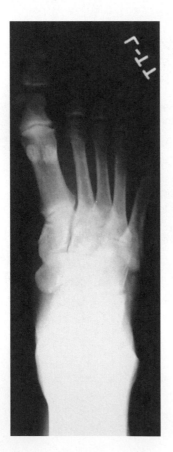

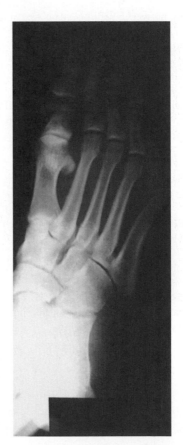

Complications of Fractures and Orthopedic Injuries

Fat embolism syndrome

Fat embolism syndrome is a potentially life-threatening complication of long-bone trauma, blunt trauma, and intramedullary manipulation. This syndrome may present 4 hours to several days after trauma or orthopedic surgery. Fat globules can occlude blood vessels of the brain, kidneys, lungs, and other organ systems.

■ **SIGNS AND SYMPTOMS**

General

Elevated temperature

Tachycardia

Restlessness

Pulmonary

Chest pain

Dyspnea

Cough

Petechiae over the anterior chest and neck

Rales

Pulmonary edema

Cerebral

Change in LOC

Hemiparesis

Tetraplegia

■ **THERAPEUTIC INTERVENTIONS**

Aggressive respiratory support

Immobilization of injured part

Monitor ABGs

Controversial therapies

   Steroids

   Heparin

   Low molecular weight dextran

Osteomyelitis

Osteomyelitis is an infection of the bone, occurring most commonly by direct contamination secondary to open fractures, penetrating wounds, or surgical procedures. The most common organism is *Staphylococcus aureus.*

■ **SIGNS AND SYMPTOMS**

Fever

Pain and tenderness over area

Edema

Redness/erythema

Exudate

Elevated sedimentation rate and WBCs

■ **THERAPEUTIC INTERVENTIONS**

Immobilization of the extremity

Culture

IV antibodies

Bone scan

Surgical incision and drainage

Debridement

■ **COMPLICATIONS**

Septic arthritis

Growth disturbances

Chronic osteomyelitis
Pathological fractures

Compartment syndrome

Compartment syndrome develops when the muscle compartment pressures exceed the intraarterial hydrostatic pressure, causing collapse of capillaries and venules and subsequent tissue necrosis. Loss of pulse distal to the affected area is a late sign.

■ **MECHANISM OF INJURY**

External

Prolonged or inappropriate application of PASG, casts, splints, or wraps
Skeletal traction

Internal

Crush injury
Burns
Spider bites
Frostbite

■ **SIGNS AND SYMPTOMS**

A hallmark sign of developing compartment syndrome is a severe "boring" pain
Pain increases with muscle stretching
Delayed capillary refill
Decreased sensation in distal aspect
Decreased function
Myoglobinuria
Renal failure
Compartment pressures greater than 20 mm Hg

■ **THERAPEUTIC INTERVENTIONS**

Removal of all forms of external compression
Do not elevate.
Do not apply ice.
Urinalysis for myoglobinuria
Fasciotomy

Volkmann's ischemic contracture

Though usually associated with supracondylar fractures, Volkmann's ischemic contracture can occur with fractures of the forearm, wrist, tibia, and femur. The etiology of the ischemia is the same as that of compartment syndrome. In addition there is an ischemic fibrosis that causes a contracture of the extremity. If left untreated, this condition can cause permanent nerve damage, pain, deformity, and even amputation of the extremity.

■ **SIGNS AND SYMPTOMS**

Pain—characterized as deep and poorly localized
Pain is aggravated by stretching.
Sensory loss distal and sometimes proximal to the injury.
Distal pulse is rarely obliterated.
Wrist or foot drop

■ **THERAPEUTIC INTERVENTIONS**

Do *not* elevate but maintain in a neutral position
Do *not* apply cold
Contracture may form within 12 hours from onset of symptoms
Immediate decompressive fasciotomy

DISLOCATIONS AND SEPARATIONS

Dislocation occurs when a joint exceeds its range of motion. A dislocation is a complete disruption of a joint so that the articular surfaces are no longer in contact. Dislocations can cause injury to the adjacent vasculature and nerve supplies. For this reason, dislocations should be reduced as soon as possible.

Severe spasm of the muscles surrounding the dislocation frequently occur. Intravenous muscle relaxants (that is, Valium) are usually needed for successful reductions.

Subluxations are minor disruptions of joints where articular surfaces contact remains. This is frequently seen in children in the radial head.

■ SIGNS AND SYMPTOMS
Severe pain
Deformity at the joint
Inability to move the joint
Swelling
Point tenderness

■ THERAPEUTIC INTERVENTIONS FOR ALL DISLOCATIONS
General emergency management of orthopedic injuries
Specific attention to neurovascular status distal to dislocation
Evaluation for concurrent fracture
Reduction
Re-evaluation of neurovascular status distal to dislocation
Postreduction radiograph

■ IMMOBILIZATION
See Table 28-2.

Specific Dislocations/Separations

Acromioclavicular separation

■ MECHANISM OF INJURY
Common athletic injury produced by a fall or a force on point of shoulder.

■ SIGNS AND SYMPTOMS
Great pain in joint area
Inability to raise arm or bring arm across chest
Deformity
Point or area tenderness
Swelling
Hematoma

■ THERAPEUTIC INTERVENTIONS
Therapeutic interventions for dislocations
Sling and swath

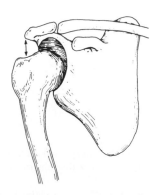

TABLE 28-2   Common Dislocations

BODY AREA	TYPICAL MECHANISM OF INJURY	CLINICAL FINDINGS	TREATMENT
Shoulder Anterior	Fall on outstretched arm or direct impact on shoulder	Arm abducted, cannot bring elbow down to chest or touch opposite ear with hand	Splint in position of comfort; reduce as soon as possible
Posterior	Rare; strong blow in front of shoulder; with violent convulsions or seizures	Arm held at side, unable to externally rotate	As above
Elbow—radius and ulna	Fall on outstretched hand with elbow in extension	Loss of arm length, painful motion, and rapid swelling: nerve lesions may occur	As above Surgical repair if dislocation is associated with fracture to radial head or olecranon
Radius—head (children)	Pulled, or nursemaid's elbow caused by sudden pull, jerk, or lift on child's wrist or hand	Pain, refusal to use arm; limited supination; can flex and extend at elbow; may have no deformity	Reduce, place in sling; advise parents that this may recur until age 5 years
Hip—usually posterior	Blow to knee while hip is flexed and adducted (sitting with crossed knees); common in passengers seated in front seat	Hip flexed, adducted, internally rotated, and shortened; may have associated fracture of femur; sciatic nerve injury (lies posterior)	Splint in position of comfort; reduce as soon as possible
Patella	May be spontaneous	Knee flexed, can palpate patella lateral to femoral condyle	Reduce (may occur spontaneously), immobilize with cast or splint
	Associated with other trauma	Excessive swelling, tenderness, and palpable soft tissue defect	Surgical repair of soft tissue injury or fractures
Knee (rare)	Direct severe blow to upper leg or forced hyperextension of knee	Ligamentous instability (requires disruption of structures to occur); inability to straighten leg; peroneal nerve and popliteal artery injury common—must assess distal neurovascular function	Immediate neurovascular assessment; reduce
Ankle	Ankle is complex joint, with multiple ligaments providing stability; dislocation is usually associated with other injury such as fracture and soft tissue trauma	Swelling, tenderness, and loss of alignment and function	Splint; usually necessitates open reduction because joint has complex motion and must have accurate alignment

Shoulder dislocation

■ **MECHANISM OF INJURY**

Anterior dislocation: usually an athletic injury from a fall on an extended arm that is abducted and externally rotated, resulting in head of humerus locating anterior to shoulder joint. Commonly, this is a recurrent injury.

Posterior dislocation: a rare form of dislocation, usually found in seizure patients in which extended arm is abducted and internally rotated.

■ **SIGNS AND SYMPTOMS**
Severe pain in shoulder area
Inability to move arm
Deformity (difficult to see in posterior dislocation)

■ **THERAPEUTIC INTERVENTIONS**
Support in position found or position of greatest comfort
Therapeutic interventions for dislocations
Swing/swath

■ **COMPLICATIONS**
Soft-tissue damage
Axillary nerve damage
Rare axillary artery damage
Rare brachial plexus damage

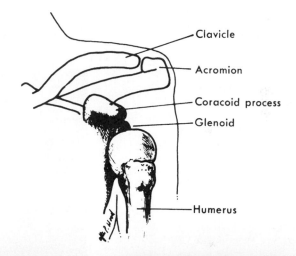

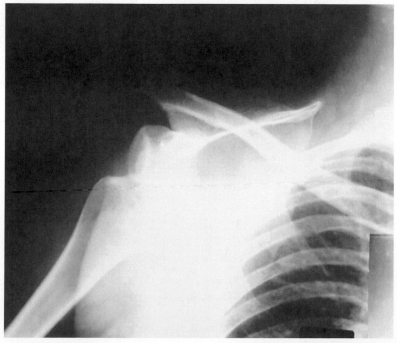

Elbow dislocation

■ **MECHANISM OF INJURY**
  Fall on an extended arm

■ **SIGNS AND SYMPTOMS**
  Pain
  Swelling
  Deformity or lateral displacement
  May feel locked
  Severe pain produced by movement

■ **THERAPEUTIC INTERVENTIONS**
  General emergency management of orthopedic
    injuries and dislocations
  Sling/swath
  Possible surgical repair

■ **COMPLICATIONS**
  Neurovascular compromise

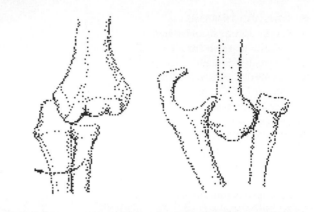

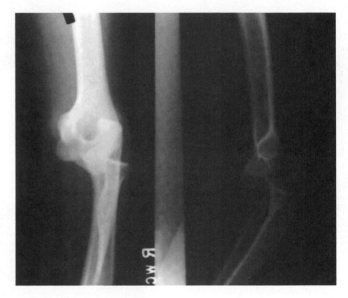

Wrist dislocation

- **MECHANISM OF INJURY**
  Fall on outreached arm and hand
- **SIGNS AND SYMPTOMS**
  Pain
  Swelling
  Point tenderness
  Deformity
- **THERAPEUTIC INTERVENTIONS**
  General emergency management of orthopedic injuries
     and dislocations
  Splint
  Sling and swath
- **COMPLICATIONS**
  Median nerve damage
- **SPECIAL NOTES**
  Median nerve damage is demonstrated by inability to
  pinch and loss of sensation in index and middle fingers.

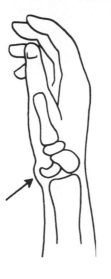
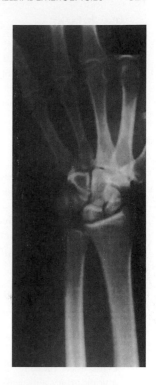

Hand or finger dislocation

- **MECHANISM OF INJURY**
  Fall on outstretched hand or finger
  Direct trauma or "jamming" force on fingertip
- **SIGNS AND SYMPTOMS**
  Pain
  Inability to move joint
  Deformity
  Swelling
- **THERAPEUTIC INTERVENTIONS**
  Therapeutic interventions for dislocations

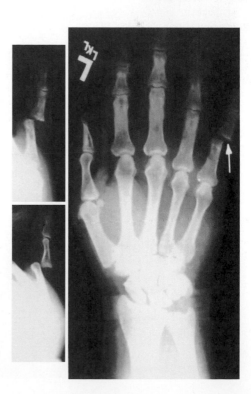

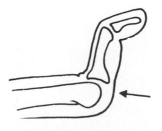

Hip dislocation

- **MECHANISM OF INJURY**

  Usually major trauma (with extended leg and foot on brake pedal before impact or with knee hitting dashboard)

  Falls

- **SIGNS AND SYMPTOMS**

  Pain in hip area

  Pain in knee

  Hip flexed, adducted, and internally rotated (posterior dislocation)

  Hip slightly flexed, abducted, and externally rotated (anterior dislocation)—a rare injury

  Joint feeling locked

  Inability to move leg

- **THERAPEUTIC INTERVENTIONS**

  General emergency management of orthopedic injuries

  Emergent surgical reduction

- **COMPLICATIONS**

  Sciatic nerve damage

  Femoral artery and nerve damage

  Relocation within 24 hours or necrosis of femoral head may occur.

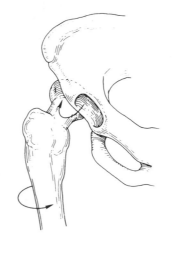

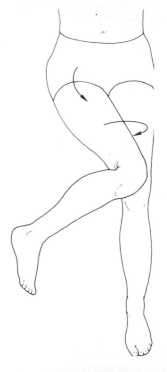

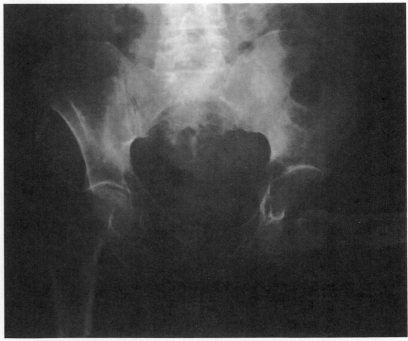

Knee dislocation

This is a true orthopedic emergency. Emergent reduction is needed to ensure salvage of limb.

■ **MECHANISM OF INJURY**

Major trauma

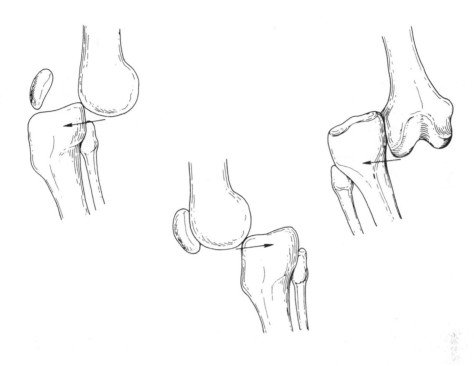

■ **SIGNS**
AND SYMPTOMS

Severe pain
Gross swelling
Deformity
Inability to move joint

■ **THERAPEUTIC INTERVENTIONS**

General emergency management of orthopedic injuries and dislocations
Splint in position of comfort
Immediate reduction (within 24 hours) to avoid arterial damage
Admission

■ **COMPLICATIONS**

Peroneal nerve damage
Posterior tibial nerve damage
Popliteal artery damage

Patellar dislocation

- **MECHANISM OF INJURY**
  Spontaneous
  Direct trauma
  Rotation injury on planted foot
- **SIGNS AND SYMPTOMS**
  Pain
  Knee usually in flexed position with inability to function
  Tenderness
  Swelling
- **THERAPEUTIC INTERVENTIONS**
  Emergency management of orthopedic injuries and dislocations
  Spontaneous reduction
  Splint or cast and crutches
- **COMPLICATIONS**
  Bleeding into knee joint (hemarthrosis)

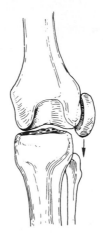

Ankle dislocation

- **MECHANISM OF INJURY**
  Usually associated with a fracture
- **SIGNS AND SYMPTOMS**
  Pain
  Swelling
  Deformity
  Inability to move joint
- **THERAPEUTIC INTERVENTIONS**
  Emergency management of orthopedic injuries and dislocations
  Splint in position of comfort
  Possible surgical reduction
  Splint or cast and crutches
- **COMPLICATIONS**
  Neurovascular compromise

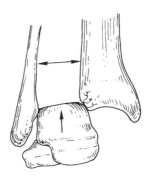

Foot dislocation

- **MECHANISM OF INJURY**
  Rare injury
  Usually automobile or motorcycle accident
  Usually associated with open wound
- **SIGNS AND SYMPTOMS**
  Pain
  Tenderness
  Swelling
  Deformity
  Inability to use foot
- **THERAPEUTIC INTERVENTIONS**
  Emergency management of orthopedic injuries and dislocations
  Sterile dressing on open wound
  Possible surgical reduction
  Splint or cast and crutches

■ **COMPLICATIONS**
Neurovascular compromise

REPETITIVE MOTION DISORDERS

Tendinitis

Tendinitis is a painful inflammation of the tendinous insertions into the bone. It is frequently seen in the shoulder (rotator cuff), elbow (lateral epicondyle), wrist (De Quervain's tenosynovitis), knee, and heel (Achilles).

■ **MECHANISM OF INJURY**
Excessive continued stress
Sudden hyperextension
Inflammation can be acute or chronic
Unknown

■ **SIGNS AND SYMPTOMS**
Aching pain that increases with motion
Swelling
Point tenderness with palpation

■ **THERAPEUTIC INTERVENTIONS**
Immobilization
Avoid activity that may be causative.
Ice acutely; heat may be beneficial in chronic phase.
Compressive dressing
Elevate
Nonsteroidal antiinflammatory medication
X-rays may show calcification.
Anesthetic and corticosteroid infiltrations (never used in Achilles tendon)

■ **COMPLICATIONS**
Synovitis
Muscle tears
Arthritis
Nerve entrapment

Bursitis

Bursitis is an inflammation of the bursa or sac that covers a bony prominence between bones, muscles, and tendons. Usually involves the elbow, shoulder, knee, heel, or hip.

■ **MECHANISM OF INJURY**
Result of trauma, direct blow or a chronic injury
Infection
Chronic occupational stress
Repetitive athletic stress
Degenerative changes

■ **SIGNS AND SYMPTOMS**
Gradual onset of symptoms
Red and warm over the injury
Aching pain that increases with motion
Gross swelling in trauma
Radiation of pain
Crepitus of joint

■ **THERAPEUTIC INTERVENTION**
Immobilize
Pad area
Ice in acute traumatic injuries
Local heat
Steroids
Bursal injection or incision if caused by infection
Gram stain and culture of aspirate

■ **COMPLICATIONS**
Synovitis
Muscle tears
Arthritis
Nerve entrapment

Nerve entrapment syndrome

Nerve entrapment (carpal tunnel) syndrome is an upper extremity problem that has an increasing incidence and poorly understood causes.[11] The syndrome involves compression of the median nerve in the carpal canal. Diagnosis remains based on clinical symptoms and signs.

■ **MECHANISM OF INJURY**
Overuse of extremity
Repetitive use of the extremity
Occupational or athletic stresses

■ **SIGNS AND SYMPTOMS**
Pain along nerve
Pain may radiate to the shoulder
Paresthesia
Numbness
Limited range of motion
Atrophy of surrounding muscles
Weakness of the extremity

■ **THERAPEUTIC INTERVENTIONS**
X-ray examinations are of limited benefit.
Splinting
Antiinflammatory medication
Steroid injections
Electrodiagnostic studies
Surgical relief of nerve entrapment

■ **COMPLICATIONS**
Synovitis
Muscle tears
Arthritis
Nerve entrapment

TRAUMATIC AMPUTATIONS

Causes of Traumatic Amputations*

Traumatic amputations are often incurred in the workplace. They are frequently seen in people who work with machines, such as farm workers, industrial workers, and mechanics; however, a substantial number of traumatic

*From Wohlstadter T: Amputations, *JEN* 5(4):36, 1979.

amputations are caused by automobile and motorcycle accidents. Power lawn mowers and motor vehicle accidents account for a large portion of amputations in the pediatric population.[12]

Emergency personnel must take steps to enhance the viability of the severed part. General emergency management of the patient with orthopedic injuries should be instituted as rapidly as possible.

Care of the Stump

Control bleeding by direct pressure, elevation, or slightly inflated blood pressure cuff.
Do *not* use clamps or tourniquet.
Remove gross debris; do *not* scrub or use cleaning solutions.
Splint.
Radiograph stump and severed part.
Administer antibiotics.
Prepare patient for surgery to debride the stump and repair vascular damage or replant the severed part.

Management of the Severed Part

1. Attempt to find the severed part if not brought to the emergency department.
2. Using sterile gloves, remove any gross foreign matter.
3. Wrap the part in a sterile gauze (for digit, ear, etc.), towel, or clean sheet (for larger limbs).
4. Wet the wrapping with sterile normal saline or Ringer's lactate, or rinse part with saline.
5. Place the part in a suitably sized bag or container and seal shut. (Do not immerse part in a solution bath!)
6. Place bag or container inside another container in iced bath.
7. Label the bag with the patient's name, the date, and the time.
8. Transport severed part with the patient, if possible, as soon as the patient's condition is stabilized.
9. A reminder: do not compromise patient care. Life-saving procedures *always* take priority over management of the severed part.

What *not* to do

Do not   Place part in tap, distilled, or sterile water
Place in soapy water, formalin, or antiseptic solution
Apply a tourniquet
Freeze or allow in direct contact with ice
Make a judgment as to the viability of the part; this is the physician's decision
Immerse part completely in solution bath (this would cause the part to become water-logged)

Survival time

The quality of the preservation of the amputated part will greatly influence its survival time. A well-preserved part without a large amount of muscle tissue (which necroses quickly) can be replanted up to 24 hours after the trauma. However, a nonpreserved part can remain viable for 6 hours at the most.

PATIENT EDUCATION/DISCHARGE INSTRUCTIONS

Aftercare Instructions for Patients with Casts

Return to the emergency department, the orthopedic clinic, or your private physician in 24 hours for follow-up care.
Keep the cast dry.
Keep the limb elevated above the level of the heart for 24 hours after the injury.
Do not place sharp objects (for example, coat hangers, knitting needles) down cast. If skin itches, blow cool air (hairdryer) down the cast or scratch the other extremity.

If any of the following abnormalities are present, return to the follow-up clinic immediately:

Check the temperature of the digits; it is abnormal if they are very cold or very hot.

Check the color of the digits; it is abnormal if they are blue.

Check if there is feeling in the digits; it is abnormal if there is no feeling, tingling, or decreasing sensation.

Wiggle the digits at least once each hour.

If a foreign object is dropped into the cast, call the follow-up care facility immediately.

Return to the follow-up clinic if the cast becomes too tight or if a foul odor is present.

CRUTCH AND CANE FITTING

In fitting crutches, measure with the shoe the patient will be wearing, preferably a low-heeled, rubber-soled, tie shoe.

Axillary Crutches

Length

Arm piece should be 2 inches from axilla (no weight on axilla).

Tips should be 6 to 8 inches to side and front of foot at 25-degree angle.

Hand piece

Elbow should be at 30-degree angle of flexion.

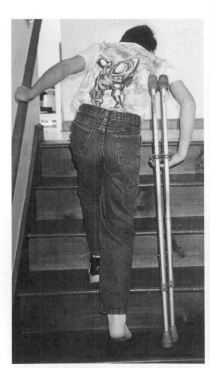 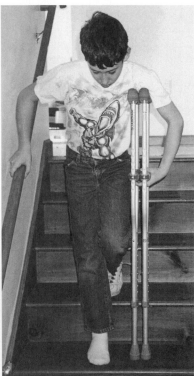

FIGURE 28-3. **A,** Going upstairs with railing and crutches. **B,** Going downstairs with railing and crutches.
(Courtesy Emilie Goudey, Lenox, Mass)

Loftstrand Crutches

Length
  Tips should be 6 inches to side and front of foot at 25-degree angle.
Hand piece
  Elbow should be at 30-degree angle of flexion.

GAIT TRAINING

Have the patient stand and balance.
Have the patient hold the crutches 4 inches to the side of the foot and 4 inches in front of the foot.
All weight is carried on the hands by straightening the elbows. Instruct the patient *not* to place any weight on the axillae, even while resting.
In the emergency department, a three-point gait is usually taught, as this type of gait is used when little or no weight bearing is desired.
Be sure to include stair climbing (Figure 28-3, A and B), sitting, and standing instructions.

INJURY PREVENTION STRATEGIES

Emergency nurses are in the foreground of prevention. Become involved in community and legislative initiatives to decrease death and disability caused by orthopedic injuries and trauma. Below are just a few injury prevention strategies that would decrease the number of orthopedic injuries each year.
Encourage parental supervision of infants and young children.
Promote safety and child passenger laws.
Educate on firearm safety.
Encourage enforcement of existing alcohol and drug use laws.
Support traffic safety enforcement.
Support playground redesign.
Support lawn mower and snow blower redesign.
Encourage the use of wrist guards, knee pads, and helmets in sporting activities such as skating, skiing, and bicycling.
Take a break from work at a repetitive task every hour.
Maintain OSHA and workplace standards.
Do not wear loose clothing or jewelry around machinery.

REFERENCES

1. Alonso JE et al: The management of complex orthopedic injuries, *Surg Clin North Am* 76(4):879-903, Aug 1996.
2. Emergency Nurses Association: Orthopedic emergencies. In *Emergency nursing core curriculum,* ed 4, Philadelphia, Saunders.
3. Martin DP et al: Development of a musculoskeletal extremity health status instrument: the musculoskeletal function assessment instrument, *J Orthop Res* 14(2):173-181, March 1996.
4. Simon RR, Koenigsknecht SJ: Emergency orthopedics: the extremities, ed 2, Norwalk, Conn, 1987, Appleton & Lange.
5. Levin LS et al: Management of severe musculoskeletal injuries of the upper extremity, *J Orthop Trauma* 4(4):432-440, 1990.
6. Rockwood CA, Green DP: *Fractures in adults,* ed 2, Philadelphia, 1984, Lippincott.
7. Butt WD: Fractures of the hand: II statistical review, *Can Med Assoc J* 86:775-779, 1972.
8. Cwinn AA: Pelvic and hip. In Rosen P et al, editors. *Emergency medicine: concepts and clinical practice,* ed 3, St Louis, 1992, Mosby.

9. DeLee JC: *Fractures and dislocations of the ankle: surgery of the foot and ankle,* ed 6, St Louis, 1993, Mosby.

10. Wilson JN: *Watson-Jones fracture and joint injuries,* ed 5, vol 2, London, 1976, Churchhill, Livingston.

11. VonSchroeder HP, Botte MJ: Carpal tunnel syndrome, *Hand Clin* 12(4):643-655, 1996.

12. Trautwein LC, Smith DG, Rivara FP: Pediatric amputation injuries: etiology, cost, and outcome, *J Trauma* 41(5):831-838, 1996.

SUGGESTED READINGS

Molitor L: A 72-year-old woman with a hip fracture, *J Emerg Nurs* 23(3):284, 1997.

Shea SS: Radiologic assessment of the injured elbow, *J Emerg Nurs* 24(2):161-164, 1998.

Ziglar MK, Parnish RS: An 18-year-old male patient with multiple trauma including open pelvic fracture, *J Emerg Nurs* 20:265-7, 1994.

Multiple Trauma

Joan Elaine Begg-Whitman

Each year, one out of three Americans sustains a traumatic injury.[1] Trauma is a major cause of disability in the United States and accounts for approximately 140,000 deaths annually.[2] It is the leading cause of death in people under the age of 44,[3] accounts for half the deaths in children under age 4, and 80% of deaths in persons aged 15 to 24 years old.[4] In any emergency department one must be prepared to care for the critically injured trauma patient.

THE ABC⁴ PRIMARY TRAUMA SURVEY

The ABC⁴ Primary Trauma Survey is an organized format for use in the rapid assessment and intervention of the multiply traumatized patient. It provides a systematic approach, whereby a multiply traumatized patient can be initially assessed for life-threatening injuries in approximately 2 minutes. As life-threatening problems are identified, interventions must be initiated. The ABC⁴ primary trauma survey is as follows:

A = Airway
B = Breathing
C^1 = Circulation
C^2 = Cervical Spine
C^3 = Chest
C^4 = Consciousness

A = Airway

Assessment of the patient's airway is the first step in the primary trauma survey.

Assessment of the airway should be a "reflex reaction"—it should *always* be done first. The method of airway management should be based on patient findings; treat each patient individually. Airway management includes the following:

Supplemental oxygen

All multiple-trauma patients should receive supplemental oxygen through the appropriate delivery device and at the correct concentration.

Head and neck position

Always assume that the patient has a cervical spine injury until it can be ruled out by a cervical spine x-ray series or other diagnostic tool.

If head and neck position becomes essential in airway management, begin with a modified jaw thrust maneuver, maintaining the cervical spine in a neutral position.

Airway adjuncts

The use of airway adjuncts may become necessary in the management of the patient's airway. Use adjuncts according to their availability, indications, and contraindications.

■ **OROPHARYNGEAL AIRWAY**

Use the oropharyngeal airway only in patients who are unconscious and who do not have a gag reflex.

■ **NASOPHARYNGEAL AIRWAY**

The nasopharyngeal airway may be used on conscious patients who have an intact gag reflex. It is particularly useful in patients with facial trauma, where edema may rapidly ensue and airway obstruction is possible.

■ **ESOPHAGEAL OBTURATOR/ESOPHAGEAL GASTRIC TUBE AIRWAY**

This airway should only be used in patients who are apneic and without a gag reflex. It may be considered when airway management and maintenance are essential and endotracheal intubation cannot be accomplished.

■ **ENDOTRACHEAL TUBE**

Consider placement of an endotracheal tube when total airway management is essential.

In general, orotracheal intubation is recommended in the trauma victim.[5] One must be particularly cautious not to hyperextend the cervical spine in the trauma patient. One method of accomplishing endotracheal intubation without hyperextension of the C-spine is by using a technique known as *tactile* or *digital intubation,* where the epiglottis is palpated with the index and middle fingers of the nondominant hand and the tube is placed with the dominant hand and guided with the fingers of the nondominant hand. This should only be performed on deeply comatose patients.

Nasotracheal intubation may also be considered.

More detail on the use of airway adjuncts can be found in Chapters 4 and 5.

■ **CRICOTHYROTOMY**

Cricothyrotomy is a technique that should be used only when airway management by other means cannot be accomplished and the patient has an upper airway obstruction, such as occurs with a fractured larynx.

Two methods used to maintain the airway in this case are:

Needle cricothyrotomy

Surgical incision through the cricoid membrane and tube placement

Suction

Ensure that adequate suction is readily available. As a backup device, a plastic turkey baster is often quite useful for suction when other devices prove to be inadequate.

B = Breathing

The function of ventilation and perfusion is to bring oxygen to the alveoli and to carry carbon dioxide and other waste products from the alveoli. Adequate breathing and ventilation are essential to the trauma victim whose status may be compromised as a result of a ventilation or perfusion defect. Monitor O_2 saturations and blood gases.

Several methods of providing assisted positive pressure ventilation are:

Mouth-to-mask

Using a mask with a nonbackflow valve and breathing into the mask rather than directly into the patient's mouth provides a barrier between the rescuer and the victim. This device offers several advantages: It is far more palatable than mouth-to-mouth for most rescuers; it reduces the likelihood of infectious disease transmission; and supplemental oxygen may be added to a port on the mask, increasing the amount of oxygen concentration delivered to the patient.

Bag-valve-mask device

With supplemental oxygen and tubing attached to add a dead space, this device is capable of delivering up to 95% oxygen. The caregiver is also able to sense lung compliance. One of the problems with this device is that it is difficult for one rescuer to achieve an adequate seal.

Demand valve

A demand valve delivers 100% oxygen at 100 L/min. The rescuer must be particularly cautious because there is a possibility of overventilation and development of or further increase of tension pneumothorax. It should not be used on a small child because the flow is too great and may be harmful.

Ventilator

If a ventilator is used, the caregiver should maintain constant observation of the patient and the ventilator. A variety of ventilators can be used on trauma victims, but a volume-cycled ventilator is most commonly used.

C^1 = Circulation

Circulatory status can be assessed by first checking for the presence and quality of a carotid and/or femoral pulse. Peripheral pulses may be absent as a result of direct injury or sympathetic nervous system response as a compensatory mechanism, which causes peripheral vasoconstriction.

Assess the patient's vital signs, including pulse, respirations, blood pressure, temperature, and skin vitals (color, temperature, and moisture) and capillary refill.

Assessing for pulses should be done at three points: first try radial, then femoral, then carotid

If radial pulse present,	estimate BP at 80 mm Hg
If femoral pulse present,	estimate BP at 70 mm Hg
If carotid pulse present,	estimate BP at 60 mm Hg

If no pulses are felt then institute CPR, BLS, and ACLS measures.

Hypovolemic shock

Hypovolemic shock occurs when oxygen and nutrients cannot be transported to the cells and waste products cannot be transported from the cells because blood volume is decreased and adequate pressures cannot be maintained. This results in a reduced amount of available hemoglobin, decreased cardiac output, and low blood pressure.

The average 70 kg (154 lb) person has a blood volume of approximately 5 liters. In a person who was healthy before suffering a traumatic incident and who has normal compensatory mechanisms:
- Mild shock results from a 10% to 20% blood loss (0.5 to 1.0 liters).
- Moderate shock results from a 20% to 40% blood loss (1.0 to 2.0 liters).
- Severe shock results from greater than 40% blood loss (2.0 liters).
- Hypovolemia is the most common cause of shock in pediatric trauma victims.
- Children *are not* small adults.
- Children can lose up to 25% of their blood volume before exhibiting hypotension. Tachycardia, poor pulse quality, cold extremities in a warm environment, increased diastolic blood pressure, restlessness, and delayed capillary refill are the clearest indicators of impending shock in these patients. Hypotension is a late sign of blood loss in children.
- Children have significantly less circulating blood volume than adults, therefore relatively minor injuries can cause significant blood loss, and resultant shock.

■ SIGNS AND SYMPTOMS

Restlessness and anxiety
Cool and clammy skin
Tachycardia
Delayed capillary refill
(If greater than 2 seconds, assume shock until proven otherwise.)
Hypotension
Tachypnea
Decreased level of consciousness

Patient complaint of being cold
Patient complaint of being thirsty

■ COMPENSATORY MECHANISMS

There are several compensatory mechanisms in shock that will activate an attempt to salvage the brain, heart, and lungs:

Sympathetic nervous system activation. Sympathetic nervous system activation causes the release of epinephrine and norepinephrine, providing alpha and beta stimulation; this causes the heart rate and peripheral resistance to increase. Peripheral vasoconstriction will occur, causing the patient to have cool, clammy skin and cool distal extremities. Because of the peripheral vasoconstriction, the patient, if awake, may complain of being cold.

Renin-angiotensin mechanism activation. When blood flow through the renal arteries decreases, renin angiotensin I and angiotensin II are released. These cause the release of aldosterone, which causes the kidneys to reabsorb sodium and thereby water. As a result of this compensatory mechanism, as well as a decreased renal blood flow, urinary output will decrease.

Antidiuretic hormone release. When hypovolemic shock ensues, antidiuretic hormone (ADH) is released. This causes the kidneys to reabsorb water. This will also be a cause of decreased urinary output.

Intracellular fluid shift. In shock states cell walls become permeable to fluids. Fluids leave the cells and fill the intravascular space. This may also cause the patient, if alert and oriented, to complain of being thirsty, as the cells "dehydrate."

Jugular (neck) veins in shock. If a patient is in shock, assess the jugular veins: Distension may indicate a tourniquet effect on the chest contents, decreasing blood return to the right side of the heart and backflow into the jugular veins. Think about the possibility of a pericardial tamponade or a tension pneumothorax and treat accordingly. Be sure to check neck veins periodically, especially when a cervical collar is in place and the jugular veins are not readily visible.

If neck veins are flat, consider the possibility of hypovolemia and assess further for this condition.

■ THERAPEUTIC INTERVENTIONS

100% oxygen. Oxygen may often be required under positive pressure. If positive pressure is used, be alert to the development of a tension pneumothorax. As soon as possible, obtain arterial blood gases to ensure accurate evaluation of oxygenation status.

Pneumatic antishock garment (PASG). The pneumatic antishock garment has fallen out of favor with most providers of trauma care.

IVs

Start two large-bore (14 gauge, if possible) IV lines using a warmed crystalloid solution.

Lines may be started in the antecubital space, jugular veins, or any other large vein site.

Run solutions at a rate that will maintain systolic pressure above 100 mm Hg.

Send a blood specimen for type and cross-match.

Consider using large bore "trauma" tubing or a rapid infusion device.

Control bleeding. Use direct pressure whenever possible. Consider using pressure points and clamping or tourniquets when bleeding is uncontrolled and the situation is life-threatening.

C^2 = Cervical Spine

A cervical spine injury should be considered present in all multiple-trauma patients until it can be proven negative on full cervical spine x-ray series or other diagnostic tools, such as CT. If x-ray is to be used to clear the C-spine, four views are necessary:

Cross-table lateral (must visualize to T-1)
Anterior-posterior
Lateral
Open-mouth odontoid
Flexion/extension views (to check for soft-tissue damage)

Protect the cervical spine by using a stiff cervical collar, rolled blanket, adhesive tape across the eyebrows and onto the backboard, backboard, or other acceptable C-spine protection device. Be sure to protect the thoracic, lumbar, and sacral spine as well by immobilizing from the top of the head to the hips.

C³ = Chest

Five types of chest injury should be ruled out in the primary survey. If they are detected, it is important to initiate *immediate* therapeutic intervention because any of these conditions may be immediately life threatening. In-depth discussion of each of these conditions can be found in Chapter 26.

Tension pneumothorax

Air entry into the pleural cavity.
■ **SIGNS AND SYMPTOMS**
Cyanosis
Distended jugular veins
Dyspnea
Deviated trachea (away from the tension)
Cough
Diminished or absent breath sounds
Chest pain
Mediastinal shift (seen on x-ray)
Tachycardia
Decreasing blood pressure
■ **THERAPEUTIC INTERVENTIONS**
Needle thoracostomy or chest tube placement

Flail chest

Fracture of two or more adjacent ribs in two places or sternal fracture, creating a detached chest wall segment that disrupts chest wall integrity.
■ **SIGNS AND SYMPTOMS**
Paradoxical movement of the chest wall
Dyspnea
Cyanosis
Tachycardia
■ **THERAPEUTIC INTERVENTIONS**
Selective endotracheal intubation (if respiratory rate is less than 23, Pao_2 is less than 60 on 50% oxygen, and/or tidal volume is less than 5 ml/kg)
100% oxygen under positive pressure
Careful fluid administration
Analgesia
Consider stabilization of the flail segment

Pericardial tamponade

Accumulation of fluid, most commonly blood, within the pericardial sac.
■ **SIGNS AND SYMPTOMS**
Increased heart rate
Decreased blood pressure ⎫
Muffled heart sounds   ⎬ Beck's Triad
Distended jugular veins   ⎭
Dyspnea
Kussmaul's respirations

Paradoxical pulse

Cyanosis (periorbital and peripheral)

■ **THERAPEUTIC INTERVENTIONS**

Oxygen at high flow rate

High Fowler's position

IV line

Pericardiocentesis or pericardial window

Open chest wound (sucking chest wound)

An open chest wound is a chest wall defect that allows air to enter the pleural space. An open pneumothorax occurs as positive-pressure atmospheric air rushes into negative-pressure pleural space on inspiration.

Usually seen after penetrating chest trauma.

■ **SIGNS AND SYMPTOMS**

Sucking sound

Dyspnea

Diminished or absent breath sounds

Tachycardia

Hypotension

Signs of tension pneumothorax

■ **THERAPEUTIC INTERVENTIONS**

If the wound is less than two thirds the size of the trachea (the mainstem bronchus), one can safely care for the patient without using an occlusive dressing.

Cover a larger defect with an occlusive dressing, such as petroleum-impregnated gauze taped on three sides.

Watch closely for the development of signs and symptoms of tension pneumothorax.

If signs and symptoms of tension pneumothorax appear, immediately remove occlusive dressing and consider immediate chest tube placement.

Provide supplemental oxygen.

Massive hemothorax (more than 1500 ml of blood)

Collection of blood in the pleural space.

■ **SIGNS AND SYMPTOMS**

Same as those for hypovolemic shock (see Chapter 9)

■ **THERAPEUTIC INTERVENTIONS**

Same as those for hypovolemic shock (see Chapter 9)

Oxygen

IV lines for fluid and blood replacement

Chest tube(s)

Large bore (36 French)

Possible autotransfusion

Possible emergency thoracotomy

C^4 = Consciousness

Assess neurologic status using the Glasgow Coma Scale and DERM mnemonic (see Chapter 12).

A brief neurologic assessment can be as simple as eye opening, response to asking patient's name, hand squeezing, and pupil check.

Glasgow Coma Scale

BEST MOTOR RESPONSE

Obeys simple commands	6 points
Localizes noxious stimulus	5 points
Flexion withdrawal	4 points
Abnormal flexion	3 points
Abnormal extension	2 points
No motor response	1 point

BEST VERBAL RESPONSE

Oriented	5 points
Confused	4 points
Verbalizes/exclamatory or disorganized	3 points
Moans/groans	2 points
No vocalization	1 point

EYE OPENING

Spontaneously	4 points
To speech	3 points
To noxious stimulus	2 points
No eye opening	1 point

Coma is defined as no response and no eye opening or a score of 7 or less. If the patient is intubated and being ventilated, verbal response should be recorded as a "T" (for tubed). For example, a patient who has flexion withdrawal, is intubated and ventilated, and opens eyes to noxious stimuli would have a GCS of 6T. The Glasgow Coma Scale may not be useful in patients who are severely hypovolemic or intoxicated.

DERM mnemonic

D = Depth of coma
Use stimulus/response. Example: Responds to painful stimulus with flexion withdrawal.
E = Eyes
Check pupillary response.
R = Respiration
Describe rate, rhythm, and depth of respirations
M = Motor/movement
Check extremity movement; if it is present, describe whether it is unilateral or bilateral.

The caregiver may wish to calculate a trauma score for outcome prediction. One that is frequently used is the Champion Trauma Score (CTS).[6] In the Champion Trauma Score the Glasgow Coma Scale and a trauma-scoring method are tabulated as follows:

GLASGOW COMA SCALE SCORE

Point conversion for use with CTS

14-15	=	5
11-13	=	4
8-10	=	3
5-7	=	2
3-4	=	1

THE SECONDARY SURVEY

Following a primary survey, where life-threatening conditions are identified and treated, a more thorough secondary survey should be performed. Begin by reevaluating the patient's airway. It is also at this point that fractures should be splinted.

The secondary survey is a rapid head-to-toe survey, starting at the head.

A complete set of vital signs is assessed here. In patients with major or suspected chest trauma the apical and radial pulses should be compared. The blood pressure should be taken in both arms. These vital signs will be used as a baseline for continual reassessment.

The patient's general appearance should be assessed: body positioning, guarding, odors present (such as alcohol, gasoline, feces, urine)

This is the process where *all* injuries are assessed, not just the obvious ones, by inspection, auscultation, and palpation. Remember to prevent heat loss and keep patient warm.

Head

Systematically assess and treat the head and neck for lacerations, fractures, and deformities.

Hyperventilate major head trauma patients to lower P_{CO_2} to approximately 28 torr (no less).

Administer mannitol and/or furosemide for major head trauma patients.

Consider computerized axial tomography (CT scan) or skull x-rays.

Suture lacerations.

Check all areas for bruises, discoloration, lacerations, deformities.

Do a rapid systemic evaluation of the following:

Neck

Recheck airway

Check for:

Fractured larynx (anterior neck subcutaneous emphysema)

Wounds/hematomas

Neck vein distension

Pulses

Deformities

Pain

Penetrating objects

Midline trachea

Subcutaneous emphysema

If a C-spine injury is present, administer methylprednisolone (solumedrol in accordance with protocol)

Face

Check for:

Airway problems

Symmetry

Obvious fractures

Dental step-defects or malocclusion

CSF rhinorrhea

Eyes

Check for:

Pupillary response

Trauma

Periorbital ecchymosis

Ears

Check for:
CSF otorrhea
Ruptured tympanic membrane

Mouth

Check for:
Foreign bodies
Obstruction/lacerations

Chest

Check for wounds/abrasions/deformities/penetrating objects/holes.
Check heart sounds.
Check lung sounds.
Check chest wall symmetry.
Obtain arterial blood gases.
Obtain a 12-lead ECG.
Obtain a chest x-ray, if not already done.

Abdomen

Check for:
Bowel sounds
Rigidity
Pain
Tenderness
Wounds/abrasions/hematomas
Penetrating objects
Eviscerations
Distension

Spine

Check for:
Deformities
Pain on palpation
Abrasions/bruises

Pelvis/hips

Check for:
Fractures
Deformities
Femoral pulses and distal pulses
Abnormal rotation and/or flexion of legs

Extremities

Check for:
Pulses
Neurologic status distal to injury
Fractures/dislocations/crepitus
Movement
Skin color and temperature
Capillary refill

Perineum

Check for:
Bleeding
Urine extravasation

Buttocks

Check for:
Wounds
Abrasions

General management

Following the completion of systemic assessment:
Cover open wounds.
Repair lacerations.
Never remove an impaled object; secure and stabilize it until it can be surgically removed.
Remember to assess the posterior side of the patient, maintaining C-spine immobilization.
Administer appropriate IV fluids, blood products, medications.
Ensure that appropriate specimens have been sent to the lab.
Remember tetanus prophylaxis.
Order further appropriate diagnostic tests, such as x-rays, CT scans, peritoneal lavage, pericardiocentesis, serum and urine laboratory tests.
Obtain appropriate consults.
Prepare the patient for possible surgery.
Care for patient and family/significant others' psychological needs.

UNDRESSING THE PATIENT

Undressing the trauma patient is a vitally important step in performing a complete evaluation. Without exposing the patient it is impossible to make a systematic assessment of all of the patient's obvious and occult injuries. Although it appears to be a straightforward task, it can be difficult to remove some pieces of clothing, particularly the protective garb that is worn in sports.

Helmets

A variety of helmets are available for those sports that recommend head protection—motorcycle, bicycle, kayak, football, hockey, and auto racing are just a few. The careful removal of this gear is imperative in protection of the potential cervical spine injury.

Procedure

1. Never attempt to remove a helmet alone; airway protection can be achieved with the helmet on, and the potential for complicating an injury with a difficult removal is great.
2. One person should apply inline traction by placing his hands on each side of the helmet with his fingers on the patient's mandible and exerting general pulling; loosen or cut the chin strap to remove.
3. A second person should then receive the weight of the patient's head by placing one hand behind the head, resting on the occiput, and the front hand on the angles of the mandible, thumb on one side, fingers on the other (the second person is now in control of the head and neck).
4. The first person should then remove the helmet by pulling laterally on the sides and sliding it off.

NOTE: If the helmet has full face protection, special consideration must be given to the eye covering, which must be removed first; if it cannot be removed, tilt the helmet (not the head) back to pass the face protector over the patient's nose.

Boots

Heavy boots create a problem if the patient has sustained an unstable injury to the foot or lower leg. Some simple techniques make the process of removal less painful. REMEMBER: Boots are usually very expensive, and removal without cutting is generally appreciated.

Procedure

1. Inform the patient of each step of the removal process as it is about to occur; employ the patient's cooperation.
2. Place the patient supine; unlace boot and open the boot as freely as possible.
3. Have one person slip both hands on the lateral and medial sides of the patient's lower leg, into the boot; support the ankle and foot as one unit with both hands.
4. Have the second person remove the boot, pulling the toe of the boot in a cephalad direction to gently release the heel (which is being stabilized by the first person).

Rear Entry Ski Boots

To remove rear entry ski boots follow the procedure above, but keep in mind that with the entry in the back the leg must be elevated enough to accommodate the rear flap opening and the need for pulling before the heel is released is exaggerated.

Neoprene Wet Suit/Stretch One-Piece Ski Racing Suits

Wet suits and one-piece stretch ski racing suits pose a special problem when the patient is a victim of trauma. In most cases the suits can be rolled and pulled off the patient, being turned inside out in the removal (usually requiring more than one undresser). If this is not an option in the emergency setting, they must be cut off. However, consider their great expense and cut along seams if necessary.

Down Clothing

Do not ever cut!

■ **GENERAL GUIDELINES FOR UNDRESSING THE PATIENT**
1. Preserve as much clothing as possible without wasting time.
2. Undress the uninjured extremity first, then the injured limb.
3. Dress in the reverse of #2; injured limb first, uninjured extremity last.
4. Don't forget to look for teeth, contact lenses, and prosthetics.
5. Consider the chain of evidence if foul play was involved with the patient and if the clothes or their contents may be used in court.
6. Remove jewelry and deposit (witnessed) it in a valuables protection envelope in a designated safe, or release it to family. Record this transaction on patient's chart.
7. Consider religious clothing when undressing if situation permits, and consult patient or family about its removal and safekeeping.
8. When clothing must be cut away from patient, try to cut on seams.

TRAUMA FLOW SHEET

It is essential, in trauma, to carefully document all events and findings. Use of a specifically designed flow sheet (Figure 29-1) facilitates this and ensures that important items are not forgotten.

Care of the multiply traumatized patient presents us with an enormous challenge. An organized, systematic, and rehearsed approach will prove most beneficial to the patient. Remember, trauma care is a team effort!

EMERGENCY DEPARTMENT TRAUMA CHART

Age:	Sex: ☐M ☐F	DATE:
Approx. Time of Injury:		Other Hospital:
Time of Arrival at DHMC:		MODE: ☐AMB ☐AIR ☐CAR

(Addressograph)

MECHANISM _____

SAFETY DEVICES:
☐ Shoulder Belt   ☐ Helmet
☐ Lap Belt   ☐ Air Bag
☐ Lap & Shoulder Belt   ☐ Other: ___

FOR MVC:
☐ Driver   ☐ Rear Pass Ⓜ
☐ FS Passenger   ☐ Rear Pass Ⓡ
☐ Rear Pass Ⓛ   ☐ Pedestrian

☐ *TRAUMA ALERT*   ☐ *TRAUMA NINE*

E.D. TEAM

Nurse #1 _____
Nurse #2 _____
ED Attending _____
ED Resident _____
Other _____

REVIEW

☐ YES   ☐ NO

SCENE DATA

LOC:
☐ Awake / Alert
☐ Confused
☐ Responds Pain
☐ No Response
☐ > 20 min extrication

Last vitals
BP _____
P _____
R _____
☐ Assisted

TREATMENTS:
Airway   O2 @ ___ L ☐PASG
☐ OP / NP   ☐ C.Collar   ☐ IV#1
☐ EOA   ☐ Backboard   ☐ IV#2
☐ ET / NT   ☐ Other
☐ Other _____

TRAUMA TEAM	**Name**	**Called**	**Arrived**
Trauma Resident			
Trauma Attending			
Anesthesiologist			
Radiology Tech			
Radiologist			
Social Worker / Chaplain			
Other			
Other			
Other			
Other			
Other			

PREVIOUS HOSPITAL

AIRWAY	*TREATMENTS & DIAGNOSTICS*	*MEDICATIONS*
☐ OP / NP	☐ C Collar ☐ Chest Tube	☐ Narcotics
☐ EOA	☐ Backboard ☐ DPL	☐ Paralytics
☐ ET / NT	☐ PASG ☐ CT ___	☐ Dexamethasone
☐ O2 @ ___ L	☐ IV#1 ☐ XRAYS ☐ C-SPINE	☐ Antibiotics
☐ Assisted	☐ IV#2 ☐ CHEST	☐ Tet Tox
	☐ LABS	☐ Other ___

HISTORY

Meds: _____

Allergies: _____ Ht: ___ Wt: ___ Last Tetanus: ___ LMP: ___ Food: ___

Time:	Notes	Time	Notes

RELATIVE NOTIFIED: ☐Yes ☐No   Relationship: _____   LOCATION: _____   BELONGINGS GIVEN TO: _____

DISPOSITION: ☐PACU   ☐OR   ☐PICU   ☐FLOOR   ☐STEP DOWN ___   ☐ICU   ☐MORGUE

TIME OF DEATH: _____

ME NOTIFIED: ☐Yes ☐No   AUTOPSY: ☐Yes ☐No

TRANSFER TIME: _____

ORGAN / TISSUE DONATION REQUESTED: ☐Yes ☐No

FIGURE 29-1. Trauma flow sheet.

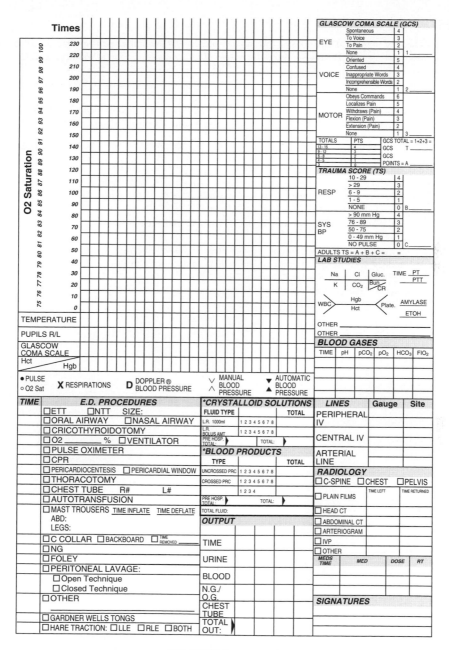

Times

O2 Saturation: 75 76 77 78 79 80 81 82 83 84 85 86 87 88 89 90 91 92 93 94 95 96 97 98 99 100

230 220 210 200 190 180 170 160 150 140 130 120 110 100 90 80 70 60 50 40 30 20 10 0

TEMPERATURE

PUPILS R/L

GLASGOW COMA SCALE

Hct / Hgb

● PULSE   ○ O2 Sat   **X** RESPIRATIONS   **D** DOPPLER® BLOOD PRESSURE   ∨∧ MANUAL BLOOD PRESSURE   ▼▲ AUTOMATIC BLOOD PRESSURE

GLASGOW COMA SCALE (GCS)

EYE	Spontaneous	4
	To Voice	3
	To Pain	2
	None	1	1 ____
VOICE	Oriented	5
	Confused	4
	Inappropriate Words	3
	Incomprehensible Words	2
	None	1	2 ____
MOTOR	Obeys Commands	6
	Localizes Pain	5
	Withdraws (Pain)	4
	Flexion (Pain)	3
	Extension (Pain)	2
	None	1	3 ____

TOTALS	PTS	
13 - 15	4	GCS TOTAL = 1+2+3 =
9 - 12	3	GCS
6 - 8	2	GCS T ____
4 - 5	1	POINTS = A ____
3	0	

TRAUMA SCORE (TS)

RESP	10 - 29	4
	> 29	3
	6 - 9	2
	1 - 5	1
	NONE	0	B
SYS BP	> 90 mm Hg	4
	76 - 89	3
	50 - 75	2
	0 - 49 mm Hg	1
	NO PULSE	0	C

ADULTS TS = A + B + C =   =

LAB STUDIES

Na | Cl | Gluc.   TIME   PT ____
K | CO2 | Bun/CR   PTT ____
WBC   Hgb/Hct   Plate.   AMYLASE
                          ETOH

OTHER ____
OTHER ____

BLOOD GASES

TIME	pH	pCO2	pO2	HCO3	FIO2

TIME	E.D. PROCEDURES
	□ETT □NTT SIZE:
	□ORAL AIRWAY □NASAL AIRWAY
	□CRICOTHYROIDOTOMY
	□O2 ___ % □VENTILATOR
	□PULSE OXIMETER
	□CPR
	□PERICARDIOCENTESIS □PERICARDIAL WINDOW
	□THORACOTOMY
	□CHEST TUBE R# L#
	□AUTOTRANSFUSION
	□MAST TROUSERS TIME INFLATE TIME DEFLATE
	ABD:
	LEGS:
	□C COLLAR □BACKBOARD □TIME REMOVED ____
	□NG
	□FOLEY
	□PERITONEAL LAVAGE:
	□Open Technique
	□Closed Technique
	□OTHER ____
	□GARDNER WELLS TONGS
	□HARE TRACTION: □LLE □RLE □BOTH

*CRYSTALLOID SOLUTIONS

FLUID TYPE		TOTAL
L.R. 1000ml	1 2 3 4 5 6 7 8	
L.R. BOLUS AMT	1 2 3 4 5 6 7 8	
PRE HOSP. TOTAL:	TOTAL:	

*BLOOD PRODUCTS

TYPE		TOTAL
UNCROSSED PRC	1 2 3 4 5 6 7 8	
CROSSED PRC	1 2 3 4 5 6 7 8	
	1 2 3 4	
PRE HOSP. TOTAL:	TOTAL:	
TOTAL FLUID:		

OUTPUT

TIME
URINE
BLOOD
N.G./O.G.
CHEST TUBE
TOTAL OUT:

LINES

LINES	Gauge	Site
PERIPHERAL IV		
CENTRAL IV		
ARTERIAL LINE		

RADIOLOGY

□C-SPINE □CHEST □PELVIS
□PLAIN FILMS   TIME LEFT   TIME RETURNED
□HEAD CT
□ABDOMINAL CT
□ARTERIOGRAM
□IVP
□OTHER

MEDS TIME	MED	DOSE	RT

SIGNATURES

FIGURE 29-1. continued.

REFERENCES

1. American College of Surgeons/Committee on Trauma: *Optimal care of the injured patient,* Chicago, 1998, ACS.
2. US Department of Health and Human Services: *Healthy people 2000 summary report,* Washington, D.C., 1992, US Government Printing Office.
3. US Department of Health and Human Services, Division of Trauma and Transplantation: *Model trauma system care plan,* Washington, D.C., 1993, US Government Printing Office.
4. American College of Surgeons/Committee on Trauma: *Advanced trauma life support manual,* Chicago, 1997, ACS.
5. Shea J: Lecture presentation at Emergency Nurses Association Annual Meeting, Orlando, Florida, Sept 1992.
6. Champion HR et al: Trauma score, *Crit Care Med* 9(9):672, 1981.

SUGGESTED READINGS

Cardona VD et al: *Trauma nursing: from resuscitation through rehabilitation,* ed 2, Philadelphia, 1993, Saunders.

DeMaria EJ: Evaluation and treatment of the elderly trauma victim, *Clin Gen Med* 9:461, 1993.

Emergency Nurses Association: *Trauma nurse care course, student manual,* Chicago, 1994, the Association.

Hill DA, Abraham KJ, West PH: Factors affecting outcomes in the resuscitation of severely injured patients, *Australia N Z J Surg* 63(8):404, 1993.

Laskowski-Jones L: Managing hemorrhage: taking the right steps to protect your patient, *Nurs 97* 27:36-41, 1997.

Ottara, Speert M, Mullaby S: Nursing care of the patient with a complete scalp avulsion, *J Emerg Nurs* 22:552-559, 1996.

Schmidt J, Moore GP: Management of multiple trauma, *Emerg Med Clin North Am* 11(1):29051, 1993.

Sheehy SB et al: *Manual of clinical trauma care: the first hour,* ed 3, St Louis, 1999, Mosby.

Trauma notebook, bimonthly feature, *J Emerg Nurs* 1992-present.

Burn Trauma

Joan Elaine Begg-Whitman

It is estimated that over 60,000 people are hospitalized for burn injuries and 10,000 people die from burn injuries each year. The most common cause of death from burn injuries in the first 48 hours is respiratory problems.

Burns are injuries to the tissues caused by:
- Intense heat or flame (thermal burns)
- Acids or alkalis (chemical burns)
- Electrical current (electrical burns)
- Overexposure to sun or x-rays (radiation burns)
- Friction (friction burns)

The severity of the burn is determined by:
- The amount of body surface area (BSA) involved
- The degree (depth) of the burn (Table 30-1)
- The patient's age
- Previous medical or surgical condition
- Current underlying trauma
- Complications from the original burn injury

CLASSIFICATION OF BURNS

First-Degree Burns (Partial Thickness Burn)

Burns through the epithelial layer of skin
Appear as areas of erythema.

Second-Degree Burns (Partial Thickness Burn)

Burns that include a partial thickness of the dermal layer of the skin
Appear as erythematous areas with blisters.

Third-Degree Burns (Full Thickness Burn)

Full thickness burns of the dermal layer of the skin
Appear white and leathery and may or may not blister.
Thrombosed vessels can sometimes be visualized beneath these burns.
Some burns extend to muscle and bone.
May have a charred appearance.

TABLE 30-1   Classification of Burn Injury

DEPTH OF BURN	SENSITIVITY	APPEARANCE	HEALING TIME AND RESULTS	TREATMENT
Partial thickness				
First-degree				
Epidermal	Hyperalgesia	Erythema	3-5 days; no scarring	Moisturizers
Superficial dermal	Hyperalgesia	Blisters, pink to red, moist	6-10 days; minimal scarring	Topical antibacterial agents or biologic dressings required
Second-degree				
Moderate dermal	Normal algesia	Blisters, pink, moist	10-18 days; some scarring	Topical antibacterial agents or biologic dressings required
Deep thermal	Hypoalgesia or analgesia	Blisters, opaque, with less moisture	>21 days; maximal scarring if not excised and grafted	Topical antibacterial agents and early excision and grafting
Full thickness				
Third-degree				
Loss of all dermal elements with extension into fat, muscle, and bone	Analgesia	White, opaque, brown, or black, occasionally deep red; very dry, leathery; may or may not have blisters or thrombosed veins	Never heals if area is larger than 3 cm². The longer the wound is open, the more hypertrophic the scar	Topical antibacterial agents and early excision and grafting

From Sheehy SA, Marvin JA, Jimmerson CL: *Manual of clinical trauma care: the first hour,* St Louis, 1989, Mosby.

Rule of 9s

Burns are categorized as major, moderate, or minor. The extent of burns may be assessed using the Rule of 9s (Figure 30-1) and/or the Lund and Browder Chart (Figure 30-2).

Major burns

A second-degree burn over more than 25% of BSA *or*

A third-degree burn over more than 10% of BSA in an adult

A second-degree burn over more than 20% of BSA in a child

Any third-degree burn in a child

Burns involving the hands, face, eyes, ears, feet, or perineum

All inhalation burns

All electrical burns

Any deep, circumferential burn

Burns with associated major trauma

Burns in any poor-risk patient (age over 55 years, underlying medical problems, for example, diabetes, heart diseases, renal failure)

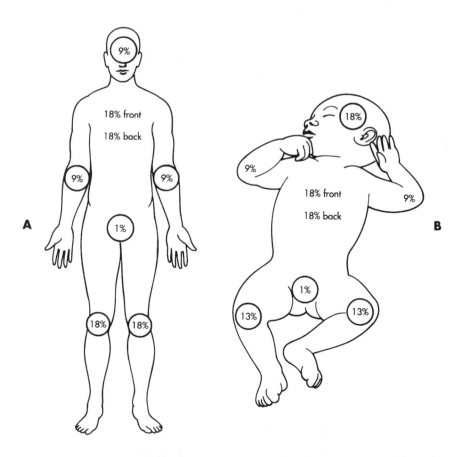

FIGURE 30-1. Rule of Nines. **A,** Adult. **B,** Child.

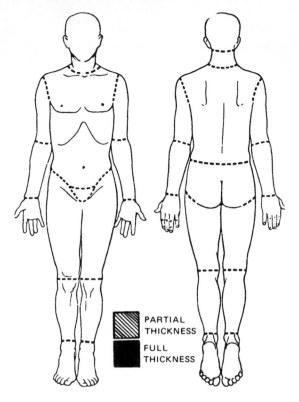

Percent Surface Area Burned

AREA	1 YEAR	1-4 YEARS	5-9 YEARS	10-14 YEARS	Y 15 YEARS	ADULT	2°	3°
Head	19	17	13	11	9	7		
Neck	2	2	2	2	2	2		
Ant. Trunk	13	13	13	13	13	13		
Post Trunk	13	13	13	13	13	13		
R. Buttock	2½	2½	2½	2½	2½	2½		
L. Buttock	2½	2½	2½	2½	2½	2½		
Genitalia	1	1	1	1	1	1		
R. U. Arm	4	4	4	4	4	4		
L. U. Arm	4	4	4	4	4	4		
R. L. Arm	3	3	3	3	3	3		
L. L. Arm	3	3	3	3	3	3		
R. Hand	2½	2½	2½	2½	2½	2½		
L. Hand	2½	2½	2½	2½	2½	2½		
R. Thigh	5½	6½	8	8½	9	9½		
L. Thigh	5½	6½	8	8½	9	9½		
R. Leg	5	5	5½	6	6½	7		
L. Leg	5	5	5½	6	6½	7		
R. Foot	3½	3½	3½	3½	3½	3½		
L. Foot	3½	3½	3½	3½	3½	3½		
TOTAL								

FIGURE 30-2. Lund and Browder formula.

(From Artz CP, Moncrief JA: *The treatment of burns*, ed 2, Philadelphia, 1969, Saunders.)

Moderate burns

A second-degree burn over 15% to 25% of BSA in an adult
A second-degree burn over 10% to 20% of BSA in a child

Minor burns

A second-degree burn over less than 15% of BSA *or*
A third-degree burn over less than 2% of BSA in an adult
A second-degree burn over less than 10% of BSA *or*
A third-degree burn over less than 2% of BSA in a child

Hospital admission is recommended for patients with:
    Second- or third-degree burns over greater than 10% of BSA
    Burns of hands, feet, and perineum
    Circumferential burns
    Electrical or chemical burns
    Burns associated with multiple or significant trauma
    Burns associated with suspected child abuse

BURN CARE

Burn care should be initiated by the first person to arrive at the scene of the incident.

Care of Minor to Moderate Burns

Stop the burning process.
Remove smoldering material.
Remove restrictive clothing and jewelry.
Initiate cooling efforts (saline soaked dressings).
Avoid use of ice or cold fluids because this could produce hypothermia.
Avoid hypothermia.
Assess extent of burn.
Shave hair surrounding wound, but do not shave eyebrows.
Debride devitalized tissue.
Leave blisters intact.
Cover wound with antimicrobial agent and bulky dressing.
Check for tetanus prophylaxis.
Consider antibiotics.
Provide aftercare instructions.
    Keep dressing clean and dry.
    Elevate burned extremity for 24 to 48 hours.
    Give prescriptions or instructions for analgesia.
    Provide follow-up care; check wound in 2 days.

Care of Moderate to Major Burns

Prehospital

Rescuer should protect self against flames, noxious gases, smoke, explosions, falling debris, and so on.
Flush chemicals from the surface or remove victim from electrical source.
ABCs (especially in those with facial and neck burns).

Check for signs of smoke inhalation (flames in a closed space, carbonaceous sputum, facial and neck burns, hoarse voice, coughing).

Check for other injuries (especially victims involved in explosions, motor vehicle accidents, or jumping from a burning building).

Remove smoldering clothing (if nonadherent to skin).

Control bleeding.

Remove restrictive clothing and jewelry.

Make brief neurologic exam (include level of consciousness, pupils, motor and sensory function).

Splint fractures.

Initiate an intravenous line of Ringer's lactate (if the burn is less than 30% of body surface area, run at a rate of 3 to 4 ml/lb/hr; if burn is greater than 30% body surface area, run at rate of 6 to 8 ml/lb/hr). Later, use Baxter's formula.

Control pain (if burn is not associated with trauma, administer morphine sulfate or meperidine hydrochloride intravenously).

Estimate extent of burn.

Cover burned area with clean, dry, sterile (if possible) sheet. Do not wrap large burns in saline-soaked dressings because cool dressings will reduce body temperature.

Check vital signs (do not avoid taking blood pressure because the limb is burned).

Administer humidified oxygen at 100% concentration.

Pay strict attention to airway and suctioning.

In the emergency department

Continue fluid resuscitation.

Repeat vital signs every 15 minutes.

Obtain arterial blood gases.

Endotracheal intubation if PO_2 is less than 50 mm Hg.

Consider analgesia.

Use nasogastric tube to decompress stomach; avoid possible aspiration of gastric contents.

Have the patient assume a comfortable position.

Obtain chest x-ray film.

Start additional IV lines.

Insert Foley catheter; send urine to lab to check for myoglobulinuria and/or hemoglobinuria.

Initiate hourly urine measurements.

Start arterial line if blood pressure is difficult to obtain.

Lab: Complete blood count, prothrombin time, electrolytes, calcium, magnesium, blood urea nitrogen, creatinine, glucose, bilirubin, phosphorus, alkaline phosphatase, total protein, carboxyhemoglobin, and toxicology screen, if indicated

Get type and cross-match if indicated.

Monitor cardiac rhythm.

Take 12-lead ECG.

Weigh.

Consider burn unit admission or referral to burn center.

Airway Management

Inhalation injuries occur frequently with burn injuries. They may occur in three phases. Most inhalation injuries are a combination of these types:

Carbon monoxide toxicity

Upper airway obstruction

Injury of lower airway and lung parenchyma by chemicals

Because of the potential for obstructive edema, establish a patent airway.

It may be necessary to initiate a nasopharyngeal or endotracheal tube.

If there is airway obstruction, it may be necessary to perform emergency cricothyrotomy.

Sometimes pulmonary damage is not evident in the early prehospital and emergency department phases.

Always anticipate pulmonary complications and have equipment readily available so that intervention can take place readily and rapidly.

When a patient gives a history of exposure to smoke or other toxic products of combustion, assume and anticipate pulmonary complications and pulmonary damage until it is proven otherwise.

■ **SIGNS AND SYMPTOMS OF SMOKE INHALATION**

Soot in the nostrils

Singed nasal or facial hair

Carbonaceous sputum

Hoarse voice

Drooling

Stridor

Cough

Burns around mouth

■ **THERAPEUTIC INTERVENTIONS**

Oxygen at high flow by mask or nasopharyngeal or endotracheal tube

Obtain a carboxyhemoglobin level; this may help to predict pulmonary complications and allow for preventive therapeutic interventions early in the course of treatment.

Pain Management

Remember *not* to cool the entire burn area all at once if extensive surface area is burned; doing so may cause severe hypothermia.

If an analgesic is given, administer it through the IV route to ensure uniform, timely distribution throughout the body. The most common analgesic agent administered is morphine sulfate, given in 2 to 4 mg increments slowly and titrated to achieve the desired analgesic effect. Pay close attention to respiratory status; morphine sulfate may cause respiratory depression.

An alternative to morphine sulfate administration is nitrous oxide gas, which the patient can self-administer.

IV Fluid Replacement

Problems with fluid and electrolyte balances are directly proportional to the extent of the burn injury.

Place a Foley catheter and carefully measure hourly urine output.

Calculate fluid replacement in accordance with the extent of the burn, using one of the major burn formulas as a guideline.

Start fluid replacement therapy from time of injury, not from time of arrival to hospital or initiation of IV.

The Baxter (Parkland) formula

First 24 hours—give Ringer's lactate 4ml/kg of body weight multiplied by the percentage of burned BSA:

Give half the calculated amount in the first 8 hours.

Give the remaining half over the next 16 hours.

Second 24 hours—give D_5W to maintain serum sodium at less than 140 mEq/L.

Give potassium supplement to maintain normal serum potassium level.

Give plasma or plasma substitute to maintain adequate circulating volume.

The modified Brooke formula

First 24 hours—give 2 ml/kg of body weight multiplied by the percentage of burned BSA.

Give half of the calculated amount in the first 8 hours.

Give the other half over the next 16 hours.

Second 24 hours—D_5 and NS or NS to maintain adequate urine output.

Give colloids—0.3 ml/kg of body weight multiplied by the percentage of burned BSA.

Blood and blood products are not given in the initial phases of the burn injury unless the patient is hypovolemic from associated trauma.

Fluid amounts may be adjusted in accordance with pulse, blood pressure, urine output, urine glucose, level of consciousness, and the presence of nausea and vomiting or a paralytic ileus.

Standard fluid guidelines are not used when an electrical injury has occurred. Ringer's lactate should be administered at a rate of 1 to 2 L/hr until the patient demonstrates that he or she is being adequately resuscitated. This is evidenced by a urine output two to three times normal (so that myoglobin can be excreted rapidly). Urine output should be between 75 and 100 cc/hour.

Escharotomy

Escharotomy is performed if circumferential burns are constricting the chest wall, causing respiratory compromise or constriction of arteries and venous structures of the extremities and impairing circulation. The most common sites for escharotomies are:

Fingers	Chest
Hands	Legs
Arms	Toes

These may be performed in the early phases of emergency department care if there is a threat to life or limb from the impairment. Escharotomy is done by simply cutting through all the layers of the skin with a sterile scalpel and blade, allowing for separation of the tissue and for circulation to be reestablished. Incisions are made in the areas shown in Figure 30-3.

Special Management of Specific Burns

Chemical burns

Chemical burns occur when the patient comes in direct contact with a caustic chemical agents such as an acid or alkali substances. Alkalis usually cause a more serious burn.

All chemical burns should be flushed copiously. Chemical burns need to be irrigated with water or normal saline for 30 to 60 minutes. All clothing and jewelry should be removed. Powdered chemicals should be brushed from the skin before irrigation. Consult a poison control center should you encounter any unusual or unfamiliar chemical. Neutralizing agents are contraindicated because the chemical reaction may produce more heat. Resultant burns should be treated as thermal burns.

If there are chemical burns of the eye, irrigate the eyes with copious amounts of normal saline solution or water for at least 20 to 30 minutes. Immediately after irrigation, but before fluorescein staining and slit-lamp examination, obtain results of visual acuity examination. Chemical burns of the eyes usually require ophthalmologic consultation.

Electrical burns

Sometimes an electrical burn may appear very minor because of the lack of ability to visualize the damage. Entrance and exit sites may be small, but destruction of underlying tissue may be extensive. This destruction is caused by the intense heat that results from the passage of electrical current through the tissues. The direction and the extent of electrical burns may not be evident for 7 to 10 days.

A common complication of an electrical burn injury is ventricular fibrillation caused by the passage of electrical current through the myocardium. If ventricular fibrillation occurs, initiate cardiopulmonary resuscitation immediately and accomplish defibrillation as soon as possible. In this instance, prolonged resuscitation efforts are often successful.

Other important considerations in management of electrical burn victims include:

Avoid direct contact with the victim.

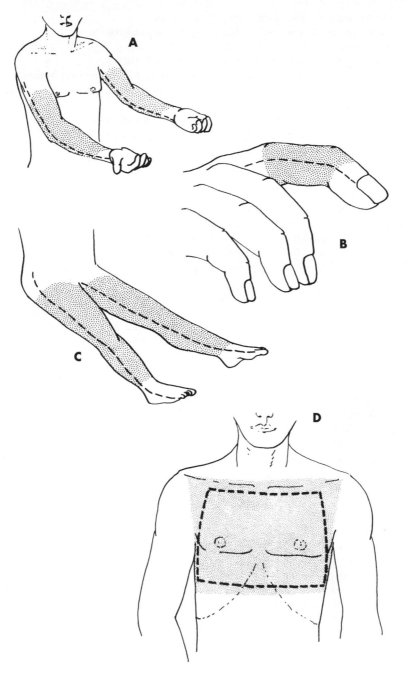

FIGURE 30-3. Proper sites for escharotomy. **A,** Arms. **B,** Fingers. **C,** Legs. **D,** Anterior thorax.

Remove the victim (carefully) from the source of the current.

Use a nonconductive object to remove the source of the electrical current *or*

Turn off the electrical current.

Initiate ABCs immediately if patient has no pulse and is not breathing.

Check for concurrent trauma and apply appropriate life-saving therapeutic intervention.

Notify the receiving hospital as soon as possible, because they may have to make arrangements for:

    A burn-unit bed *or*

    Transfer of a patient to a burn center once the patient is stabilized

An ECG is indicated if the current appears to have passed through the chest. Hospital admission is essential for electrical burn victims who have demonstrated:

Major burn injury

Loss of consciousness

Cardiac dysrhythmias

Radiation burns

Radiation burns are usually caused by overexposure to the sun. Sunburn cases are typically first degree and sometimes second-degree burns. The most comforting measure for this patient is the application of cool, moist compresses. If fever and chills are present, administer antipyretic agents such as aspirin or acetaminophen.

Tar burns

Tar burns usually result from roofing tar or asphalt and usually involve the face, head, neck, hands, and arms. Cooling should be initiated immediately. No attempts should be made to peel off the tar. Instead, it should be softened and loosened with mineral oil, vaseline, or a solvent made especially for this purpose. The resultant burns should be treated as thermal burns.

Friction burns

Friction burns are also known as "brush burns," "floor burns," and "road burns." This type of burn is caused by heat produced by friction. Friction burns are frequently seen in athletes who fall on gymnasium floors, tennis courts, or artificial-surface football fields or running tracks, and in motorcycle riders not wearing protective clothing who are involved in accidents.

Remove foreign bodies or debris (cinders, dirt particles, and so forth). This often requires administration of a topical local anesthetic or nitrous oxide gas.

Scrub the wound with a surgical soap solution and a soft brush.

Ensure that all particles are removed to avoid permanent scarring known as tattooing.

SUGGESTED READINGS

Edlich RF: Thermal burns. In Rosen et al, editor: *Emergency medicine*, ed 4, St Louis, 1998, Mosby.

Froman P: Wound care—burns. In Hamilton G, editor: *Presenting signs and symptoms in the emergency department: evaluation and treatment,* Baltimore, 1993, Williams & Wilkins.

Meyer A, Salber P: Burns and smoke inhalation. In Saunders C, Ho M, editors: *Current emergency diagnosis and treatment,* ed 4, Norwalk, Conn, 1992, Appleton & Lange.

Newbury L, Emergency Nurses Association: *Sheehy's emergency nursing*, St Louis, 1998, Mosby.

Special Populations

Sexual Assault

Patricia M. Speck

Sexual assault is a felony crime that two thirds of all victims will not report. Females are victimized most often, and two thirds of all victims know their assailant.

During assault: Victims may fear for their lives.

After the assault: Victims may feel disbelief, followed by a period of confusion.

Feelings of guilt, self-blame, shame and embarrassment, and fear with extreme vulnerability and helplessness are common. Victims may experience an overall sense of personal violation.

Emergency departments are mandated by federal law to have policies and procedures in place for providing care to victims of sexual assault. The primary focus of emergency department staff members is:

1. to minimize the physical and psychological trauma to the victim
2. to maximize the probability of the collection and preservation of physical evidence (blood, sperm, saliva, hair, clothing, debris, documentation, and so forth) for use in the criminal justice system

Under many state laws, when the victim discloses a rape or sexual assault, emergency department staff members will be required to report the crime. Reporting without the patient's permission is controversial, given the stigma of rape. Laws may require reporting sexual assault but allow the adult victim to decide about giving information or evidence to the police. Adult victims have many valid reasons for not wanting to participate in the criminal justice process. Their wishes should be respected. In all states the child victim or parents are not given a choice about participating in investigations that involve child abuse or child sexual assault. Emergency department staff members do not decide whether any patient is telling the truth or has been a victim of rape or sexual assault. Their responsibility is to *first* provide for the medical health and safety of the patient while providing emotional support and privacy. After the health and safety of the patient are ensured, then staff members become responsible for collecting or preserving evidence for law enforcement and making referrals to appropriate and available community agencies.

TRIAGE

Medically Nonurgent Patient

Most victims of sexual assault do not require urgent or emergent medical care in the emergency department. When appropriate the patient and any family or friends should be ushered to a private, quiet, and comfortable area away from the routine of the emergency department. A nursing assessment should occur at that time (see *Nursing Assessment*). Registration and consent for medical treatment can take place in this quiet, private environment, and the nurse can initiate the emergency department's sexual assault procedure to call law enforcement. The nurse may call the Sexual Assault Nurse Examiner (SANE) and call law enforcement, if appropriate. Every attempt should be made by the emergency department nurse to ensure that the patient is not left alone. A designated professional support person (that is, the SANE, a social worker, a rape crisis counselor, or an advocate) "on call" can provide critical psychologic intervention.

SANE programs provide crisis intervention, evidence collection, physical evaluation, health information and recommendations, medical and psychological referral, and prophylactic medications. A rape crisis counselor or advocate can collaborate with the SANE and emergency department personnel in explaining procedures and providing issue-oriented counseling for the patient, family members, and significant others. In addition, the "on-call" professional support person can provide information regarding the criminal justice process. The professional support person can also provide community referrals and information regarding victim compensation.

When the evidentiary examination will occur in the hospital, the RN taking the initial history should be the nurse who remains with the patient either throughout the entire emergency department visit or until the SANE arrives. When the evidentiary examination will occur in an area outside the emergency department or in a community-based SANE program, the emergency department RN should remain with the patient either until law enforcement arrives to transport the patient or the patient is medically discharged from the emergency department. When there is no SANE program available, emergency department personnel should carefully document care procedures to help explain the reason evidence is lacking.

Medically Urgent/Emergent Patient

For the 1% to 3% of all sexually assaulted patients who are medically urgent or emergent, consideration of the effect on the forensic evidence should accompany every procedure. The emergency department procedure for reporting sexual assault should be initiated as soon as possible.

NURSING ASSESSMENT

Nursing assessment for rape and sexual assault victims should occur as follows:
- Assess for serious trauma, particularly if the history indicates possible neck injuries, blunt trauma, choking, or that drugs or objects were used during the assault. Serious trauma should always be treated before or during evidence collection. With minor injuries, treatment can usually wait until after the evidence collection process.
- Assess the general physical appearance of the patient for evidence of force.
- Assess the general emotional state for evidence of acute rape trauma syndrome.
- Obtain a complete set of vital signs.
- Assess immunization status, particularly tetanus and hepatitis B.
- Assess medical history including the following:
  Age of first menarche or menopause
  Tanner stage (children only)
  Gravity/parity and whether currently pregnant
  Allergy to medication
  Hospitalization history
  Mental Health history
  Medical history
  Surgical history
  Present illness, if any
  Present medications (that is, contraceptives, over-the-counter medications, prescribed medications)

BASIC PRINCIPLES OF RAPE AND SEXUAL ASSAULT EVIDENCE COLLECTION

The following lists basic principles of rape and assault evidence collection:
- To maintain the chain of evidence, all evidence collected from a victim will remain with the collector or be locked in a secure area until released to law enforcement.
- All items collected or released by any emergency department professional involved in the care of a sexual assault victim must be documented in the medical chart.
- All evidence collected should be placed and sealed in containers provided in the rape kit, which is packaged under FDA regulations.

- All containers of evidence should be labeled with the following information:
  the chart number assigned by the hospital emergency department
  the law enforcement case number
  the patient's full name
  the patient's birth date
  the date and time of the rape
  the date and time of evidence collection
  the examiner's name and credentials
  a description and condition of the evidence (for example, underpants—light blue nylon, size 8, stained in crotch, elastic pulled from posterior waist area)
- All objects, for example, knives, bullets, or clothing (that is, shirts, pants, underwear) that are removed, must be placed by the collector in individual paper collection devices, sealed, and labeled as described above.
- Whenever possible, any clothing removed should be unbuttoned and/or unzipped and removed; if clothes must be cut off, do not cut through any stains, holes, tears, or buttonholes.
- When moisture is needed to collect biologic samples, do not saturate the cotton tip. Rather, slightly moisten the cotton-tipped swab. Moisture dilutes biologic samples, thereby reducing the chance of detecting scant DNA when present. Then the samples should be dried and placed in a separate, labeled envelope obtained from the rape kit.
- All physical evidence of the crime collected from the victim should be air dried, folded without shaking (taking care not to cross-contaminate the surfaces), and then placed by the collector in individual paper collection devices, sealed, and labeled as described above.
- The collector should obtain a sample of evidence from a site before any activity or procedure that will result in washing away biologic evidence of the crime (that is, catheter insertion, voiding, eating, smoking, drinking). Then the samples should be dried and placed in a separate, labeled envelope obtained from the rape kit.
- After drying, all cotton-tipped applicators are placed bulb first in a separate, labeled envelope obtained from the rape kit and then properly sealed.
- Do *not* place any moist evidence in plastic or glass containers. Heat and moisture promote growth of organisms and mold that destroy evidence.

SEXUAL ASSAULT EVIDENCE COLLECTION: OTHER CONSIDERATIONS

Who

The collection of the physical evidence may be completed by a SANE, advanced practice nurse or nurse, or physician in accordance with the emergency department policy and procedure.

Consent

Permission for medical treatment of sexual assault victims is covered by the routine emergency department permission signed on entering an emergency department. An additional, written informed consent or informed refusal from the adult client or guardian for the evidentiary examination must also be explained and obtained. This permission should also contain a clause consenting to the release of physical evidence to law enforcement. This physical evidence includes samples, clothing or objects, and written documentation.

What

Rape kits made specifically for sexual assault or abuse evidence collection packaged under FDA regulations are available and should be used for this procedure. Hospital laboratories generally do not have procedures that guarantee the chain of evidence for specimens.

When

All supplies should be gathered or available in the examination room *before* the start of evidence collection. The kit should be opened *after* the examiner is certain that the evidence collection process can be continued without interruption until the kit is resealed. If the examiner leaves the room, it is considered an abandonment of the process of evidence collection and is a breach in the chain of evidence.

How

Patients who have survived a sexual assault deserve to have professional nursing care, including retaining some control over treatment. Introduction to the nurse and the SANE role (if SANE program is available in your community), explanation about the process of evidence collection, or education about health risks may answer questions for the patient before the patient thinks about them. Answering patient concerns as they arise and using statements such as "I'm sorry this happened to you," can also comfort the patient during this process. Staff members who feel uncomfortable performing these professional nursing skills should delegate the care of victims.

EVIDENCE

Forensic Interview

Verbal history of the crime

"Tell me what happened to you tonight" is an example of an open-ended statement that can be used to begin the forensic interview. Closed questions that require answers of "yes" or "no" are discouraged but may be used to clarify unclear statements given by the patient. "Did Billy rape you tonight?" is an example of a closed question.

Information that should be gathered includes the following:
- Date and time of the assault
  History of assault beginning with:
  1. method of approach by assailant
  2. if the assailant is known or unknown to the victim
  3. number of assailants
  4. race and gender of assailant(s)
  5. weapon use (for example, blunt objects, sharp objects, gun, knives)
  6. type of force used (for example, physical force, verbal threats, implied weapon or threat)
  7. assault details (for example, oral, vaginal, and/or anal penetration, kissing, touching, or exposure)
  8. penetrating object (for example, finger, penis, tongue, object)
  9. oral contact by assailant and where
  10. erection and/or ejaculation by assailant
  11. condom or lubricant use
  12. any patient activities after assault that may have affected retrieval of evidence (for example, brush teeth, bathe, vomit, change clothes, douche, defecate, urinate, eat, drink, smoke)
- During the forensic interview, key answers should be documented and quoted whenever possible.
- After the forensic interview, the examiner should explain the evidence collection process *before* each procedure begins and as needed throughout the evidence collection process.

Photography

The following lists considerations when photographing forensic evidence:
- The 35-mm camera is preferred in forensic photography.

- At the beginning of the 35-mm film roll, document the identifying information about the case, indicating that it is the beginning of the roll.
- Photograph the appearance of the patient before the evidence collection process begins.
- Color and height references should be included in the photographs of the patient, and the background of the photograph should be uncluttered.
- Any visible injury or evidence of force should be serially photographed.
- At the end of the 35-mm film roll, document the identifying information about the case indicating that this is the end of the case photographs.
- Digital videography with photographic print capability is an acceptable alternative to using a 35-mm camera. Follow the guidelines for forensic photography as previously indicated.
- Although not recommended in forensic photography, if Polaroid is the only camera available, or if there are no provisions for chain of evidence when film is developed, follow the guidelines for forensic photography as previously indicated.

Clothing collection

The purpose of clothing collection is to demonstrate force (that is, tears, cuts) or to evaluate for the presence of biologic evidence (for example, stains, debris). Semen places the offender with the victim; debris places the victim at a crime scene. It is difficult to prevent cross-contamination during disrobing, but the following collection techniques may help:
- Place a large clean paper sheet as a barrier on the floor.
- Place a second clean paper sheet on top of the barrier. A sheet may be packaged in the kit for this purpose.
- Have the patient stand in the center of the sheet and undress slowly, one item at a time.
- Place the clothing on the sheet or a clean drying rack and allow the clothing to dry, if moist.
- If you are concerned about cross-contamination between different stains on the clothing, fold the sheet so that the sheet covers the entire piece of clothing. If the item is too large, place another clean paper sheet over the item. Then fold the paper and clothing together to avoid cross-contamination between different sections of the same piece of clothing. Place each piece of folded clothing in a separate, labeled paper bag.
- If clothing has evidence of force (for example, ripped clothing), cross-contamination is not an issue; therefore, place each folded piece in a separate, labeled paper bag.
- Seal the bags with evidence tape. Sign the evidence tape noting the date and time.
- Repeat this process for each piece of clothing secured from the victim as evidence.
- When the victim steps off the paper sheet, brush any debris to the center of the second clean paper sheet. Fold the paper in half, then in thirds, then in quarters and place the debris in the envelope labeled "miscellaneous" that is provided. Seal the envelopes as instructed in the kit. Discard the barrier sheet.

Other clothing collection tips include the following:
- Clothing collection from the rape victim is rarely so detailed as when the victim's clothing has evidence of stains, cuts, debris, or force.
- Underpants put on by the victim after the rape may be the only evidence needed to prove the offender was present at the crime scene.
- In this case, underpants can be removed, dried, folded, placed in the labeled envelope and sealed. Cross-contamination is not an issue with this type of evidence.
- Minimize shaking or disturbing the clothing because valuable trace evidence may be lost.
- Do not use staples to hold items together because the staples may pose a biohazard risk for persons handling the evidence.

Wood's lamp or alternate light source screening

When available, Wood's lamps or alternate light sources (for example, infrared, ultraviolet) are used to screen the body and clothing for biological stains and injury. Photography using 35-mm film or digital videography of the areas of illumination should be documented when possible.

Foreign material collection

Debris collection devices provided in the kit should be used when collecting leaves, dirt, rocks, hair, and so on. When these devices are absent, brush the debris to the center of a clean paper sheet. Fold the paper in half, then in thirds, then in quarters and place the debris in the envelope labeled "miscellaneous" that is provided. Seal the envelope as instructed in the kit.

Biologic Evidence Collection

Blood, saliva, or semen identified outside the vaginal, oral, or anal areas should be collected either by using a two-step, cotton-tip swab method or a general swab on the identified area as follows:

- In the first method, the cotton tip is slightly moistened with distilled water, and the identified area is lightly swabbed. The second cotton-tip applicator is dry and used to lightly swab the moisture from the first applicator.
- In the second method, two cotton-tip applicators are slightly moistened with distilled water, and both are used to lightly swab the identified area.
- With each method, the specimen must be dried and placed in the envelope labeled "miscellaneous."
- Seal the envelopes as instructed in the kit.
- Check with the state's forensic laboratory to determine the preferred method of collection.

Fingernail collection

When the patient reports scratching the assailant, the examiner should attempt to collect samples from the fingernails. The following two methods are currently in use:

1. The examiner uses a plastic device to scrape under the tips of the nails.
   The examiner should avoid scraping the patient's skin under the nail.
   The plastic scrape and the debris collected is placed in a labeled envelope and sealed.
2. The second method requires cutting the exposed nail tip and placing the nail clipping in the labeled envelope or container.
   Consult with the state's forensic laboratory to determine the preferred method.

Examination for physical evidence

The physical examination should be conducted considering the forensic history of the crime and with an unbiased search for all physical evidence of the crime. The physical evaluation should include inspection of the entire body for subtle or overt injury, including abrasions, lacerations, bruising, or pattern injury. When the patient complains of tenderness or pain, the examiner should fully document the finding, including location, description of palpation, visibility of injury, and perception of the patient. Remember, the patient may not know the cause of every visible injury.

■ ORAL SPECIMEN COLLECTION

- Determine and document the patient's activities after the assault, that is, if the patient has rinsed the mouth, had anything to drink, or smoked.
- Ask if he/she has spit out the oral contents; if so, where. Collect the object, or advise the law enforcement officer of the same.
- Obtain slide, swabs, and oral swabs envelope from the rape kit.
- Using the two sterile swabs, swab the buccal area, posterior sublingual area, oral pharynx, and gum line.
- If the patient has dentures, swab the superior and anterior denture palate and crevices also.
- Using both swabs, prepare one slide.
- Air dry the smear and swabs before placing in envelopes.
- Place the swab in the labeled envelope and the smear in the labeled container provided.
- At this time, the patient can be offered a toothbrush, tooth paste, and mouthwash as a comfort measure.

■ NASAL EVIDENCE COLLECTION

Occasionally during an oral assault, the victim chokes or retches. Some victims may even vomit the ejaculate. The gastric reflux forces evidence into the nasal pharynx and this evidence may be collected using one of several methods.

1. If the patient is crying and has blown the contents into Kleenex, collect the Kleenex, dry, and place in an envelope labeled "miscellaneous".
2. Instruct the patient to blow his/her nose into a sterile 2 × 2. Dry and place in an envelope labeled "miscellaneous".
3. If no mucus is visible, sterile saline can be used to moisten the nasal passages and wash seminal products from these areas. Although distilled water may be preferred, the saline buffers the pain of the nose drops. Remember, this method may require considerable effort on the part of the victim.
4. Using distilled water and the two-swab method, cotton-tipped applicators can be used to swab the external nasal passages.

■ SALIVA STANDARD COLLECTION

The known saliva sample may be collected using one of several methods. Remember, eating, drinking, and smoking are discouraged 30 minutes before collection of the saliva standard.

1. One method uses a folded filter paper packaged in the kit. The half-circle on the filter paper is placed on the tongue and saturated with saliva with the mouth closed. The patient should be instructed not to bite the paper. This item is dried before being placed in the labeled envelope provided in the kit.
2. Another method uses cotton-tip applicators that are placed on the tongue and saturated by the patient. This item is dried before being placed in the labeled envelope provided in the kit.
3. A third requires the victim to spit into a sterile collection device packaged in the rape kit. The device should be sealed and contents refrigerated until transfer to the forensic laboratory.

■ BLOOD STANDARD EVIDENCE COLLECTION

The blood standard evidence collection is as follows:

- Collection tubes for the patient's blood standard are usually included in the rape kit.
- They may include one or a combination of the following: an EDTA lavender top, an ACD yellow top, or a silicone-coated red top.
- Each tube must be labeled with the following minimum information: the patient's name, law enforcement case number, hospital record number, date collected, and collector's name and credentials.
- Whole blood placed in rape kits must be packaged to avoid breakage, and must be refrigerated after collection.
- If unclaimed by law enforcement, the rape kit may be kept in a secured refrigerator.

    Check with the state's forensic laboratory for acceptable temperature ranges and time frames for storage. In some states the blood collected from the victim is immediately transferred to a sterile DNA filter-paper card provided in the kit.

- Procedures for transferring the victim's blood to the filter-paper card must be in place to prevent contamination of the DNA sample with extraneous or examiner DNA.
- After saturation of the filter-paper card, the sample is closed and dried.
- Next the DNA filter-paper card is put in the labeled envelope, which is then sealed.
- In states where rape kit storage is mandatory, and funds are scarce, or in states where the number of victims is large, procedures for whole blood transfer to the DNA filter-paper card at the time of collection reduce or eliminate the following:

1. likelihood of cross-contamination with other evidence if blood tubes break in transfer to the forensic laboratory
2. biohazard risk for personnel if the blood tubes break during transfer
3. costly storage in laboratory refrigerators or freezers mandatory for whole blood storage
4. problem of expiration dates on whole blood tubes

    Occasionally victims of rape may refuse blood collection because they fear needles or just do not want to do it when they are in the emergency department. Keep in mind that blood can be drawn from the victim at a later time.

■ BLOOD COLLECTION FOR MEDICAL SCREENING TESTS

Drug screening may be indicated if there is medical concern, if the victim may have been drugged, or if it is routine protocol. Some programs have found that alcohol levels are helpful in court (for example, if victims are impaired they are unable to consent to sexual relations). There is also the potential for damaging a case. With the patient's permission, proper counseling, and provision for follow-up counseling, baseline testing for hepatitis B, syphilis, or HIV can occur at the same time the blood standard is collected. There is controversy regarding any STD testing, given the potential for insurance repercussions and extensive attention to the victim's sexual history or lifestyle in court.

■ HEAD AND PUBIC HAIR EVIDENCE COLLECTION

Step 1

Assailant hair is presumed to be mingled with victim hair during the sexual assault. Whether collecting head or pubic hair, the towel provided in the kit is placed *under* the head or buttocks. The victim's hair is combed so that any loose hair or debris will fall onto the towel. If there is matting with blood, semen or feces, the hair and debris mat is cut and placed in the towel, and then the hair is combed again. The towel is folded with the debris and comb, placed in the envelope marked "Hair Combing," labeled, and placed in the kit.

Step 2

Fifteen to 50 hairs are cut close to the skin from several areas of the scalp and the pubic area. The hair is placed in a labeled envelope and sealed.

Most clinicians have discontinued plucking hairs unless and until it is needed for comparative analysis at a later date.

■ VAGINAL (AND VULVAR) SPECIMEN COLLECTION FROM ADULT ESTROGENIZED FEMALES

Collection of biological evidence from the adult female reproductive tract should be done as follows:

- Obtain the sterile cotton-tip applicators and slide from the kit, and place the items near the examination table and specimen dryer.
- Label the collection devices and containers with identifying information (see basic principles for labeling listed on p. 565).
- Inspect the external structures of the perineum for injury using magnification, that is, colposcope with halogen lighting.
- Using the methods described on p. 565, swab the vulvar area with cotton-tip applicators.
- Using a plastic speculum with illumination, gently insert and distend the vaginal vault inspecting for injury; do *not* use lubrication.
- Locate the cervix, and remove the cervical mucus with a sterile cotton swab; if the history dictates, dry and label properly, and then send this swab to the forensic laboratory for analysis.
- Place the cotton-tip applicators in the fluid pool located in the posterior fornix of the vagina and swab the entire surface of the vagina.
- Prepare the slide smear as directed by the forensic laboratory.
- Air dry all vulvar and vaginal swabs and slides in the specimen dryer, and place in the separate, labeled envelopes provided.

■ MEDICAL SCREENING FOR SEXUALLY TRANSMITTED DISEASES

During the vaginal examination, and with the patient's consent, collect cultures and other screening tests after evidence collection at the site is complete. These tests may include cultures or DNA probes for *N. gonorrhea* and *Chlamydia trachoma* or a wet mount to look for trichomonads, bacteria, blood or yeast. Any medical test that has the potential for tissue injury (for example, Pap smear) is discouraged at this time. When properly collected from adults, these tests are considered baseline medical testing. Positive cultures are generally not considered to be the result of the rape. Although screening is not recommended on asymptomatic children, positive STD results in children are reportable to the state's department of children's services.

■ ANAL SPECIMEN COLLECTION

Collect biological evidence from the anal area as follows:

- Obtain the sterile swabs and slide from the kit, and place the items near the examination table and specimen dryer.
- Label the collection devices and containers with identifying information (see basic principles for labeling listed on p. 565).
- Inspect the external structures of the anus for injury using magnification, that is, colposcope with halogen lighting.

- Inspect the internal structures of the anus for injury and dilation; if available, use an anoscope to inspect the internal structures of the distal rectal ampullae. Do *not* use lubrication.
- If an anoscope is used during inspection, air dry the swabs and send to forensic laboratory in the separate, labeled envelopes provided.
- Using the sterile cotton-tip applicators, swab the external anal area.
- Using the sterile cotton-tip applicators, gently swab the anal verge and distal rectal ampullae.
- Prepare the slide smear as directed by the forensic laboratory.
- Dry all anal swabs and slides, and place them in the separate, labeled envelopes provided.

■ PENILE SPECIMEN COLLECTION

In the event of an assault involving a male victim's penis, collection of biological evidence from the penile area is facilitated by following these steps:

- Obtain the sterile swabs and slide from the kit, and place the items near the examination table and specimen dryer.
- Label the collection devices and containers with identifying information (see basic principles for labeling listed on p. 565).
- Inspect the external structures of the penis for injury or disease using magnification, that is, colposcope with halogen lighting.
- Using the sterile cotton-tip applicators, thoroughly swab the penile shaft and glans area. If the assault included oral copulation of the male, also swab along the penile shaft hair line and scrotal sack for saliva.
- Prepare the slide smear as directed by the forensic laboratory.
- Dry all penile swabs and slides and place in the separate, labeled envelopes provided in the kit.

DOCUMENTATION

Rape and sexual assault documentation should include:

Subjective: The subjective portion of the history summarizes the chief complaint and quotes the patient's statements and the interviewer's questions directly whenever possible.

Objective: The objective portion is observed medical fact, that is, injury character and location. This portion may include drawings, photographs, and any medical laboratory test with the results of the test. Pregnancy tests should be performed to assess for existing pregnancy. Screening for STDs should be performed to assess for existing disease. When these tests are positive, treatment plans must be altered by the provider.

Assessment: The assessment should avoid legal terms, such as rape, sexual assault, or child abuse. Courts may actually prohibit the entry of documentation as evidence where foregone legal conclusions are documented on the medical or evidentiary record. In addition, if the legal outcome does not support the medical assessment of "rape" or "child abuse," the provider may be found liable for misdiagnosis or even malpractice. For the same reason, some prosecutors prefer that the word "patient" rather than "victim" be used.

Plan: The plan should include medical treatment and referral.

Medical Treatment

Medical treatment includes the following:

- Prophylaxis for disease and pregnancy is recommended after a screening procedure for contraindications.
- The CDC Guidelines (1998) recommend treating rape victims with:
  125 mg Cephtriaxone IM in a single dose plus 1g Azithromycin PO in a single dose or 100 mg Doxycycline PO BID × 7 days plus 2 gm Metronidazole PO in a single dose
- In addition, patients should be up to date or immunized with tetanus and hepatitis B.
- Emergency contraception is the "morning after" pill.
- The most common "morning after" pill (Ovral) is a combination estrogen and progesterone birth control pill and is most commonly prescribed "Take 2 now and 2 in 12 hours PO." The "morning after" pill is given within 72 hours of the rape to menstruating females of childbearing years who have no contraindication to its usage.

• Patients should be tested for pregnancy and negative results received before the patient takes the pregnancy interception medication.

Follow-up Recommendations

Consider the following when recommending follow-up care:
• After a rape, victims have historically been difficult to follow up for medical concerns and counseling.
• If the patient seeks care later, some may omit the rape history making it difficult for the provider to assess the health and well-being of the client.
• The emergency department or sexual assault nurse examiner is in the best position to offer comprehensive education, immediate support, and allay concerns over follow-up (for example, refer patients to anonymous HIV testing centers or free STD clinics).
• Follow-up information should include *written* instructions.
• The nursing instructions should:
   Teach STD and pregnancy risks following sexual assault.
   Teach signs and symptoms of infection and medication reactions.
   Advise no intercourse without condoms until all screening tests for STDs return negative.
   Teach perineal or other injury care.
   Refer to health care systems.
   Advise about community resources including rape crisis, court advocacy, or victim's compensation.
   Advise medical follow-up in 2 to 4 weeks to repeat STD assessment including *N. gonorrhea,* Chlamydia trachoma, and a wet mount for bacterial or parasitic infection. (This assessment may be deferred if the patient has received prophylactic antibiotic therapy and has no symptoms.)
   Advise medical follow-up in 3 months for repeat serological screening tests, including syphilis and HIV.
   Advise medical follow-up in 6 months for serological test for HIV.

SECURING AND TRANSFERRING THE EVIDENCE

When securing and transferring the evidence, be aware of the following:
• All packaged evidence should be kept in a separate and secure location that is temperature controlled.
• If whole blood is in the kit, keep the kit refrigerated in a separate and secure location until transfer.
• All evidence collected by the examiner can be transferred to the forensic laboratory by the investigating law enforcement officer or authorized agent of the jurisdiction.
• To maintain the chain of evidence, have all parties sign the evidence label; date and time the exchange; and copy the documentation for your record.

TESTIMONY

Remember the following points regarding testimony:
• Each person involved in the process of evidence collection after the complaint of a felony, such as rape, is subject to the court of jurisdiction where prosecution is a possibility.
• A fact witness is not an expert but may testify to items about which they have "personal knowledge."
• Personal knowledge is obtained by actual observation obtained while participating in or witnessing an event.
• Fact witnesses can be compelled to testify about matters personally observed.
• An expert witness is a qualified person who provides unbiased and neutral opinion.
• The expert's opinion is scientifically sound regarding the evidence or fact.
• The expert is qualified singularly by each court that considers experience, training, or education about the subject to which the expert's testimony relates.
• An expert cannot be compelled to testify about his/her opinion.

Other tips when called to give testimony are:
- Before testimony, actively prepare by meeting with the attorneys to discuss the facts of the case, review the written record, review your deposition, and educate the attorneys.
- During testimony, use correct terms, but explain these terms.
- Do not be pressured to answer any question. You have the right to respectfully address the judge, and, with the judge's permission, explain your answers.
- Do not show emotion or take questions personally.

SUGGESTED READINGS

Aiken MM, Speck PM: Confidentiality in cases of rape: a concept reconsidered, *J Clin Ethics* 2(1):63, 1991.

Aiken MM, Speck PM: Sexual assault and multiple trauma: a sexual assault nurse examiner (SANE) challenge, *J Emerg Nurs* 21(5):466, 1995.

Aiken MM, Burgess A, Hazelwood R: False rape allegations. In Hazelwood R, Burgess A: *Practical aspects of rape investigation: a multidisciplinary approach,* ed 2, Boca Raton, Fla, 1995, CRC Press.

Bureau of Justice Statistics, US Department of Justice: *Criminal victimization in the United States, 1994,* NCJ-162126, May 1997.

International Association of Forensic Nurses: *Sexual assault nurse examiner standards of practice,* 1996. (in press)

Ledray L: The sexual assault nurse clinician: a fifteen year experience in Minneapolis, *J Emerg Nurs* 18(3):217, 1992.

Ledray L: The sexual assault examination: overview and lessons learned in one program, *J Emerg Nurs* 18(3):223, 1992.

Ledray L: *SANE development and operation guide 1998,* Washington DC, 1998, Office for Crime Resource Center. (1-800-627-6872)

Ledray L: SANE programs, *J Emerg Nurs* 22:460-465, 1996.

Lipscomb GH et al: Male victims of rape, *JAMA* 287(22):3064, 1992.

Muram D et al: Adolescent victims of sexual assault, *J Adolesc Health* 17:372, 1995.

Office of Victims of Crime, US Department of Justice: *Sexual assault nurse examiner: SANE operations manual,* 1998 (in press).

Sexual assault: clinical issues, bimonthly feature, *J Emerg Nurs,* 1996-present.

Sexual assault and STD, *MMWR* 47(RR-1), January 23, 1998.

Simmelink K: Lessons learned from three elderly sexual assault survivors, *J Emerg Nurs* 22: 619-621, 1996.

Speck PM, MM Aiken: Memphis sexual assault resource center: 20 years of community nursing service, *The Tennessee Nurs* 58(2), 1995.

Speck PM: Memphis sexual assault resource center: consent for pregnancy prevention, *J Emerg Nurs* 22(3):253, 1996.

CHAPTER 32

Domestic Violence

Susan Mathias

In the United States, 8 to 12 million women are at risk for domestic abuse by their current or former intimate partners.[1] Battered women account for 1 in 4 women who attempt suicide, 1 in 4 women who are pregnant, and 1 in 10 women seeking care for any reason in the emergency department.[2] Domestic violence is the single largest cause of injury to women, more than motor vehicle accidents, muggings, and rapes combined.[3] Chronic medical and mental health conditions, minor and serious injuries, and death are results of domestic violence.[4]

Domestic violence is defined as a pattern of assaultive and coercive behaviors of an individual against their current or former intimate partner to achieve control over the victim.[4] Most circumstances involve women being abused by their male partners. However, violence against men by their female partners, and violence against one partner in same-gender relationships can also occur.[4,5]

Domestic violence can take many forms, such as intentional physical abuse, psychologic and emotional abuse, sexual abuse, and economic control.[4,5,6] Although only one type of abuse may be experienced, battered women have reported that all categories of abuse will occur over time if the situation remains unchanged.[6]

Physical abuse is usually repetitive, and increases in frequency and severity. Examples of physical abuse include pushing, shoving, slapping, kicking, choking, restraining, leaving the victim in a dangerous place, and refusing to help when sick or injured. Emotional abuse may occur either before physical abuse, or in conjunction with physical violence. Psychologic abuse is used to control by fear or terror. The victims are made to feel guilty, responsible, alone, powerless, and helpless. Examples of psychologic abuse include threats of harm, physical and social isolation, extreme jealousy, intimidation, humiliation, degradation, and economic deprivation.[4,5,6]

It is important to understand that domestic violence occurs in all socioeconomic, racial, religious, educational and age groups. There is no specific personality type, occupation, or sexual orientation profile for victims.[2,4] Most victims are not identified unless the health care provider directly and sensitively asks about the possibility of domestic abuse.

INDICATIONS OF DOMESTIC VIOLENCE

Victims of domestic violence present with a multitude of complaints ranging from direct trauma to physical and mental health symptoms related to the stress of abuse. Headaches, asthma, lupus, nonulcer dyspepsia, irritable bowel syndrome, dyspareunia, vague pelvic pain, preterm labor, chronic musculoskeletal pain, fatigue, anxiety, depression, post-traumatic stress disorder, insomnia, and hearing loss can all relate to injuries or stress associated with domestic violence.[1,4]

Indications of domestic violence include:[4,7]

1. The patient admits to past or present physical or emotional abuse as a victim or *witness*.
2. The patient denies physical abuse, but presents with unexplained bruises, whiplash injuries consistent with shaking, areas of erythema consistent with slap injuries, grab marks on arms or neck, lacerations, burns, scars, fractures or multiple injuries in various stages of healing, fractured mandible, or perforated tympanic membranes.

3. Common sites of injury in battering are areas hidden by clothing or hair (that is, face, head, chest, breasts, abdomen, and genitals). Accidental injuries usually involve the extremities, whereas domestic violence often involves both truncal and extremity injuries.
4. Extent or type of injury is inconsistent with the explanation offered by the patient.
5. There are multiple injuries or injuries at various stages of healing.
6. The woman is pregnant. Violence often begins with the first pregnancy and with injuries to the breasts or abdomen.
7. The patient presents evidence of sexual assault or forced sexual actions by her partner.
8. The patient is the mother of an abused child.
9. The partner (or suspected abuser) accompanies the patient, insists on staying close to the patient, and may try to answer all questions directed to her.
10. The patient indicates fear of returning home and concern for the safety of children.
11. Substantial delay exists between the time of injury and presentation for treatment. The patient may have been prevented from seeking medical attention earlier or may have had to wait for the batterer to leave.
12. The patient describes the alleged "accident" in a hesitant, embarrassed, or evasive manner, or avoids eye contact.
13. The patient has "psychosomatic" complaints such as panic attacks, anxiety, choking sensation, or depression.
14. Complaints of chronic pain (back or pelvic pain) with no substantiating physical evidence often signify fear of impending or actual physical abuse.
15. Psychiatric, alcohol, or drug abuse history in the patient or partner; for example, eating disorder, self-mutilation.
16. History of suicide attempts or suicidal ideation. Battering accounts for one in every four suicide attempts by all women and half of all suicide attempts by black women.
17. Review of medical records reveals repeated use of emergency department or other medical and/or social services. Medical history reveals many "accidents" or remarks by nurse or physician indicating that previous injuries were of suspicious origin, or frequent visits with vague complaints.

ASSESSMENT AND INTERVENTION

The Emergency Nurses Association recommends the development of routine protocols and procedures for assessment and identification of domestic violence.[8] Many battered women will acknowledge abuse if questioned in a nonhumiliating manner and safe environment. If not asked directly, however, many women are hesitant to bring up the subject.[4]

Intervention goals for victims include: 1) proper medical care for the presenting complaint or injury, 2) emotional support, 3) establishment of a safety plan and available options, 4) legal protection including proper documentation, and 5) information on support services and community resources.[4]

It is imperative to provide a quiet, safe, private environment to assess the victim. The patient should be interviewed privately, not in the presence of family members or other accompanying individuals. Have the patient undress completely so that any hidden injuries will be exposed. Assess mental and emotional status also (including substance abuse, suicidal ideations, or homicidal ideations).

It is important to understand the psychologic effect of being battered. The victim usually is made to feel ignorant and worthless by the abuser. She may have been repeatedly told that no one cares or wants to hear, and that if she reveals the abuse, more violence will follow. Therefore, it can be extremely difficult for victims to take that first step. Breaking through that barrier of silence and denial begins the process of effective healing (physically and psychologically).

Take a careful medical/physical history.

Ask nonthreatening questions:
1. You seem frightened of your partner. Has he ever hurt you?
2. Sometimes patients tell me they have been hurt by someone close to them. Could this be happening to you?

3. Does your partner consistently control your actions or put you down?

4. Your partner seems very concerned and anxious. Was he responsible for your injuries?

5. I noticed you have a number of bruises. Could you tell me how they happened? Did someone hit you?[7]

The acronym SAFE will help recall questions to ask in a nonjudgmental way. Here are some examples of questions:

Stress/Safety: What stress do you experience in your relationships? Do you feel safe in your relationship/marriage? Should I be concerned for your safety?

Afraid/Abused: Are there situations in your relationships where you have felt afraid? Has your partner ever threatened or abused you or your children? Have you been physically hurt or threatened by your partner? People in relationships/marriages often fight. What happens when you and your partner disagree?

Friends/Family: Are your friends aware that you have been hurt? Do your parents or siblings know about the abuse? Do you think you could tell them and do you think they would be able to give you support? (Assess the degree of social isolation.)

Emergency Plan: Do you have a safe place to go and the resources you (and your children) need in an emergency? If you are in danger now, would you like help in locating a shelter? Would you like to talk with a social worker/counselor/me to develop an emergency plan?[9]

It is *very* important to assess the patient's safety to help reduce the danger she might face after discharge. Let the patient know that domestic violence is against the law and that she can choose to make a police report. She can also get a temporary restraining order.

Questions to ask:

1. Where is the abuser now?
2. Does he know that you are here?
3. Has the abuser ever used or threatened to use weapons?
4. Are weapons available to the abuser?
5. Has the abuser been drinking or taking drugs?
6. Has the abuse been increasing in severity and/or frequency?
7. Do you have children?
8. Are they safe now?
9. Are they being abused? (Refer to your child abuse protocol.)
10. Does the abuser verbally threaten you?
11. Has the abuser threatened your friends or relatives?
12. Has the abuser threatened to commit suicide if you leave?

Explain to the patient the physical and emotional sequelae of chronic battering.

Stress the importance of follow-up for medical, legal, and social support.

Emphasize to the patient that she *can* break the cycle of violence.[10]

ADVOCACY/SUPPORT SERVICES

The role of the advocate is an important one. Advocates receive special training and are usually volunteers. Their role is to be available to help and support the patient when needed, from the initial visit in the emergency department through the critical days or months ahead.

The advocate's role is to offer the victim opportunities to explore the various options available (for example, crisis intervention, safe home network, and legal advocacy). Advocates make no judgments and work with the victim in *support* of choices she makes, regardless of whether the advocate agrees with the choice. There are many times when the victim/patient actually returns home to an unsafe and potentially violent environment. Victims are frequently not prepared to separate from violent partners for a variety of complex, psychosocial reasons (that is, low self-esteem, guilt, fear, loneliness, lack of support systems, lack of money, and so forth). It is the role of the advocate to provide *unconditional* support so that the victim can feel that she is no longer alone.

When someone presents to the emergency department as a victim of domestic violence, local women's advocacy/support services should be notified to initiate contact and support while the patient is in the emergency department. Know your area's hotline numbers for abused women/children. Often social services will be contacted to assist the patient through the various programs/options available to her.

KNOW YOUR LEGAL OBLIGATIONS

It is important to know the law in the state in which you live regarding the reporting of domestic violence injuries:

1. Do you report life-threatening injuries (that is, gunshot wounds, strangulation, and so forth)?
2. Do you report if the patient has been drinking or has a history of alcohol or drug abuse?

Every state has some legislation that offers protection to domestic violence victims. Be aware of state laws and services for abuse victims in your area.[1]

CHARTING

I. Accurate and concise documentation is essential for future medical and legal assessments. Clearly document:
   A. 1. Time, date, place, and witnesses to assault/"accident"
      2. Name, badge number, and telephone number of law enforcement officer accompanying the patient
      3. Assessment of the patient's safety
   B. Avoid long descriptions and quotes that deviate from the medical problem (for example, "He was angry at me because I let the kids go to the movies."). This type of information is inadmissible in court and could be counterproductive if inconsistent with court testimony.
   C. If the patient states abuse as the cause of injury, prepare patient's explanation by writing: "Patient states . . . ." This protects the patient and yourself since you cannot be held liable for recording a patient's statement or the medical facts of your expert medical opinion. For example you would record, "Patient states she was hit in the face by her husband's fist."
II. Avoid subjective data that might be used against the patient (for example, "It was my fault he hit me because I didn't have the kids in bed on time.").
III. If patient denies being assaulted, write, "The patient's explanation of injuries is inconsistent with physical finding" or "injuries are suggestive of battering."
IV. Record size, pattern, estimated age, description, and location of all injuries.
   A. Use body injury map to locate injuries.
   B. Be specific, for example, "multiple contusions and lacerations" will not convey a clear picture to a judge or jury, but "contusions and lacerations of the throat" will back up allegations of attempted strangling. Record nonbodily evidence of abuse, such as torn clothing and jewelry (Domestic Violence protocol, Dartmouth-Hitchcock Memorial Hospital).[7]
   C. Use color photographs whenever possible. Take at least two pictures of major trauma areas. Photograph the same injury from different angles. Include pictures of full body, midrange, and close ups, if possible.[1]

REFERENCES

1. American Medical Association: *Diagnostic and treatment guidelines on domestic violence,* Chicago 1994, American Medical Association.
2. American Medical Association Council on Scientific Affairs: Violence against women: relevance for medical practitioners, *JAMA* 267, 1992.
3. *National women's health report* 13(4), Fall 1991.
4. Warshaw C, Ganley AL: *Improving the health care response to domestic violence: a resource manual for health care providers,* ed 2, New York, March 1996, The Family Violence Prevention Fund and Pennsylvania Coalition Against Domestic Violence.

5. Center on Crime, Communities, and Culture: *Pathfinder on domestic violence in the United States,* New York, 1997, The Center on Crime, Communities, and Culture of the Open Society Institute.

6. Varvaro FF, Cotman PG: *Domestic violence: a focus on the emergency room care of abused women,* Pittsburgh, 1986, Women's Center and Shelter of Greater Pittsburgh.

7. Krasnoff M. *Dartmouth-Hitchcock domestic violence protocol,* Lebanon NH: 1993 Dartmouth-Hitchcock Medical Center Publication, May 1993.

8. Emergency Nurses Association, position statement, 1997.

9. Ashur ML: Asking about domestic violence SAFE questions, *JAMA* 269(18):2367, 1993. (letter)

10. Campbell JC, Sheridan DJ: Emergency nursing interventions with battered women, *Clinic Articles* 15(1):12, 1989.

SUGGESTED READINGS

Berlinger JS: "Why don't you just leave him?" *Nurs 98* 28(4):35-40, 1998.

Campbell JC et al: Correlates of battering during pregnancy, *Res Nurs Health* 15:219, 1992.

Ganley AL: Understanding domestic violence. In Lee D, Durborow N, Salber PR, editors: *Improving the health care response to domestic violence: a resource manual for health care providers,* San Francisco, 1995, The Family Violence Prevention Fund.

Miller TR, Cohen MA, Wiersema B: *Crime in the United States: victim costs and consequences* (final report to the National Institutes of Justice), Washington, D.C., 1995, The Urban Institute and The National Public Services Research Institute.

Salber PR, Taliaferro E: Domestic violence. In Rosen et al: *Emergency medicine,* ed 4, St Louis, 1998, Mosby.

Stark E, Flitcraft A: Killing the beast within: women battering and female suicidality, *Int J Health Sci* 25(1):43, 1995.

Obstetric and Gynecologic Emergencies

Marybeth Murphy

Patients with obstetric and gynecologic emergencies are frequent visitors to the emergency department. There are many varieties of OB/GYN emergencies; some of the more common ones are referenced in this chapter. For additional information, the reader is referred to one of the many OB/GYN reference texts listed at the end of this chapter.

CHILDBIRTH

■ **MEDICAL CONSIDERATIONS**
The Consolidated Omnibus Reconciliation Budget Act (COBRA) of 1989 was inspired by an "inappropriate" obstetric transfer. COBRA identifies women in labor as having a condition too unstable for transfer.

Although usually one of the most natural occurrences on earth, the imminent birth of a baby can frighten the best of us. The most important thing to remember is to remain calm and organized.

■ **DEFINITIONS**
labor   The process by which the fetus, placenta, and membranes are expelled from the uterus. This usually occurs 40 weeks after conception.
gravida   The number of pregnancies, including the present.
para   The number of pregnancies that have gone to at least 20 weeks of gestation, regardless of whether the infant was dead or alive at birth.
primigravida   Pregnant for the first time.
nullipara   Woman who has not carried a pregnancy to viability.
primipara   Woman who has carried one pregnancy to viability.
multipara   Woman who has carried more than one pregnancy to viability.

■ **EXAMPLES**
Gravida 3, Para 1   Woman in her third pregnancy; she has delivered one viable child.
Gravida 4, Para 0   Woman in her fourth pregnancy; she has carried none of them to viability.
Gravida 2, Para 2   Woman in her second pregnancy; she has delivered two viable children (twins).

COMPLICATIONS OF PREGNANCY

Bleeding in Pregnancy

Placenta previa

Placenta previa is defined as implantation of the placenta in the lower uterine segment in advance of the fetal presenting part. The previa may be complete or partial and is further distinguished in reference to the cervical dilation before the onset of labor. All forms are potentially associated with life-threatening hemorrhage.

■ **SIGNS AND SYMPTOMS**
Sudden *painless* bleeding (usually after 7 months of gestation)
Bright red blood from the vagina
Shock (decreased blood pressure and elevated pulse)

■ **THERAPEUTIC INTERVENTIONS**
Insert large-bore IV line and infuse Ringer's lactate solution.
Draw sample for CBC and type/hold.
Maintain patient in left lateral recombant position and/or Trendelenburg.
Defer vaginal examination until ultrasound indicates placental location.

Abruptio placentae

Abruptio placentae is a major cause of bleeding in the last trimester of pregnancy. It is caused by separation of the placenta from the uterine wall before the actual birth process. This usually occurs after 20 weeks of gestation.

■ **SIGNS AND SYMPTOMS**
Painful uterine contractions
Uterine rigidity
Sudden colicky pain
Frank, bright red bleeding or concealed bleeding
Increased pulse rate
Decreased blood pressure
Fetal heart tones may be absent
If a large area of the placenta is separated, fetal heart tones may not be present

■ **THERAPEUTIC INTERVENTIONS**
Begin large-bore IV line with bolus of lactated Ringer's solution.
Administer oxygen at 8 ml/min via nasal cannula.
If unstable from a cardiovascular standpoint, fluid replacement is first priority.
Mark the level of the uterus on the abdomen.
Transport rapidly to obstetrical setting.

Pregnancy-Induced Hypertension

Preeclampsia

One form of pregnancy-induced hypertension (PIH) is preeclampsia. Preeclampsia is a hypertensive, multisystem disorder associated with hypertension, proteinuria, edema, CNS irritability, and at times coagulation or liver function abnormalities.

■ **SIGNS AND SYMPTOMS**
Elevated blood pressure (systolic pressure of greater than 140 mm Hg, diastolic pressure of greater than 90 mm Hg, or an increase in the systolic blood pressure of greater than 30 mm Hg and a diastolic pressure increase of 15 mm Hg over first trimester baseline.)
Albuminuria (2+ dipstick on catheter specimen or clean catch)

Oliguria
Edema of face, hands, sacrum
Increased weight gain of greater than or equal to 2 pounds per week
Visual changes
Facial puffiness
Headaches
Nausea
Epigastric or URQ pain
Increased DTRs with clonus

■ **THERAPEUTIC INTERVENTIONS**
Give supportive care.
Schedule obstetric consultation immediately.
Initiate magnesium sulfate therapy as ordered.
Transfer for obstetrical care.

Eclampsia

Eclampsia represents the convulsive phase of preeclampsia. Approximately 5% of preeclamptic patients will become eclamptic. Significant maternal and fetal mortality is associated with eclampsia.

■ **SIGNS AND SYMPTOMS**
Seizures
Symptomatology of preeclampsia
Elevated blood pressure (systolic pressure of 140 to 200 mm Hg, diastolic greater than 90 mm Hg)
Albuminuria (2+ dipstick on catheter specimen or clean catch)
Oliguria
Edema of face, hands, sacrum
Increased weight gain
Vision changes
Facial puffiness
Headaches
Nausea
Epigastric or URQ pain
Increased DTRs with clonus
Decreased fetal heart tones particularly during seizure and postictal for as long as 15 to 20 minutes

■ **THERAPEUTIC INTERVENTIONS (FOR SEIZURE CONDITION)**
Maintain airway
Give oxygen at 8L/min by mask or cannula
Maintain left lateral positioning
Magnesium sulfate administration for seizure prophylaxis[1]
    4g to 6 g bolus over 15 minutes followed by maintenance dose
    1 to 3 g/hr by continuous infusion pump
Monitor BP, Resp rate, and DTR every hour or as indicated
Transfer to appropriate obstetrical service

Gestational Trophoblastic Disease

Gestational trophoblastic disease includes hydatidiform mole and gestational trophoblastic tumors.

■ **SIGNS AND SYMPTOMS**
Bright red or brownish bleeding/spotting
Enlarged uterus
Very high human chorionic gonadotrophing (hCG) levels

Often absence of fetal heart tones (FHT) at 12 weeks or greater
"Snowstorm" pattern with ultrasound
Signs of preeclampsia at an early gestational age
■ **THERAPEUTIC INTERVENTIONS**
Monitor vital signs carefully if bleeding is heavy.
Prepare for dilation and curettage (D & C) uterine evacuation if bleeding is heavy.
Monitor pulmonary status carefully if D&C is performed.
Observe for signs and symptoms of preeclampsia.

Ectopic Pregnancy

An ectopic pregnancy follows implantation of a fertilized egg outside the endometrial cavity, usually in the fallopian tube. Of all ectopic pregnancies, 98% are tubal, with cervical, abdominal, and ovarian implantations accounting for the remaining 2%. As the fetus grows, the fallopian tube will eventually rupture.

■ **SIGNS AND SYMPTOMS**
Abnormal uterine bleeding
Severe sudden onset of unilateral pelvic pain
Abdominal tenderness and guarding
Positive pregnancy test
Suspected pregnancy (full breasts, late period, and so forth)
Missed menstrual period or "late" for period
Syncope
Woman feels that she would feel better if she could have a bowel movement
Adnexal mass
Shoulder pain

> **If ruptured**
> Decreasing blood pressure
> Elevated pulse
> Decreasing level of consciousness
> Cold, clammy skin
> Delayed capillary refill

■ **DIAGNOSIS**
HCG levels
Hematocrit and hemoglobin
Pregnancy test
Ultrasound
Culdocentesis

■ **THERAPEUTIC INTERVENTIONS**
Administer oxygen at 8 L/min by nasal cannula.
Initiate IV therapy with Ringer's lactate.
Administer antibiotics.
Consider applying the pneumatic antishock garment (PASG) if indicated and in accordance with local protocol.
Prepare the patient for surgery.
Give $Rh_o(D)$ immune globulin (RhoGAM) if indicated.

Ruptured Ovarian Cyst

Ovarian cysts may be asymptomatic until hemorrhage, rupture, or torsion occurs. A ruptured ovarian cyst may be confused with an ectopic pregnancy because signs and symptoms are quite similar.

■ **SIGNS AND SYMPTOMS**

Lower abdominal pain—sudden, sharp, unilateral

Nausea and vomiting

Peritoneal irritation

Irregular menstrual cycle

Adnexal mass

Low-grade temperature

Hemoperitoneum

■ **THERAPEUTIC INTERVENTIONS**

Administer oxygen at 8 L/min by nasal cannula.

Initiate IV therapy with Ringer's lactate.

Place the patient in shock position.

Consider applying the PASG if indicated and in accordance with local protocol.

Give antibiotics.

Surgery is required for removal of the cyst.

STAGES OF LABOR

Stage I—Dilation Stage

From the onset of regular uterine contractions to complete cervical dilation. Average time: 12.5 hours in a primipara; 7 hours in a multipara.

Stage 2—Expulsion Stage

From the time of complete dilation until the baby is delivered. Average time: 80 minutes in a primipara; 30 minutes in a multipara.

Stage 3—Placental Stage

From the time immediately following delivery of the baby until the expulsion of the placenta. Average time: 5 to 15 minutes.

EMERGENCY DELIVERY

■ **SIGNS AND SYMPTOMS OF IMPENDING DELIVERY**

If the following signs and symptoms are present, prepare for immediate delivery. When assisting with a delivery, attempt to maintain sterile technique if possible. If delivery is imminent, do not delay to maintain sterility at the risk of endangering both the mother and the infant.

Heavy, bloody show

Frequent contractions

Desire to "bear down" by the mother

Mother stating that she is going to defecate or that the "baby is coming"

Bulging membranes from the vulva

Crowning of the fetal head (Figure 33-1)

Fetal bradycardia

■ **EQUIPMENT**

Basin or plastic bag

Scissors or scalpel (sterile) to cut cord

2 cord clamps or 2 Kelly clamps

1 bulb syringe

Sterile gloves

Heated Isolette (if possible) or warm blankets

Identification bands for mother and infant

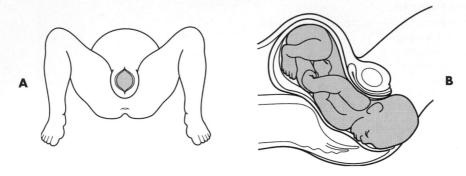

FIGURE 33-1. Childbirth sequence. **A,** Crowning. **B,** Cross-section view of crowning.

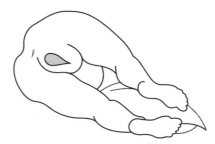

FIGURE 33-2. Side-lying position.

■ **PROCEDURE**

1. Prepare the mother by placing her in a prone position with her knees bent or in a side-lying position (Figure 33-2). Delivery of the anterior shoulder is often easier if mother is side lying. This implies someone supporting her upper leg.
2. Take vital signs (including fetal heart tones) if time permits.
3. Offer much verbal support; explain what is going on.
4. Put on sterile gloves.
5. Place a fluid-absorbent pad under mother.
6. Have the mother pant with each contraction or push gently.
7. Place gentle pressure on the fetal head when it crowns to avoid rapid expulsion of the fetus. Support the perineum with a towel (Figure 33-3).
8. Support the head with both hands, but allow it to rotate naturally (Figure 33-4, Figure 33-5).
9. Check for the cord around the infant's neck.
     If it is there, attempt to slip it over the infant's head.
     If it is too tight, immediately clamp the cord in two places and cut the cord between the clamps.
10. If the membranes are still intact, quickly snip them at the nape of the neck, and peel them away from the face.
11. Suction the infant. Suction mouth first in order to clear the oropharynx. Suction nose second. Suctioning the nose often stimulates the baby to gasp—you want the mouth cleared when this happens. (Remember that newborns are obligate nose breathers.)
12. Deliver the shoulders by guiding the head downward to deliver the anterior shoulder and then upward to deliver the posterior shoulder.
13. The remaining parts of the infant deliver quickly. You may need to apply gentle traction (Figure 33-6, *A*).
14. Note the time of birth.

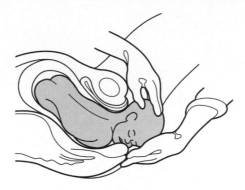

FIGURE 33-3. Perineal support.

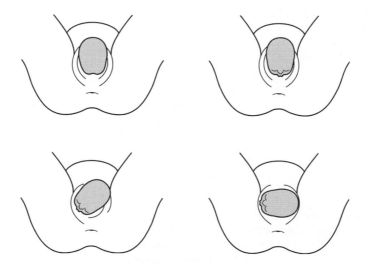

FIGURE 33-4. Birth and rotation

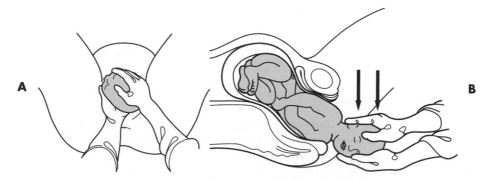

FIGURE 33-5. **A,** Delivery of head. **B,** Cross-section view of delivery of head.

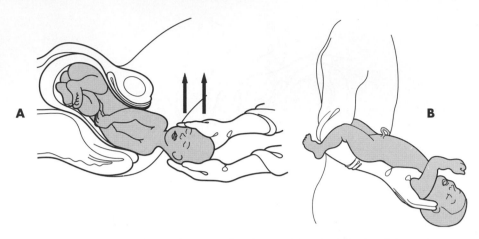

FIGURE 33-6. **A,** Delivery of the rest of body. **B,** Holding the baby, head dependent.

TABLE 33-1 Apgar Score Chart

	0	1	2
Heart rate	0	Less than 100	More than 100
Muscle tone	Limp	Some flexion	Well flexed
Reflexes (catheter in nose)	No response	Grimace	Cough or sneeze
Color	Blue, pale	Pink body, blue extremities	Pink

15. Hold the infant along the length of your arm with the head dependent and suction the mouth and nose once again or place the infant on the surface of the bed (Figure 33-6, *B*).
16. Clamp the cord and cut between the clamps using sterile scissors.
17. Dry the baby immediately and thoroughly. Assess for evidence of respiratory effort as you are drying the baby.
18. The infant should make a first effort to breathe by crying spontaneously. If spontaneous breathing still does not occur, initiate positive pressure ventilation.
    Check heart rate after 30 minutes of positive pressure ventilation. If heart rate is below 80, initiate chest compressions and neonatal CPR.
19. Determine an Apgar score at 1 minute and again at 5 minutes (Table 33-1).
20. Keep the infant warm by wrapping it in a blanket and/or placing it in a heated Isolette. If an Isolette is not available, have the mother hold the infant, using skin-to-skin contact.

Delivery of the Placenta

Placental separation occurs, on average, within 3 to 5 minutes; however, it may also be delayed for as long as 30 minutes. Patience is indeed a virtue here. The consequences of impatient interventions are catastrophic.

■ **SIGNS AND SYMPTOMS OF IMPENDING DELIVERY OF THE PLACENTA**
The umbilical cord advances 2 to 3 inches farther out of the vagina.
The fundus rises upward in the abdomen.
The uterus becomes firm and globular.
A large gush of blood comes from the vagina.

■ **PROCEDURE**
1. Instruct the mother to "bear down."
2. Do *not* exert traction on the cord. Keeping the umbilical cord slightly taut, gently lift the uterus cephalad with the other hand.
3. Massage the fundus immediately after delivery of the placenta.
4. Once the placenta is delivered, inspect it for missing sections.
5. Save the placenta in a basin or plastic bag and send it with the mother to the obstetrical unit.
6. Oxytocin 10 u per 500 cc of lactated Ringer's is effective in reducing bleeding.

Care of the Mother

Wipe the perineal area gently with a clean dry towel.
Place a sanitary napkin or towel in the perineal area.
Massage the fundus while applying suprapubic pressure.
Initiate IV therapy (usually Ringer's lactate or Ringer's lactate with 5% dextrose) at approximately 150 ml/hr (faster if bleeding is excessive).
Administer oxytocic agents in accordance with the facility policy or in accordance with physician's orders (usually pitocin).
Keep the mother warm.
Observe closely; monitor the vital signs frequently (every 15 minutes) until they are stable.
Put an infant identification band on the mother's wrist.

Care of the Infant

Dry the infant.
Keep the infant warm.
Maintain the infant's airway by placing the infant on its side.
Apply erythromycin or silver nitrate eye prophylaxis (in accordance with facility policy).
Administer phytonadione (Aquamephyton) for hypoprothrombinemia prophylaxis (in accordance with facility policy).
Observe the cord for bleeding.
Put an identification band on both the wrist and ankle.
Observe closely and monitor vital signs.

Normal Newborn Vital Sign Range

Pulse: 100-160	Respirations: 40-60	Temperature: >36.5° C

COMPLICATIONS OF DELIVERY

Meconium-Stained Fluid

■ **SIGNS AND SYMPTOMS**
Meconium-stained amniotic fluid. (Fluid will be green or dark yellow. It can also be very thick.)
■ **THERAPEUTIC INTERVENTIONS**
Apply oxygen.
Attempt to have mother blow with contractions as if she were "blowing out a candle."
Prepare equipment to intubate the baby at birth. (A size 3.0 or 3.5 tube is needed.) If possible, have a pediatrician present.

When equipment is available, encourage mother to push with contractions if she feels pressure or the urge to push.

Suction the baby's mouth and nose thoroughly after delivery of the head and before delivery of the body.

If intubation is possible, visualize the vocal cords immediately after birth. If meconium is visible below the cords, insert an endotracheal tube (ET) and apply suction as the ET tube is removed. This requires the use of a meconium aspirator.

Repeat this procedure before encouraging the baby to breathe (hopefully no longer than 20 to 30 seconds).

Fetal Bradycardia

■ **SIGNS AND SYMPTOMS**

Decreased fetal heart rate (less than 100 beats per minute)

Fetal heart rate baseline via electronic fetal monitor less than 100 beats per minute.

■ **THERAPEUTIC INTERVENTIONS**

Encourage mother to push if she feels the urge to push.

Administer oxygen at 8 L/min via nasal cannula or mask.

Place the mother in a side-lying position.

Check for prolapsed cord.

Initiate IV therapy with Ringer's lactate.

Follow steps for normal vaginal delivery or rapid transport for cesarean section.

Be prepared to administer neonatal resuscitation.

Breech Position of Fetus

In 3% of all births the fetus presents in the breech position, with either the buttocks first or a foot first (known as a footling breech). These positions are dangerous for the fetus because of the increased likelihood of a prolapsed cord and of a difficult delivery. Delivery of the fetus in these states is best accomplished by cesarean section. If delivery is progressing, apply the following therapeutic interventions:

Support the legs and buttocks of the baby.

When the mother has a contraction, pull gently on the baby. Placing a towel around the baby helps to grasp the infant.

Insert your finger into the vagina—deliver one shoulder, then the other (Figure 33-7).

Do *not* pull on the baby. This may cause the cervix to clamp tighter around the baby's head. Work with the mother's contractions.

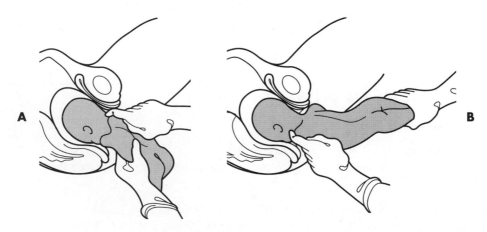

FIGURE 33-7. **A,** Extraction of anterior arm. **B,** Extraction of posterior arm. Breech-shoulder delivery.

Deliver the head by supporting the baby's chest with your arms and hands.

Place your finger into the posterior vagina and find the baby's mouth.

As mother pushes with contractions, reach into baby's mouth, grasp the chin and apply gentle upward pressure to head and shoulders (Figure 33-8).

It may be necessary to apply suprapubic pressure as well.

Prolapsed Cord

A prolapsed cord is a state in which the cord precedes the infant. This is an acute emergency (Figure 33-9).

■ **SIGNS AND SYMPTOMS**

Visible cord protruding from vagina

Fetal heart rate less than 100

■ **THERAPEUTIC INTERVENTIONS**

Elevate the mother's hips or place in knee-chest position.

Administer oxygen at 8 L/min by nasal cannula.

Keep the mother warm.

Place a gloved hand into the vaginal canal and elevate the fetus's head to relieve pressure on the cord; once this has been accomplished, leave your hand in place.

Leave the cord as it is; do not attempt to place it back in the vagina.

Feel whether the cord is pulsating, *but* handle it as little as possible to prevent spasm of the cord vessels.

Notify the appropriate personnel and transport the patient so that an immediate cesarean section can be performed. If transport time is prolonged, keep cord moist with saline-moistened towels.

Postpartum Hemorrhage

Postpartum hemorrhage is defined as excessive bleeding from the genital tract at any time after the birth and up to 6 weeks after delivery. If it occurs within 24 hours, it is called *primary postpartum hemorrhage*. If blood loss reaches 500 ml, it must be treated as a postpartum hemorrhage.

■ **SIGNS AND SYMPTOMS**

Steady flow of bright red blood

Decreasing blood pressure

Increasing pulse

Pale, clammy skin

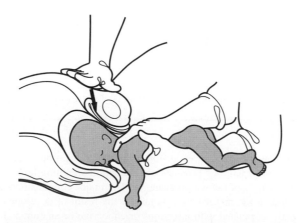

FIGURE 33-8. Delivery of arms and shoulders. Breech-head delivery.

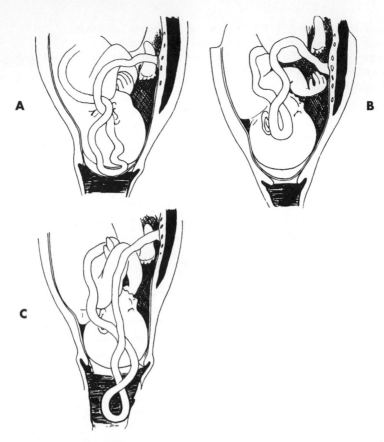

FIGURE 33-9. **A,** Cord prolapsed at the inlet. **B,** Cord prolapsed in the vagina. **C,** Cord prolapsed through the introitus.
(From Dickason E: *Maternal-infant nursing care,* ed 2, St Louis, 1994, Mosby.)

Nausea
Signs of hypovolemia
■ **THERAPEUTIC INTERVENTIONS**
Massage the uterus while applying suprapubic pressure.
Apply manual pressure to tears if present.
Give oxygen at 8 L/min by nasal cannula.
Place the mother in Trendelenburg's position.
Begin IV therapy with Ringer's lactate with oxytocin (Pitocin, Syntocinon).

ABORTION

The term *abortion* is defined as the death or expulsion of the fetus or products of conception before the twenty-fourth week of pregnancy, with the products of conception weighing less than 500 grams. The frequency of abortion is 10% to 15% of known pregnancies. The major complications of abortion are hemorrhage and infection. Pregnancy loss in the first trimester is largely the result of developmental defects of the embryo. Later loss is more frequently associated with infections or endocrine or anatomic abnormalities within the maternal reproductive organs.

Types of Abortions
Threatened abortion

A threatened abortion is said to occur in cases where early symptoms of abortion, such as episodic, painless uterine bleeding and mild cramping are present. The cervical os is closed, the uterus is enlarged and soft, and the pregnancy test is positive.

■ THERAPEUTIC INTERVENTIONS
Bed rest
Pelvic rest
Mild sedatives
Ultrasound confirmation

Inevitable abortion

Increased pain, cramping, and bleeding occurs, and the cervical os is dilated 3 cm or more.

■ THERAPEUTIC INTERVENTIONS
Bed rest
Analgesics/narcotics
Patient may have D & C at provider's and patient's discretion
RhoGAM if indicated

Incomplete abortion

In an incomplete abortion, bleeding is heavy, cramping is severe, and the cervical os is open. The uterus is enlarged and the pregnancy test is positive. Some tissue has been passed, but some products of conception have been retained.

■ THERAPEUTIC INTERVENTIONS
Oxygen at 8 L/min by nasal cannula
IV therapy with Ringer's lactate
Oxytocic agents
Surgery for currettage
RhoGAM if indicated

Complete abortion

In complete abortion there is a small amount of bleeding, cramping is mild, all tissue has been passed, and the cervical os is closed.

■ THERAPEUTIC INTERVENTIONS
Observation

Missed abortion

A loss of pregnancy in which the products of conception remain in the uterus for an extended period after the fetus has died. In addition, the characteristic symptoms of bleeding and cramping are absent.

■ THERAPEUTIC INTERVENTIONS
Some providers may send the patient home for expectant management.
Possible dilation and curettage

Septic abortion

Infection after abortion occurs occasionally in patients who had a complete abortion without dilation and curettage. More frequently it occurs in patients with delayed treatment of incomplete abortion or as a result of an earlier elective termination of pregnancy. The organisms most frequently responsible are alpha- and beta-hemolytic strep, gram-negative aerobes such as *E. coli,* and occasionally *Clostridium welchii,* all of which are often the normal flora of the vagina.

Particular concern must be directed toward *Clostridium,* an anaerobic organism capable of producing gas gangrene, tissue necrosis, and tissue sloughing in the uterus. Prompt treatment is essential and if improvement does not occur after dilation and curettage, hysterectomy is indicated.

■ **SIGNS AND SYMPTOMS**

Foul discharge

Constant pain

Temperature elevation

Chills

Uterine tenderness

■ **THERAPEUTIC INTERVENTIONS**

To avoid significant morbidity and mortality the treatment of septic abortion must be immediate and aggressive antibiotics appropriate to infecting agent

Oxytocin infusion

Dilation and curettage

Observe for signs of endotoxic shock: hypotension, renal failure, and tachycardia

Postabortion Considerations

The patient should be given the following information after abortion.

Vaginal bleeding may last 1 to 2 weeks. The bleeding should get progressively lighter until it subsides.

Slight cramping is normal for several days.

No douching, tampons, and intercourse for at least 2 weeks or until her follow-up visit.

Rest for 2 to 3 days.

Take temperature morning and evening for 5 days.

Contact provider for:

Temperature above 100° F

Excessive bleeding

Severe cramps

Chills

Severe nausea and vomiting

If the patient receives a dilation and curettage with anesthesia, give appropriate information regarding effects of medication.

Many women and men find the loss of their child, even very early in pregnancy, devastating.

Comfort as appropriate.

Determine what information the patient needs regarding causes of abortions.

Refer the patient to experts for more information.

Refer the patient to support groups such as Compassionate Friends or SHARE. The obstetrical unit may have a list of resources.

Refer patient to counseling as needed, especially if patient has a history of depression or concurrent stresses.

VAGINAL BLEEDING

Abnormal uterine bleeding is one of the most common gynecologic complaints. Causes of uterine bleeding are many and varied. Particular concern for the welfare of the fetus exists if the patient is pregnant.

To assist in establishing a firm diagnosis, it is important to obtain a good history from the patient. Important questions to answer are:

Are the vital signs stable? Is the hematocrit stable? If not:

Initiate IV therapy with Ringer's lactate.

Have the PASG standing by.

Is the patient pregnant? Do a 2 minute and 2 hour pregnancy test.

If the patient is pregnant, is she aborting?

Do *not* do a vaginal examination if the patient is more than 20 weeks gestation.

Before doing a vaginal exam on a pregnant patient who is bleeding, it is important to rule out placenta previa by ultrasound.

If the patient is not pregnant or is under 20 weeks, a vaginal exam should be performed.

Is the cervical os open or closed? If it is closed, abortion may be threatening. Patients may experience bleeding caused by trauma, cervical or vaginal lesions, or cervical or vaginal polyps. Treatments center around the immediate concern for the patient's well-being with a recommendation for follow-up gynecologic consultation.

Dysfunctional Uterine Bleeding

The most common cause of dysfunctional uterine bleeding (DUB) is a disturbance in the cyclic pattern of the endometrium. This can be caused by a variety of abnormalities in the patient's hormonal patterns.

■ THERAPEUTIC INTERVENTIONS

Treatment for immediate concerns related to bleeding

IV therapy/volume support

Long-term therapy: either progestin alone, oral high-dose estrogen-progestin birth control pills, or estrogen alone

Recommendation for follow-up gynecologic consultation

GYNECOLOGIC INFECTIONS

Pelvic Inflammatory Disease

Pelvic inflammatory disease (PID) is a commonly used term that implies infection in the pelvis: the uterus, fallopian tubes, ovaries, pelvic peritoneum, or some combination of these sites. The term can obscure diagnosis and treatment. Three clinically identifiable subgroups of PID are: endometritis-salpingitis, pelvic peritonitis, and tuboovarian abscess.

Pelvic inflammatory disease occurs as a result of upward migration of bacteria. PID involves many organisms: those that are sexually transmitted, and those that are normal flora of the lower genital tract. The bacteria most often isolated are gonococci (involved in 25% to 80% of cases), streptococci, *E. Coli, Proteus, Klebsiella-enterobacter,* Clostridia, and *Chlamydia.* There are several predisposing factors. Among these are an IUD, trauma, multiple intercourse partners, or history of recent abortion. PID may be the cause of chronic abdominal pain, ectopic pregnancy, or infertility. The presenting symptoms and treatment options are outlined in Table 33-2.

Toxic Shock Syndrome

Toxic shock syndrome is characterized by the abrupt onset of pyrexia, myalgias, and a diffuse rash with edema, and blanching erythema. Less frequent symptoms are vomiting, diarrhea, and hypotension. The etiologic bacteria is usually *Staphylococcus aureus,* which can be isolated from local sites of skin disruption.

Menstrual toxic shock syndrome is most often associated with use of tampons and the contraceptive sponge. However, it has also been associated with tubal ligation, hysterectomy, and carbon dioxide laser vaporization of genital condyloma.

■ THERAPEUTIC INTERVENTIONS

Eliminate source of toxin

Supportive therapy for septic shock

Blood pressure support

TABLE 33-2   Diagnosis and Management of Symptomatic Pelvic Inflammatory Disease

HISTORY AND PELVIC EXAMINATION	LABORATORY TESTS	TREATMENT
Pain and tenderness	Gram stain and culture genital tract Complete blood count Possible culdocentesis or laparoscopy	Oral antibiotics Pain medication
Pain, tenderness, and fever <102.5° F	As above	As above; may need hospitalization and intravenous antibiotics
Pain, tenderness, and fever >102.5° F or nausea and vomiting	As above plus blood culture	Hospitalization and intravenous antibiotics
All the above plus pelvic mass	As above plus culdocentesis if cul de sac is bulging	Surgery if mass does not resolve on antibiotics
Septic shock in addition to any of the above	As above plus central venous pressure monitor	As above plus steroids and cardiovascular medications

From Kase N, Weingold A, Gershenson O: *Principles and practice of clinical gynecology,* New York, 1990, Churchill Livingstone.

Respiratory support
Penicillin
Corticosteroids
Contact isolation

Infections of External Genitalia

Recognition and diagnosis of external genitalia infections are made through visual observation. Some of the more common ones are:

INFECTION	THERAPEUTIC INTERVENTIONS
Scabies	Kwell lotion or shampoo
Vulvar abscess	Incision and drainage Antibiotics Sitz baths
Simple cyst	Sitz baths
Bartholin's cyst (infected)	Antibiotics Sitz baths Later, incision and drainage Urination via Foley catheter Check for gonorrhea
Condyloma (genital warts)	Local application of podophyllin Trichloracetic acid Large lesions surgically removed or treated with laser
Herpes	Acyclovir Analgesics

Vaginal Infection

If the ecology of the vagina is disturbed, vaginal infection may occur. Vaginal infection is not usually an emergency situation but is a frequently seen complaint in the emergency department because it is an annoyance to the patient. The four most common types of vaginal infections are described in Table 33-3.

TABLE 33-3   Gynecologic Emergencies:
Differential Diagnosis of Common Vaginal Infections

ORGANISM	OCCURRENCE	COLOR	ODOR	CONSISTENCY	OTHER	LAB TEST(S)	THERAPEUTIC INTERVENTION
Hemophilus vaginalis	31% of all vaginal infections	Whitish-gray	Foul	Watery		Wet mount culture and Gram's stain to exclude other organisms	Sultrin, 1 applicatorful 2 times a day for 4 to 6 days
Bacterial (nonspecific) vaginitis	27% of all vaginal infections	Yellow	Foul	Water/creamy	May be caused by retained foreign body	Wet mount culture and Gram's stain to exclude other organisms	Antibiotics (type-specific); remove foreign body
Candida albicans	26% of all vaginal infections	White	Odorless	Cheesy; heavy flow	Causes monilial vaginitis	Pseudohyphae from KOH wet mount	Nystatin (Mycostatin) vaginal tablets 1 to 2 times daily for 7 to 14 days or clotrimazole (Gyne-Lotrimin) vaginal tablets once a day for 7 days
Trichomonas vaginalis	16% of all vaginal infections	Yellowish-gray	Fishy	Creamy; bubbly	Frequently, erythema around cervical os	Wet mount shows motile protozoa	Metronidazole (Flagyl) 250 mg po 3 times daily for 7 days. Male partner must also be treated with same drug and dosage. If woman is pregnant, substitute Tricofuron

From Budassi SA: Differential diagnosis of vaginal discharge, *JEN* 6(3):35, 1980.
Other causes of vaginal discharge include: cancer of cervix or uterus, IUD, pelvic inflammatory disease, rectal or bladder fistula, and senile vaginitis.

ABDOMINAL/PELVIC PAIN

Endometriosis

The condition in which endometrial tissue cells are found growing outside the uterus is known as endometriosis. This tissue reacts to hormonal changes just as normal endometrial tissue does. As menstruation occurs, endometrial tissue sloughs; this may be the cause of the chief complaint of pelvic pain.

■ **SIGNS AND SYMPTOMS**
Depends on the extent of the disease
Dysmenorrhea
Episodic pelvic pain
Dysuria/hematuria
Dyspareunia
Infertility

■ **DIAGNOSIS**
Clinical visualization by laparoscopy
Biopsy

■ **THERAPEUTIC INTERVENTIONS**
Hormone (exogenous)
Danazol (Danocrine)
Oral contraceptive agents
Consider surgery

SEXUAL ASSAULT

Sexual assault is covered in detail in Chapter 31.

CONTRACEPTIVE EMERGENCIES

Occasionally a patient with a contraceptive emergency will present to the emergency department. Table 33-4 lists some of the more common contraceptive emergencies.

Because of increasingly difficult access to care for some women, the emergency department serves as the only option for health care. When emergencies arise around pregnancy, it is a stressful and frightening time. A

TABLE 33-4   Contraceptive Emergencies

TYPE	PROBLEM	THERAPEUTIC INTERVENTION
Diaphragm	Unable to remove	Remove with ring forceps
IUD	Unable to remove	Remove with ring forceps
	Lost string	X-ray or ultrasound to determine position; may be removed with IUD hook
	Partial expulsion	Remove; consider alternate form of contraception
	Migration to abdominal cavity	X-ray or ultrasound to determine position; may require exploratory laparotomy
Oral contraceptives	Thrombophlebitis	Bed rest; local heat; anticoagulation
	Pulmonary embolus	ABCs; oxygen, IV, analgesia, bronchodilators, heparin, reassurance
	Cerebrovascular accident	ABCs; oxygen IV

sympathetic, capable caregiver who offers scientifically based information without awkwardness can be very important to families.

REFERENCE

1. Repke JT: *Intrapartum obstetrics,* New York, 1996, Churchill Livingstone.

SUGGESTED READINGS

Abbott J: Acute complications related to pregnancy. In Rosen et al: *Emergency medicine*, ed 4, St Louis, 1998, Mosby.

Barnhart K et al: Prompt diagnosis of ectopic pregnancy in an emergency department setting, *Obstet Gynecol* 84:1010, 1994.

Benrubi G: *Obstetric and gynecologic emergencies,* Philadelphia, 1994, Lippincott.

Brenner PF: Differential diagnosis of abnormal vaginal bleeding, *Am J Obstet Gynecol* 175:766, 1996.

Cunningham FG et al: *Williams Obstetrics,* ed 18, New York, 1993, Appleton & Lange.

DeCherney AH, Pernole M: *Obstetric and gynecologic diagnosis and treatment,* ed 8, Norwalk, Conn, 1994, Appleton & Lange.

Kase N, Wiengold A, Gershenson D: *Principles and practice of clinical gynecology,* New York, 1990, Churchill Livingstone.

Ledger WJ: The management of pelvic inflammatory disease, *Hosp Phys* 10:45, 1982.

Long CA: Evaluation of patients with abnormal uterine bleeding, *Am J Obstet Gynecol* 175:784, 1996.

Lubarsky SL et al: Late postpartum eclampsia revisited, *Obstet Gynecol* 83:502, 1994.

Morrison LJ: Unique concerns of pregnancy. In Rosen et al: *Emergency medicine,* ed 4, St Louis, 1998, Mosby.

Newton E, Solomon RH: Vaginal bleeding unrelated to pregnancy. In Rosen et al: *Emergency medicine*, ed 4, St Louis, 1998, Mosby.

Pansky M et al: Nonsurgical management of tubal pregnancy, *Am J Obstet Gynecol* 164:888, 1993.

Ryan KR, Berkowitz RS, Barbrieri RL: *Kistner's gynecology: principles and practice,* ed 6, St Louis, 1995, Mosby.

Weinman S: Nonsurgical treatment of an ectopic pregnancy with methotrexate *J Emerg Nurs* 22(6):597-599, 1996.

Pediatric Medical Emergencies

Anne Cassels Turner

This chapter presents a broad overview of pediatric problems commonly seen in the emergency department. Because there is not enough space to detail every possible emergency condition, the reader is referred to the list of suggested readings at the end of the chapter.

GENERAL APPROACH TO THE PEDIATRIC PATIENT

Most health care personnel are not used to working with large numbers of sick children on a daily basis. As a result, it is normal to feel a bit anxious when a pediatric patient arrives in the emergency department, especially a very sick child. It is important to remain calm and to have self-confidence. There are a few basic rules to follow when dealing with a sick child:

- Be gentle but firm.
- Use common sense.
- Speak directly to the child.
- Be honest with the child; if something is going to hurt, say that it is going to hurt.
- Tell the child what is about to be done.
- Tell the child what is being done while it is being done.
- Remember that parents may be very anxious, too:

    Allow the parents to be with the child whenever possible.

    If for some reason the parents cannot be with the child, be sure that someone is available to stay with them or at least to keep them informed periodically about the child's condition.

    Between examinations, allow the child to sit on the parent's lap if possible.

    Some procedures are more easily accomplished if the parent holds the child (for example, examinations of a child's ear), but a parent should never be asked to hold a child for a painful procedure.

Table 34-1 provides a description of theories of child development and emergency department interventions according to age.

PEDIATRIC TRIAGE

Pediatric triage begins with the visual assessment: "Does the child look sick?" The level of activity, skin color, and breathing pattern are the key signs to consider in the initial visual assessment. Is the child extremely pale, ashen, or mottled? Is the child markedly tachypneic with grunted or shallow respirations? Visual triage must be more than a simple peek through the blankets.

TABLE 34-1   Theories of Child Development and Suggested Interventions

	BIRTH-18 MO	19 MO-2 YR	3 YR-5 YR	6 YR-11 YR	12 YR-18 YR
Theories of child development					
Erikson	Trust vs mistrust	Autonomy vs shame and doubt	Initiative vs guilt	Industry vs inferiority	Identity vs role confusion
Freud	Oral-sensory	Anal	Phallic	Latency	Genital
Piaget	Sensorimotor egocentrism	Preoperational, beginnings of perceptual constancy	Preoperational, prelogical reasoning	Concrete operations	Formal operations
Task mastery	Differentiate self and nonself	Toilet training	Use of language	Logic	Abstract thinking
Pain perception	Physical but possibly not cognitive pain perceived, in younger patients	Primarily egocentric: "Here and now" May see pain as punishment	Pain as punishment Overextension of causality Fear and fantasy	Beginning of understanding of true causality Fear of destruction and death	Concept of emotional and physical pain Understanding of root causes of pain
Suggested interventions	1. Involve caretaker in care of child. 2. Keep child warm. 3. Keep room quiet. 4. Provide comfort measures (for example, pacifier). 5. Keep child on caretaker's lap during physical examination. 6. Return child to caretaker as soon as possible after procedures; allow caretaker to comfort child.	1. Prepare caretaker for procedures. 2. Tell caretaker that he or she may assist in normal care. 3. Give child a familiar toy or blanket as a transitional object. 4. Use child's name. 5. Restrain child as little as possible. 6. Avoid covering child's face. 7. Describe sensations and talk with child during the procedures. 8. Praise, smile, and have a cheerful attitude.	1. Explain procedure *immediately before* performing it. 2. Allow child to see and touch samples of equipment. 3. Be honest: "This will sting." 4. Use simple distractions and talk to child. 5. Allow child to see under bandages. 6. Use praise, adhesive bandages, and small rewards.	1. Explain procedure beforehand. 2. Enlist cooperation. 3. Ask about simple preferences. 4. Give alternatives (for example, child may yell but not move). 5. Identify sensations and personnel. 6. Use distraction and counting games. 7. Include child in discharge instructions. 8. Use rewards, stickers, badges, and praise.	1. Give *full* explanations. 2. Encourage child's participation. 3. Allow time for questions. 4. Provide *privacy.* Child may want to exclude parents. 5. Avoid teasing and embarrassing child. 6. Allow as much control as possible. 7. Provide discharge instructions to patient. 8. Reassure child that his or her behavior was appropriate.

From Barkin R et al: *Pediatric emergency medicine: concepts & clinical practice*, ed 2, St Louis, 1996, Mosby.

Triage Criteria

I. Primary Survey
   A. Airway
      1. Patency
   B. Breathing
      1. Rate—tachypnea/slow respirations
      2. Quality
      3. Breath sounds—wheezing, stridor
      4. Mechanics—retractions, grunting
   C. Circulation
      1. Skin color: mottled, ashen pallor, cyanotic, dusky, flushed
      2. Capillary refill time—delayed >2 seconds
      3. Skin temperature
      4. CNS perfusion—response to parents, response to threatening stimuli (nurse), response to pain
II. Vital Signs (Table 34-2)—note any deviation from normal
   A. Age of child
   B. Temperature—any temperature associated with abnormalities of activity, respiration pattern, or dermal warning signs
      1. Fever, greater than 105° F
      2. Hypothermia
         a. Less than 96° F (infant)
         b. Less than 95° F (toddler, child)
   C. Heart rate
         a. Greater than 200 beats/minute (infant)
         b. Greater than 180 beats/minute (toddler)
         c. Greater than 160 beats/minute (child)
         d. Profound bradycardia in any age group
            (Note that sinus arrhythmia is normal in most pediatric patients.)

TABLE 34-2 Average Vital Signs and Weight by Age

AGE	HEART RATE AVERAGE (BEATS/MIN)	RANGE	SYSTOLIC BLOOD PRESSURE AVERAGE (mm Hg)	RANGE	RESPIRATORY RATE (BREATHS/MIN)	WEIGHT (kg)
Preterm	140	120-180	50	40-60	55-65	2
Term newborn	140	90-170	72	52-92	40-60	3
1 mon	135	110-180	82	60-104	30-50	4
6 mon	135	110-180	94	65-125	25-35	7
1 yr	120	80-160	94	70-118	20-30	10
2 yrs	110	80-130	95	73-117	20-30	12
4 yrs	105	80-120	91	65-117	20-30	16
6 yrs	100	75-115	96	76-116	18-24	20
8 yrs	90	70-110	99	79-119	18-22	25
10 yrs	90	70-110	102	82-122	16-20	30
12 yrs	85	60-110	106	84-128	16-20	40
14 yrs	80	60-105	110	84-136	16-20	50

From Barkin R et al: *Pediatric emergency medicine: concepts & clinical practice*, ed 2, St Louis, 1996, Mosby.

D. Respiratory rate
  a. Greater than 60 breaths/minute (infants)
  b. Greater than 40 breaths/minute (toddlers)
  c. Greater than 30 breaths/minute (child)
E. Blood pressure—any BP associated with poor capillary refill
  1. Systolic
    a. Less than 50 systolic (infants)
    b. Less than 60 systolic (toddlers)
    c. Less than 70 systolic (child)
F. Weight, less than third to fifth percentile for age

MEDICATION ADMINISTRATION

Pediatric dosages of medications are given in accordance with the child's weight (see Table 34-2). Total pediatric dosage should never exceed adult dosage. An infant and standing scales should be available in the department for accurate weights for assessment of dehydration and medication administration.

INTRAVENOUS THERAPY IN PEDIATRICS

The most difficult aspects of starting an IV on an infant or child are finding a vein, controlling the patient during puncture, and anchoring the needle to prevent infiltration and mechanical irritation to the vessel. The most significant aspect of the procedure is supporting the patient and the parents emotionally and performing so efficiently that little pain results. The most underrated aspect of this procedure is the fear and discomfort the clinician experiences when establishing an IV on a tiny child, particularly when the clinician has not used the skill frequently enough to be precise and efficient.

Young children tend to have deep veins well covered with subcutaneous tissue, and in the presence of volume depletion may not evidence peripheral veins even with a tourniquet applied. If the volume is severely depleted and the child is thus compromised, do not attempt peripheral extremity lines. Such cases are emergencies of the highest magnitude; to avoid a time delay, intraosseous access, central lines, or a cutdown by an experienced clinician would be best.

In cases where time is not of the essence, scalp veins or veins on the dorsum of the hand or foot may be used to place a 24-gauge or larger over-the-needle catheter.

Sites to Avoid

Antecubital fossa (clinical lab technicians will need access to these areas)
Veins over joints
Veins that might need to be used for cutdown (femoral, saphenous)
Bruised, fractured, or burned areas
The favorite hand of a thumb-sucking child

Criteria for Selection of Large Veins

Large quantities of fluid must be administered
Blood products must be administered
Solution is hypertonic

Equipment Needed for Peripheral Vein IV

24-gauge or larger over-the-needle catheter (with syringe attached)
Alcohol or iodinated solution (CAUTION: may obscure vein in poor light)

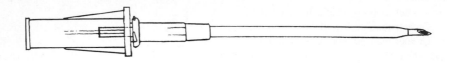

FIGURE 34-1. Catheter-over-needle.

(From Newbury L, Emergency Nurses Association: *Sheehy's emergency nursing: principles and practice* ed 4, St Louis, 1998, Mosby.)

IV extension tubing attached to a 100 ml volume control chamber, connected to an IV solution and properly flushed, attached to infusion pump

Armboard padded

Tourniquet

Silk tape, cut in strips, or clear occlusive dressing (Tegaderm)

Technique for Inserting Over-the-Needle Catheter into Peripheral Vein

Explain the procedure to the child and parents. If time permits, a topical anesthetic such as Emla will help reduce pain and anxiety, especially in an older child. Emla must be applied 45 minutes before the procedure for optimal relief of pain.

Select a vein and restrain all extremities before beginning. You will need assistance in holding, especially a toddler or infant. If time permits, apply a warm compress over selected insertion site to promote vasodilation. Prep the area per your hospital's guidelines.

Make the puncture with the bevel away from the vein and the point toward the vein; the indirect method is preferred (entering from the side and at a slight angle to the vein) when using an over-the-needle catheter (Figure 30-1) to avoid flattening the vein or piercing the posterior wall.

Once the skin and vein are entered, realign the needle and advance slightly. Blood will generally appear in the flashback chamber, but may not in a neonate. If a small syringe is attached before puncture, slight negative pressure can be applied to the plunger to elicit a flashback of blood.

On flashback of blood, stop advancing the needle. Stabilize with one hand while the thumb and forefinger of the other hand disengage the catheter from the needle and advance it into the vein as far as possible.

Release the tourniquet, remove the needle, and begin the flow of IV fluid.

Apply adhesive bandage over insertion site, apply tape in chevron pattern over catheter. Place three rows of tape over site or an occlusive clear dressing (Tegaderm), add tension loop of tubing. Wrap rolled gauze dressing over IV site for added protection.

INTEROSSEOUS INFUSION

See Chapter 6.

AIRWAY

Hypoxia is not an uncommon finding in children. Children have higher metabolic rates than adults. Oxygen consumption is 50% greater in a child than in an adult. With each degree of temperature increase there is an associated oxygen consumption increase of 7%. Pay close attention to this and to the patency of the child's airway.

The most common cause of respiratory distress in children is airway obstruction. The four main areas of airway obstruction are the basopharynx, the oropharynx, the larynx and upper trachea, and the lower airway. If the child is in respiratory distress but is moving some air, try to identify the cause of the obstruction. Perform a rapid assessment for:

Level of consciousness, irritability, lethargy

Signs of hypoxia (for example, circumoral or general cyanosis, increasing respiratory rate)

Breath odor

Lung sounds (for example, wheezes, rhonchi, stridor, rales)

Midline trachea

Distended neck veins

Skin vital signs (color, temperature, moistness)

Use of accessory muscles of respiration

Decreased air movement

Vital signs (be sure to include temperature)

Dehydration

Nasal flaring

Nasopharynx Obstruction

Nasopharynx obstruction may occur as a result of foreign bodies, edematous adenoids, edema from trauma, or carcinomas.

■ **SIGNS AND SYMPTOMS**

Mouth breathing (remember that very small infants are obligate nose breathers; a nasal obstruction in an infant may be life-threatening)

Cyanosis

■ **THERAPEUTIC INTERVENTIONS**

Turn the child on his or her side.

Insert an oropharyngeal airway.

Administer oxygen.

Oropharynx Obstruction

Obstruction of the oropharynx may be caused by facial trauma with swelling of the tongue or by foreign body aspiration.

■ **SIGNS AND SYMPTOMS**

Noisy breathing (gargling or snoring sounds) or absence of breath sounds

Neck extended "like a turtle"

Insistence on sitting up

Cyanosis

Difficulty speaking

Difficulty swallowing

■ **THERAPEUTIC INTERVENTIONS**

Insert an oropharyngeal airway if epiglottitis has been ruled out.

Administer oxygen therapy.

Keep patient calm.

If the patient is moving air, do not attempt to remove the foreign body and do not change the patient's position.

If there is no air movement, hold the infant prone with head lower than the trunk, administer five back blows, followed by up to five downward chest thrusts (Figure 34-2).

Once again, attempt to ventilate the infant.

If the child is unable to cough or breathe effectively, a series of up to five subdiaphragmatic abdominal thrusts is recommended.

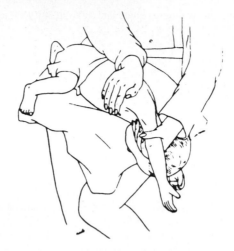

FIGURE 34-2. Child is placed in head down position while up to five firm back blows are applied.

Larynx Obstruction

Epiglottitis

Epiglottitis is a life-threatening bacterial infection of the epiglottis and the surrounding structures. The infection is usually caused by *Hemophilus influenzae* type B.

■ **SIGNS AND SYMPTOMS**

Massive swelling of epiglottis (usually from a bacterial infection)
Commonly seen in 2- to 5-year-old children, but may be seen even in adults
Pallor
Inspiratory stridor
Elevated temperature (above 103.1° F [39.5° C])
Abrupt onset
Anxious appearance
Tachycardia
Sore throat
Respiratory difficulty
Muffled voice
Refusal to change to other than a sitting position (Never place a child on his or her back.*)
Neck extended (like a turtle)
Profuse salivation
Dysphagia
No cough
Hypoventilation
History of infection, ingestion of a hot beverage, or steam inhalation

■ **THERAPEUTIC INTERVENTIONS**

Keep the child as calm as possible; crying can cause laryngospasm and airway obstruction.
Do not attempt to look into the child's mouth; doing so may cause respiratory arrest.*
Make ENT/anesthesia evaluation—most safely done in the operating room with intubation/tracheostomy equipment available.

*Inserting a tongue blade into the mouth or having the child lie down may induce respiratory arrest.

Parent and child should be wheeled together to the OR in the company of an anesthesiologist, ambu bag with age appropriate mask, endotracheal tube size for age and a size smaller plus an oxygen tank.

Consider an emergency needle cricothyrotomy.

Administer steroids.

Croup

Croup is a viral infection of the trachea and larynx—it may extend to the bronchi—that causes edema and inflammation of the lining of the trachea and larynx.

■ SIGNS AND SYMPTOMS

Child usually 3 months to 3 years of age

History of increasing nocturnal distress for several days resulting from an upper respiratory infection

Usually active, appears well

Low-grade fever

Loud "barking" cough

Hoarse voice

Inspiratory stridor

Sternal retraction

Tachypnea

Tachycardia

■ THERAPEUTIC INTERVENTIONS

Cardiac monitor

Humidified oxygen to maintain transcutaneous saturation above 95%

Normal saline nebulizers

L. Epinephrine or racemic epi via nebulizer if in respiratory distress

Laryngospasm

Laryngospasm is not common, but when it occurs, it can be life threatening. It is difficult to distinguish from a foreign body airway obstruction. It may be caused by anaphylaxis.

■ SIGNS AND SYMPTOMS

Vomiting	Bronchospasm
Urticaria	Hypotension
Periorbital edema	Absence of breath sounds

■ THERAPEUTIC INTERVENTIONS

Ensure airway management, consider intubation.

Administer oxygen therapy.

Perform emergency needle cricothyrotomy if the airway cannot be opened.

Administer epinephrine if caused by anaphylaxis.

Administer antihistamines if indicated.

Administer bronchodilators if indicated.

Administer steroids if indicated.

Lower Airway Obstruction

Asthma

Asthma is a recurrent reactive airway disease associated with reversible airway obstruction caused by bronchospasm, mucous gland hypertrophy, and mucus plugging.

■ SIGNS AND SYMPTOMS

Expiratory wheezes (sometimes inspiratory also)

Possibly no expiratory sounds if there is no air movement

Coughs

Retractions
Prolonged expiration
Tachycardia
Dyspnea

■ **THERAPEUTIC INTERVENTIONS**

Administer oxygen as tolerated to maintain transcutaneous oxygen saturation above 95%.
Cardiac monitor
Administer beta-2 specific nebulized bronchodilator.
Administer antibiotics if needed.
Administer corticosteroids for moderate to severe episodes.
Consider epinephrine.

Status asthmaticus

Status asthmaticus is asthma that fails to respond to conventional therapy. It will lead to respiratory failure if therapeutic intervention is not applied.

■ **THERAPEUTIC INTERVENTIONS**

Administer beta-2 specific nebulized bronchodilator every 20 minutes until resolution of bronchospasm.
Administer humidified oxygen therapy according to arterial blood gas values/transcutaneous oxygen saturation.
Establish an IV line—consider hydration to maintain adequate volume status.
Administer corticosteroids.
Consider IV aminophylline for patients who do not respond to inhaled beta agonists.
Treat fluid and electrolyte imbalances according to laboratory values.
Be prepared to handle respiratory arrest.

Bronchiolitis

Bronchiolitis is a viral infection of the lower respiratory tract that occurs in children less than 2 years old, most often in children under 1 year. It is most often caused by respiratory syncytial virus.

■ **SIGNS AND SYMPTOMS**

Poor feeding
Rhinorrhea
History of mild respiratory infection
Respiratory difficulty
Wheezing, dyspnea
Frequent coughing
Prolonged expiratory phase
Intercostal and subcostal retractions
Nasal flaring

■ **THERAPEUTIC INTERVENTIONS**

Monitor transcutaneous oxygen saturation.
Nasal washing for RSV culture
Administer beta-2 specific nebulized bronchodilator.
Humidified oxygen to keep sats > 95%
Corticosteroids
Contact precautions unless RSV cultures are negative.
IV hydration only if not taking adequate liquids.

Pneumonia

Pneumonia is an inflammation of the lung parenchyma caused by a variety of infectious agents, including viruses and bacteria.

Viral

Most commonly respiratory syncytial and parainfluenza viruses.

■ **SIGNS AND SYMPTOMS**
Gradual onset over a few days, preceded by upper respiratory infection
Cough
Low-grade fever
Rales
Tachypnea
Wheezing
Apnea episode in infant

■ **THERAPEUTIC INTERVENTIONS**
Hydration as necessary
Antipyresis
Oxygen as needed
Nasal aspiration for RSV titer

Bacterial

■ **SIGNS AND SYMPTOMS**
More abrupt onset
Fever
Tachypnea, tachycardia
Grunting respirations
Decreased breath sounds
Meningismus with upper lobe pneumonia
Older children may complain of abdominal pain with lower lobe pneumonia

■ **THERAPEUTIC INTERVENTIONS**
Same as with viral
Antimicrobial therapy

FEVERS

An elevated temperature is probably the single most common cause for which a parent brings a child to the emergency department. Fevers have various causes, most commonly infection, but also can result from poisonings, dehydration, and collagen–vascular diseases.

■ **SIGNS AND SYMPTOMS**

Rapid pulse	Flushed skin
Tachypnea	Agitation
Diaphoresis	

■ **THERAPEUTIC INTERVENTIONS**
Give forced fluids (clear liquids).
Dress the child in lightweight clothing.
Give antipyretic medication: acetaminophen (Tylenol), 15 mg/kg initially and/or Ibuprofen, 10 mg/kg; avoid
   Ibuprofen if newborn or child has been vomiting. Do not use aspirin in a child under 12 years of age.
Give tepid bath or shower.
Treat the cause of the fever.
Fever without a known cause in the infant under 3 months of age should receive fever work-up, including
   lumbar puncture, blood cultures, and urine culture.

SEIZURES

The most common etiology of seizures in children is fever. Febrile seizures usually occur between the ages of 3 months and 5 years. They occur in association with a febrile illness, most often of viral etiology. Two thirds of children who have had seizures will not have another. Frequent causes of seizures are central nervous system infections, poisoning, epilepsy, and head injury.

Refer to Chapter 12, Neurologic Emergencies, for further information on seizure disorders.

POISONING

Pediatric poisoning can be difficult to diagnose in the field and the emergency department. It is important, on the telephone as well as in person, to obtain a good history from the child's parents, relatives, friends, or neighbors.

What drug or product did the child take?

How much did the child take?

When did the child take it?

Is the child having any symptoms at present?

Is the child having difficulty breathing?

What medication does the child take routinely?

Has the child ever done this before?

Request that the product or product container, even if empty, be brought to the emergency department.

Calls concerning poisoning should be referred to the nearest poison control area for management. Pediatric signs and symptoms and therapeutic interventions for poisoning are similar to those in adults. Please refer to Chapter 16, Toxicologic Emergencies, for this information.

Poisoning Statistics

According to the annual report of the American Association of Poison Control Centers, children younger than 3 years of age were involved in 44% of the cases; and 59% occurred in children less than 6 years.[1] A male predominance is found among poison exposure victims younger than 13 years, but the gender distribution is reversed in teenagers. Children younger than 6 years of age comprised only 4.1% of the fatalities. Children younger than 6 years are more likely to ingest nontoxic substances or minute amounts of toxic substances. The majority of preschoolers' ingestions are done because they are curious; adolescents' ingestions are most often suicide attempts.

"Red Flag" Drugs and Products

The following drugs and products can cause serious toxicity in children (often with a very small dose or amount).

Clonidine—signs and symptoms occur within 30 minutes. Decreased blood pressure, decreased respirations (apnea), bradycardia, and coma.

Clozapine (Clozari)—one half tablet has caused respiratory arrest in a child.

Cyclic antidepressants.

Lomotil (Diphenoxylate)—requires 24-hour hospitalization in children.

Isoniazid causes seizures—causes pyridoxine deficiency. Pyridoxine (Vitamin B_6) is antidotal.

Chloroquine (antimalarial drug) has a quinidine-like effect on the heart and vasodilatory properties.

Super nail glue removers—contain a product converted to cyanide.

Oil of wintergreen—contains methyl salisalate 98% 1 ml—1365 mg of salycylate.

Propoxyphene (Darvon) causes CNS and cardiovascular decrease, coma, and seizure. Sudden respiratory arrest within 15 to 30 minutes.

Nicotine causes sudden onset seizures in 15 to 90 minutes.

Camphor-containing products cause sudden onset seizures within 5 minutes.

Organophosphate pesticides cause CNS decrease, dyspnea, and coma.

Calcium channel blockers—children with one tablet of the sustained-release variety have developed bradycardia and hypotension 16 to 24 hours after ingestion. Admit.

Chloral hydrate—deep coma occurs rapidly.

Highest frequency of substances ingested by children:

1. Over-the-counter drugs
2. Prescription drugs
3. Cleaners
4. Cosmetics
5. Plants

Button Battery Ingestion

There are several hundred button battery ingestions by children in the United States every year. X-ray localization should be done in all button battery ingestions, regardless of whether the child is symptomatic or not. If the battery is retained in the esophagus, removal is indicated to prevent esophageal burns and more serious sequelae, such as death. If the battery is not in the esophagus and child has no peritoneal signs, discharge to home. Parents are instructed to search stool to recover battery and to contact Poison Control Center for further information.

Iron Ingestion

Iron ingestion is the primary cause of pediatric poisoning deaths. It is rapidly absorbed in the small intestine. Excess iron is directly caustic to the gastrointestinal mucosa, causing hemorrhage with resulting hypovolemia and shock.[2]

Aftercare Instructions for Parents (Table 34-3)

Discuss:

  Follow-up care

  Prevention

See Table 34-3 for key prevention concepts compiled by the New Hampshire Poison Information Center.

THE UNCONSCIOUS CHILD

Evaluation of the unconscious child must be rapid, systematic, and thorough.

Ensure ABCs.

Monitor transcutaneous oxygen saturation by pulse oximetry; administer oxygen as necessary; consider intubation.

Cardiac monitor

Full vital signs, rectal temp

Make neurologic assessment, including Pediatric Glasgow Coma Scale (Table 34-4).

Obtain history from family.

Initiate IV, nasogastric tube, Foley catheter.

Laboratory evaluation: CBC, lytes, BUN, CR. Consider when indicated LFTs, ammonia and toxicology screen, ABG, ETOH level, lumbar puncture, CT scan of head.

Chest x-ray

Keep examining room warm and child covered whenever possible to prevent heat loss.

TABLE 34-3   Key Prevention Concepts Compiled by the New Hampshire Poison
Information Center

POISON PROOF YOUR HOME	MEDICINE SAFETY	PESTICIDE SAFETY	PROTECT YOUR CHILD
Throw away antidote charts. Most charts are outdated. Call the Poison Center for information instead.	Do not take medicines in front of children. They tend to mimic adults.	Read and follow label directions before using a pesticide.	Put products away immediately after they are used.
Ammonia—mix with water only.	Do not refer to medicine as candy.	Remove food and dishes before treating a kitchen area. Wait for shelves to dry before replacing items.	Do not leave a child and poison alone "for a second." A considerable number of poisonings occur while a parent is on the telephone.
Perfumes, colognes, and aftershaves—store them as you would medicine.	Do not give medicine in the dark or without reading the label.	Keep children and pets away from sprayed area for 24-48 hours.	If you have young children, crawl on your hands and knees to see if there are any hazards. This puts you at their eye level and you may spot a possible hazard. Brightly colored containers and objects, especially red, attract a child's attention.
Insecticides, weedkillers, gasoline, and turpentine—lock up in a cabinet.	Lock medicines in a cabinet. Clean out medicine cabinet twice a year. Flush old or outdated medicine down the toilet.	Avoid breathing the fumes. Ventilate the inside of the house well before re-entering.	
Ashtrays—empty and keep cigarettes and butts out of the reach of children.	Keep grandmother's pocketbook on a high shelf when she is visiting. Elderly frequently carry pills in their purse without childproof caps.	Wear washable clothing that covers your arms, legs, and feet. (Suede, leather, boots and jewelry cannot be decontaminated.)	Destroy berries and mushrooms from any areas on your property that are accessible to children.
Medications and vitamins—keep safety caps securely on and out of the reach of children.		Never spray outdoors on a windy day.	
Know the names of your plants both indoors and outdoors.		Avoid breaks, spills, and splashes from container.	
Post local regional poison centers number near telephone		Store pesticides in their original container in a locked cabinet.	
Keep all medicines in original containers with child-proof caps		When finished, take a thorough shower, washing hair and skin twice with soap. Wash contaminated clothing separately.	
		Mixing or diluting should be done outside in a well-ventilated area.	
		Lock up poisons in a specific cupboard or in a tackle box!	

TABLE 34-4   Pediatric Glasgow Coma Score (PGCS)

GLASGOW COMA SCORE (GCS)	PEDIATRIC MODIFICATION	
Eye opening	**Eye opening**	
≥1 year	*0-1 year*	
4 Spontaneously	Spontaneously	
3 To verbal command	To shout	
2 To pain	To pain	
1 No response	No response	
Best motor response	**Best motor response**	
≥1 year	*0-1 year*	
6 Obeys command		
5 Localizes pain	Localizes pain	
4 Flexion withdrawal	Flexion withdrawal	
3 Flexion abnormal (decorticate)	Flexion abnormal (decorticate)	
2 Extension (decerebrate)	Extension (decerebrate)	
1 No response	No response	
Best verbal response	**Best verbal response**	
>5 years	*2-5 years*	*0-2 years*
5 Oriented and converses	Appropriate words and phrases	Cries appropriately, smiles, coos
4 Disoriented and converses	Inappropriate words	Cries
3 Inappropriate words	Cries/screams	Inappropriate crying/screaming
2 Incomprehensible sounds	Grunts	Grunts
1 No response	No response	No response

A score is given in each category. The individual scores are then added (range 3-15). A score <8 indicates severe neurologic injury.
From Barkin R: *Pediatric emergency medicine,* St Louis, 1992, Mosby.

Causes of Unconsciousness in a Child

Central nervous system

Trauma
Infection
Seizures

Cardiovascular

Congestive failure
Congenital heart disease
Infection

Respiratory

Acute respiratory failure/obstruction/hypoxia
Trauma
Allergy
Infection

Shock

Septic
Hypovolemic

Neurogenic
Cardiogenic
Anaphylactic

Gastrointestinal

Vomiting and diarrhea
Dehydration

Metabolic

Ketoacidosis
Hypoglycemia
Toxic ingestions
Reye's syndrome

Endocrine

Addisonian crisis

MENINGITIS

Meningitis is an inflammation of the meninges of viral or bacterial etiology. The most common bacterial organisms are *H. influenzae*, *S. pneumoniae*, and *N. meningitidis*. The clinical presentation of meningitis varies with the age of the child and the severity of the illness.

■ **SIGNS AND SYMPTOMS**

Neonate
Irritability
Lethargy
High-pitched cry
History of fever is variable in neonates
Bulging anterior fontanelle
Poor feeding
Seizures

Infants
Irritability
Fever
Vomiting
Seizures
Nuchal rigidity
Lethargy
Apnea
Hypothermia

Children
Coma
Fever
Vomiting
Nuchal rigidity
Headache
Altered mental status

■ **THERAPEUTIC INTERVENTIONS**

Ensure ABCs
Lumbar puncture—see Figure 34-3 for positioning child LP.
An alternate position for infants is sitting upright with neck flexed forward.

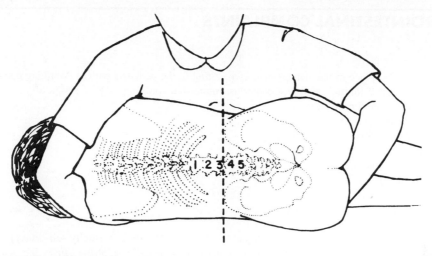

FIGURE 34-3. Position for pediatric lumbar puncture.
(From Barkin R et al: *Pediatric emergency medicine: concepts & clinical practice*, ed 2, St Louis, 1997, Mosby.)

IV line for fluid maintenance and IV antibiotics
Antipyretics for fever
Monitor vital signs and oxygen sat.
Isolation precautions

MENINGOCOCCEMIA

Meningococcemia is caused by *Neisseria meningitidis* and death can result within hours.

■ **SIGNS AND SYMPTOMS (rapid onset)**
Fever
Chills
Rash—maculopapular, petechial, or purpuric
Possible headache
Hypotension
Disseminated intravascular coagulation

■ **THERAPEUTIC INTERVENTIONS**
Immediate treatment
Cardiac monitor
O_2 saturation
Careful monitoring of vital signs
Isolation precautions
LP, septic work-up, CBC, electrolytes, glucose, ESR
Urinalysis, DIC screen
IV access
Prompt initiation of appropriate antibiotic therapy

GASTROINTESTINAL COMPLAINTS

Vomiting

Antiemetics have no place in the management of vomiting in the pediatric patient. Vomiting can have many causes, most often self-limiting viral gastroenteritis. Intractable vomiting may be a sign of:

Increased intracranial pressure
Reye's syndrome
Gastrointestinal reflux
Pyloric stenosis
Viral gastroenteritis
Bowel obstruction

Diarrhea

Diarrhea is commonly defined as 3 or more liquid stools a day. Diarrhea is usually self-limiting and caused by viral gastroenteritis. Bacteria and parasites can be other causes. Regardless of the cause, diarrhea should stop in less than a week.

If serious episodes of diarrhea occur, they may be accompanied by voluminous stools, bloody diarrhea, and/or vomiting.

■ THERAPEUTIC INTERVENTIONS

One half cup of oral rehydration solution after each stool or every hour. The solution should be taken in small amounts so it is easily absorbed.
Breastfeeding and eating solid foods should continue, especially carbohydrates and protein.
Avoid sugary drinks and salty soups.

Dehydration

Vomiting and diarrhea are the most common causes of dehydration in a child.

Approximately 60% of a child's body weight and 78% of a newborn's weight is fluid, 25% of which is extracellular and thus unstable. This fact, coupled with the child's high metabolic rate (with a high fluid turnover) and kidneys that are inefficient (producing a large amount of dilute urine), predispose the child to dangerous dehydration when large amounts of fluid are lost rapidly through fever, vomiting, or diarrhea.

Table 34-5 provides estimation of dehydration.

■ SIGNS AND SYMPTOMS

Dry mucous membranes
Decreased urination
Weight loss
Depressed anterior fontanelle
Thirst
Absence of tears
Reduced skin turgor
Listlessness
Sunken eyeballs
Orthostatic hypotension

■ THERAPEUTIC INTERVENTIONS

Obtain electrolytes, BUN, urine specific gravity. Give initial bolus of 20 ml/kg RL or NS over 20 minutes. If no improvement, repeat 20 mg/kg bolus or RL or NS, then hydrate according to weight and percentage of dehydration.
Mild to moderate dehydration:
Orally rehydrate with solutions such as Pedilyte or Ricelyte.

TABLE 34-5   Estimation of Dehydration

CLINICAL MANIFESTATIONS	DEGREE OF DEFICIT			
	5%	10%	15%	20%
Heart rate	Normal range	Compensatory tachycardia	Noncompensatory tachycardia	Morbid tachycardia Bradycardia
Blood pressure	Normal range	Normal range	Low normal	↓Blood pressure
Quality of pulses	Normal	2+ peripheral 3+ central	1+ peripheral 2+ central	0 peripheral 1+ central
Capillary refill	2-3 sec.	>3 sec.	>4 sec.	>5 sec.
Urinary output	<2 ml/kg/h	<1 ml/kg/h	<0.5 ml/kg/h	None
Level of consciousness	Irritable	Irritable/lethargic	Obtunded	Obtunded/coma
Color/temperature	Pink/warm	Pale/cool	Cyanotic/cold	Ashen/cold
Mucous membranes	Moist	Dry	Dry	Parched
Fontanel	Flat	Slightly depressed	Sunken	Sunken
Weight	↓5%	↓10%	↓15%	↓20%

From Jackson DB, Saunders R: *Child health nursing,* Philadelphia, 1992, Lippincott.

Frequent small amounts of fliud (5 to 10 cc) are tolerated best.
Monitor urine output.
Severe dehydration
Establish IV access.
Initial fluid bolus of 20 ml/kg RL or NS more than 20 minutes
If no improvement, repeat bolus.
Then hydrate according to weight and percentage of dehydration.
Monitor level of consciousness.
Careful record of I & O

ABDOMINAL PAIN

A definite cause for abdominal pain in the ambulatory pediatric patient is not always found. The most common cause of abdominal pain in children is viral gastroenteritis. Constipation is a frequent cause. Other causes of pediatric abdominal pain include pneumonia, lead intoxication, diabetic ketoacidosis, poisoning, and foreign body ingestion. Children should be evaluated appropriately to rule out the more serious causes of abdominal pain. Abdominal surgical emergencies will be discussed in the next chapter. Common tests to evaluate abdominal pain are complete blood count and urinalysis.

VARICELLA (CHICKENPOX)

Varicella is caused by the same organism that causes herpes zoster. There is a 14- to 21-day incubation period. Varicella is contagious from 1 day before the appearance of the rash until all lesions begin to crust, approximately 5 days. Children with varicella appear mildly sick. The level of illness seems to parallel the amount of rash involved. The rash, which consists of macules, papules, and vesicles, occurs primarily on the trunk and extremities, although it is not uncommon to find some amount of rash on the face. Children with varicella usually develop a rash as the first sign of the disease. Occasionally they will have a slight fever for 1 or 2 days before the rash appears. If a child is immunosuppressed, danger of severe illness is great. Hospital admission is required.

Therapeutic intervention includes administration of antipyretics, antihistamines, and lots of oral fluids as well as other supportive therapy. Avoid aspirin. Oatmeal baths may help relieve itching. The caregiver should be sure that the child's fingernails are short to avoid bacterial infection when the child scratches the lesions.

SUDDEN INFANT DEATH SYNDROME

Sudden infant death syndrome (SIDS), or crib death, is the sudden, unexpected death of an apparently healthy baby for which no adequate cause of death can be found on autopsy. It usually occurs in infants between the ages of 1 month and 1 year, with peak incidence being at 2 to 4 months. There are several theories as to why SIDS occurs. The most prominent, though unproved, of these are that SIDS is caused by:

Disorder (apnea) of sleep
Nasal congestion (infants are obligate nose breathers)
Laryngeal spasms

On postmortem examinations of SIDS victims, some of the more common findings are:

Frothy sputum in the mouth and nose
Emesis
Small height and weight for age
Empty bladder and rectum
Intrathoracic petechiae
Pulmonary congestion
Dilated right heart

■ **THERAPEUTIC INTERVENTIONS**

Usually nothing can be done to save the infant despite rigorous resuscitation efforts. Most therapeutic intervention will be directed toward the grieving parents. The most common reaction by parents of a child who dies of SIDS is complete devastation. There are many guilty feelings and much self-blame or blame of one parent by the other parent, especially if one parent is away at the time of the infant's death. The incidence of divorce is very high among parents with infants who have died from SIDS.

It is important, after some preparatory counseling, to state that the baby is dead and has died from SIDS. Let the parents know that SIDS is a common cause of death in infancy and that there was nothing they could have done to prevent it. It is important to let them know that it is *not* a hereditary disease.

Arrange for an autopsy and inform the parents that they will be notified of the cause of death within 48 hours. Once the parents receive notification of the official cause of death, schedule another counseling session with them. If this is beyond the capabilities of your staff, refer the family to the National Foundation for Sudden Infant Death Syndrome, 8240 Professional Place, Landover, MD 20785. The number of a local SIDS parent group can be obtained from the national group or local phone directory.

REFERENCES

1. Litovitz TL: 1992 Annual report of the American Association of Poison Control Centers National Data Collection System, *Am J Emerg Med* 9:497, 1993.
2. Barkin R et al: *Pediatric emergency medicine,* St Louis, 1996, Mosby.

SUGGESTED READINGS

Austin P: The pediatric patient: general approach and unique concerns. In Rosen et al: *Emergency medicine,* ed 4, St Louis, 1998, Mosby.
Flaherty L: Neonates and premature infants: overview of differences and ED management, *J Emerg Nurs* 22(2):120-124, 1996.
Henderson D, Peckham D: Summer surfing, indoors: the Emergency Medical Services for Children (EMSC) website, *J Emerg Nurs* 22(4):347-349, 1996.
Keddington R: A triage vital sign policy for a children's hospital emergency department, *J Emerg Nurs* 24(2):189-192, 1998.
Kelley SJ: *Pediatric nursing,* ed 2, New York, 1997, Appleton & Lange.
Losek JD: Intossusception: don't miss the diagnosis! *Ped Emerg Care* 9:46, 1993.
Pediatric update, bimonthly column, *J Emerg Nurs,* 1991-1999.
Strawser D: Pediatric bacterial meningitis in the emergency department, *J Emerg Nurs* 23(4):310-315, 1997.
Todres ID, Fugate JH: *Critical care of infants and children,* Philadelphia, 1996 Lippincott.
Zaritsky AL, Luten RC: Pediatric resuscitation. In Rosen et al: *Emergency medicine,* ed 4, St Louis, 1998, Mosby.

Pediatric Trauma and Surgical Emergencies

Anne Phelan Bowen

More than half of all childhood deaths (ages 1 to 14) result from injury. Mechanisms of injury causing pediatric deaths include unintentional injuries, such as motor vehicle incidents, falls, drowning and burns, as well as intentional injuries, such as homicide, suicide, and child abuse. Thousands of children require emergency department treatment annually as a result of trauma, many of whom suffer permanent disability.

The principles of trauma assessment and management are the same for the child victim as the adult. However the caregiver should be familiar with some issues unique to children. The vast majority of pediatric trauma results from blunt trauma (approximately 85%) as opposed to penetrating injury (approximately 15%). The injured child is best cared for in an emergency department prepared to meet his or her unique needs, with appropriate personnel and equipment.[1] A quick reference system for identifying the right-sized equipment for children can save precious minutes. The Broselow tape and color coded boxes are the most frequently used system (Figure 35-1).

PRIMARY SURVEY

This rapid initial assessment is used to identify and treat life-threatening injuries.

Airway (with Full Spine Immobilization)

■ **DEVELOPMENTAL/ANATOMIC CONSIDERATIONS**
Oral cavity is small in comparison to tongue size.
Young infants under 3 months are obligate nasal breathers.
The narrowest portion of a child's airway is the cricoid cartilage.

■ **ASSESSMENT**
Assure patency of airway.
Look for oral foreign bodies.
Maintain full spine immobilization.

■ **THERAPEUTIC INTERVENTIONS**
Use the jaw thrust maneuver to open the airway in an unconscious child.
Suction any obstructing matter, such as blood, emesis, or secretions from the airway.
Oral airways, when required, are inserted using a forward motion with the tongue depressed outward.
Rotation of the airway is contraindicated because it may cause trauma to the soft tissues of the palate and hypopharynx.
Nasal airways are better tolerated by the conscious child. These are to be used in the absence of maxillofacial injuries.

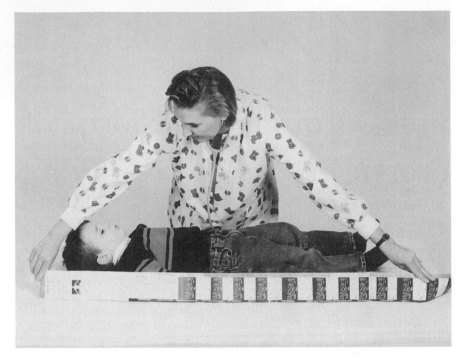

FIGURE 35-1. The Broselow tape system is one way to organize pediatric resuscitation equipment. The child's length is measured against the tape measure. This leads the team to a color-coded pack or code cart drawer containing the appropriate sizes of equipment for that child.
(Courtesy Armstrong Medical Industries, Lincolnshire, IL.)

Intubation is recommended when respiratory distress or poor ventilation persist, or when the child has a Glasgow coma score (GCS) of 8 or less. Use an uncuffed tube for children younger than 8 years old to avoid cord trauma, subglottic edema, and pressure necrosis.

Breathing

Because children have a high metabolic rate, they also have a higher rate of oxygen consumption than adults. When breathing becomes inadequate, hypoxemia occurs more rapidly.

■ **ASSESSMENT**

Observe respiratory rate, depth, symmetry, and quality.

Observe for signs of respiratory distress or air hunger; grunting, nasal flaring, retractions, head bobbing, or shoulder lifting.

Auscultate breath sounds for equality and adventitious sounds.

Palpate the position of the trachea gently, noting the presence of any crepitus.

Check the integrity of the chest wall.

■ **THERAPEUTIC INTERVENTIONS**

Administer 100% oxygen to all children, at least during the initial assessment.

Monitor oxygen saturation, via pulse oximetry, noting that readings are unreliable in children with poor peripheral perfusion.

Provide assisted ventilation with bag-valve-mask or positive pressure ventilation.

Decompress suspected tension pneumothorax with needle thoracostomy and prepare for chest tube insertion.

Prepare for intubation for optimal long-term aggressive airway management.

Circulation

Children have a circulating blood volume of approximately 80cc/kg and a strong young heart muscle. In the presence of a decrease in circulating blood volume, their primary mechanism to increase their cardiac output is to increase their heart rate. Hypotension is a late sign of shock in children, usually occurring after a circulating blood loss of about 25%.

■ **ASSESSMENT**

Check capillary refill time.

Observe for areas of external hemorrhage.

Palpate the quality and effectiveness of a peripheral and central pulse.

Observe skin color and temperature.

■ **THERAPEUTIC INTERVENTIONS**

If pulseless, initiate CPR and follow pediatric advanced life support protocols.

If pulse is present but ineffective, obtain vascular access using 2 large-bore IV catheters (or obtain intraosseous access) and administer a 20 cc/kg bolus of warmed Ringer's lactate or normal saline. If response is unsatisfactory, repeat the bolus and administer 10cc/kg of packed RBCs (type specific or O negative) to prevent coagulopathies.

Apply direct pressure to areas of uncontrolled external hemorrhage.

Disability—Neurologic Evaluation

Children's large head size in relation to body size, accompanied by more lax neck muscles, make them more susceptible to head injuries. Head injuries are the leading cause of traumatic death and disability in children.

■ **ASSESSMENT**

Assess pupillary size, shape and response.

Determine level of consciousness using the GCS or AVPU scale.

A- alert and oriented

V- responsive to verbal stimuli

P- responsive to painful stimuli

U- unresponsive

■ **THERAPEUTIC INTERVENTIONS**

Consider pharmacologic intervention to improve mental status in selected cases, such as narcan or D25.

Restrict IV fluids to ⅔ maintenance only when the child is hemodynamically stable.

SECONDARY SURVEY

After completing the primary survey and resuscitation, perform a secondary survey to identify all injuries present. The child's respiratory, circulatory, and neurologic status are also frequently reassessed. Because the remaining injuries are not immediately life threatening, the following interventions identified in the secondary survey are performed at the end of the assessment:

Expose the child by undressing so that a complete assessment can be performed.

Warm the child. Children lose body heat more quickly than adults, so they should be kept warm by blankets, radiant warmers, and warmed IV fluids.

Get a full set of vital signs, including a blood pressure and rectal temperature.

Obtain a history from the caregiver and EMS personnel. The history should include: mechanism of injury, treatment before arrival, past medical history, allergies, medications, immunization status, and last food/fluid intake.

Perform a head-to-toe assessment in detail, including both anterior and posterior body surfaces.

Interventions after the secondary survey may include:

Sending trauma labs

Preparing for trauma imaging

Dressing lacerations or debriding burn wounds

Splinting suspected fracture sites

Placing Foley catheter and/or naso/orogastric tube

SELECTED INJURIES

Head Trauma

Head injuries are very common in children primarily because of their large head size in relation to body mass. Most childhood head trauma is blunt in nature, and head injuries account for most of the permanent disabilities seen.

- A great volume of blood can be lost via scalp laceration.
- An infant can have a severe enough intracranial bleed to become hypotensive and shocky, but brainstem herniation is rarer than in older children. Observe the infant for bulging anterior fontanelles up to approximately age 12 to 18 months.
- Occasionally depressed skull fractures may be palpable. Boggy crepitant swellings associated with subgaleal hematoma is often felt over linear skull fractures.
- Seizures sometimes occur as a result of head injuries. Children with significant intracranial bleeds or diffuse cerebral edema are often given prophylactic anticonvulsant medications.
- Cerebral perfusion pressure is calculated by subtracting the intracranial pressure (normal is less than 15mm Hg) from the systolic blood pressure. If the systolic blood pressure is low and the intracranial pressure is high, cerebral perfusion pressure will be low and the brain will not receive an adequate supply of oxygen and nutrients.
- Children often suffer cerebral hyperemia following significant head injuries. The etiology of this increased cerebral blood flow is not known. One method of decreasing the amount of blood flowing to the brain is to hyperventilate the child to a PCO_2 of 30 to 35mm Hg.
- In children with penetrating neck injuries, careful attention must be paid to ongoing assessment of their airway. The bleeding and swelling resulting from this trauma often cause airway compromise.

Blunt Abdominal Trauma

The intraabdominal organs in children are less protected by an immature cartilaginous rib cage and less firm musculature than adults.

- The most common sites of injury in the abdomen are the liver, spleen, and intestines.
- Blunt abdominal trauma in children is difficult to assess. Use of CT scan is advisable. Ultrasound imaging is also emerging as a valuable assessment tool.
- Early placement of a nasogastric tube will decompress the stomach, reduce diaphragmatic irritation, and improve respiratory effort. The stomach can often become distended when children swallow air while crying.
- In the absence of blood at the urinary meatus, insertion of a Foley catheter will enable the nurse to carefully monitor urinary output.
- Measurement of the abdominal girth at the level of the umbilicus will enable the team to detect more subtle abdominal distension.

Extremity Trauma

Sprains, strains, and limb fractures are frequent childhood injuries.

- Comparison views of the uninjured side may be required.
- Fractures occurring near the epiphyseal (growth) plates require specialized attention.

- Always obtain x-rays of the joint above and below a subtle suspected fracture site in children not yet able to communicate the pinpoint level of their pain to the caregiver.
- Document the peripheral neurovascular assessment after any manipulation or splinting of the injured extremity.

COMMON TRAUMA LAB TESTS IN CHILDREN

Type and cross-match	Prothrombin time
CBC + differential	Partial thromboplastin time
Serum electrolytes	Glucose
BUN	Arterial blood gases
Amylase	

(Should be able to run all the specimens listed above with 7 to 10 ml of blood.)

STANDARD TRAUMA X-RAYS

Cervical spine
Chest
Pelvis
CT scan as indicated

PEDIATRIC SURGICAL EMERGENCIES

Appendicitis

Appendicitis is common in adolescents and young adults. It is the most common cause of abdominal surgery in children. It is often difficult to diagnose in the early stages of inflammation in infants and toddlers. The incidence of rupture in children under 6 years of age exceeds 50%, possibly because of the thickness of the appendiceal wall in these younger patients.[2]

■ **SIGNS AND SYMPTOMS**

Starts as periumbilical pain, then localizes in right lower quadrant—McBurney's point
Anorexia—if not present, appendicitis unlikely
Vomiting
Decrease in activity level
Guarding of right lower quadrant
Pain with movement
Mild temperature elevation
With rupture—high fever, rigid abdomen, tachycardia, dehydration

■ **THERAPEUTIC INTERVENTIONS**

Maintenance of NPO
Hydration
Abdominal x-ray film*
CBC
Urinalysis to rule out other causes
Abdominal ultrasound if difficulty obtaining diagnosis
Antibiotic therapy
Early operative intervention

*Febrile children should also get a chest x-ray. Lower lobe pneumonias often cause diaphragmatic irritation. Pain is referred to the lower abdomen, mimicking appendicitis pain, especially in school-age children.

Intussusception

Intussusception is the telescoping of one segment of bowel into another. It most commonly occurs between the ages of 3 to 12 months with a male predominance. The usual location is the ileocecal valve.

■ **SIGNS AND SYMPTOMS**

May have had respiratory infection or viral gastroenteritis.

Episodic abdominal pain, comfortable between episodes

Vomiting after onset of pain occurs in 50% of cases.

Passage of "currant jelly" stool with bloody mucus in ⅓ of children with intussusception

Early exam may be normal except colic.

Later in course: fever, tachycardia, dehydration, lethargy

■ **THERAPEUTIC INTERVENTIONS**

Maintenance of NPO

CBC, BUN, electrolytes

IV hydration

Abdominal x-ray film

Barium or air contrast enema for attempted reduction for hemodynamically stable child

Operative intervention if enema reduction failed, unstable child, or the intussusception recurs.

Incarcerated Inguinal Hernia

An inguinal hernia becomes incarcerated when viscera becomes entrapped in the hernial pouch. It occurs most often in infants under 1 year of age. With prolonged incarceration, there is increased edema and pressure, causing strangulation and tissue ischemia.

■ **SIGNS AND SYMPTOMS**

Cramping abdominal pain

Irritability

Vomiting

Firm to fluctuant mass in groin

Edema, erythema over mass with strangulated hernia

■ **THERAPEUTIC INTERVENTIONS**

Reduction in emergency department if not strangulated, with sedation

If strangulated, operative intervention

Malrotation with Midgut Volvulus

Malrotation is a congenital anomaly in which abnormal rotation and attachment of bowel to the mesentery occurs. The midgut, which consists of the duodenum, small intestine, and ascending to the midtransverse colon, then becomes vulnerable to twisting (volvulus) and infarction.

■ **SIGNS AND SYMPTOMS**

Bilious vomiting

Abdominal pain, distension

Bloody stools

Hematemesis

Later—shock, sepsis

■ **THERAPEUTIC INTERVENTIONS**

Stable—hydration, upper GI series, then operative intervention

Unstable—antibiotic therapy, emergency operative intervention

Testicular Torsion

Testicular torsion is the twisting of the spermatic cord causing venous obstruction, swelling, arterial ischemia, and testicular infarction. It often occurs in patients with a congenital abnormality of the spermatic cord, most often a bell clapper deformity. The adolescent age group is most commonly affected.

- **SIGNS AND SYMPTOMS**
  Usually acute onset of pain
  Swelling, tenderness, erythema of scrotum
  Enlarged testes
  Possible association with nausea, vomiting
  No urinary symptoms
  "Blue dot" sign, visible scrotal discoloration
- **THERAPEUTIC INTERVENTIONS**
  Doppler ultrasound if diagnosis uncertain
  Timely surgical correction to prevent testicular infarction

AERODIGESTIVE FOREIGN BODIES REQUIRING SURGICAL INTERVENTION

Ingestion and aspiration of foreign bodies occurs most frequently among infants, toddlers, and preschool children. Symptoms vary; the child can be asymptomatic or have acute airway compromise.

Airway Foreign Bodies

- **SIGNS AND SYMPTOMS**
  Witnessed episode of choking or gagging
  Dyspnea
  Cough
  Decreased breath sounds
  Stridor
  Wheezing
  Cyanosis
- **THERAPEUTIC INTERVENTIONS**
  Assess ABCs.
  Obtain chest x-ray film.
  Consider lateral decubitus view by fluoroscopy.
  Nasal foreign bodies may be treated with the oral insufflation technique or balloon catheter extraction.
  Depending on location of foreign body, removal by laryngoscopy or bronchoscopy.
  Assess for presence of a second foreign body.

Esophageal Foreign Bodies

Refer to Figure 35-2
- **SIGNS AND SYMPTOMS**
  Can be asymptomatic
  Drooling
  Inability to swallow food
  Vomiting
  Pain in neck or throat

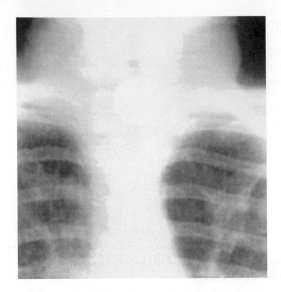

FIGURE 35-2. Coin in esophagus appears round. If lodged in trachea, it would look like a slit.
(From Silverman F, Kuhn J: *Coffey's pediatric x-ray diagnosis: an integrated imaging approach*, ed 9, vol 1, St Louis, 1993, Mosby.)

■ **THERAPEUTIC INTERVENTIONS**

Assess ABCs.

Obtain PA and lateral x-rays of the chest and neck.

All esophageal foreign bodies must be removed, usually by esophagoscopy.

If recent ingestion, some esophageal foreign bodies can be removed under fluoroscopy.

Gastrointestinal Foreign Bodies

■ **SIGNS AND SYMPTOMS**

History of ingestion

Usually asymptomatic

Exam usually benign

Rare perforation

■ **THERAPEUTIC INTERVENTIONS**

Chest x-ray film

Most often conservative treatment

If ingested object is very large or has sharp edges, child will require hospitalization.

Operative intervention is required when there is significant bleeding, peritoneal signs are present, or there is failure to progress through GI tract.

REFERENCES

1. Seidel J, Tittle S, Henderson D et al: Guidelines for pediatric equipment and supplies for emergency departments, *J Emerg Nurs* 22:1-4, 1996.
2. Ashcraft K, Holder T: *Pediatric surgery,* ed 2, Philadelphia, 1993, Saunders.

SUGGESTED READINGS

Baker S: Advances and Adventures in Trauma Prevention, *J Trauma* 42(3):369, 1997.
Buntain W: *Management of pediatric trauma,* Philadelphia, 1995, Saunders.

Cardona V et al: *Trauma nursing: from resuscitation through rehabilitation,* ed 2, Philadelphia, 1994, Saunders.

Girotti M: Reengineering trauma care: the challenge of the nineties, *J Trauma* 40(6):855, 1996.

Givens T: Pediatric cervical spine injury: a three year experience, *J Trauma* 41(2):310, 1996.

Hulka F et al: Influence of a statewide trauma system on pediatric hospitalization and outcome, *J Trauma* 42(3):514, 1997.

Moront M et al: The injured child an approach to care, *Pediatr Clin North Am* 41(6):1201, 1994.

Pieper P: Pediatric trauma, an overview, *Nurs Clin North Am* 29(4):563, 1994.

Ravenscraft K: Psychological considerations for the child with acute trauma. In Randolph JC et al, editors: *The injured child: surgical management,* Chicago, 1979, Year Book Medical Publishers.

Rhoads J: Trauma care, trauma prevention, and the role of the American Trauma Society, *J Trauma* 41(3):375, 1996.

Scaletta T, Schaider J: *Emergent management of trauma,* New York, 1996, McGraw-Hill.

Child Abuse and Neglect

Deborah Parkman Henderson

Although child maltreatment has always been present, western culture recognized it as a problem only with the publication by Kempe and associates in 1962.[1] It is now estimated that there are 652,000 cases of child maltreatment in the United States each year.[2] Of the *known* cases 49% are reported by hospitals (personnel in emergency departments and pediatric units) and physicians, 23% by police, 12% by schoolteachers, nurses, and guidance counselors, and 16% by others (neighbors, friends, and even parents themselves).[3]

Child maltreatment is defined as any harm that occurs to a child as a result of physical, emotional, or sexual abuse. It can take many forms. Many children are the victims of more than one type of abuse.

TYPES OF ABUSE

Physical Neglect

Failure to provide basic needs, such as food, shelter, clothing, schooling, and medical care

Emotional Neglect/Abuse

Failure to provide a secure, loving, trusting, nurturing environment[4]
Actions or words by another that cause damage to a child's psychologic well-being

Physical Abuse

Nonaccidental trauma inflicted on a child

Sexual Abuse

Molestation of a child by an older child, an adolescent, or an adult, which can include violent acts and "non-touching" acts such as pornographic photography. (See Chapter 31).

DUTY TO REPORT

The duty to report actual or suspected child maltreatment exists in all 50 states. It must be reported to the local police and/or social service agency. Anyone who reports child maltreatment is immune from prosecution, Remember: The reporter does not have to prove child maltreatment to report it. If there is a suspicion, it should be reported.

FACTORS THAT MAY CONTRIBUTE TO CHILD MALTREATMENT

Sociologic Situations

Unemployment
Inadequate housing
Dangerous environment
Profound poverty[5]
Low self-esteem

Caretaker Stressors

Single parenting
Young mother[6]
Illness (especially chronic illness) of child
Many small children
Premature child
Child with feeding difficulty
Hyperactive child
Psychiatrically or physically ill parent[7]
Child with developmental disability
Child with physical disability
Addicted child (mother abused drugs during the prenatal period)
Parental alcohol or drug abuse

Situational Responses

Substance abuse by parent or significant other of parent
Parent/significant other competing with child for attention
Lack of impulse control

Parental Factors

History of abuse of the parent as a child
Belief that corporal punishment is an acceptable form of punishment
Inability to provide nurturing love
Domestic abuse of a parent

SIGNS AND SYMPTOMS OF CHILD MALTREATMENT

Neglect

- Unkempt appearance
- Unclean appearance
- Malnourished
- Poor dentition
- Inappropriate dress for weather conditions
- Failure to thrive
- Severe cradle cap
- Severe diaper rash

- Bald patches on scalp
- Attention-seeking behavior
- Usually passive or aggressive behavior

Physical Injury

What to pay attention to

- Lack of parental concern for injured child
- Manipulative behavior of the child
- Child seems unusually sad or depressed
- Confusing/conflicting stories
- Unexplained injury
- Injury inconsistent with history
- Evasive answers to questions
- Nonbelievable history
- History that does not fit the growth and development level of the child
- Frequent or repeated injuries
- Frequent emergency department visits for nonspecific problems
- No explanation of the injury
- Anger toward the child for being injured
- Use of many different emergency departments (to prevent discovery) (that is, "doctor shopping")
- The child's belief that punishment is deserved
- The child's fear of adults
- Low self-esteem in the child
- Attention-seeking behavior of the child

What to look for

■ **BRUISING**
abrasions/ecchymosis/lacerations in various stages of healing, hand prints, marks that take on the shape of the object, such as an extension cord, a rope, or a belt buckle

■ **BITE MARKS**
(human bite marks)

■ **FRACTURES**
Especially in children less than 3 years old
When the story is inconsistent with the type of fracture
Fractures in various stages of healing

■ **HEAD INJURIES**
Unexplained unconsciousness
Unexplained cardiopulmonary arrest
Subgaleal hematoma
Traumatic alopecia
Hair growing in various lengths in different spots
Subdural hematoma
If a subdural hematoma is found, it should be assumed to be caused by child maltreatment until proven
    otherwise
If a subdural hematoma is found in an infant, it may have been caused by severe shaking
Displaced nasal cartilage
Bleeding from nasal septum
Fractured mandible

- **MOUTH**
  Lacerated frenulum of upper lip, lower lip, under tongue
  Loosened or missing teeth not age appropriate
  Burns of lips or tongue
- **EYES**
  Hyphema
  Periorbital ecchymosis ("black eye")
  Retinal hemorrhage
  Detached retina
- **EARS**
  Ruptured tympanic membrane, bruising behind ear, injuries to external auricle (ear)
- **PETECHIAE**
  Choking may cause petechiae to form on the face and head
  May be caused by twisting the skin
- **TRUNCAL INJURIES**
  Bruising
  Burns
  Lacerations
- **GENITALIA AND PERINEAL INJURIES**
- **LIMB INJURIES**
  Fractures (metaphyseal, transverse, or oblique fractures, as well as rib fracture and skull fracture)
  Dislocations
- **BURNS**
  Unusual burn patterns
  Cigarette burns branding burns, hot object burns
  Submersion and immersion (stocking burns, glove burns) burns
  Scald burns
  Iron burns
  Chemical burns
  Electrical burns
  Microwave burns
- **POISONING**
  The story does not fit the findings
  The child has ingested alcohol or illegal drugs
  "Morning after" poisoning (drinks left over from party the night before)
- **MUNCHAUSEN'S-BY-PROXY**
  The history and symptoms have been fabricated by the caregiver to gain medical attention

Emotional Abuse
By the parents

Verbal abuse
Verbal threats
Constant criticism
Expectations that are outrageous
Use of a child to play husband against wife and vice versa
Extreme behaviors (anger, passivity)
Lack of affection shown toward the child
Use of child for bargaining between parents

The child may demonstrate

Withdrawal
Eating disorders
Head banging
Rocking
Learning disorders
Enuresis
Suicidal behavior
Self-destructive or risk-taking behavior

THE INTERVIEW

The initial interview in the emergency department will most likely set the tone for the entire evaluation process. This is a very preliminary interview *not* a forensic interview. Excessive questioning for fine details and directive questions should be avoided. The primary goal of therapeutic intervention in the emergency department is to care for the immediate medical needs of the child, to prevent further harm to the child, and to assist the child and the family to deal with this crisis.

The caregiver(s) and child should be interviewed separately. This will allow the caregiver(s) to become emotional without worrying about what their child will think while this is going on. Methods to interview a child will vary, depending on the child's growth and development age. It is always best to have one single interviewer talk to a child. Attempt to make the child feel comfortable.

- Ask open-ended questions at first.
- Avoid questions that deal directly with the assault at first.
- Be sure to use language that the child can understand.
- If the child does not speak with you, see if role reversal may help. Ask the child to pretend that he or she is the nurse and you are the child.
- Ask how many times this has happened before.
- Ask when this happened this time.
- Ask if this has happened to his or her brothers or sisters or any other children.
- Ask if the child knows the person who did it and who that person is.

THE EXAMINATION

Undress the child completely, providing for the child's modesty needs. Always take the time to explain what you are about to do. Perform:

- A primary and secondary survey
- A skeletal survey (performed on children who are younger than 3 years old or are unable to talk and have suspicious injuries)
- A hematological survey, if indicated
- A visual acuity examination, if indicated
- An eye examination
- A neurological examination
- A chest examination
- An abdominal examination (including a rectal examination); do not insert an instrument into the rectum or pelvis
- An assessment of growth and development level
- Check for other physical injuries.
- Toxicology screening

Be sure to carefully document all findings and to preserve evidence so that the chain of custody of the evidence is not broken. Record facts only—no speculation! Include quotes from the child and describe behaviors of the child. Document any strange reactions of the child. Use body maps to locate and document injuries (or findings). Describe any diagnostic tests that were done and any treatments that were given. Document any statements about when and where the abuse occured.

If photographs are taken, they must be labeled with the date and time they were taken, the child's name and medical record number, and the name of the person taking the photograph.

Following the examination, ask the child if he or she has any questions. Keep the caregiver(s) informed of the physical findings. Make sure to emphasize that follow-up appointments are very important to keep.

THE REPORT TO AUTHORITIES

The report will depend upon your institution's policies and procedures. In general, the following should be reported:

- The child's name (and possible other names used)
- The child's address and phone number
- The child's birth date
- Where the assault occurred
- The reason for your suspicion
- The cause of the injury
- The extent of the injury
- The circumstances surrounding the injury
- The name of the child's mother and father
- The name of the suspect
- The suspect's address and phone number
- Your name, work address, and work phone number
- A description of the child
- The location of the child when the abuse occurred
- Where the child lives now

Be sure to document to whom this information was reported and the date and time it was reported.

OTHER CONDITIONS THAT MIMIC CHILD MALTREATMENT

There are several other conditions that may mimic child maltreatment. Some common conditions are:

- Sudden infant death syndrome
- Failure to thrive
- Several coagulation disorders
- Blood dyscrasias
- Mongolian spots
- Ethnic practices that produce physical marks
  - Cupping and moxibustion (Chinese)
  - Coin rubbing (Vietnamese)
  - Scarring (East African)
- Reyes syndrome

PREVENTION OF CHILD MALTREATMENT

The key to a reduction in child maltreatment is prevention. Prevention can be accomplished to some extent by intensive education. Children must know that it is not OK to hurt anyone. Teenagers must know this also. And, most important, parents and other adults must understand that it is not OK to hurt a child. Families who are at high risk must receive education to learn how to cope with stress, to understand normal growth and development patterns, to know where to find help and support. Schoolteachers and guidance counselors should receive special education to identify families and children at risk and to identify a child who has been maltreated. An objective of the *Healthy People 2000* project is to reduce the incidence of child maltreatment to less than 25.2 per 1000 children.[8]

Hospital personnel, and emergency care personnel in particular, must be familiar with identification of the maltreated child and must be encouraged to report all suspected cases for the welfare of the child. In some states, education about child abuse is mandatory for certain professionals.

REFERENCES

1. Kempe CH et al: The battered child syndrome, *JAMA* 181:17-24, 1962.
2. US Department of Health and Human Services *2000: Summary report,* Washington, D.C., 1992, US Government Printing Office.
3. Ards S, Harkell A: Reporting of child maltreatment: a secondary analysis of the National Incidence Surveys, *Child Abuse Negl* 17(3):337, 1993.
4. Garbino J: Psychological child maltreatment: a developmental view, *Prim Care* 20(2):307, 1993.
5. US Department of Health and Human Services, National Center on Child Abuse and Neglect: *National study of the incidence and severity of child abuse and neglect: executive summary,* Washington, D.C., 1982, US Government Printing Office.
6. Stier DM et al: Are children born to young mothers at increased risk of maltreatment? *Pediatrics* 91(3):642, 1993.
7. Helfer RE, Kempe CH: *Child abuse and neglect,* Cambridge, Mass, 1970, Harper & Row.
8. US Department of Health and Human Services *2000: Summary report,* Washington, D.C., 1992, US Government Printing Office.

SUGGESTED READINGS

American Association of Pediatrics: Guidelines for the evaluation of sexually abused children, *Am Assoc Pediatr News,* Nov 1990.

Herman-Giddens ME: Vaginal foreign bodies and child sexual abuse, *Arch Pediatr Adolesc Med* 148:195, 1994.

Fountain K, Pierce B: Child abuse and neglect. In Emergency Nurses Association: *Sheehy's Emergency nursing,* ed 4, St Louis, 1998, Mosby.

Kelley SJ: Child abuse and neglect. In Kelley SJ: *Pediatric emergencies,* ed 2, Norwalk, Conn, 1996, Appleton & Lange.

Kelley SJ: Interviewing the sexually abused child, *JEN* 11:5, 234, 1985.

Kelley SJ: Critical communications for the sexually abused child, *Pediatr Nurs* 11:421, 1985.

Ladebauche P: Childhood trauma: when to suspect abuse, *RN* 60(9):38-43, 1997.

Tercier A: Child abuse. In Rosen et al: *Emergency medicine,* ed 4, St Louis, 1998, Mosby.

CHAPTER 37

Psychiatric Emergencies

Gail E. Polli

The goal of emergency care of the patient who has a psychiatric or psychologic crisis is to understand the etiology of the patient's acute distress and/or presenting problem and to intervene with short-term management and/or referral.

GENERAL MANAGEMENT TECHNIQUES

Identify the nature and severity of the patient's presenting problem. Often one must rely on the patient's family or friends for this information. There are certain key questions that should be answered:

Why is this person coming for help *now?*

Is the patient a danger to himself, herself, or others?

What were the events that led up to this condition?

Was there some thing or event that triggered it?

Who brought the patient in?

What does the patient expect from this visit?

What medication is the patient taking?

In the interview with the patient:

Appear calm and nonjudgmental.

Set firm limits, if necessary.

Encourage the patient to remain as focused as possible.

Be sure that help is nearby should the patient become physically dangerous; do not allow the patient to come between you and the door.

Try to decrease the patient's anxiety.

Do not argue with the patient or try to talk the patient out of how he/she is feeling.

Be clear in your explanations to the patient.

Be honest with the patient about your therapeutic plan.

MENTAL STATUS EXAMINATION

Patients who come to the emergency department with a chief complaint that may represent a psychiatric problem should have a mental status examination that includes the following parameters:

General

General appearance

Level of consciousness (for example, alert, lethargic, stuporous)

Orientation to time, place, person, reason for being there

Behavior and psychomotor activity

Attitude, the manner in which the patient relates (for example, hostile, cooperative, passive)

Speech

Rate
Tone
Fluency
Pressured

Mood

What is the subjective, internal emotion the patient is feeling? (Ask the patient.)

Affect

What is the patient's external range of expression (for example, flat, blunted, restricted, broad)?
Is this mood appropriate?

Intellect

Use of vocabulary
Level of education
Fundamentals of knowledge

Memory

Assess short-term, recent, and remote memory

Thought processes

Are there flights of ideas, loosening of associations, tangential thinking, or thought blocking?
Is the patient's thinking disorganized, rambling, or incoherent?

Content of thoughts

Does the patient have phobias?
Is the patient constantly repetitious?
Is the patient obsessive, compulsive, suicidal, preoccupied, or delusional?

Perception

Assess for the presence of hallucinations or illusions (type and content)

Insight and judgment

Understanding of problems, illness, and/or need for help or treatment (insight)
Ability to make sound decisions (judgment)

STRESS

Stress is a state that is intensified when there is a change or threat with which the individual must cope. Stress as a motivating force can help both the patient and the health care provider. Unchanneled stress can be inhibiting and debilitating.

Stress is:
Essential for life and growth
Always present to some degree, since every individual is continually adapting to internal and external environmental changes
A response to living
Subject to individual response and stimulus specificity
Displayed as specific signs and symptoms
Measurable qualitatively and quantitatively
Growth-promoting or growth-impeding

Considered psychologic when it focuses on the meaning of a stimulus and its anticipated capacity to produce harm

Considered physiologic when it focuses on the harm or disturbance to tissue structure or function that has already occurred

A stressor is a factor or agent that is perceived as a threat to existence or lifestyle and thereby causes an increase in the stress state. Assumptions regarding stressors include that they are:

A source of motivation for change

Categorized by origin: social, psychologic, or physical

Uniquely perceived by each individual

The product, and not the cause, of perception

A condition that imposes a demand on the individual for adjustment

Some generalized sources of stressors can be identified:

Sense of helplessness

Sense of hopelessness

Diminished ability to meet expectations of self or others

Diminished ability to function

Sense of isolation or alienation

Threat to identity through altered body image (real or imagined)

Loss of control (real or imagined)

Pain (emotional or physical)

Change in status (real or imagined)

Loss of someone or something important (a person, pet, home, job, or health)

Factors that influence stress response include:

Cognitive activity	Genetic influences
Personality traits	Past coping patterns
Past experiences	Situational factors
Cultural learning	Environmental factors
	Biologic variables

Classes of response to stressors include:

Affective

Motor-behavioral

Alteration of cognitive functioning

Physiologic changes

All responses to stressors (mental, emotional, cognitive, and somatic) consume energy. There is no correlation between the intensity of the stressor and the coping behavior used by an individual.

Assessment of Stress Level

Assessment of an individual's stress state is made by observation, interaction data, and clinical data. People respond to stress in a holistic manner, but the central nervous system and endocrine system create the most specific physiologic indices. Baseline information about blood pressure, pulse rate, and respiratory rate provide parameters for assessment of stress level, but an ongoing comparison of these parameters is needed, because none of them shows an absolute increase or decrease during periods of increased stress.

Observational and interaction data

■ IDENTIFICATION OF STRESSOR

Origin

Number

Duration

■ **ASSESSMENT OF PATIENT**
Degree of perceived threat
Past experience with comparable stressor
Physical and psychologic energy reserve
Resources, capabilities, and potential
Personality variables
Levels of anxiety
Appearance and physical history
■ **EVALUATION OF ENVIRONMENT**
Situational constraints
Cultural restraints
Social controls
Support system available

ANXIETY

Anxiety is a diffuse response that alerts an individual to an impending threat, real or imagined. Fear is a natural psychologic and physiologic response to an actual threat. Fear is object-focused, but anxiety is "faceless fear"—no identifiable object can be isolated.

The cause of anxiety is any perceived threat to the security of an individual. The origin may be the result of:
- Biologic factors:
  Alteration in homeostasis
  Lack of food, water, shelter, clothing
  Fear of illness, injury, surgery, old age, pain
- Psychologic factors:
  Decreased self-esteem
  Death or loss of a loved one or thing
  Pain
  Real or imagined rejection or abandonment
- Sociologic factors:
  Inability to meet expectations of role, status, values
  Inability to maintain sense of belonging
■ **THERAPEUTIC INTERVENTIONS**
The goal is to promote an environment in which the patient can achieve an adequate degree of self-control.
To decrease the patient's feelings of anxiety:
Provide general support.
Encourage the patient to talk.
Keep calm and appear calm.
Direct the patient toward reality.
Assist the patient in setting priorities.
Help the patient identify the source of anxiety.
Let the patient have some control of the situation.
Consider use of antianxiety medication (for example, Ativan).
Use consultations and referrals when necessary.

Levels of Anxiety
Mild
Mild anxiety is usually a productive state; use this situation as an information-sharing relationship.

Moderate

Moderate anxiety may be productive, but expends more energy than is necessary; use this as a directive-supportive relationship.

Serious

Serious anxiety is usually nonproductive and even counterproductive; the caregiver must take control of the situation. Give direct commands in short, simple sentences, and focus on intellectual functioning.

Severe

Severe anxiety is crippling to witness and experience, and rapidly becomes contagious. Isolate the individual from others (use physical restraints if needed). Do not leave the patient alone. Be supportive but firm.

Terror

Terror is a "do-or-die" situation; assume total responsibility for the patient. Take over total care.

Psychiatric and Psychologic Emergencies

The health team's most important function is to establish the feeling that capable assistance to establish self-control is available. Some individuals lack self-control and are out of contact with reality. The primary concern of the emergency physician is not to specify an etiology or label the presenting syndrome, though this can be helpful, but to facilitate an evaluation of the degree of dysfunction and amount of contact with reality so that immediate treatment is made or referral to another resource for more extensive treatment is accomplished (Box 37-1).

GENERAL APPROACH TO THE MENTALLY DISTURBED PATIENT

Remember that illness has three components:
- Physical
- Psychologic
- Sociologic

In dealing with the patient with mental illness:

Establish good rapport.

Establish eye contact.

Appear relaxed.

Let the patient know he or she is really cared about as a patient.

Listen well, but redirect the patient gently when necessary to keep the interview focused.

Establish a chief complaint.

What is the patient asking for?

Why is the patient asking for it at this time?

What precipitated this visit?

What usually precipitates it?

What has helped in the past?

Speak clearly and without jargon.

Recognize regression—encourage independence and participation in decision making whenever possible.

Be honest.

Expect safe behavior and state this clearly.

Anticipate the emotional component.

Explain procedures to the patient.

Take the patient seriously.

Validate feelings.

BOX 37-1 Management Strategies to Use with the Angry/Belligerent Patient

1. Why do people get angry?
   A. *The helpless child:* Under stress (such as pain or illness), many people feel as helpless a child. They then become angry with "parental" figures (for example, physicians and nurses), who they see as not taking care of them.
      Strategy: Decrease the stress by telling the patient that you are interested in taking care of him or her.
   B. *The temper tantrum:* Many persons have learned that anger will get them what they want. For example, a child throws a temper tantrum to get ice cream, and his mother gives it to him just to stop the screaming. The child learns he will get his ice cream if he yells loud enough. (You can see how this might apply to the patient who demands pain medication.)
      Strategy: Point out to the patient that his anger will not get him what he wants, but will in fact make it more difficult for those trying to help him.
   C. *Scapegoating:* Sometimes when you are feeling angry with one person, you end up taking it out on another. Patients do the same thing.
      Strategy: If patients' anger seems out of proportion to the situation, you might ask if they are angry at something or someone else.
   D. *Inadvertent provocative behavior:* Sometimes, without realizing it, you may be talking in such a way as to provoke someone's anger toward you
      Strategy: Do not exhibit body language or talk in a demeaning, patronizing, authoritarian, or careless manner.
2. Additional tools.
   A. *Bullfight technique:* Agree with the reality aspects of the patient's anger. ("You have a point there; you have been waiting for the doctor for a long time.")
   B. *Engage the patient as an ally in his own treatment.* ("Given the realistic limitations we are under, how do you think we can best help your situation?") Ask the patient for suggestions.
   C. *Show your jugular.* ("I, like you, am upset when patients aren't seen quickly.")
   D. *Make yourself a person, not an impersonal target.* ("It's difficult to take care of someone who is as angry as you are. It rattles me, and I don't function well.")
   E. *Suggestion box technique:* ("Let me give you the name of an administrator to whom you can write or talk.")
   F. *Set firm limits and expectations of behavior.* Point out clearly the consequences to the patient of not keeping within those limits. ("If you yell this loudly, we will have to call the security guards.")
   G. *Time-out:* Give the person a private place to get angry and hostile and tell him to come back when he has cooled off.

Courtesy Dr. Regina Pally, Los Angeles.

Do not be afraid to ask for help.
Do not be afraid to admit to not knowing something.
Include the family or significant others in the patient's life whenever possible.

NONPSYCHOTIC SITUATIONS

Acute Anxiety Attack

An acute anxiety attack typically lasts from a few minutes to several hours. The individual does not lose contact with reality, but judgment and insight are impaired. The major management focus is on preventive aspects through teaching self-management.

■ SIGNS AND SYMPTOMS
Hyperactivity
Dry mouth
Fidgety movement of hands
Precordial discomfort (sense of pressure in chest)

Choking sensation

Dysphagia or inability to swallow

Feelings of "impending danger," "dying," or "going crazy"

Literal attempts to escape

Hyperventilation: breathlessness, paresthesias, and acute restlessness

Sweaty palms

Tachycardia

Tremors

Profuse sweating

Urinary frequency

■ **THERAPEUTIC INTERVENTIONS**

Rule out hyperventilation syndrome.

After a thorough physical examination with attention to the cardiopulmonary system, if no physical cause is
   found, emphasize to the patient the importance of seeking mental health treatment on a nonemergency basis
   to work on the underlying cause of anxiety.

Avoid false or excessive reassurance; give supportive, reassuring attention during the attack.

Acute Grief

Grief is the expected response to a significant loss, such as the loss of a loved one, loss of one's health, loss of
a job or way of life, major financial loss, and so on. The mourning process is influenced by a person's cultural
background, personality style, and past history of losses, as well as other individual factors.

■ **SIGNS AND SYMPTOMS**

Initially shock, disbelief, and/or denial may be present

Emotional lability with overt tears or moaning

Diminished and slowed speech

Inability to concentrate

Anger, sadness, and/or guilt may be present

Thought content focused on "lost object"

Feelings of helplessness

Vital signs within normal limits

Anorexia or change in appetite and weight

Sleep disturbance may be present

■ **THERAPEUTIC INTERVENTIONS**

Accept the individual's behavior and provide supportive dialogue.

Encourage expression of feelings, especially sadness and loss.

Provide privacy in a room with normal lighting but decreased environmental stimuli.

Teach the importance of proper nutrition and fluid intake, even if the desire to eat is diminished.

Encourage the individual to seek out a close friend or family member or bereavement group to discuss feelings
   of grief.

Depression

Depressive disorders are commonly encountered in emergency settings, have a high prevalence in the general
population, and result in significant morbidity and mortality. Normal sadness, grief, and emotional responses to
life's difficulties must be distinguished from a depressive disorder. A sad or depressed mood is only one of the
signs and symptoms of a clinical or major depression.

■ **SIGNS AND SYMPTOMS**

Feelings of worthlessness, loneliness, helplessness, and sadness

Diminished interest in usual activities

Guilt

Physical fatigue, especially in the morning

Psychomotor retardation or agitation

Sleep disturbance

Indecisiveness

Psychotic symptoms may be present in the most severe forms.

Weight change, loss of appetite, and easy fatigability

Reduced facial animation

Possible diuretic, antidepressant drug, and minor tranquilizer side effects

Wringing of hands

Suicidal ideation

Decreased libido

Constipation

Pacing

■ **THERAPEUTIC INTERVENTIONS**

Do not isolate the patient.

Avoid excessive environmental stimuli or forced decision-making.

Provide safety and psychologic security.

Reality test while encouraging the expression of feelings, especially underlying anger.

Help the patient express grief at loss of a loved one; point out that this is normal.

Explore sources of emotional support.

Involve family members and social network for continued support.

Assess the risk of suicide.

Refer the patient for psychiatric evaluation to include psychotherapy and medications, if indicated

SUICIDE

More than 30,000 people commit suicide each year, or 80 each day. In addition to completed suicides, there are over half a million unsuccessful attempts each year—1,300 each day, or 1 each minute.

Assessing Suicide Potential

SEX	Females attempt suicide three times more often than males.
	Males are three times more successful at suicide than females.
	There are 6 suicides per 100,000 females.
	There are 18 suicides per 100,000 males.
	Females tend to use drugs (that is, overdose).
	Males tend to use firearms.
AGE	Suicide potential increases with age.
	Younger people try more often.
	Older people die more often on the first attempt.
RACE/ETHNIC GROUPS/MINORITIES	Suicide rate in the United States is higher in foreign-born people.
	There is a high rate of suicide among homosexuals.
	Moslems have the lowest suicide rate of any religious group, followed by Catholics, Jews, and Protestants.
MARITAL STATUS	Married people have the lowest rate.
	Risk is high in the widowed or divorced group.
	Singles commit twice as many suicides as married people.
FAMILY HISTORY	If family history of suicide attempts is high, there is increased risk of suicide.
	Risk is high if there have been previous attempts (40% to 80% of people who are successful at suicide have made previous attempts).
SEASONAL	More suicides occur in spring and fall.
	More suicides occur on Wednesdays and Saturdays; fewest on Sundays.

OTHER | Substance abuse (alcohol, drugs) greatly increases risk.
Risk is more serious if the plan is well thought out or the patient has a weapon.
Do *not* be afraid to ask if the patient is planning suicide.
Mental illness increases the risk.
Debilitating physical illness increases the risk.
History of serious emotional loss increases the risk (at the time of the loss or on anniversary of the loss).

■ **SIGNS AND SYMPTOMS**

Feelings of worthlessness, hopelessness, helplessness, confusion
Restlessness
Agitation
Irritability
GI complaints
Insomnia
Fatigue
Indifference
Decreased physical activity
Actual suicide attempt that was unsuccessful

Approach to the Suicidal Patient

The approach to the suicidal patient has as its goal establishing a psychologically and physically protective environment. It is also important to establish an empathetic rapport.

■ **PROBLEM SOLVING**

Suicidal thoughts are attempts by the patient to solve problems. Try to find out what the patient thinks the problem is. This must be done after intervention for the crisis, such as care for the patient after overdose or wrist slashing. Common areas for problems include:

Work problems	Illness (mental and physical)
Financial problems	Alcohol abuse
Family problems	Drug abuse
Interpersonal problems	Unrelenting physical pain
	Chronic illness with little to no hope of improvement

■ **EVALUATE WITH THE PATIENT**

Look for alternatives for the patient.
If the patient is unsure of possible alternatives or has no alternatives, hospitalization is mandatory.
If there are alternatives, be specific about them.
Try to involve the family or friends whenever possible in the decision-making and/or planning.
When in doubt, obtain a psychiatric consultation.
If this is not available, admit the patient to the hospital for observation.
The patient may require sedation.

POST-TRAUMATIC STRESS DISORDER

Post-traumatic stress disorder is a reaction to a witnessed or experienced catastrophic event, such as war, rape, injury, etc. These individuals usually demonstrate emotional, physical, behavioral, and psychologic impairment.

■ **SIGNS AND SYMPTOMS**

Guilt/blame/self-punishment
Experiencing flashbacks of the event

Dissociation

Depersonalization

Psychogenic amnesia

Psychogenic fugue

Difficulty in concentrating and problem solving

Emotional lability

Sleep disturbances

Sexual dysfunction

Suicide ideations

Substance abuse

Impaired relationships: relating to mistrust, betrayal, or rejection

■ **THERAPEUTIC INTERVENTIONS**

Remain calm and relaxed.

Develop and utilize a support system.

Identify the traumatic event.

Prescribe antidepressant medications, when indicated.

Prescribe antianxiety medications, when indicated.

Assess the risk of suicide.

Assess the potential for violence.

Consider consultations and referrals.

ACUTE PSYCHOTIC REACTIONS

A psychosis is the deterioration of a person's thought process, affective response, and ability to be in touch with reality, to communicate, and to relate with others. Deterioration continues to the point at which the patient cannot deal with the processes of daily living and loses contact with reality. Do not agree with reality distortion, but avoid arguing in your approach to guiding the individual in reality testing. This patient should be treated in a quiet, sparsely decorated room. If the patient is extremely violent or has the potential to become so, restraints or a locked room may be considered. Undress the patient and place him or her in a hospital gown (remove clothing or other objects that may conceal weapons).

Schizophrenia

■ **SIGNS AND SYMPTOMS**

Delusions

Auditory hallucinations

Difficulty with associations

Disordered thought with clear sensorium

Combative or assaultive behavior

Withdrawn or catatonic behavior

Bizarre gesturing

■ **THERAPEUTIC INTERVENTIONS**

Establish a history of previous hospitalization and/or use of antipsychotic medication that the patient voluntarily stopped or was told to stop taking.

Use simple, concrete expressions and brief sentences.

Avoid figures of speech that are subject to misinterpretation.

Use a confident manner to help assure the patient of your ability to control yourself and the environment.

Listen as the patient talks of delusions to gain clues regarding thinking distortions.

If the patient is paranoid, avoid closed doors or blocked doorways; allow the patient to feel "uncornered."

If antipsychotics are given, observe for postural hypotension and dystonia side effects.

Consider hospital admission.

Paranoia

Paranoia can be a syndrome of schizophrenia or other conditions. A paranoid person demonstrates a loss of reality contact through a delusional system, generally of persecution or excessive religious statements. The paranoid patient can be dangerous because of feelings that either specific people or unnamed forces are "out to get me."

■ **SIGNS AND SYMPTOMS**

Delusions of a projective nature
Feelings of uniqueness going toward grandiosity
Auditory hallucinations
Difficulty with association
Illogical thought process
Obsessive thinking
Combative or assaultive behavior
Restlessness
Agitation

■ **THERAPEUTIC INTERVENTIONS**

Avoid psychologic and physical threats or challenges while providing limits and reality testing.
Use simple, concrete expressions.
Remain calm and authoritative.
Move slowly and quietly to avoid appearing intrusive.
Sit or stand on the same level with the patient to avoid a "power" position.
Allow the patient to be close to the slightly open door.
Allow the patient to verbalize distorted or illogical thinking.
If the patient threatens violence or aggression against a particular person or group, notify them or the authorities. (This is often legally required.)
Avoid trying to convince the patient that the delusions are erroneous and avoid adding validity to any false belief.

Hypomania/Manic Psychosis

Hypomanic or manic patients usually have recurrent episodes of either mood elevation or depression. Medication levels should be measured immediately in those patients who have been on lithium, tegrerol, or depahote therapy.

■ **SIGNS AND SYMPTOMS**

Elation or increased mental excitement that is unstable
Irritability, sometimes irrational anger
Pressured speech (difficult to interrupt the patient because the speech is often so rapid)
Increased motor activity (restless, increased energy)
Decreased need for sleep
Demanding or euphoric manner
Grandiose ideas
Loud voices
Sexual acting out or content focused on sex
Loud-colored clothing, bright-colored makeup (overdone)

■ **THERAPEUTIC INTERVENTIONS**

Assume an authoritative, nonthreatening manner.
Guard the patient, caregivers, and environment against physical harm.
Decrease environmental stimulation.
Provide an unencumbered, safe, and private room to allow pacing or ritualistic motor activity.
Do *not* encourage the patient to talk; ask succinct questions.

Respond in an unhurried, simple speech pattern.

Avoid mechanical restraints if possible.

HOMICIDAL AND ASSAULTIVE BEHAVIOR

Homicidal and assaultive behavior is experienced in acute intoxication, paranoia, or mania, or is seen in socio-pathic individuals. Extreme caution should be used to protect oneself and others in the environment.

■ **THERAPEUTIC INTERVENTIONS**

Approach the individual with an obvious show of force (group of people).

Confiscate all real or potentially harmful objects.

Physically restrain and establish psychologic and physical controls on behalf of the individual.

Establish one person as a liaison who assumes a calm, authoritative, and unhurried manner.

Speak in simple, direct sentences.

Separate the individual from the family and/or the intended victim; if the victim is not present, emergency personnel are responsible for making sure that the person is warned of the patient's ideations.

Observe for suicidal as well as homicidal attempts; suicide may follow homicidal attempts because of generally impaired judgment.

"PSYCHIATRIC" SYMPTOMS RESULTING FROM A MEDICAL OR NEUROLOGIC ILLNESS

When a patient presents to an emergency setting with a seemingly "primary psychiatric disorder," it is important to rule out all possible medical/neurologic etiologies. (*Organicity* is a term used in the past to describe this.) Patients with a variety of medical conditions (from cerebral emboli to allergic reactions) may present initially with psychiatric or behavioral symptoms. A thorough medical/neurologic work-up including lab and radiological testing is often indicated. Key indicator of organicity is that patients' symptoms/behavior are completely out of character and/or are fluctuating.

Dementia and delirium are two frequently encountered neurologic conditions in emergency settings. They can be seen separately or together.

Dementia

Dementia is a diffuse disruption and impairment of the functioning capacity of brain tissue from a variety of causes, such as Alzheimer's disease, brain tumor, vascular dementias. There is a development of multiple, cognitive deficits; usually nonreversible and chronic. Neurologic consultation is necessary for patients with new or recent onset of symptoms.

■ **SIGNS AND SYMPTOMS**

Decreased orientation

Decreased memory

Decreased judgment

Decreased ability to calculate, figure, plan, and organize

Shallow affect

Acute Delirium

Acute state of confusion

■ **CAUSES**

Biochemical disturbances, for example, electrolyte imbalance, hypoglycemia, uremia, porphyria, or hepatitis

Metastatic neoplasm

Systemic infection

Cerebral hypoxia

Drug withdrawal
Heavy metal toxicity
Hypothermia
Head injury
Polydrug use

■ **SIGNS AND SYMPTOMS**

Delusions
Illusions
Disorientation
Frightening dreams
Highly distractable
Fluctuating levels of consciousness
Outbursts of rage
Difficulty in retention and recall
Hyperventilation
Tachycardia
Tremors
Restlessness

■ **THERAPEUTIC INTERVENTIONS**

Identify and remove any toxic substance.
Orient the patient to reality by making simple repetitive statements.
Simplify the environment.
Maintain normal lighting (keep lights on at night).
Have a responsible person stay with the patient.
Avoid physical restraints, which only increase confusion, disorientation, and general agitation.

DRUG-RELATED PSYCHIATRIC EMERGENCIES

The function of emergency personnel in an acute drug-induced crisis is one of clinical intervention, critical observation, and supportive therapeutic communication.

■ **SIGNS AND SYMPTOMS**

Central nervous system depression
Respiratory depression
Increased temperature, pulse, and respirations, and decreased BP
Increased or decreased pupil size
Decreased muscle tone
Tremors
Gastrointestinal symptoms
Decreased level of consciousness
Distortion of mood/thought patterns
Track marks

■ **QUESTIONS TO ASK**

What type of drug was taken?
How much?
What has happened since the drug was taken?
What other drugs have been used (drug history)?
At what time was the last dose of the drug taken?
At what time did the patient start abusing the drug?
How was the drug taken (orally, subcutaneously, by injection, by inhalation)?
Where was the drug obtained?
Was alcohol consumed?

Categories of Drugs

Belladonna alkaloids

Over-the-counter hypnotic drugs such as Nytol and Sominex contain scopolamine. Taken in large amounts, they produce an atropine-like psychosis. Phenothiazines, tricyclic antidepressants, and antihistamines are potent anticholinergic drugs. Some plants also contain belladonna alkaloids. The classic description of belladonna effects is "blind as a bat, dry as a bone, red as a beet, and mad as a hatter."

■ SIGNS AND SYMPTOMS

Delirium

Mental confusion

Intense thirst and dry mouth

Dysphagia

Restlessness

Talkativeness

Thought blockade

Dilated pupils

Inability to visually accommodate

Flushed, hot, and dry skin

Rapid and weak pulse

Hoarse, raspy voice

Urinary retention or slow, painful urinary stream

■ THERAPEUTIC INTERVENTIONS

Give frequent sips of water.

Use a saline flush to moisten the eyes.

Insert urinary bladder catheter if needed.

Provide a calm environment in subdued lighting.

Serve as a calm, nonjudgmental listener, but *do not* encourage talking.

Opiates and related compounds

Included in the opiate group are heroin, morphine, hydromorphone (Dilaudid), pentazocine (Talwin), methadone (Dolophine), and propoxyphene (Darvon). The list is in order of intensity of euphoria and diminished sensorium.

■ SIGNS AND SYMPTOMS

State of sluggishness

State of euphoria

Somnolence

Track marks (popliteal fossa, ankles, forearm veins, sublingual)

Constricted pupils

Decreased blood pressure

Decreased heart rate

Decreased body temperature

■ THERAPEUTIC INTERVENTIONS

ABCs

Dextrose 50%

Naloxone 0.8 mg IV or IM

Observe for withdrawal syndrome: coryza, yawning, lacrimation, increased pulse and respiratory rate, perspiration, and tremors (these start 6 to 12 hours after the last dose).

Observe in addition for insomnia, severe abdominal cramps, vomiting and diarrhea, tachycardia, and hypertension (these start 12 to 48 hours after the last dose).

Observe for respiratory depression and impending heroin pulmonary edema if that drug is suspected.

If naloxone (Narcan) has been given, be alert for agitation and aggressive behavior as the patient withdraws from the opiate.

Hallucinogens

Hallucinogens are psychedelic drugs such as LSD and DMT (acid), peyote, mescaline, STP, psilocybin, and phencyclidine (PCP, angel dust). Individuals on a "bad trip" are especially sensitive to the environment and are suspicious of people. Subjective symptoms wax and wane.

■ **SIGNS AND SYMPTOMS**

Grossly impaired judgment
Intense visual or auditory hallucinations
Unusual changes in self-perception
Rapid mood swings
Flight of ideas
Lack of coordination
Loss of control that comes in waves
Panic state
Increased blood pressure and pulse rate
Pupil dilation
Chills and shivering
Increased muscle tension
Tremors
Nausea (especially with mescaline)
Convulsions

■ **THERAPEUTIC INTERVENTIONS**

1. Provide a one-on-one presence by a supportive person (a trusted, responsible friend or one particular staff person).
   a. Give simple, repetitive statements.
   b. Do *not* challenge the patient's values, beliefs, life-style, or distorted thinking.
2. Use "talk down" techniques. (Do *not* use "talk down" with PCP.)
   a. Establish verbal contact to allay fears.
   b. Encourage the patient to talk.
   c. Encourage expressions of perceptions and feelings.
3. Reality test on a continuous basis.
   a. Focus on physical characteristics of the room.
   b. Repeatedly identify person(s) in the room.
   c. Have the patient focus on inanimate, stationary objects in the room as a center of orientation.
   d. Encourage the patient to keep his or her eyes open.
4. Provide a protective, quiet, and nonthreatening room.
   a. Normal lighting.
   b. Decreased visual and auditory stimuli.
5. Guard yourself against spontaneous aggressive behavior.
6. Be alert for suicidal behavior.

Phencyclidine (angel dust)

Phencyclidine is classified as an analgesic and a hallucinogenic agent. It can be taken by inhalation, ingestion, or intravenously.

■ **SIGNS AND SYMPTOMS**

Severe anxiety, agitation, drowsiness, or coma
Psychosis (acute onset)
Constricted pupils
Increased then decreased respirations, followed by respiratory arrest

Elevated then decreased blood pressure
Vertical nystagmus
Ataxia
Euphoria
Increased then decreased deep tendon reflexes
Nausea and vomiting
Clonus
Increased then decreased urinary output
Tremors followed by seizures
Amnesia
Opisthotonos
Distorted images and thought processes
Depersonalization
Hallucinations
Dysrhythmias

■ **THERAPEUTIC INTERVENTIONS**
Reduce external stimuli (quiet, dim room).
Decrease the number of people present.
Use restraints and total observation.
Do *not* attempt to talk the patient down.
Give haloperidol (Haldol) IV (but remember that haloperidol has a shorter half-life than PCP) *or* diazepam
  (Valium).
Consider hospital admission.

Central nervous system stimulants

All psychostimulants produce excitation of the central nervous system. Tolerance develops rapidly and is sometimes accompanied by psychologic dependence. A physical withdrawal syndrome is unlikely, but a real letdown feeling accompanies discontinuation of the drug.

Amphetamines

■ **SIGNS AND SYMPTOMS**
Increased rate of speech
Extraordinary hyperactivity
Rapid flight of ideas
Mood swings
Irritability and hostility
Aggressiveness
Unexplained fear and jitteriness
Talkativeness
Hallucinations (auditory or visual)
Clear sensorium and memory
Delusions of persecution
Increased blood pressure, pulse rate, and temperature
Dilated pupils
Insomnia
Twitching muscles
Nausea or vomiting
Severe abdominal pain
Grand mal seizures

Cocaine or crack

■ **SIGNS AND SYMPTOMS**

Euphoria and feeling of mental agility

Formication (sense of insects crawling under skin)

Loose association

Paranoid delusions

Perforated nasal septum

Elevated body temperature

Dilated pupils

Skin pallor

■ **THERAPEUTIC INTERVENTIONS**

Place the patient in a quiet, secure, large room.

Reduce environmental stimuli.

Allow the patient to move about.

Observe vital signs, especially temperature.

Allow the patient to "talk down."

Be alert to violent or aggressive tendencies and protect caregivers and the environment.

Be aware of repetitious compulsive behavior.

A period of "crash" is followed by marked depression, which can lead to suicidal behavior; therefore, use precautions to prevent suicide.

Central nervous system depressants

Depressants are most dangerous in terms of acute overdose and withdrawal morbidity. Withdrawal represents a medical emergency of the first order. Tolerance develops rapidly; the shorter the half-life, the more physiologically addicting the drug. Alcohol and barbiturate intoxication are similar in signs and symptoms.

Acute alcohol intoxication

■ **SIGNS AND SYMPTOMS**

Slowed thinking

Impaired memory and judgment

Labile emotions

Disinhibited behavior

Inattention and distractibility

Euphoria or depression

Slurred speech

Agitation or extreme compliance

Unsteady gait

Smell of alcohol on the breath

Nausea and vomiting

Tremors

Flushed or pale face

Systolic hypertension

Tachycardia

Muscle weakness

■ **THERAPEUTIC INTERVENTIONS**

Observe the patient carefully.

Monitor vital signs, especially blood pressure and heart rate.

Place patient in a quiet, protected area.

Guard against aspiration and physical injury.

Speak in a calm, authoritative manner.

If a sedative or barbiturate drug is given, be alert to respiratory depression.

If a major tranquilizer is given, be alert to hypotension.

Obtain an ingestion history, including alcohol, in combination with other drugs.

See Chapter 15 for measurement of alcohol withdrawal symptoms, because the patient who stops drinking may precipitate a withdrawal crisis in increasingly serious stages.

See Chapter 15 for medical management.

Barbiturates

The main danger of overdose is stupor and cardiorespiratory collapse. Because of their ability to depress CNS functioning, there is an extremely high incidence of barbiturate use for intended or gestured suicide.

■ **SIGNS AND SYMPTOMS**

Muscular incoordination	Postural hypotension
Slurred speech	Hypothermia
Paranoid ideation	Depressed respiration
Restlessness	Nausea
Clouded sensorium progressing to coma	Convulsions
Wide-based ataxic gait	Tremors
Irritability	Hyperreflexia
Dilated pupils	Muscular weakness

■ **THERAPEUTIC INTERVENTIONS**

Management generally includes withdrawal of the abused drug under inpatient conditions for close monitoring of misuse of drugs.

Provide a quiet, secure room.

Carefully observe and record signs and symptoms.

Be especially alert for convulsions, which can progress to status epilepticus, and respiratory distress.

Avoid physical restraints.

A withdrawal syndrome appears within 10 to 15 hours: apprehension, muscle weakness, hypotension, seizures, and psychosis may occur.

Bromides

Bromides are more likely to produce chronic poisoning than an acute overdose.

■ **SIGNS AND SYMPTOMS**

Gradual increase in drowsiness without release by sleep

Depression

Confusion

Hallucinations (visual)

Delusions of paranoid nature

Hypomanic state

Acneform skin eruptions (especially on the face and around the hair roots)

Serum drug level above 75 mg/100 ml

Heavily fixed tongue

Foul breath

■ **THERAPEUTIC INTERVENTIONS**

Provide a quiet, secure room.

Ascertain the source of bromide intake; many patients are unaware of the poison-like effect of over-the-counter sleep agents.

Reality test regarding delusions and hallucinations.

Marijuana

The most common complication of marijuana is that the user experiences an anxiety attack.

■ **SIGNS AND SYMPTOMS**

Elevated blood pressure	Apprehension
Tachycardia	Restlessness
Tachypnea	Feeling of doom

■ **THERAPEUTIC INTERVENTIONS**

Psychologic support

Reassurance

Diazepam by mouth if the reaction is severe

Antipsychotic dystonic reactions

Phenothiazine dystonic reactions may be caused by prochlorperazine (Compazine), trifluoperazine (Stelazine), chlorpromazine (Thorazine), fluphenazine (Prolixin), and haloperidol (Haldol), as well as most other antipsychotic medication. Signs and symptoms of dystonic reactions are often mistaken for hypocalcemia, seizure disorders, and tetany. Be sure to ask about a medication history when a patient comes to the emergency department with these signs and symptoms.

■ **SIGNS AND SYMPTOMS**

Signs and symptoms usually appear 4 to 5 days after ingestion.

Oculogyric crisis	Facial grimaces
Protruding tongue	Opisthotonos
Torticollis	Tortipelvic crisis

■ **THERAPEUTIC INTERVENTIONS**

Diphenhydramine (Benadryl) IV or

Benztropine (Cogentin) or

Trihexyphenidyl (Artane)

Adverse central nervous system reactions to antipsychotic drugs

Sometimes the drug of choice in treating a psychiatric condition produces more stress than relief for the patient. One such instance is the severe extrapyramidal side effects of some major tranquilizers. These reactions are more likely to occur during the *initial* phase of psychotropic drug therapy. The appearance of undesirable side effects can be anxiety-provoking for the patient and the family. The potential hazard and the sudden onset of the symptoms can cause the patient to refuse to take any type of prescribed medicine that could be effective in decreasing psychotic symptoms. Emergency personnel can do much to help the individual realize that use of antipsychotic drugs requires patience in obtaining a satisfactory therapeutic response.

Medical management to counteract adverse reactions is quickly achieved in most instances by anticholinergic drugs such as diphenhydramine (Benadryl) or antiparkinsonian drugs such as benztropine mesylate (Cogentin) or trihexyphenidyl (Artane).

Parkinsonism usually develops within 20 days of the initial drug therapy. Symptoms include muscular rigidity, resting tremors, a masklike face, and drooling. Dystonia usually develops within 1 hour to 5 days.

■ **THERAPEUTIC INTERVENTIONS**

Educate the patient to the fact that untoward symptoms will disappear rapidly with proper medication, usually go away even if untreated, and usually are completely reversible.

Provide a quiet, darkened room for the patient to lie down until the antagonist drug takes effect.

Have a nonthreatening person stay with the patient until the undesirable symptoms have subsided (generally within 1 hour after administration of an antagonist drug IM).

Disposition of the patient

The major question that arises with the therapeutic intervention of the psychiatric patient is whether he or she should be hospitalized. One important factor is the presence or absence of a solid support system in terms of family or friends and their willingness to observe or supervise the patient.

When to hospitalize the patient involuntarily:

If the patient is a physical threat to himself or herself (suicidal)

If the patient is a physical threat to others (homicidal)

If the patient is completely unable to care for him or herself in the community by reason of mental illness resulting in a serious imminent risk to health and safety.

(Involuntary hold criteria differ in each state, but most states have included some form of these criteria)

The hold is usually placed by a psychiatrist or psychiatric consultant. These holds are usually for a limited time (72 hours in most states).

SUMMARY

By definition, a psychiatric emergency occurs when a person's adaptive capacity is ineffective in coping with life's stressors. Psychiatric emergencies require careful listening and a great deal of common sense. It is not easy to remain calm, appear authoritative, and thereby be therapeutic when the entire situation is anxiety-provoking. Self-sufficiency and self-control should be the goal of any intervention. The most powerful strategy in helping the individual establish a sense of self-control (power) is to show an attitude of decisive action (authority) and compassion (care).

In psychiatric emergencies the signs and symptoms of the health problem are sometimes so obvious in the individual's bizarre behavior or thinking that it is often easier to evaluate what is wrong than to assess what is right. The strengths to build on are as important as isolating the impairments causing the dysfunction. A complete evaluation includes the patient's strengths as well as weaknesses. The treatment process is based on the individual's strengths that have been identified and validated through the assessment process. Emergency personnel need to develop an understanding of people and their coping behaviors. This basic knowledge of human behavior synthesized with medical and surgical knowledge should provide the needed tools of sensitivity and knowledge to meet the patient's immediate needs.

SUGGESTED READINGS

Aguilera D: *Crisis intervention theory and methodology,* ed 7, St Louis, 1994, Mosby.

The care of psychiatric patients in the emergency department, *J Emerg Nurs* 19:375-472, 1993.

Fauman BJ, Fauman MA: *Emergency psychiatry for the house officer,* Baltimore, 1981, Williams & Wilkins.

George JE, Quattrone MS, Goldstone M: Suicidal patients: what is the nursing duty to prevent a patient's self-inflicted injuries? *J Emerg Nurs* 22(6):609-614, 1996.

Gorton JG, Partridge R: *Practice management of psychiatric emergency care,* St Louis, 1982, Mosby.

Harrahill M: Giving bad news compassionately, *J Emerg Nurs* 23(5):496-498, 1997.

Lego S: *Psychiatric nursing: a comprehensive reference,* ed 2, Philadelphia, 1996, Lippincott.

Rund DA, Hutzler JC: *Emergency psychiatry,* St Louis, 1983, Mosby.

Smith J: Organic brain syndrome. In Rosen et al: *Emergency medicine,* ed 4, St Louis, 1998, Mosby.

Stuart G, Sundeen: *Principles and practice nursing,* ed 4, St Louis, 1991, Mosby.

Stuart G, Sundeen: *Principles and practice psychiatric nursing,* ed 4, St Louis, 1991, Mosby.

Special Considerations for the Geriatric Patient

Andrea Novak

Elderly persons (over age 65) represent a growing population in the United States today. Currently they comprise 11.3% (that is, more than 25.5 million people) of the population, and that number is expected to reach 20% by the year 2030.[1] This is of significance to emergency nursing because perhaps one out of every four patients seen could be aged 65 or over. Caring for these patients requires not only knowledge surrounding the ABCs of emergency care, but an understanding of the normal physiologic changes associated with aging. For the purpose of this text, geriatric or elderly will be defined as those patients over the age of 65.

Geriatric emergency patients account for only 15% of emergency department visits, but comprise 43% of all hospital admissions and 48% of all intensive care admissions from the emergency department.[2] The length of stay in the emergency department for the elderly patient is nearly 20% longer than that for younger patients and the elderly have a higher rate of diagnostic testing than their younger counterparts.[2]

A thorough history and physical assessment are important. Special attention should be given to the patients' past medical and surgical history, preexisting conditions, and medications they are currently taking. A family member or spouse may be needed to assist in obtaining a history if the patient is not an accurate or reliable witness, and all medical records should be obtained if available. The hallmark of aging is a general decline in the functional reserve capacity of major organs and systems and a limited range of adaptability.[2] Table 38-1 reflects the physiologic changes associated with aging. These changes will directly affect the patient's ability to recover and recuperate from untoward events. They are essential to providing quality of care and must be incorporated into the nursing process. This will ensure the best outcomes for the geriatric emergency department patient.

PHYSIOLOGIC CHANGES ASSOCIATED WITH AGING

Physical Assessment

A head-to-toe assessment needs to be accomplished on any emergency patient, but it is of particular importance to the elderly patient. Observation, auscultation, and palpation are sometimes the only ways an abnormality can be identified. Because the elderly may be less able to hear high-pitched sounds, nurses should lower the pitch of their voices and speak clearly.

General observations/pertinent questions

The nurse should observe for and discuss the following when performing the assessment:
Speech or hearing impairments
Mood disturbance or difficulty with thought processes
Differences between patient's chief complaint and that of the family

TABLE 38-1   Structural and Functional Changes as a Result of Aging

BODY SYSTEM	ALTERATION
Tissues	Decreased number of active cells
	Reduced tissue elasticity
Cardiovascular	Decreased distensibility of blood vessels
	Increased systolic blood pressure
	Increased systemic resistance
	Decreased cardiac output
	Slow response to stress
Pulmonary	Decreased strength of respiratory muscles
	Limited chest expansion
	Decreased number of functioning alveoli
	Decreased elastic recoil, small airway collapse
	Decreased resting oxygen tension
	Diminished protective mechanisms
Neurologic	Decreased number of functional neurons
	Decrease in nerve conduction velocity
	Short-term memory loss
	Reduced cerebral blood flow
	Decreased visual acuity and speed of dark adaptation
	Decreased pupillary response and accommodation
	Increased auditory tone threshold
	Diminished sensation and touch acuity
Gastrointestinal/genitourinary	Decreased peristalsis
	Diminished acid secretion and thickened mucosa
	Decreased total nephron count
	Decreased glomerular filtration rate
	Diminished concentrating ability
Musculoskeletal/integumentary	Narrowing of intervertebral disks
	Bone loss, increased risk for fracture
	Increased wear on joints
	Decreased number of muscle cells
	Loss of muscle strength
	Loss of skin thickness

From Andrews JF: Trauma in the elderly, *Forum Medicum, Postgraduate Studies in Trauma Nursing,* 1990.

Living arrangements, activities of daily living, socioeconomic circumstances and the physical layout of the home, that is, if stairs are present, and so forth.

Thorough review of all of the patient's medications. Look for possible adverse reactions, drug interactions, and toxic or subtherapeutic levels. Many elderly patients are on numerous medications and this polypharmacy may be the cause of their present problem. Proper medication dosing, interactions, and scheduling should be discussed with the patient, or if appropriate a visiting nurse association referral made to set up such a schedule.

Dietary history—what the patient eats, how often, who shops, if there are difficulties associated with shopping, and smell or taste impairments, any problems with chewing, swallowing, and presence or absence of dentures and how well they fit.

Urinary incontinence, changes in bowel habits

Depression or anxiety. Poor appetite, change in sleep patterns and constipation are common in the elderly, but may also be symptoms of depression. Ask about suicidal thoughts and crying spells. Ask about over-

the-counter medications and alcohol intake. Alcohol and over-the-counter medications can interact together and/or with prescribed medications to cause psychologic and physiologic problems.

Sexual problems or difficulties. Elderly men may have a problem with impotence or unreliable erections and
women may have vaginal dryness. Remind them that it is not abnormal to still have sexual feelings.

A thorough, head-to-toe physical exam should be performed.

Head

Observation

Palpation for pain, bleeding, or fractures

Elicit history of a fall, recent or weeks ago

Elicit history of neurologic changes, changes in mental status, or history of loss of consciousness

Subdural hematomas are more frequent in the elderly as a result of anatomic changes associated with aging and
may be acute or chronic.

Prepare patient for CT and/or operating room admission.

Chest

Observation for equal, bilateral expansion, and abnormalities

Auscultation for bilateral breath sounds, presence or absence of adventitious breath sounds, and heart sounds

Palpation for pain, fractures, crepitus

Monitor O_2 sat (low 90s may be their normal)

Monitor ability to handle and clear secretions

Check for gag reflex and coughing ability

Respiration—Hypoventilation may be the patient's normal

Check for jugular vein distension (JVD)

Observe for use of accessory muscles, nasal flaring

ABGs

If ETT placement is warranted monitor for the development of pneumonia, ARDs

Abdomen

Abdominal pain in the elderly may be vague but often reflects very serious pathology.

Observe for surgical scars, distended abdomen.

Auscultate for bowel sounds

Elicit bowel elimination pattern; slowed peristalsis associated with aging tends to predispose these patients to
constipation.

Prepare for KUB—flat and upright.

Elicit urination pattern; men are predisposed to urinary dribbling and women to stress incontinence. Note
amount, color, specific gravity, and any odor of urine.

Assess for pain, guarding, or tenderness on palpation

Obtain urinalysis/urine culture.

Check skin around perineum for evidence of excoriation and breakdown.

Rectal exam, guaiac stool for occult blood, prostate exam

Extremities

Observe for deformities, bruising, normal and abnormal coloring.

Assess for pain, tenderness

Look for shortening of leg and external rotation of the foot when a fall has occurred or hip fracture is suspected.

Palpate pulses.

Assess range of motion.

Monitor vital signs frequently because fractures cause bleeding in the bones, which can cause shock in the elderly.

Assess for fractures with no history of trauma—suspect elder abuse.

Skin

Observe for turgor, intact skin, skin tears, bruising—old and new, burns—old and new, rashes, areas of breakdown, temperature, and color.

Inquire about bruises, skin tears, and burns.

Give diphtheria/tetanus inoculation if needed.

Dress tears using paper tape and nonstick dressings.

Gently clean areas of breakdown and apply protective ointment.

Take temperature. Less body fat and muscle mass makes the elderly more prone to hypothermia. Warm IV fluids, apply warmed blankets, pad bony prominences.

Inquire as to who cares for the patient if bruising and tears are not caused by falls or bumps. Suspect elder abuse. Use nonjudgmental approach and contact social services if suspicion is high.

GERIATRIC EMERGENCY

The challenge of caring for the geriatric emergency patient is related to many of the factors discussed earlier, including the effects of the aging process on the body, polypharmacy, and atypical presentations that complicate diagnosis. In addition, the elderly may not exhibit the same signs and symptoms of pain found in their younger counterparts. In the elderly, the severity of pain may not be a reliable indicator as to the severity of the condition. It is not uncommon for pain to be referred to another site.[3] The elderly are at great risk for developing serious complications and death as well. Trauma is the fourth leading cause of death in persons over 55 and the fifth leading cause of death for those over age 70.[4] Geriatric trauma patients have a higher mortality rate than younger patients for less severe injuries.[5]

Elderly patients will often have a more tenuous homeostasis. They are more prone to infections, more likely to have atypical presentations of myocardial infarction and difficult-to-assess abdominal pain. More diagnostic tests are necessary because of the increased likelihood of problems and because accurate diagnoses can be more important.

Falls

Falls are the leading cause of death in elderly trauma victims, and more than half of all deaths as a result of falls involve persons aged 75 or older. Predisposing factors include: poor vision and hearing, gait disturbances, diminished muscle strength, osteoporotic bones, and associated frailty. Medical conditions contributing to falls include cardiac arrhythmias, dizziness, seizure disorder, and arthritis. Environmental factors such as loose carpets, improper footwear, inappropriate furniture (for example, too low, sharp corners), awkward stairways, poor lighting, and unfamiliar surroundings can contribute to falls.[4] These falls contribute to fractures, head injuries, and internal injuries such as splenic rupture, and are compromising to both the previously healthy and not so healthy patient.

■ **PREVENTION**

See Box 38-1.

1. Removal or securing of loose carpeting
2. Improved lighting
3. Handrails and siderails where needed
4. Moving furniture with sharp edges or padding the sharp edges
5. Shoes with flat heels

BOX 38-1   Injury Prevention Activities for the Elderly

Remove or tack down all scatter rugs.
Check all staircases for stability, and install handrails whenever possible.
Apply nonslip strips on stairways.
Carpet areas that are prone to spills or slipperiness.
Reduce clutter and open clear pathways through all rooms.
Pad wooden or metal edges on furniture.
Install bright lights in hallways and entrances.
Place nonslip mats in bathtub and shower.
Install grab bars near all bathrooms.
Install smoke detectors and check them at regular intervals.
Investigate assistive cooking devices, such as burner shields, long-handled utensils, and protective hand gear.
Do not wear loose-fitting garments while cooking.
Use rear stove burners rather than front ones, and avoid storing goods you may need over the stove.
Check central furnace and space heaters frequently to ensure proper functioning.
Reduce thermostatic setting on water heater, and clearly label all hot water faucets.
Review directions for operating major appliances annually.

From Andrews JF: Trauma in the elderly, *Forum Medicum, Postgraduate Studies in Trauma Nursing,* 1990.

6. Assistance in the home if possible
7. Knowledge of 9-1-1 access
8. Caution about getting up too quickly after sitting or lying down.
9. Proper use of assistive devices (for example, walker).

Burns

Diminished neurologic sensation, impaired vision and hearing, and psychomotor delay may leave the elderly unable to avoid the hazards of heat and flames. Burns may be more severe than they initially appear because of thinning, aging skin.

Treatment can be found and is the same as treatment discussed in Chapter 30, however careful consideration must be made for the elderly burn victim as physiologic changes do compromise their healing and recovery.

■ **PREVENTION**
1. Short sleeved, non-nylon shirts and pajamas
2. Discourage smoking, especially while resting
3. Smoke detectors and fire extinguishers easily accessible with ease of operation
4. Assistance with cooking, as needed; extra care when cooking with gas
5. Discourage use of hot water bottles and heating pads, or have patient monitor temperature with a thermometer or set at the low setting
6. Knowledge of 9-1-1 access

Motor Vehicle Crash

Visual and hearing disturbances, decreased reaction time, and increased traffic all play a part in motor vehicle events involving the elderly. Motor vehicle crashes account for 21.5% of injuries to the elderly population.[5]

Trauma management essentially remains the same for these patients as trauma management for younger patients. Structural and functional changes associated with aging will affect care and patient recovery, however. See Chapter 29 for treatment.

■ **PREVENTION**
1. Minimal night driving if patient has night blindness
2. Encourage seat belt use
3. Have patient drive only in familiar areas, avoiding highly congested areas or areas under construction
4. If they or others are concerned with their driving abilities, encourage contacting state licensing agencies to inquire about "Over 75 Refresher Courses."

Elder Abuse

Awareness and understanding of elder abuse is becoming more apparent. Although assessment of elder abuse is often difficult and time consuming, its role cannot be stressed enough. Emergency nurses can play a large part in this role. They are usually the first persons the elderly patient encounters in the emergency department setting. Knowledge of a sympathetic, nonjudgmental approach often will elicit information from the patient.

■ **CLUES**
Unexplained fractures or bruising, burns, or internal injuries can be the presenting problems.
"Noncompliance" with medications or treatment plans.
History of being "accident prone" or multiple emergency department visits.
Fear response to caregiver.
Poor hygiene, malnutrition, dehydration, and poor skin care.
Unexplained delays in seeking treatment and differing accounts of what happened by the patient and family members can be reason to suspect elder abuse, as are unusual injury locations and unusual patient-family interactions.
   The patient may be hesitant to speak about abuse as he or she relies on that family member for care and shelter. Frustration, economic difficulties, lifestyle changes, and inability to care for the elderly patient are some reasons that elder abuse exists. If suspected, the social services division of the hospital needs to be notified to offer information and follow-up or referral.

Elder Abandonment—"Granny Dumping"

This is an alarming and growing phenomenon in emergency departments. Family members are usually the caregivers and may find it frustrating and difficult to fulfill the role of caring for a chronically ill or disabled family member. They turn to the emergency department for help when they become overwhelmed. The emergency department is the place for this abandonment because it is open 24 hours a day, 7 days a week. They come to the emergency department for support, compassion, and for a break from their caregiving role.
   With the advent of DRGs, hospitals are less likely to admit patients for "social disposition," yet with abandonment they may have little other choice. Social services must then intervene to discuss other options for the caregiving families, or to provide services to give them a respite from care, and possibly placement of these patients.
   As improvements are made in health care and preventive services, people are now living longer and more active lives. People over the age of 65 are more mobile and productive, thus putting them at higher risk for experiencing health care emergencies.
   As emergency care providers, we need to have the knowledge, skills, and understanding necessary to provide quality emergency nursing care to this growing population.

REFERENCES
1. US Bureau of the Census: *Statistical abstract of the United States: 1990,* ed 110, Washington DC, 1990, US Government Printing Office.
2. Saunders AB: *Emergency care of the elder person,* St Louis, 1996, Beverly Cracom Publishers.
3. Eliopoulos C: *Gerontological nursing,* ed 3, Philadelphia, 1993, Lippincott.
4. Loftis P, Glover, Talar: *Decision making in gerontologic nursing,* St Louis, 1993, Mosby.

5. DeKeyser F, Carolan D, Trask A: Suburban geriatric trauma: the experiences of a level I trauma center, *Am J Crit Care* 4(5):379-82, 1995.

SUGGESTED READINGS

Andersen GP: Assessing the older patient, *RN* 61:47-56, 1998.

Beers MH, Storrie M, Lee G: Potential adverse drug interactions in the emergency room, *Ann Intern Med,* 112:61, 1990.

Burke M, Walsh M: *Gerontologic nursing holistic care of the older adult,* St Louis, 1997, Mosby.

Castro JM et al: Home care referral after emergency department discharge, *J Emerg Nurs* 24(2):127-132, 1998.

Eliopoulos C: *Gerontological nursing,* ed 3, Philadelphia, 1993, Lippincott.

Molitor L: An elderly man with acute ataxia, *J Emerg Nurs* 23:651-652, 1997.

Sanders AB: *Emergency care of the elder person,* St Louis, 1996, Beverly Cracom Publications.

Sanders AB: Care of the elderly in the emergency department: where do we stand? *Ann Emerg Med* 21:792, 1992.

Vitiello MV, Bliwise DL, Prinz PN: Sleep in Alzheimer's disease and the sundown syndrome, *Neurology* 42(suppl)6:83, 1992.

While P: Pearls for practice, polypharmacy and the older adult, *J Acad Nurs Practit* 7(11):545-548, 1995.

Zietlow SP et al: Multisystem geriatric trauma, *J Trauma* 37:985, 1994.

Organ and Tissue Donation

Susan Budassi Sheehy

Each year thousands of life-saving and life-enhancing organ and tissue transplants are performed. Almost 50,000 children and adults are waiting for donor organs. In addition, more than 500,000 people are waiting for tissue allografts. These patients receive gifts of life, sight, mobility, and independence. An average of seven patients die each day waiting for an organ transplant to occur. Many attempts have been made to ease the profound shortage of donor organs and tissues.

In 1968 the passage of the Uniform Anatomical Gift Act (UAGA) allowed persons to indicate their intent to donate after death by signing an organ donor card. If there was no indication of prior intent, the UAGA permitted the legal next of kin to give consent after death. The Omnibus Budget Reconciliation Act of 1986 (OBRA) required that hospitals write policies and protocols to assure that families were given information regarding their right to donate and that potential donors would be identified and referred to a local Organ Procurement Organization (OPO).

Regardless of efforts being made to increase the supply of organs and tissues available for transplant, it is important to reflect on the needs of a grieving family. Many families find comfort in making a donation and feel strongly about their right to make that choice for their loved one.

ROLE OF THE EMERGENCY DEPARTMENT NURSE

Become familiar with donation criteria and the hospital's policy on determination of brain death.
Contact the local organ procurement organization to determine medical suitability whenever a death is imminent.
Discuss the possibility of donation with the primary physician.
Look for an organ donor card among patient's belongings.
Obtain permission for donation from medical examiner or coroner.
Offer family the option of donation in conjunction with the organ procurement organization.
Assist with donor management.
Provide bereavement support to family members.

TISSUE DONATION (CARDIORESPIRATORY DEATH)

Almost anyone who dies can be a tissue donor. Eye, heart for valve, and skin recovery can be performed in the morgue. Bone and saphenous vein recovery must be done in an operating room. Donor criteria vary. Avoid ruling someone out before making a referral.

General Tissue Donor Criteria

Do not rule out any potential donors. Consult with your local organ bank because donors change frequently. Each potential donor is evaluated by a procurement specialist. The evaluation includes a medical and social history. The following tissue and bone may be transplanted:

Eyes	Pericardium
Cornea	Fascia
Heart valves	Veins
Bone	Dura
Skin	Tendons
Saphenous vein	Cartilage

Minimum Exclusion Criteria

Unresolved septicemia
Metastatic cancer (not a rule out for eye donation)
Injectable drug abuse
HIV positive or history of high-risk group for HIV (per U.S. Public Health Service guidelines)

Management

If the patient is to be an eye donor, follow this procedure before sending the body to the morgue:
Elevate the head of the bed.
Tape the eyelids shut with paper tape.
Apply ice packs to the eyelids.
Other tissue donations do not require specific management by nursing staff.

ORGAN DONATION (BRAIN DEATH)

A potential organ donor is a previously healthy individual who has suffered "irreversible cessation of all brain functions, including the brain stem."[1] Brain death criteria are determined by state legislation based on standard medical practice.

General Organ Donor Criteria

Age: newborn to 80 years
Brain death (see *brain death criteria* below)
Intact cardiorespiratory system
Apneic, on ventilator (see *apnea test* on p. 662)
Remember, avoid ruling out a potential donor before discussing the case with the donation coordinator who is on call at the local organ procurement organization. Donor criteria may vary and change frequently based on current medical practice and the day-to-day needs of critically ill patients on the waiting list.
The following are general criteria. Each hospital has its own policy and procedure based on state law and accepted medical practice.

Brain death criteria[2]

NOTE: These criteria are determined by hospital policy.

Known etiology
Diagnosis made in absence of hypothermia (temperature less than 32.2° C), central nervous system depressants, or metabolic abnormalities
Cerebral unresponsiveness
Areflexic, except for simple spinal cord reflexes
Pupillary, extraocular, gag, and cough reflexes are absent
No spontaneous respiration

Condition irreversible (duration of observation depends on clinical judgment)
Flat EEG (if performed)
Cerebral angiography
Absence of blood flow by cerebral radionuclide scan or arteriogram (if performed)

Apnea test[2]

- Preoxygenate.
- Disconnect ventilator, give O_2 at 8 to 12 L/min by tracheal cannula.
- Observe for spontaneous respirations.
- After 10 minutes, draw ABG.
- Reconnect the ventilator.
- The patient is apneic if the $P_{CO_2} > 60$ mm Hg and there is no respiratory movement.
- If hypotension and/or dysrhythmias develop, immediately reconnect the ventilator. Consider other confirmatory tests.

Minimum Exclusion Criteria

Metastatic cancer
HIV positive or AIDS

Management*

In the majority of cases organ donor evaluation and management will be carried out in an intensive care unit because of the amount of time that it takes to complete the process. However, there will be those instances when the donation process will be initiated in the emergency department setting. Your local organ procurement organization is your primary and most valuable resource at this time.

In general the initial evaluation of a potential organ donor includes the following data:
- Age and past medical history
- Assessment of family dynamics
- Accurate bedscale weight
- Blood type
- CBC with differential, full chemistry profile including liver function tests
- ABGs on current ventilator settings
- Frequent monitoring of vital signs including urine output
- Monitoring for evidence of septicemia

While individual organ systems are being evaluated, the donor's care must be carefully managed to optimize organ perfusion and to minimize the development of infection. Thus sterile technique, when applicable, should be maintained.

The "Rule of 100s" can be used as a guideline for management:
- Maintain a systolic blood pressure of 100.
- Maintain an arterial P_{O_2} of 100 on the minimal F_{IO_2}
- Maintain an hourly urine output of 100 cc.

With the loss of cerebral function comes the potential for complications. Some of the most common complications seen in the brain dead individual include:

Neurogenic diabetes insipidus

- Caused by pituitary dysfunction and loss of endogenous ADH
- Diagnosed by hypernatremia, hypokalemia, urine outputs of greater than 500 cc per hour, hyperosmolar serum, hypo-osmolar urine
- Treatment includes the use of low-dose vasopressin infusion or DDAVP

*Courtesy of Katie Dunn, RN, BS, CPTC, Donation Coordinator, New England Organ Bank, 1994.

Neurogenic pulmonary edema
- Frequently seen in donors with a traumatic cause of death
- Mechanism of injury not well understood
- Diagnosed by CXR and deteriorating ABGs
- Treatment includes use of PEEP, of colloids vs. crystalloids, and Lasix

Neurogenic shock
- Caused by loss of vasomotor tone and dehydrational therapy
- Treatment includes volume restoration and use of vasoconstrictors. Dopamine is usually the drug of choice for hypotension. Other drug therapies may include: dobutamine, neosynephrine, and epinephrine.

Neurogenic hypothermia
- Caused by loss of hypothalamic temperature control
- May lead to ECG changes, cardiac dysrhythmias
- Proactive treatment the best choice: use of warming blankets, lights, blood and fluid warmers

BODY DONATION

Most people who desire body donation have made prior arrangements with a medical school. Call the local organ procurement organization for instructions.

HOW TO REFER A POTENTIAL DONOR

Call the organ procurement organization (OPO) assigned to your area to refer a potential donor or to ask questions regarding medical suitability. A donation coordinator will assist you with the evaluation of a potential donor and, if requested, will provide on-site services that may include obtaining consent, donor management, and organ and tissue recovery. "It is important to note that, before a declaration of death, the Organ Procurement Organization coordinator will provide advice consistent with the medical and nursing goals (i.e., survival of the patient.)."[3]

If you do not know the name or telephone number of the local organ procurement organization, call the United Network for Organ Sharing (UNOS) at 1-800-292-9537. There are 11 designated regions in the United States and within those regions there are one or more organ procurement organizations providing service (Figure 39-1).

Call the organ procurement organization every time a death occurs to assure that all families are given the option of choosing donation.

When you call the organ procurement organization be prepared to give the following information:
- Patient's name, age, sex, race, and medical record number
- Diagnosis and hospital course
- Status of brain death determination
- Whether or not the family has been approached about donation and their response

The importance of an early referral cannot be overemphasized. Placing the call when death is imminent allows you to give the family the most accurate information about the donation possibilities, decreases the time required to complete the process, and therefore increases the likelihood of a successful outcome.

Some hospitals have in-house coordinators or donor nurses whose responsibility it is to act as liaison with the local organ procurement organization and to facilitate one or more stages of the donation process. Find out what your hospital's policy and protocol are on organ and tissue donation.

MEDICAL EXAMINER CASES

In certain cases you must ask the medical examiner or coroner to release the body for donation. It is wise to obtain this permission before speaking to the patient's family, because the medical examiner may restrict the donation or may refuse to allow any organs or tissues to be recovered.

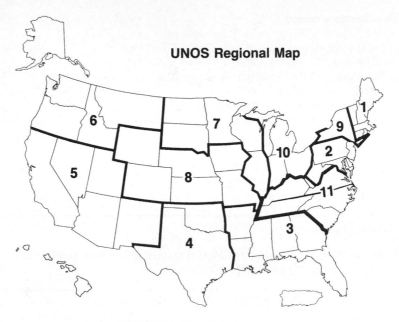

FIGURE 39-1. UNOS regional map.

A medical examiner's or coroner's case may include:
- Homicide or suspicion of homicide
- Suicide or suspicion of suicide
- Death by accident, trauma, or poisoning

CONSENT

"A thorough evaluation of donor potential before discussion with the family can prevent the situation in which a family readily embraces the opportunity to donate only to be informed later that this option does not exist for them."[3]

By Whom

Any health care professional who is caring for the patient, who has a positive attitude about donation, and who is familiar with the process. This may be the organ procurement organization's donation coordinator or the donor hospital's physician, nurse, pastoral caregiver, or social worker.

Those family members authorized to give consent, and the order in which they have this authority, is specified in each state's Uniform Anatomical Gift Act. The health care proxy's ability to direct care on the patient's behalf ends at the death of the patient. He or she therefore may not consent to donation unless authorized to do so under the UAGA.

How

Give the family time to acknowledge the loss of the loved one.

Provide a private space for grieving and discussion.

Assess the family's understanding of what the physician has told them.

Identify the patient's legal next-of-kin and key support persons.

Assess the family's understanding of brain death.

Explain brain death in terms they can understand.

Ask the family to reflect on what their loved one would have wanted.

Provide facts about donation essential to helping them make their decision.

Give them as much time as possible to discuss it among themselves.

Allow time to say goodbye to their loved one.

Provide support whether or not they choose to donate.

Document your discussion with the family in the patient's medical record.

Facts

The patient will be tested for HIV and other transmissible diseases.

There is no cost to the donor family.

The family should contact the donor hospital or organ procurement organization if there is a question about billing.

All major religions support organ and tissue donation.

The organ procurement organization will provide general follow-up information about the recipients.

There is no disfigurement as a result of a donation.

The quality of medical care will not be compromised if donation is considered.

BEREAVEMENT SUPPORT

Some organ procurement organizations provide bereavement support services. Contact your hospital's Social Service Department to inquire about what services are available locally.

WHY SHOULD WE OFFER FAMILIES THE DONATION OPTION?

Many health care professionals worry that offering the option of donation to a grieving family causes them to suffer more than they already have. However, most families take comfort in making this gift and they have the right to make that decision. *If we do not ask, we have made that decision for them.*

The best reason for offering families the donation option is expressed eloquently by Maggie Cooligan, a critical care nurse and donor mother: "It is true that in the sudden or traumatic death of our loved one, we are experiencing one of the most difficult types of loss. You observe us in a state of shock, a state of anger and/or guilt, and a state of denial. You do not want to increase the hurt. You do not want to expose your own feelings of mortality. You do not want to ask. However, your request presents us with hope when we have lost all hope. You present us with an option when we have no other options. We have already experienced the pain of death. What more can you say to hurt me when you have already said, 'your child has died.' Potential donor families have a right to be offered the option to donate. We have a right to alleviate some of the pain we will experience in grieving. We have the right to make some sense out of a usually senseless death. We have a right to be part of allowing another person to live."[4]

REFERENCES

1. UNOS: *Vital connections,* Washington DC, 1996, US Department of Health and Human Services, Health Resources Administration.
2. Report of the medical consultants on the diagnosis of brain death to the President's Commission for the Study of Ethical Problems in Medicine and Biomedical and Behavioral Research: guidelines for the determination of death, *JAMA* 246:2184, 1981.
3. Willis R, Skelley L: Serving the needs of donor families: the role of the critical care nurse, *Crit Care Nurs Clin North Am* 4(1):63, 1992.
4. Cooligan M: Katie's legacy, *Am J Nurs* 87:483, 1987.

SUGGESTED READINGS

Bragman KL et al: The organ donor, *Crit Care Clin* 6(4):821-839, 1990.

Cho YM et al: Transplantation of kidneys from donors whose hearts have stopped beating, *N Engl J Med* 338(4):221-225, 1998.

Kennedy AP et al: Utilization of trauma-related deaths for organ and tissue harvesting, *J Trauma* 33(4):516-519, 1992.

Morris JA, Jr, Wilcox TR, First WH: Pediatric organ donation: the paradox of organ shortage despite the remarkable willingness of families to donate, *Pediatrics* 89(3):411-415, 1992.

Seminoff LA, Arnold RM, Caplan AL: Health care professional attitudes towards donation, *J Trauma* 39(3):553-559, 1995.

Waller JA et al: Potential availability of transplantable organs and tissues in fatalities from injury and nontraumatic intracranial hemorrhage, *Transplantation* 55(3):542-546, 1993.

Forensic Nursing

Suzanne L. Brown

FORENSIC NURSING: MEDICOLEGAL CASES

According to Taber's *Cyclopedic Medical Dictionary* the term *forensic* is defined as "pertaining to the law." Whenever the medical field and the legal system overlap, a medicolegal case occurs.

- Forensic nurses may be hospital, clinic, or independently based, employed with the medical examiner or law enforcement agencies.
- Forensic nurses may work with forensic cases that involve the living or the dead.
- Proper collection of evidence in medicolegal cases is a legal, ethical, and professional responsibility.

Examples of medicolegal cases include the following:

- Gunshot wounds
- Sexual assault
- Domestic violence
- Equivocal deaths
- Child abuse
- Elder abuse
- Suicide attempts
- Accidents
- Stab wounds

Scope of practice of forensic nurses includes the following roles:

- Sexual assault nurse examiners
- Nurse coroners/death investigators
- Forensic nurse educators
- Forensic pediatric nurses
- Forensic photographers
- Forensic geriatric nurses
- Forensic psychiatric nurses
- Emergency/trauma nurses
- Correctional nurses

The forensic nurses are considered experts in their specialty based on education, experience, and training. As a result, they may be called on to serve as expert witnesses in court.

Forensic nursing organizations include the following:

- The International Association of Forensic Nurses (IAFN) was established in 1992
- The American Nurses Association endorsed forensic nursing as a nursing specialty in 1996
- The Emergency Nurses Association (ENA) supports forensic nursing

THE MULTIDISCIPLINARY APPROACH

Nurses must work with other medical personnel, police jurisdictions, and other legal services to help collect, preserve, and identify evidence in possible medicolegal cases. The forensic nurse should be familiar with hospital protocols, victim rights, forensic guidelines, and appropriate referral agencies.

Reporting to Police/Medical Examiner

Nurses need to be aware of the laws regarding the reporting of crimes in a particular state. In all states, registered nurses are mandated reporters for any suspicion of abuse of children. Most states require the reporting of all violent injuries; some may require reporting only if a case involves gunshot or stabbing wounds. All deaths that are sudden, unexpected, or questionable are to be reported to the authorities.

Terms

- *Cause of death* is the injury or disease that resulted in death (that is, cause of death was a stab wound)
- *Manner of death* can only be one of five categories:
  accidental
  homicide
  suicide
  natural
  undetermined
- *Mechanism of death* is a physiologic state that was not compatible with life (that is, cardiac arrest, cardiopulmonary arrest, and so forth).

Therefore, if a patient comes into the emergency/trauma center with a stab wound, the cause of death would be a stab wound to the aorta, the manner of death could be homicidal, and the mechanism of death could be cardiopulmonary arrest. Many hospitals are asking for the cause of death, not the mechanism of death, on the death certificates/patient record.

PHOTOGRAPHY

Whenever possible, photographs should be taken of all injuries on medicolegal cases. Photographs can tell a story of the crime that may have just occurred. Photographs can document the exact site of the injury, date the timeframe of the injury, and help with reconstruction of the injury at a later date.

Photographs should be taken at long range, midrange and close up. The purpose of long-range photographs is to identify the person with the injury. Midrange photographs are then done to show closer photographs in relation to the area injured. Finally, close-up photographs are then done to show the exact wound. A scale or ruler should be in at least one of the close-up photographs to reflect the measurements of the injury.

- Long range:
  1. Use wide-angle lens if available
  2. Take several photographs from different angles
  3. If using 35-mm film, take Polaroids or video as backup
  4. Label each photograph (described on p. 669)
- Midrange:
  1. Gives link to overall picture and close-up picture
  2. Shows detail and perspective of injury with patient
  3. Label and identify each photograph
- Close up:
  1. Take picture as item will allow (fill camera viewfinder with item)
  2. Identify and label each photograph

3. Take at least one picture without a scale
4. Take at least one picture with a scale

Photographs should be labeled with at least the patient's name, the date and time of the photograph, and the photographer's signature. Any other identifying information that may help with recollection can also be included (that is, right or left arm). If you have a police case number, include that number on the photograph as well.

PHYSICAL EVIDENCE

Dating of Bruises

Depending on the amount of force used and the location of the injury, bruises can develop at different stages. As a result, bruises should be documented as clearly as possible with descriptive terms. The color of bruises can correlate with the age of the wound.

General guidelines for bruises:

0 to 3 days: red with crisp borders
3 to 5 days: red/blue with crisp borders
5 to 7 days: green with distinct borders
7 to 10 days: yellow with indistinct margins
More than 10 days: brown with fading borders
After 2 weeks: absent

An ultraviolet or UV light photograph can be useful to document physical injuries no longer visible to the naked eye.

Bite Marks

Bite marks need to be photographed as described in the *Photography* section on pp. 668-669. Bite marks need to be identified as animal or human bite marks, as well as child vs. adult marks. Domestic-animal bites are usually "V" shaped in appearance, and deeper in penetration (puncture marks), whereas the bite mark of an adult is more ovoid in shape.

Acute abusive bite marks need to have swabs obtained for DNA analysis. One cotton-tipped applicator should be moistened with sterile water, rubbed over the bite mark, a second dry cotton tipped applicator is then rubbed over the site. Swabs then need to be air-dried and packaged in a sealed paper bundle. Chain of custody must be maintained at all times (*see* Chain of Custody).

A forensic dentist may need to be contacted to obtain imprints/molds of the bite mark.

Fingernail Scrapings

If the patient has the potential of any blood, fibers, or debris under their fingernails from the alleged assailant, fingernail scrapings should be obtained. Each fingernail tip should be cut or scraped onto a clean piece of paper. Each hand debris should be collected separately and labeled "right hand" and "left hand."

Clothing

Any clothing that was involved in a potential medicolegal case should be properly collected and handled. In many cases, clothing that the person was wearing at the time of the crime may contain trace evidence that could link a case together.

Guidelines for collection of clothes:

• Never cut through any holes, tears, or rips in the clothing. Holes in clothing can later be matched up with a weapon or can show the distance of a gunshot based on the gunshot residue around the hole.

- Place each item in a separate *paper* bag, never plastic bags. Paper bags allow the clothing to "breathe." Plastic bags will produce moisture, which causes mold or mildew to develop, causing a breakdown or destruction of evidence.
- Do not allow fluids or stains to touch. Place protective piece of paper inside clothes, then roll or fold clothes with stain on the inside.
- Document the clothing that the patient arrived with. Document condition of clothing (that is, tears, unusual markings, and so forth).
- Do not shake clothing (this could result in the loss of trace evidence).
- Clothes should not be placed on the floor or under a stretcher (this could cause cross-contamination from other cases). If possible, bag clothing upon removal. Otherwise, clothing can be placed on a clean white hospital sheet (include this sheet in a separate paper bag when turning clothing over to police).
- Document the chain of custody of all clothing.

CHAIN OF CUSTODY

Chain of custody is the proper tracking and documentation of all evidence as it is passed on throughout the entire case. Chain of custody starts with the first person to obtain the evidence and is documented on all transfers of the evidence (Figure 40-1).

Chain of custody is maintained on clothing and personal belongings of the victim or assailant, photographs, film, collected swabs and debris, blood alcohol levels, and toxicology reports.

Chain of custody includes the following:
- Bag or container, sealed with tape.
- Initial, date, time should be placed over the seal on bag or container
- The signature of person giving and the name of person receiving item(s)

Documentation

- Document all injuries
  Site, location
  Shape
  Type of wound (see wound characteristics)
  Characteristics (for example, color, texture, etc.)
- Initiate chain of custody if not already started
- Document any specimens collected
  Site
  Packaging
  Chain of custody
- Document condition of clothing on arrival
- Document names and numbers of law enforcement officials/medical examiner/coroner who were notified.

WOUND CHARACTERISTICS

- *Blunt injuries* result from the force of impact. Examples of blunt injuries are abrasions, contusions (*see* Dating of Bruises), lacerations, and fractures. Blunt injuries can be seen in motor vehicle crashes, assaults, or accidents.
- *Sharp injuries* result from cuts in the skin. Examples of cuts are stab wounds and surgical incisions.
- *Dicing injuries* are usually caused by multiple injuries. An example of a dicing injury would be superficial cuts sustained from multiple glass fragments during a motor vehicle crash.
- *Bite marks* (*see* Bite Marks).

FORENSIC EVIDENCE CHAIN OF CUSTODY FORM

Victim name:　　　Last　　　First	Facility	Phone number
Name: _____ Signature: _____	Date/Time: _____	Facility: _____
Received from: _____	Date/Time: _____	Facility: _____
Received by: _____	Date/Time: _____	Facility: _____
Received from: _____	Date/Time: _____	Facility: _____
Received by: _____	Date/Time: _____	Facility: _____
Received from: _____	Date/Time: _____	Facility: _____
Received by: _____	Date/Time: _____	Facility: _____
Received from: _____	Date/Time: _____	Facility: _____
Received by: _____	Date/Time: _____	Facility: _____
Received from: _____	Date/Time: _____	Facility: _____
Received by: _____	Date/Time: _____	Facility: _____
Received from: _____	Date/Time: _____	Facility: _____

FIGURE 40-1. Sample chain of custody form.

- *Defensive wounds* may be sharp injuries, blunt injuries, or dicing injuries. They are usually inflicted on the backs of the lower arms, palmar surfaces of the hands, or on the victim's back (that is, whatever part of the body was used as a defense against the injury).
- *Hesitation wounds* may be sharp or dicing injuries. Hesitation injuries are usually self inflicted and seen in suicide attempts. Hesitation injuries usually have a more superficial starting and ending point, with the center of the wound being deeper. Hesitation injuries are usually linear and may be unilateral (that is, the side away from the dominant hand).
- *Gunshot wounds* (*see* Gunshot Wounds.)

DRAWING CONCLUSIONS

Gunshot Wounds

- Document/draw/describe the exact location(s) of the wound(s).
- Photograph all the wounds if at all possible.
- Document the appearance of possible entrance and exit wounds.
- Do not insert surgical devices/tubes into a gunshot wound. This may alter the wound's appearance and may destroy evidence.
- Assess for any gunshot residue on the wounds. Cover the gunshot wound with sterile gauze.
- Place paper bags on both hands until a perpetrator of the crime has been established.

Sexual Assault

See Chapter 31.

Stab Wounds

- Document/draw exact locations of wound(s).
- Photograph wounds.
- Do not insert surgical devices/tubes that may alter the wound's appearance into the wound at least until photographs are taken.
- Assess for defensive wounds on forearms/palmar surface of hands.
- Assess for blood/debris under fingernails

Suicides/"Accidents"

Hangings

- Note clothing patient was wearing at time of death. Consider possibility of an autoerotic death. Males who are accidental victims of an autoerotic death may be dressed in female underclothing. Some family members may alter the appearance of their family member on discovery because of embarrassment or concerns about "rumors."
- Assess for a suicide note. In an autoerotic death a note will not be left behind.
- Assess for pornographic magazines/paraphilia at the accident site.
- Assess the home for an "escape mechanism." In many autoerotic deaths there is a knife or scissors at the site for a quick-release mechanism.
- Check for any defensive wounds, ligature marks, or other signs of a struggle. These would also rule out an autoerotic death.

Motor vehicle crashes: rule out a possibility of a suicide attempt

- Assess for history of depression, previous suicide attempts, or a history of other single-car accidents. Some single-car accidents may be suicidal attempts.
- Assess accident site for skid or brake marks. In some suicide attempts, no skid marks may be found.

SUGGESTED READINGS

Breo DL: JFK's death: the plain truth from the MDs who did the autopsy, *JAMA* 267(20):2794, 1992.

Collins KA, Lantz PE: Interpretation of fatal, multiple, and exiting gunshot wounds by trauma specialists, *J Forensic Sci* 39(1):94, 1994.

Cumming M: Nurse-coroner to forensic consultant: one emergency nurse's experience, *J Emerg Nurs* 22:494-497, 1996.

Lynch V: Forensic nursing in the emergency department: a new role for the 1990s, *Crit Care Nurs Q* 14:3, 1991.

Lynch V: Clinical forensic nursing: a new perspective in the management of crime victims from trauma to trial, *America on Line Internet search article,* 1997, International Association of Forensic Nurses.

Payne-James JJ, Dean PJ: Assault and injury in clinical forensic medical practice, *Med Sci Law* 34(3):202, 1994.

Pasqualone G: The importance of forensic photography in the emergency department, *J Emerg Nurs* 21:566-567, 1995.

Pozzi C: Forensic and safety nursing consulting, *J Emerg Nurs* 22:536-537, 1996.

Spitz WV: *Medicolegal investigation of death,* ed 3, Springfield, Ill, 1993, Charles C Thomas.

Winfrey M: Developing a graduate forensic nursing elective, *J Emerg Nurs* 22:54-57, 1996.

Index

Page references followed by *t* or *f* indicate tables or figures; references followed by *b* indicate boxes.